Haematology and Blood Transfusion
Hämatologie und Bluttransfusion

31

Edited by
H. Heimpel, Ulm · D. Huhn, Berlin
C. Mueller-Eckhardt, Gießen
G. Ruhenstroth-Bauer, München

Modern Trends in Human Leukemia VII

New Results
in Clinical and Biological Research
Including Pediatric Oncology

Organized on behalf of the Deutsche Gesellschaft für
Hämatologie und Onkologie, Hamburg, June 21, 1986
and Wilsede, June 22–25, 1986

Wilsede Joint Meeting on Pediatric Oncology IV
Hamburg, June 27/28, 1986

Edited by
Rolf Neth, Robert C. Gallo, Melvyn F. Greaves,
and Hartmut Kabisch

With 182 Figures and 118 Tables

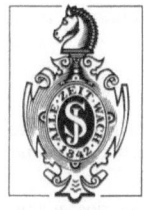

Springer-Verlag Berlin Heidelberg New York
London Paris Tokyo

Dr. Rolf Neth, Universitäts-Krankenhaus Eppendorf,
Medizinische Klinik, Abteilung für klinische Chemie,
Martinistraße 52, 2000 Hamburg 20, FRG

Dr. Robert C. Gallo, National Cancer Institute, Laboratory
of Tumor Cell Biology, Bethesda, MD 20205, USA

Dr. Melvyn F. Greaves, Leukemia Research Fund Centre, Institute of
Cancer Research, Chester Beatty Laboratories, Fulham Road,
London SW3 6JB, UK

Dr. Hartmut Kabisch, Universitäts-Kinderklinik,
Abteilung für Hämatologie und Onkologie,
Martinistraße 52, 2000 Hamburg 20, FRG

Supplement to
BLUT – Journal of Clinical and Experimental Hematology
Organ of the *Deutsche Gesellschaft für Hämatologie und Onkologie* der *Deutschen Gesellschaft für Bluttransfusion und Immunhämatologie* and of *Österreichische Gesellschaft für Hämatologie und Onkologie*

ISBN-13: 978-3-540-17754-8   e-ISBN: 978-3-642-72624-8
DOI: 10.1007/978-3-642-72624-8

Library of Congress Cataloging-in-Publication Data.
Modern trends in human leukemia VII : new results in clinical and biological research including pediatric oncology/organized on behalf of the Deutsche Gesellschaft für Hämatologie und Onkologie, Hamburg, June 21, 1986 and Wilsede, June 22–25, 1986; Wilsede Joint Meeting on Pediatric Oncology IV, Hamburg, June 22/28, 1986: edited by Rold Neth, ... [et al.].
    p. cm. – (Haematology and blood transfusion = Hämatologie und Bluttransfusion: 31)
    Includes bibliographies and index.
    "Supplement to Blut" – T.p. verso.
    ISBN (invalid) 038717754X (U.S.)
1. Leukemia – Congresses. 2. Leukemia in children – Congresses. I. Neth, Rolf. II. Deutsche Gesellschaft für Hämatologie und Onkologie. III. Wilsede Joint Meeting on Pediatric Oncology (4th : 1986 : Hamburg, Germany) IV. Blut. Supplement. V. Series: Haematology and blood transfusion: 31.
    [DNLM: 1. Leukemia – congresses. W1 HA1655 v. 31/WH 250 M68911 1987]

Typesetting, printing and bookbinding: Brühlsche Universitätsdruckerei, Giessen
2127/3130-543210

Scientific Organisation of the Sessions

New Strategies in Leukemia Diagnostic and Therapy

Greaves, Melvyn F., Leukemia Research Fund Centre, Institute of Cancer Research, Fulham Road, London SW3 6JB, United Kingdom

Waldmann, Thomas A., National Cancer Institute, Bethesda, Maryland 20892, USA

Clinical Aspects of the Treatment of Acute Leukemia

Henderson, Edward S., Roswell Park Memorial Institute, Medical Oncology, 666 Elm Street, Buffalo, New York 14263, USA

Hoelzer, Dieter, Zentrum der Inneren Medizin, Abteilung Hämatologie, Theodor-Stern-Kai 7, 6000 Frankfurt 70, FRG

Lister, Andrew T., Imperial Cancer Research Fund, Department of Medical Oncology, St. Bartholomew's Hospital, London EC1A 7BE, United Kingdom

Cell Biology

Metcalf, Donald, Royal Melbourne Hospital, Cancer Research Unit, Melbourne, Victoria 3050, Australia

Moore, Malcolm A.S., Memorial Sloan-Kettering Cancer Center, 1275 York Avenue, New York, NY 10021, USA

Immunology

Mitchison, N. Avrion, Department of Zoology, Tumour Immunology Unit, Gower Street, London WC1E 6BT, United Kingdom

Riethmüller, Gert, Institut für Immunologie, Goethestr. 31, 8000 München 2, FRG

Virology

Vogt, Peter K., Department of Microbiology, 2025 Zonal Avenue, Los Angeles, CA 90033, USA

Bister, Klaus, Max-Planck-Institut für Molekulare Genetik, Ihnestr. 63–73, 1000 Berlin 33, FRG

Wilsede Joint Meeting in Pediatric Hematology and Oncology IV

Kabisch, Hartmut, Universitäts-Kinderklinik, Abteilung für Hämatologie und Onkologie, Martinistr. 52, 2000 Hamburg 20, FRG

Winkler, Kurt, Universitäts-Kinderklinik, Abteilung für Hämatologie und Onkologie, Martinistr. 52, 2000 Hamburg 20, FRG

Local Organisation

Mannweiler, Klaus, Heinrich-Pette-Institut für experimentelle Virologie und Immunologie an der Universität Hamburg, Martinistr. 52, 2000 Hamburg 20, FRG

Neth, Rolf, II. Medizinische Universitätsklinik, Abteilung Klinische Chemie, Martinistr. 52, 2000 Hamburg 20, FRG

Schubert, Johannes, St.-Joseph-Hospital, Wiener Str. 1, D-2850 Bremerhaven, FRG

Contents

Frederick Stohlmann Jr. Memorial Lecture

New Strategies in Leukemia Diagnostic and Therapy

Participants of the Meeting

Aghib, D., Dipartimento di Genetica e di Biologia dei Microorganismi, University of Milan, Milan, Italy

Akers, David W., Polyarts, P.O. Box 326, Mountlake Terrace, Washington 98043, USA

Ambros, Peter F., St. Anna-Kinderspital, Hämatologisches Labor, Kinderspitalgasse 6, A-1090 Vienna IX, Austria

Anders, Fritz, Genetisches Institut, Heinrich-Buff-Ring 58–62, D-6300 Giessen, FRG

Asha, P.K., Friedrich Miescher-Institut, Postfach 2543, CH-4002 Basel, Switzerland

Asjö, Birgitta, Karolinska Institutet, Dept. of Virology, S-10521 Stockholm, Sweden

Bading, Hilmar, Max-Planck-Institut für Molekulare Genetik, Abt. Schuster, Ihnestrasse 73, D-1000 Berlin 33, FRG

Barin, Francis, Laboratoire de Virologie, CHRU Bretonneau, F-37044 Tours Cedex, France

Barnett, M.J., ICRF Department of Medical Oncology, St. Bartholomew's Hospital, London, United Kingdom

Bartram, Claus R., Universitätskinderklinik, Abteilung II, Prittwitzstrasse 43, D-7900 Ulm, FRG

Bassan, R., ICRF Department of Medical Oncology, St. Bartholomew's Hospital, London, United Kingdom

Berghe, Herman van den, Centrum voor menselijke erfelijkheid u.z. gasthuisberg, Herestraat 49, B-3000 Leuven, Belgium

Beug, Hartmut, Europäisches Laboratorium für Molekularbiologie, Meyerhofstrasse 1, D-6900 Heidelberg, FRG

Biberfeld, Gunnel, Karolinska Institutet, Dept. of Pathology, S-10401 Stockholm, Sweden

Biberfeld, Peter, Karolinska Institutet, Dept. of Pathology, S-10401 Stockholm, Sweden

Bister, Klaus, Max-Planck-Institut für Molekulare Genetik, Ihnestrasse 63–73, D-1000 Berlin 33, FRG

Boguslawska-Jaworska, Janina, Institute of Pediatrics, Dept. of Haematology, ul. Smoluchowskiego 32/4, PL-50372 Wroclaw, Poland

Bolognesi, Dani P., Dept. of Surgery, Surgical Visology Laboratory, Durham, North Carolina 27710, USA

Boyd, Janis, Royal Melbourne Hospital, Cancer Research Unit, Melbourne, Victoria 3050, Australia

Broder, Samuel, National Cancer Institute, Clinical Oncology Program, Bethesda, Maryland 20205, USA

Brown, G., Department of Immunology, University of Birmingham, Birmingham B15 2TJ, United Kingdom

Büchner, Thomas, Medizinische Universitätsklinik, Albert-Schweitzer-Strasse 33, D-4400 Münster, FRG

Burnett, A. K., Glasgow Royal Infirmary, Castle Street, Glasgow G4 OSF, United Kingdom

Burny, Arsene, Department de Biologie Moleculaire, Laboratoire de Chimie Biologique, Rue des Chevaux, 67, B-1640 Rhode-St.-Genese, Belgium

Caligaris-Cappio, Federico, Dipartimento di Scienze Biomediche e Oncologia Umana, Via Genova 3, I-10126 Torino, Italy

Cantrell, Doreen Ann, Cell Surface Biochemistry Laboratory, P.O. Box 123, Lincoln's Inn Fields, London, WC2A 3PX, United Kingdom

Carrasco, C. Humberto, Department of Diagnostic Radiology, The University of Texas M.D. Anderson Hospital and Tumor Institute at Houston, 67232 Bertner Avenue, Houston, Texas 77030, USA

Chen, Po-min, Veterans General Hospital, Section Medical Oncology, Taipei, Taiwan 112, Republic of China

Chermann, Jean-Claude, Institut Pasteur, 28, Rue du Dr. Roux, F-75724 Paris Cedex 15, France

Cichutek, Klaus, Dept. of Molecular Biology, Wendell M. Stanley Hall, Berkeley, California 94720, USA

Cleary, Michael L., Laboratory of Experimental Oncology, Department of Pathology, Stanford University, Stanford, California 94305, USA

Cook, Peter, Sir William Dunn School of Pathology, South Parks Road, Oxford OX1 3RE, United Kingdom

Cory, Suzanne, Royal Melbourne Hospital, Post Office, Melbourne, Victoria 3050, Australia

Creutzig, Ursula, Kinderklinik, Abt. Hämatologie und Onkologie, Albert-Schweitzer-Strasse 33, D-4400 Münster, FRG

Davis, Roger J., Dept. of Biochemistry, 55 Lake Avenue North, Worchester, Massachusetts 01605, USA

Dean, Michael, Frederick Cancer Research Facility, P.O. Box B, Frederick, Maryland 21701, USA

Derulska, Danuta, Instytut Pediatrii, Klinika Chorob Rozrostowych i Skaz Krwotocznych, ul. Marszalskowska 24, PL-00-576 Warszawa, Poland

Dexter, T. Michael, Paterson Laboratories, Christie Hospital, Dept. of Experimental Haematology, Wilmslow Road, Manchester M20 9BX, United Kingdom

Dopfer, R., Department of Pediatric Hematology and Oncology, University Children Hospital, Ruemelinstrasse 21, D-7400 Tübingen, FRG

Douer, Dan, Institute of Hematology, Sheba Medical Center, Tel Hashomer, Israel

Duesberg, Peter H., Dept. of Molecular Biology, Wendell M. Stanley Hall, Berkeley, California 94720, USA

Elstner, Elena, Universitätsklinik für Innere Medizin, Charite, Schumannstrasse 20/21, DDR-1040 Berlin, GDR

Essex, Myron, Dept. of Cancer Biology, 665 Huntingdon Avenue, Boston, Massachusetts 02115, USA

Feldman, Michael, The Weizmann Institute of Science, Dept. of Cell Biology, P.O. Box 26, Rohovot 76100, Israel

Fenyö, Eva-Maria, Karolinska Institutet, Dept. of Virology, S-10521 Stockholm, Sweden

Fisher, Amanda, National Cancer Institute, Bethesda, Maryland 20205, USA

Foon, Kenneth A., Dept. of Internal Medicine, Division of Hematology/ Oncology, 3119 Taubman Center, Ann Arbor, Michigan 48109, USA

Gaedicke, Gerhard, Universitäts-Kinderklinik, Abteilung Pädiatrie II, Prittwitzstrasse 43, D-7900 Ulm, FRG

Galili, Naomi, Dept. of Pathology, Laboratory of Experimental Oncology, 300 Pasteur Drive, Stanford, California 94305, USA

Gallo, Robert C., National Cancer Institute, Bethesda, Maryland 20205, USA

Gallwitz, Dieter, Institut für Molekularbiologie und Tumorforschung, Emil-Mannkopfstrasse 1, D-3500 Marburg, FRG

Ganesan, Trivadi S., ICRF, Dept. of Medical Oncology, St. Bartholomew's Hospital, West Smithfield, London EC1A 7BE, United Kingdom

Ganser, Arnold, Zentrum der Inneren Medizin, Abteilung Hämatologie, Theodor-Stern-Kai 7, D-6000 Frankfurt 70, FRG

Gissmann, Lutz, Deutsches Krebsforschungszentrum, Institut für Virusforschung, Im Neuenheimer Feld 280, D-6900 Heidelberg, FRG

Göttlinger, Heinz, Institut für Immunologie, Goethestrasse 31, D-8000 München 2, FRG

Goldman, John, Hammersmith Hospital, Ducane Road, London W12 OHS, United Kingdom

Greaves, Melvyn F., Leukaemia Research Fund Centre, Institute of Cancer Research, Fulham Road, London SW3 6JB, United Kingdom

Grossman, Zvi, Pittsburgh Cancer Institute, 230 Lothrop Street, Pittsburgh, Pennsylvania 15213, USA

Handgretinger, R., Universitätskinderklinik, Otfried-Müller-Strasse 10, D-7400 Tübingen, FRG

Hart, Ian R., Imperial Cancer Research Laboratories, Lincoln's Inn Fields, London WC2A 3PX, United Kingdom

Hardesty, Boyd A., Clayton Foundation Biochemical Institute, Experimental Science Building 442, Dept. of Chemistry, Austin, Texas 78712, USA

Haseltine, William A., Dana-Farber Cancer Institute, Laboratory of Biochemical Pharmacology, 44 Binney Street, Boston, Massachusetts 02115, USA

Hausen, Harald zur, Deutsches Krebsforschungszentrum, Im Neuenheimer Feld 280, D-6900 Heidelberg, FRG

Hehlmann, Rüdiger, Medizinische Poliklinik, Pettenkoferstrasse 8a, D-8000 München 2, FRG

Heisig, Volker, National Cancer Institute, Laboratory of Tumor Cell Biology, Bethesda, Maryland 20205, USA

Heit, Wolfgang, Zentrum der Inneren Medizin, Abteilung Hämatologie, Theodor-Stern-Kai 7, D-6000 Frankfurt 70, FRG

Henderson, Edward S., Roswell Park Memorial Institute, Medical Oncology, 666 elm Street, Buffalo, New York 14263, USA

Herrmann, Friedhelm, Klinikum der Johannes Gutenberg-Universität, Abteilung für Hämatologie, Langebeckstrasse 1, D-6500 Mainz 1, FRG

Hoelzer, Dieter, Zentrum der Inneren Medizin, Abteilung Hämatologie, Theodor-Stern-Kai 7, D-6000 Frankfurt 70, FRG

Hrodek, Otto, 2nd Department of Pediatrics, Charles University, V uvalu 84, CS-15006 Prague, Czechoslovakia

Hünig, Thomas, Genzentrum der Universität München, Am Klopferspitz, D-8033 Martinsried, FRG

Hui, K., Laboratory of Gene Structure and Expression, National Institute for Medical Research, The Ridgeway, Mill Hill, London NW7 1AA, United Kingdom

Hunsmann, Gerhard, Deutsches Primatenzentrum, Abteilung Virologie und Immunologie, Kellnerweg 4, D-3400 Göttingen, FRG

Hyjek, Elzbieta, Katedra Onkologii AM, ul. Gagarina 4, PL-93509 Lodz, Poland

Ihle, Rainer, Universitätsklinik für Innere Medizin, Charite, Schumann-strasse 20/21, DDR-1040 Berlin, GDR

Jackson, D. A., Sir William Dunn School of Pathology, University of Oxford, South Parks Road, Oxford OX1 3RE, United Kingdom

Janka, Gritta, Universitäts-Kinderklinik, Abteilung für Gerinnungsforschung und Onkologie, Martinistrasse 52, D-2000 Hamburg 20, FRG

Kabisch, Hartmut, Universitäts-Kinderklinik, Abteilung für Gerinnungsforschung und Onkologie, Martinistrasse 52, D-2000 Hamburg 20, FRG

Kanki, Phyllis, Dept. of Cancer Biology, 665 Huntingdon Avenue, Boston, Massachusetts 022115, USA

Karawajew, L., Central Institute of Molecular Biology, Academy of Sciences of the GDR, DDR-1115 Berlin-Buch, GDR

Kirsten, H. Werner, Dept. of Pathology, 5841 South Maryland Avenue, Chicago Illinois 60637, USA

Kisseljov, Fjodor, Institute of Cancerogenesis, Dept. of Viral Molecular Biology, Kashiskoe sh. 24, Moscow, USSR

Klener, Pavel, II. Interni Klinika, U nemocnice 2, Prague 2, Czechoslovakia

Knapp, Walter, Institut für Immunologie, Borschkegasse 8a, A-1090 Wien, Austria

Knebel-Doeberitz, Magnus von, Deutsches Krebsforschungszentrum, Institut für Virusforschung, Im Neuenheimer Feld 280, D-6900 Heidelberg, FRG

Knyazev, Peter G., N.N. Petrov Institute of Oncology, Pesochny-2, Leningrad, USSR

Koprowski, Hilary, The Wistar Institute, 36th Street at Spruce, Philadelphia, Pennsylvania 19104, USA

Kowenz, Elisabeth, European Molecular Biology Laboratory, Postfach 102209, D-6900 Heidelberg, FRG

Kramer, Gisela, Clayton Foundation Biochemical Institute, Experimental Science Building 442, Dept. of Chemistry, Austin, Texas 78712, USA

Lapin, Boris A., Institute of Experimental Pathology and Therapy, Gora Trapetziya, P.B. 66, Sukhumi, USSR

Laufs, Rainer, Institut für Mikrobiologie, Martinistrasse 52, D-2000 Hamburg 20, FRG

Lister, Andrew T., Imperial Cancer Research Fund, Dept. of Medical Oncology, St. Bartholomew's Hospital, London EC1A 7BE, United Kingdom

Löhler, Jürgen, Heinrich-Pette-Institut für Experimentelle Virologie und Immunologie, Martinistrasse 52, D-2000 Hamburg 20, FRG

Lohmann-Matthes, M.-L., Fraunhofer Institut für Toxikologie und Aerosolforschung, Nicolai-Fuchs-Strasse 1, D-3000 Hannover 61, FRG

Majdic, O., Institute of Immunology, University of Vienna, A-1090 Vienna, Austria

Mannweiler, Klaus, Heinrich-Pette-Institut für Experimentelle Virologie und Immunologie, Martinistrasse 52, D-2000 Hamburg 20, FRG

Marlink, Richard, Dept. of Cancer Biology, 665 Huntingdon Avenue, Boston, Massachusetts 02115, USA

Matioli, Gastone T., Dept. of Microbiology, 20205 Zonal Avenue, Los Angeles, California 90033, USA

Matthews, Thomas J., Department of Surgery, Duke University Medical School, Durham, North Carolina 27710, USA

McCredie, Kenneth B., Anderson Hospital and Tumor Institute, Dept. of Developmental Therapeutics, 6723 Bertner Avenue, Houston, Texas 77030, USA

Mertelsmann, Roland, Universität Mainz, Abteilung für Hämatologie, Langenbeckstrasse 1, D-6500 Mainz 1, FRG

Mes-Masson, Anne-Marie, Molecular Biology Institute, Los Angeles, California 90024, USA

Metcalf, Donald, Royal Melbourne Hospital, Cancer Research Unit, Melbourne, Victoria 3050, Australia

Mitchison, N. Avrion, Dept. of Zoology, Tumour Immunology Unit, Gower Street, London WC1E 6BT, United Kingdom

Mizutani, Shuki, Leukaemia Research Fund Centre, Institute of Cancer Research, Chester Beatty Laboratories, Fulham Road, London SW3 6JB, United Kingdom

Moore, Malcolm A.S., Memorial Sloan-Kettering Cancer Center, 1275 York Avenue, New York, N.Y. 10021, USA

Moroni, Christoph, Friedrich Miescher-Institut, P.O. Box 2543, CH-4002 Basel, Switzerland

Müller, Dorit, Boehringer-Mannheim, Biochemica Werk Tutzing, Bahnhofstrasse 9–15, D-8132 Tutzing, FRG

Munk, Klaus, Deutsches Krebsforschungszentrum, Im Neuenheimer Feld 280, D-6900 Heidelberg, FRG

Neil, James C., Beatson Institute for Cancer Research, Bearsden, Glasgow G61 1BD, United Kingdom

Neth, Rolf, II. Medizinische Universitätsklinik, Abt. Klinische Chemie, Martinistrasse 52, D-2000 Hamburg 20, FRG

Nicola, Nicos A., Royal Melbourne Hospital, Cancer Research Unit, Melbourne, Victoria 3050, Australia

Niemeyer, Charlotte M., Dana Farber Cancer Institute, Division of Medical and Pediatric Oncology, 44 Binney Street, Boston, Massachusetts 02115, USA

Novotny, J.R., Abteilung Pädiatrie II, Universitäts-Kinderklinik, Prittwitzstrasse 43, D-7900 Ulm, FRG

Oblakowski, Piotr, Instytut Hematologii, u. Chocimska 5, PL-00-957 Warszawa, Poland

Ohno, Susumu, Beckmann Research Institute, 1450 East Duarte Road, Duarte, California 91010, USA

Ottman, Oliver G., Memorial Sloan-Kettering Cancer Center, Dept. of Developmental Hematopoiesis, 1275 York Avenue, New York, N.Y. 10019, USA

Pasternak, Günter, Zentralinstitut für Molekularbiologie, Robert-Rössle-Strasse 10, DDR-1115 Berlin-Buch, GDR

Pauli, Georg, Institut für Virologie, Nordufer 20, D-1000 Berlin 65, FRG

Petrakova, Alena, Research Institute of Child Development, Dept. of Genetics, V. uvalu 84, CS-15006 Prague, Czechoslovakia

Pinkerton, R., Department of Paediatric Oncology, Centre Léon Berard, Lyon, France

Ralph, Peter, Cetus Corporation, Dept. of Cell Biology, 1400 53rd Street, Emeryville, California 94608, USA

Ratner, Lee, Division of Hematology/Oncology, Washington University, St. Louis, Missouri, USA

Rapp, Ulf R., National Cancer Institute, Viral Pathology Section, Frederick, Maryland 21701, USA

Rawle, Frances C., ICRF Human Tumour Immunology Group, University Street, London WC1E 6JJ, United Kingdom

Riethmüller, Gert, Institut für Immunologie, Goethestrasse 31, D-8000 München 2, FRG

Rohatiner, Ama Z.S., Imperial Cancer Research Fund, Dept. of Medical Oncology, St. Bartholomew's Hospital, London EC1A 7BE, United Kingdom

Rokicka-Milewska, Roma, Institute of Pediatrics, Dept. of Oncology and Haemorrhagic Diathesis, Marszalkowska 24, PL-00-579 Warszawa, Poland

Rothbard, Jonathan B., Dept. of Zoology, Tumour Immunology Unit, Gower Street, London WC1E 6BT, United Kingdom

Schilsky, Richard L., Joint Section of Hematology-Oncology, Room L-231 Blood Center, Michael Reese Hospital and Medical Center, Lake Shore Drive at 31st Street, Chicago, Illinois 60616, USA

Schimpl, Anneliese, Institut für Virologie und Immunbiologie, Versbacher Strasse 7, D-8700 Würzburg, FRG

Schmidt, Carl Gottfried, Innere Klinik und Poliklinik, Westdeutsches Tumorzentrum, Hufelandstrasse 55, D-4300 Essen

Schmidt, Reinhold E., Medizinische Hochschule Hannover, Abt. Immunologie und Transfusionsmedizin, D-3000 Hannover 61, FRG

Schneider-Gädicke, A., Deutsches Krebsforschungszentrum, Institut für Virusforschung, Im Neuenheimer Feld 280, D-6900 Heidelberg, FRG

Schreiber, Hans, La Rabiba Children's Hospital and Research Center, Dept. of Pathology, East 65th Street at Lake Michigan, Chicago, Illinois 60649, USA

Schubert, Johannes, St.-Joseph-Hospital, Wiener Strasse 1, D-2850 Bremerhaven, FRG

Smith, Geoffrey L., Dept. of Pathology, Division of Virology, Addenbrooke's Hospital, Hills Road, Cambridge CB2 2QQ, United Kingdom

Souza, Lawrence, Amgen, 1900 Oak Terrace Lane, Thousand Oaks, California 91320, USA

Stauss, Hans J., Department of Pathology, University of Chicago, Chicago, Illinois 60637, USA

Steffen, Martin, Memorial Sloan-Kettering Cancer Center, 1275 York Avenue, New York, N.Y. 10021, USA

Stehelin, Dominique, Institut Pasteur, Unité d' Oncologie Moléculaire, 1, rue Calmette, B.P. 245, F-59019 Lille Cédex, France

Testa, N.G., Department of Experimental Haematology, Paterson Laboratories, Manchester M20 9BX, United Kingdom

Topol, L.Z., Institute of Carcinogenesis, Cancer Research Center, Moscow, USSR

Trainin, Ze'ev, Kimron Veterinary Institute, P.O.B. 12, Beit-Dagan, 50200 Israel

Tsujimoto Yoshihide, The Wistar Institute, 3601 Spruce Street, Philadelphia, Pennsylvania 19050, USA

Uchanska-Ziegler, Barbara, Institut für Organische Chemie, Ob dem Himmelreich 7, D-7400 Tübingen, FRG

Urban, James L., Division of Biology, California Institute of Technology, Pasadena, CA 91125, USA

Voevodin, Alexander F., Institute of Experimental Pathology and Therapy, Gora Trapetziya, P.B. 66, Sukhumi, USSR

Vogt, Peter K., Dept. of Microbiology, 2025 Zonal Avenue, Los Angeles, California 90033, USA

Wain-Hobson, Symon, Institut Pasteur, 27, Rue du Docteur Roux, F-75724 Paris, France

Waldmann, Thomas A., National Cancer Institute, Bethesda, Maryland 20892, USA

Warner, Noel L., Becton Dickinson Monoclonal Center, 2375 Garcia Avenue, Mountain View, California 94043, USA

Weiss, Robin A., Chester Beatty Laboratories, Fulham Road, London SW3 6JB, United Kingdom

Wiedemann, Leanne M., The Leukaemia Research Fund Centre, Institute of Cancer Research, Fulham Road, London SW3 6JB, United Kingdom

Wendler, I., Deutsches Primatenzentrum Göttingen, Kellnerweg 4, D-3400 Göttingen, FRG

Willems, Luc, Département de Biologie Moléculaire, Laboratoire de Chimie Biologique, Rue des Chevaux, 67, B-1640 Rhode-St.-Genèse, Belgium

Wilson, E. Lynette, Dept. of Clinical Science and Immunology, Observatory, Cape Town, South Africa

Witz, Isaac P., Dept. of Microbiology, The George S. Wise Faculty of Life Sciences, Tel Aviv, Israel 69978

Wodnar-Filipowicz, Aleksandra, Friedrich Miescher-Institut, P.O. Box 2543, CH-4002 Basel, Switzerland

Yakovleva, L. A., Institute of Experimental Pathology and Therapy, USSR Academy of Medical Sciences, Sukhumi, USSR

Yohn, David, International Association for Comparative Research on Leukemia and Related Diseases, 410 West 12th Avenue, Columbia, Ohio 43210, USA

Yoshida, Misuaki, Dept. of Viral Oncology, Cancer Institute, 1-37-1 Kami-Ikebukuro, Toshima-ku, Tokyo 170, Japan

Young, Bryan D., Imperial Cancer Research, Lincoln's Inn Fields, London, United Kingdom

Zagury, Daniel, Université Pierre et Marie Curie, 4, Place Jussieu, F-75005 Paris, France

Zintl, Felix, Universitäts-Kinderklinik, Kochstrasse 2, DDR-6900 Jena, GDR

In Memoriam Dr. Mildred Scheel

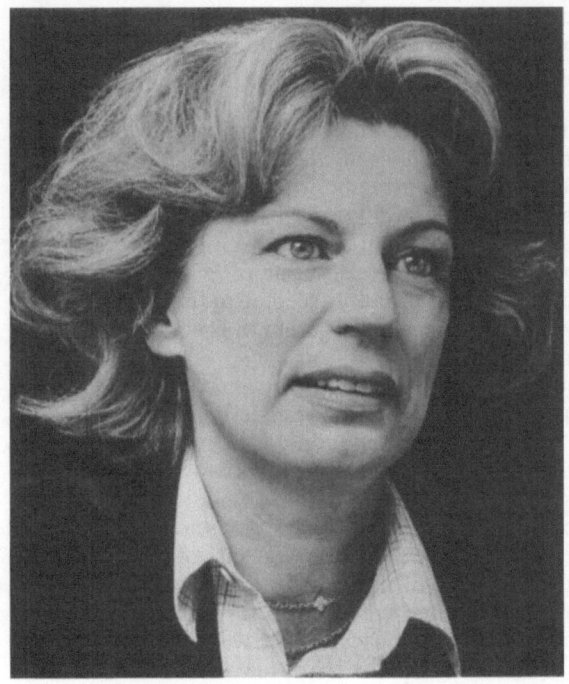

The Wilsede Meeting is also supported by the Wilsede Fellowship Programme of the Dr. Mildred Scheel Stiftung, which is part of the Deutsche Krebshilfe. Since that Foundation was established by Dr. Mildred Scheel, it is appropriate that we should reflect and comment on the great contribution which she made to cancer prevention, treatment and research. This meeting is the first Wilsede meeting since her untimely death on 13 May last year. She succumbed to cancer – the disease to whose conquest she had devoted the whole of her professional life.

Who was Mildred Scheel? What were her ideas and what did she achieve with her Foundation?

Mildred Scheel was born in Cologne in 1932, daughter of a physician and radiologist. She studied medicine and specialized in radiology. Later, she married Mr. Walter Scheel before he was appointed Minister for Foreign Affairs. When Mr. Scheel subsequently became President of the Federal Republic of Germany, she became the "First Lady" of this country. No doubt this helped her to fulfil her noble ambition to contribute to the fight against cancer. As a consequence of this, she founded the Deutsche Krebshilfe in 1974. From that time on, all her efforts were directed towards encouraging people to contribute money for this crucial purpose. During the first 10 years of the Deutsche Krebshilfe, she was able to collect more than 230 million Deutschmarks. She developed many significant ideas for organizing cancer prevention, early diagnosis and treatment that was applicable on a large scale. She initiated the establishment of the first five cancer centres in this country. Once they were functioning successfully, she was able to convince the Government to assume full responsibility for maintaining them. She then prepared to launch new undertakings. It became apparent to people that she had unique qualities that enabled her to initiate new ideas for fighting cancer, and this added significantly to her personal success. She also supported in particular the treatment of childhood cancer in many hospitals, and initiated the psychosocial after-care of patients and their families. In addition, she aided individuals who were economically affected by having cancer.

The Dr. Mildred Scheel Stiftung was established to promote and support cancer research. It supports a great number of research projects in many institutes and provides a fellowship programme for scientists to work and study at institutions abroad. Included in that programme is the Wilsede Fellowship Programme. Dr. Mildred Scheel Stiftung is now an important body in the Federal Republic of Germany for the granting of fellowships. Many of Mildred Scheel's initiatives were not broadly accepted at first, but through her continued energy they are now accepted as common practices in the oncological field in this country.

When she had a particular goal in sight, no obstacles could prevent her from reaching it. Yet, for all her tenacity, Mildred Scheel was a warm, loving and sensitive person who had special understanding for cancer patients, together with a human touch. She was always very hard-working and enthusiastic, and stimulating for all of us. None of those who, like myself, had worked with her in the Foundation for over 10 years can remember her ever missing a meeting of the board or the scientific councils of the Deutsche Krebshilfe or the Dr. Mildred Scheel Stiftung, until the last few weeks of her life. During those meetings she listened carefully to the experts, although sometimes she came to her own conclusions when she was convinced that a particular step forward had to be made. She never lost her enthusiasm for helping others, even when she realized what would be the consequence of her own illness. She always seemed to be positive in her attitude and could always stimulate others with her spirit and her personality. She could have done so much more in the future and she is sadly missed by all of us today. We all will always remember her with great devotion.

Klaus Munk
Heidelberg

Wilsede Scholarship Holders

Anger, Bernd, Abteilung Innere Medizin II, Steinhövelstrasse 9, D-7900 Ulm, FRG

Auerswald, Ulrich, Institut für Klinische Immunologie, Martinistrasse 52, D-2000 Hamburg 20, FRG

Bading, Hilmar, Max-Planck-Institut für Molekulare Genetik, Ihnestrasse 73, D-1000 Berlin 33, FRG

Brown, Geoffrey, Dept. Immunology, Vincent Drive, Birmingham B15 2TJ, England

Debatin, Klaus, Kinderklinik, Sektion Onkologie/Immunologie, Im Neuenheimer Feld 150, D-6900 Heidelberg 1, FRG

Douer, Dan, The Chaim Sheba Medical Center, Institute of Hematology, Tel-Hashomer, Israel 52621

Dührsen, Ulrich, Heinrich-Pette-Institut für Experimentelle Virologie und Immunologie, Martinistrasse 52, D-2000 Hamburg 20, FRG

Gebhardt, Angelika, National Institute for Medical Research, The Ridgeway, Mill Hill, London NW7 1AA, England

Hampson, Ian N., Paterson Laboratories, Christie Hospital, Dept. Experimental Haematology, Wilmslow Road, Manchester M20 9BX, England

Hartmann, Wolfgang, Universitätskinderklinik, Prittwitzstrasse 43, D-7900 Ulm, FRG

Heitmüller, Jens, Schauenburgerstrasse 81, D-2300 Kiel 1, FRG

Hemmering, Angelika, Max-Planck-Institut für Biochemie, Abteilung Virologie, D-8033 Martinsried, FRG

Henke, Michael, Medizinische Universitätsklinik, Hugstetter Strasse 55, D-7800 Freiburg, FRG

Hirsch, Anja, Institut für Virologie, Frankfurter Strasse 107, D-6300 Giessen, FRG

Hui, Kam Man, National Institute for Medical Research, The Ridgeway, Mill Hall, Lab. Gene Structure and Expression, London NW7 1AA, England

Kayser, Winfried, II. Medizinische Klinik, Metzstrasse 53/57, D-2300 Kiel, FRG

Kern, Peter, Bernhard-Nocht-Institut für Schiffs- und Tropenkrankheiten, Bernhard-Nocht-Strasse 74, D-2000 Hamburg 4, FRG

Köller, Ursula, Institut für Immunologie, Borschkegasse 8a, A-1090 Wien, Austria

Kojouharoff, Georgi, Institut für Immunologie und Genetik, Deutsches Krebsforschungszentrum, Im Neuenheimer Feld, D-6900 Heidelberg, FRG

Leitner, Barbara, Med. Nat. Forschungszentrum, Ob dem Himmelreich 7, D-7400 Tübingen, FRG

Lori, Alfred, Kantonsspital Basel, CH-4031 Basel, Switzerland

Mergentahler, Hans-Günther, Institut für Experimentelle Hämatologie, Landwehrstrasse 61, D-8000 München 2, FRG

Michaelis, Claudia, Am Großen Wannsee 32, D-1000 Berlin 39, FRG

Mizutani, Shuki, Leukaemia Research Fund Centre, Institute of Cancer Research, Fulham Road, London SW3 6JB, England

Neil, James C., The Beatson Institute, Garscube Estate, Switchback Road, Bearsden, Glasgow G61 1BD, Scotland

Norton, John D., Dept. Haematology, The Royal Free Hospital, Pond Street, Hamstead, London NW3 2QG, England

Ostmeier, Hermann F., Pathologisches Institut, Joseph-Stelzmann-Strasse 9, D-5000 Köln 41, FRG

Schmetzer, Helga, Medizinische Klinik III, Marchioninistrasse 15, D-8000 München 70, FRG

Schneider-Gädicke, Ansbert, Deutsches Krebsforschungszentrum, Im Neuenheimer Feld 280, D-6900 Heidelberg 1, FRG

Stauss, Hans Josef, La Rabiba Children's Hospital and Research Center, East 65th Street at Lake Michigan, Chicago, Illinois 60649, USA

Stevens, Richard F., Royal Manchester Children's Hospital, Pendlebury, Manchester M27 1HA, England

Tony, Hans-Peter, Medizinische Poliklinik, Klinikstrasse 8, D-8700 Würzburg, FRG

Melo, Junia VAZ de, MRC Leukaemia Unit, Ducane Road, London W12 0HS, England

Völkers, Bernd, Zentrum der Inneren Medizin, Theodor-Stern-Kai 7, D-6000 Frankfurt 70, FRG

Wiedemann, Leanne, Leukaemia Research Fund Centre, Institute of Cancer Research, Fulham Road, London SW3 6JB, England

Würsch, Andreas, Kantonsspital Basel, CH-4031 Basel, Switzerland

Yron, Ilana, Dept. Microbiology, The George S. Wise Faculty of Life Sciences, Tel Aviv, Israel 69978

Preface

Ideo autem omnes ad consilium vocari diximus,
*quia saepe iuniori Dominus revelat quod melius est.**

Benedictus de Nursia
Regula Benedicti, ca. 550 A. C.
Caput III,3

The Wilsede Meetings were initiated in 1973 as an unusual experiment, and in the meantime this biennial symposium has already come to constitute an established and successful tradition.

In June 1986 scientists and physicians met for the seventh time in the 300-year-old Emmenhof in Wilsede, in the heart of the Lüneburg Heath, to discuss modern trends in human leukemia.

It was Pappenheim who in 1910 prepared the first international hematology congress. It was to have been held in Berlin under the title „Der große mononukleäre Leukozyt Ehrlichs, seine Morphologie und Funktion, seine Herkunft und seine Benennung" (Ehrlich's large mononuclear leukocyte. Its morphology, function, origin, and name), which was the most important and topical question at that time. It is amazing to think that as early as 1900, thanks to the pioneering research of Maximov and the innovative staining method developed by Ehrlich, the differentiation of the blood cells had, to a large extent, already been discovered. It is a sad fact that this congress never took place due to personal controversies among leading hematologists, especially between Pappenheim and the Austrian hematologist Türk.

Fortunately the Wilsede Meetings have never incurred this type of personal controversies. On the contrary, both matter-of-fact discussions at a high scientific level and the development of personal friendships have always characterized their singular atmosphere.

The seventh Wilsede Meeting was also in this tradition, and under the active and sure-handed guidance of the chairmen an outstanding scientific program was presented, the participants contributing toward a convivial and friendly atmosphere. I would like to express my thanks for this and hope that there will be many future Wilsede's where we will all get together again.

Rolf Neth

---

* Wir haben aber deshalb bestimmt, daß alle zur Beratung einberufen werden, weil der Herr oft einem *Jüngeren offenbart,* was das Beste ist.

* But we have therefore declared that everyone should be summonded to the conference, because God often reveals to the young people which way is best.

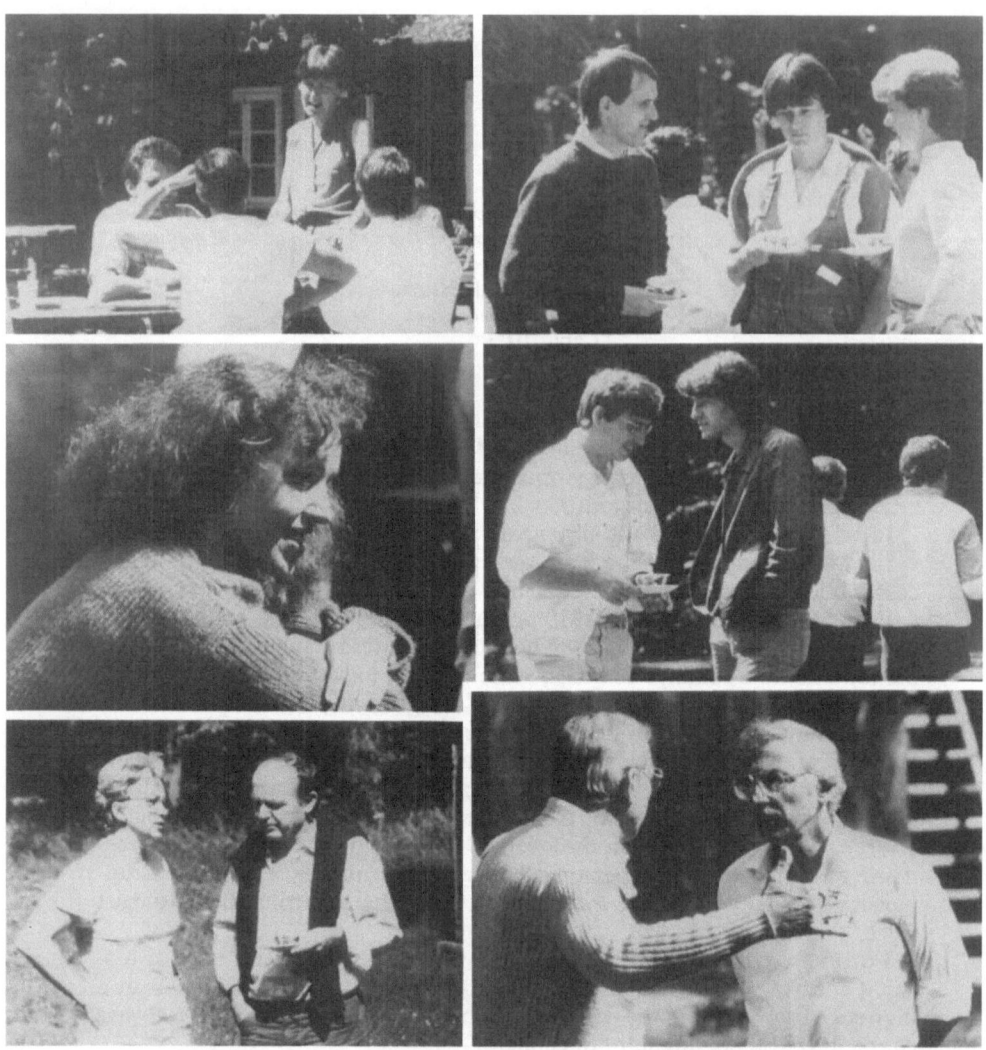

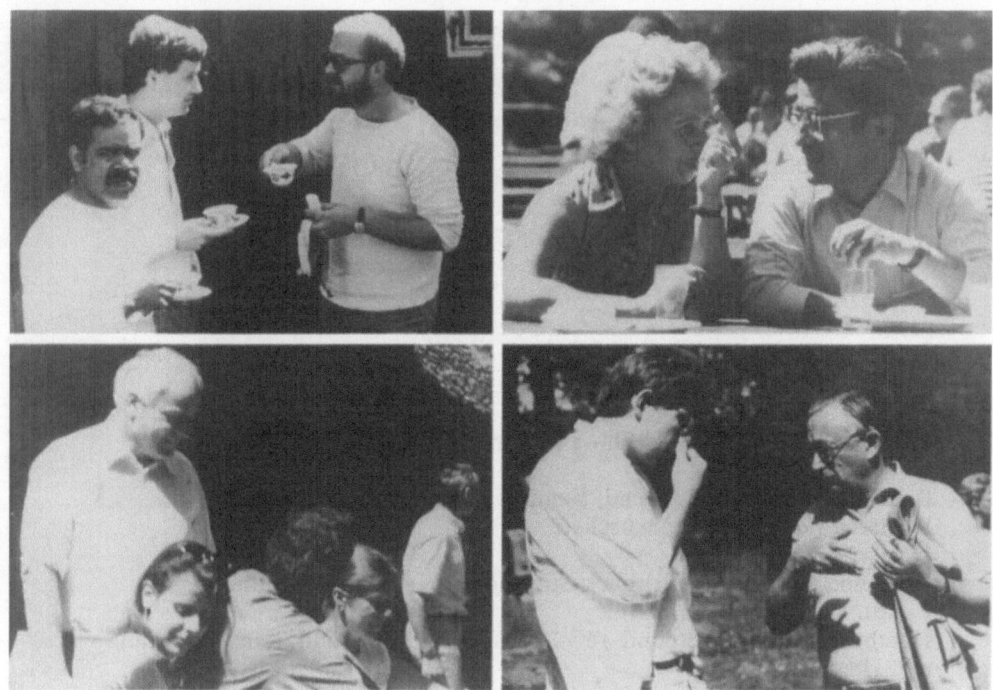

Scientific and Personal Discussion around "De Emmenhof"

Acknowledgements

We should like to thank all those who made this workshop possible:

Bundeministerium für Jugend, Familie, Frauen und Gesundheit
Deutsche Forschungsgemeinschaft
Deutsche Krebshilfe
Erich und Gertrud Roggenbuck-Stiftung zur Krebshilfe, Hamburg
Freie und Hansestadt Hamburg
Hamburger Landesverband für Krebsbekämpfung und Krebsforschung
e.V. Hamburg
Leukemia Research Fund. Great Britain
Leukemia Society of America
Paul Martini Stiftung

For their generous hospitality we thank the Stiftung F.V.S. zu Hamburg,
Verein Naturschutzpark e.V. Hamburg, the Amerikahaus in Hamburg and
the Freie und Hansestadt Hamburg.

I would like to thank Dr. Jürgen Wieczorek, Ms. Anne Clauss and Mr.
Jürgen Schaubel of Springer-Verlag for their assistance in the production of
the book. On behalf of the authors and editors: Rolf Neth

Hans Eidig Lecture

Wilsede, June 23, 8pm

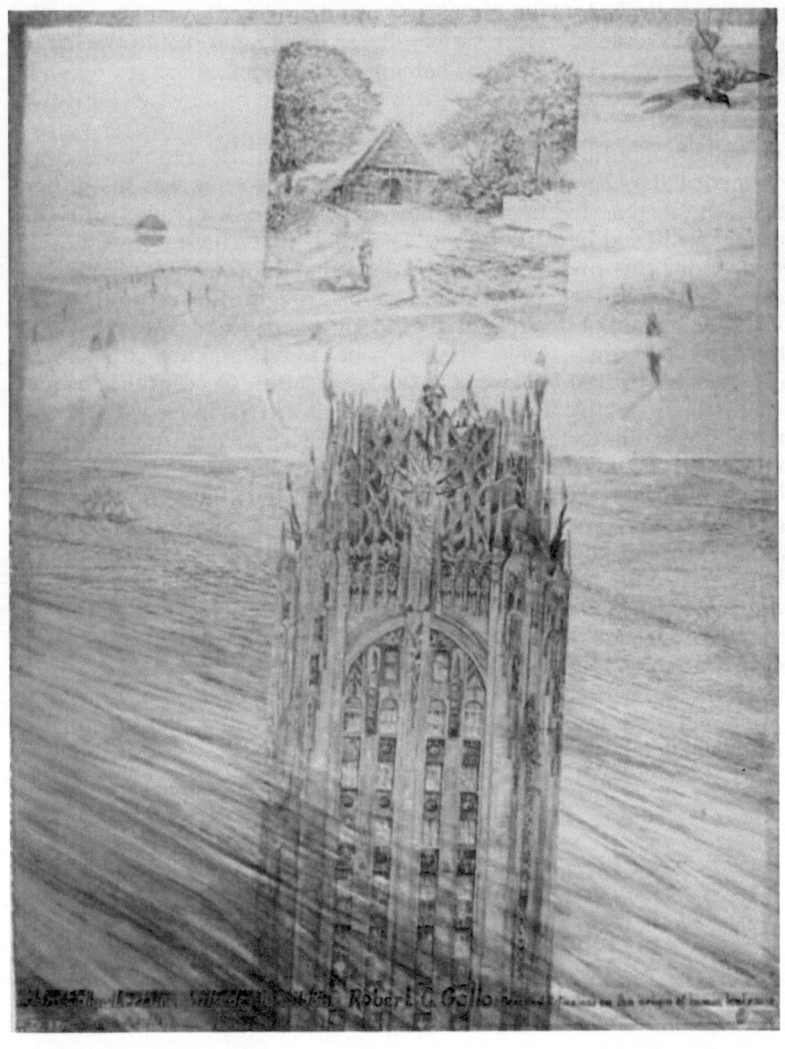

Aquarell 76 × 56 cm, 1986   Michel Weidemann

Introduction to Hans Eidig and Robert C. Gallo

An introduction to Bob Gallo, as a person and a scientist, would certainly be superflous. I would therefore simply like to draw a parallel to the life of the lectures eponym, Hans Eidig. The name of this special lecture reminds us not only of particular historical circumstances but, more importantly, of this man's life.

Hans Eidig was born in 1804 in the village of Klein Klecken. It was originally intended that he should become a forest ranger, as was his father. However the yearning for freedom and independence, which was to influence his entire life led him to become a poecher rather than a forester. He was very good at this, and there was a great demand for his services. But his desire for freedom and independence was too strong for the restraints of his way of life, not afraid of this risking his life for others, he became the Robin Hood of the Lüneburger Heide. He had good friends and advisors as well as many enemies. In 1835 he agreed to the king's offer to accept the cash reward on his head and to emigrate to America. He arrived in New York with his girlfriend, dreaming of freedom and independence. Thereafter we largely lose track of his life in the new continent. However, those of us from this region believe that he traveled to the West Coast of the United States where he discovered gold.

Although I do not know whether this legend is true, it remains very much alive here, and today's inhabitants of this village remember him as a local hero who always tried to protect our ancestors from humiliation at the hands of their feudal masters. In the New World Hans Eidig gained the freedom and independence that he had always sought.

Against the background of these words honoring the memory of Hans Eidig, I should like now to present Bob Gallo, who will explain the origin of human leukemia.

Rolf Neth

Personal Reflections on the Origin of Human Leukemia

Robert C. Gallo

Before I finish this lecture everyone else is going to be dreaming of freedom and independence. Rolf Neth wishes to link me with Hans Eidig. I may indeed have three features in common with this fellow, this Robin Hood as you call him. These are: very good friends, at least a few good enemies, and some foolishness – foolishness to give a lecture at this hour about such a topic.

First, I have been asked to give my reflections of the Wilsede meetings since their origin some 15 years ago and, then, on the virus "hot spot" theory, based on an article that I wrote for the first Wilsede meeting. That article was an attempt to counter the overused and overstated virogene/oncogene theory as it was originally proposed. We have, however, progressed far past that stage. About the beginning of the meetings.

In 1970 or 1971 I first met Rolf Neth. We walked along the Hamburg harbor and later we came to this forest he loves so much. He catalyzed (almost immediately) a similar affection from me. I told him that this would be a great place for meetings, regular meetings to promote friendly informal discussions among friends and adding new people as time went by.

By 1970 there was much activity developing in basic cancer research and all its subtopics. I felt those dealing with blood cell biology and the leukemias and lymphomas would make the greatest advances. First, because we could get our hands on such cells; secondly, because so many animal models were available, and, thirdly because there seemed to be, in general, a high caliber of people involved in research in that area of cancer. I also believed that it was time to push human studies to the point that they would be scientifically acceptable. So I though that if we had small meetings with a percentage of people always returning and then in time, adding people who get interested and who had particularly interesting information from diverse disciplines but linked by some interest in blood cells, lymphocytes and/or their malignant transformation, we could enhance development of the field.

The atmosphere of this marvelous forest was to augment the interactions. In time we hoped research in human disease would no longer be frowned on by the intellectual lights. To signal this feeling, we incorporated "human" in the meeting titles. Av Mitchison, Peter Duesberg, Rolf and Malcolm Moore and Mel Greaves gave the spark and life to the early meetings, as, of course, did the great Fred Stohlman at the first. Now forced to think back on all those years, I don't know if there's disappointment or elation in the progress the field has made nor whether we achieved our objective. The biggest disappointment I had is that at the time those meetings were organized, everyone was talking about multiple causes or primary agents or whatever we wanted to call the true causes of leukemia and lymphomas, but we all thought there would be one common mechanism at least one common, final biochemical mechanism. That doesn't turn out to be the case.

At the beginning of this century, the idea of leukemia most people pictured was that of a very wild disorder of cell proliferation. Later, with advances in the understanding of pernicious anemia (in which erythroblasts resemble malignant cells), the induction of abnormal cells to differentiate into normal cells using a simple vitamin replacement, vitamin B_{12}, came the opposite polar extreme idea that leukemia was simply a nutritional disease. One specific factor might take the whole thing away.

Certainly by the time of these meetings, a position very much in between was already in hand. Around 1950, as I remember the literature, a group in northern Italy, led by G. Astaldi and F. Gavosto and their co-workers, published a series of papers on thymidine radioautographs of labelled cells, concluding that leukemic cells do not wildly proliferate, but, in fact generally, have longer generation periods than do normal cells. By the first meeting people had already accepted the idea that leukemia was a kind of a block or a frozen state of differentiation, maybe partly reversible, maybe not. During that period of time, just before the meetings began, the concept of monoclonality had predominantly came from people who were doing chromosome studies, and made unambiguous by the studies of Phil Fialkow and his colleagues who used G-6-PD variants as X-linked enzyme markers to demonstrate monoclonality of CML. These studies were described at these meetings. So we had the concept of clonality of a partial or complete block in differentiation and presumed that a common molecular mechanism might account for all. At that time also most people thought stem cells were the only targets of a putative leukemogenic agent. This was championed, but it is not to be the case. Today we would say any cell capable of continued proliferation, even if committed, can be a target of a carcinogen or a leukemogen.

The first meeting began about 4 or 5 years after the discoveries by Leo Sachs and his co-workers and by Donald Metcalf and Bradley which led to a reproducible system of growing cultured cells in colonies and growth factors for leukocytes. The first blood cell growth factor had, in fact, already been discovered many years before by Allan Erslev, my first scientific mentor when I was a medical student. This was by the growth factor erythropoietin for red cells and was partly defined at the time of the first Wilsede. However, the field of leukocyte biology really progressed by the clonal assay systems. By the first meeting, we had the idea (at least for myeloid leukemic cells) that the block in differentiation could be overcome, at least in part. Leo Sachs talked here about the uncoupling of growth and differentiation and proposed that the molecules for these are in general separable. Both of these pioneering groups and their colleagues, especially Malcolm Moore, developed the concept that the "blocked" differentiation was not absolute and that some leukemic cells could at least be partially differentiated.

During this period, people also began to get a handle, not only on CSF and the related CSF molecules, but on other growth factors and their receptors. Not only the proteins, but eventually also the genes for some. The earliest of these was interleukin 2 (IL-2) and its receptor.

At the same time, so-called protooncogenes became defined. We should remember how those terms came about, and what an oncogene really meant, and what is has become to mean today. Perhaps the word today is used a bit too loosely. These genes were defined as ones capable of transforming a primary cell. They were first genetically and molecularly defined by groups in California, notably our own, Peter Duesberg, Peter Voigt and, also, by S. Hanafusa and Michael Bishop. Thus, the first transforming genes were being defined at the time of our earliest meeting and became a frequent topic of discussion – as they continue to be. Dominic Stehelin working with Bishop and independently some people at NIH, Edward Scolnik, Peter Fishinger, and Ray Gilden obtained data that the oncogenes of viruses were derived from the genes of normal cells, but had evolved away from those genes of normal cells. With those defined oncogenes in hand from animal viruses we could capture analogous genes from cells for the first time. Probes were now available to go into normal cellular DNA to "fish out" those homologs of retroviral oncogenes. The genes in normal cells were then called protooncogenes. We could explore the presence of these genes, what state they were in, i.e., amplified – nonamplified, rearranged or not, expressed or not and whether their coding was related to that of known genes for proteins important to growth, e.g., growth factors and their receptors. For the first time, genes and gene products suspected to be important for cell growth and/or differentiation of normal and leukemic cells could be compared. In the past 4 or 5 years or so several results have indicated that these previously independent fields will merge, because certain protooncogenes have indeed turned out to be genes for growth factors or receptors. The c-*sis* gene for the platelet-derived growth factor, the *Erb*B gene as a truncated EGF receptor, and recently the *fos* gene as the macrophage colony stimulating factor receptor are cases in point.

At the earliest meetings, I remember the good debates between Jane Rowley and Henry Kaplan on another area of leukemia/lymphoma research, relating to the relevance of chromosomal changes and whether these constitute anything other than secondary effects. As I remember it, Henry Kaplan was always asking for direct evidence that specific chromosomal changes were important for the initiation and/or progression of leukemias and lymphomas. In 1971–1973 the only clear-cut example of this available to us was that of chronic myelogenous leukemia and the Philadelphia chromosome. At about that time the concept that a balance of genes was important to control cell growth was also being widely discussed. Studies from childhood cancers with consistent chromosomal deletion and those of Fritz Anders on fish melanoma provided us with concepts of regulatory genes which control other genes that are more directly involved in cell growth.

The chromosomal changes that occur in human leukemia still raise some questions. The first problem as I see it, is why are there specific "hot spots" in human chromosomes that undergo change? In a recent review Mittelman has shown the accumulation of chromosomal breaks in a variety of human leukemias; it is evident that there are sites that must be especially fragile. Another interesting question that I rarely hear discussed is why adult tumors show progressive subclone heterogeneity? This is less common in childhood tumors, but in adult cancer we always talk about progression of the cancer and heterogeneity of subclones as though this is natural and should occur. But can anyone really explain them? It's usually said that this is due to an alteration in genetic regulation in addition to the primary chromosomal abnormality; however, this would imply that an alteration in regulators regularly occurs.

Does anything specifically cause the chromosomal change? There are at present no specific molecular mechanisms or inciting agents that have been proven to cause any of the important chromosomal changes. I believe that everyone would accept the idea that specific chromosomal changes are common and are probably very important to the pathogenesis, if not to the origin, of many human leukemias and lymphomas. In my own view, three genes deserve special discussion, for research into them seems most exciting. These are the c-*abl* gene in chronic myelogenous leukemia, the c-*myc* gene in Burkitt's lymphoma, and perhaps the chromosome 5 deletions in myeloid leukemia. The cluster of CSF genes and the receptors for CSF in one region of chromosome 5 suggests that any change in this region is likely to be important for leukemia. Obviously, when there is a specific chromosomal change occurring regularly in a certain leukemia, one would expect it to be important. When there are regions coincident with the location of genes important for the growth and differentiation of a particular cell type, we logically attach special attention to it.

The first consistently observed chromosomal abnormality, the Philadelphia chromosome, was discovered by Hungerford and Nowell in the early 1960s. This was first thought to be chromosome 21 deletion but was later shown to involve a translocation between chromosome 9 and chromosome 22. When we had a handle on the gene, several laboratories, including my own, were able to localize the c-*abl* gene to a region in chromosome 9 where the break occurs. We now know that this gene is translocated to chromosome 22, adjacent to a gene given the abbreviation BCR. Shortly thereafter Canaani at the Weizmann Institute in Israel discovered an abnormal c-*abl* messenger RNA in chronic myelogenous leukemia. This seems to be an area worthy of major investment. The study of the nature of this gene product might determine the function of the normal c-*abl*, explain why blast crisis develops, and eventually obtain evidence as to whether leukemia transformation and blast crisis are directly related to the abnormal c-*abl* product. An increase in number of chromosome 22 is common in CML blast crisis. Is this associated with an increased dosage of the c-*abl* messenger RNA? Probably so, but still, like in almost the entire field, we're left completely wanting for an explanation at the biochemical (mechanism) level of what the molecular genetics has defined.

Another approach that has been principally explored and pioneered by Carlo Croce and discussed in detail at this year's meeting, has been to examine cellular nucleotide sequences near chromosomal breaks consistently where there are no known oncogenes and, hence, no easily available or known molecular probes. This considerable endeavor is done by sequencing all around the chromosomal break point and determining which, if any, of these sequences near the chromosomal breaks are abnormally expressed. These can then be molecularly cloned and studied in detail. In other words, these sequences are not homologues of any known oncogene, nor do we have information that they code any growth factor or growth factor receptor. They are identified and worked with solely because they are sequences or genes located near a known consistent chromosomal break. This approach is logical and very likely important way to proceed. The problems are knowing what the gene product does and proving that it is important for the development of the tumor.

The last sequence I wish to discuss is that of the cellular homologue of the *myc* gene. We reported at one of the Wilsede meetings an analysis of the human c-*myc* gene. This was at a time when the abnormal chromosomes in Burkitt lymphoma were well known (generally 8 and 14). At these meetings George Klein and his associates showed that this phenomenon involves an 8:14 translocation. Independently, Carlo Croce showed that this same region of chromosome 14 involves the heavy chain loci of immunoglobulin genes. Subsequently, Riccardo Dalla Favera, a postdoctoral, cloned and mapped the human c-*myc* gene for the first time. Then together, with Flossie Wong-Staal, he formed a collaboration with Carlo Croce and then demonstrated the location of c-*myc* at the distal end of the long arm of chromosome 8. In later studies we reported that c-*myc* was translocated from chromosome 8 to chromosome 14 in each Burkitt lymphoma. The results were also presented and discussed in detail at these meetings. Now, of course, it is known that translocations also involve chromosome 8 and chromosomes 2 and 22. P. Leder, C. Adams, S. Cory, G. Klein, P. Marcu, T. Rabbits and particularly C. Croce and their colleagues have made major contributions to our understanding of the details of the various translocations and their significance.

This give me an opening to discuss a few aspects of the epidemiology of leukemias and lymphomas. Burkitt lymphoma (BL) seems to be a classical example of the multistage, multifactoral, multigenetic series of events said to be prerequisites for the development of a malignancy. We would all probably agree that the Epstein-Barr virus (EBV) plays a role in this malignancy, but the generally precise geographic limitation of BL means that its development requires at least one additional environmental factor, and holoendemic malaria is believed to be one such factor. The malarial organism apparently not only provides chronic antigenic stimulation but may also alter T-cell function in such a way that cytotropic T cells do not properly control EBV. So there appears to be three key events: the presence of EBV, the presence of chronic antigen stimulation, and possibly a change in T-cell function. Furthermore, the available evidence argues that during B-cell gene rearrangement a chance translocation of the *myc* gene occurs, and that this leads to one step in the tumor origin. The probability of this event is presumably increased by the chronic antigenic stimulation change in T-cell function and the excess replication of EBV. The last twist comes from new data that seems to argue that even this activation of the c-*myc* gene is not sufficient, and that there must be still another event. Susan Cory will present evidence at this Wilsede meeting that many cells of transgenic mice have translocated activated c-*myc* genes but a tumor arises from only one such cell. Thus, this disease demonstrates multifactoral, multistage, probably multiple genetic events in a cancer.

But can this serve as a general model? Should we think about all leukemias, lymphomas, and cancers as multifactoral, multistage and multigenetic? There are some things that bother me about this conclusion. For example, Kaposi's sarcoma occurs in a high percentage of homosexuals with AIDS. Does that mean that these people run around with multiple genetic events already in their endothelial cells just waiting for a T4 cell depression? I believe it much more likely that this is due to the requisite genetic changes occurring with one or, at most, two events; these changes probably include the addition of new genetic change from infection with a virus yet to be discovered. Another apparent exception involves cancers occurring in young girls whose mothers had received estrogen during pregnancy, and who at age 13 or 14 may develop vaginal cancers. Can we see this as multistage, multifactoral, multigenetic events? Also, what about the T-cell leukemias associated with HTLV-I? Because of the considerable time between infection and the leukemia, it is clear that there is more than one stage and probably more than one genetic event, but I know of no evidence that other exogenous factors are required. All current data argues that the virus and the virus alone is sufficient.

Regarding most other leukemias and lymphomas, looking for inciting agents or "true primary causes" has been difficult and not very productive to date. It would be disappointing if it turns out there are no initiating agents in most of the other leukemias or lymphomas, because this would mean most are chance events and mean we have nothing to do other than the laborious protein chemistry and metabolism studies like Boyd Hardesty and his colleagues have been doing and reporting at these meetings. Some epidemiological studies demonstrated the importance of radiation, e.g., the Atomic Bomb in Japan and occupational sources of radiation in mostly myeloid leukemias. Chloramphenicol and benzene exposure have also been reported to be associated with an increased incidence of some leukemias. How can we think of chloramphenicol and benzene in causing leukemia? Perhaps they alter programs of gene expression and allow some cell clones to emerge that have been genetically altered by other agents. Although these few chemicals and some forms of radiation are linked to an increased incidence of leukemia, it is, of course, only a very small fraction. For the vast majority of such cases no environmental factor(s) have yet been found.

Retroviruses in animals and also in humans (at least since 1979) have been frequently reported and passionately discussed at the Wilsede meetings from the outset; these have been the special interest of many investigators here, including myself. This interest came from the numerous and diverse leukemia-causing animal retroviruses that were already available when these meetings began. Many of us believed (and still do) that these animal models provide powerful tools for an understanding of the molecular and cellular pathogenesis of leukemias/lymphomas and of the genes involved. Some of us also believed that through studies of them we might also learn how to find similar viruses in humans if they existed.

When we recall the first meetings at the beginning of the 1970s, the retroviruses that were then discussed most thoroughly and most commonly (and those best supported financially) were the endogenous retroviruses. The genes for these viruses exist in the germ line and are present in multiple copies; and most, if not all, vertebrates and even some other species contain these genetic elements. Sometimes these are capable of giving rise to a whole virus particle. These were the major early focus of studies in leukemogenesis. For example, Henry Kaplan's first studies of radiation leukemogenesis suggested that radiation induced the expression of an endogenous virus which is critical to the development of the leukemia in this case in mice. Huebner and Todaro's original theory maintained that *all* cancer is due to the activation of these endogenous viruses, i.e., to oncogenesis, and was invariable due to expression of endogenous viral genes. This idea in its original and literal form has now been discarded. Ironically, the only retroviruses known to be involved in cancer in humans or in animals (except for a few very inbred mouse strains) are infectious (exogenous) retroviruses.

We began to focus on exogenous retroviruses in animals and humans in 1970 after the discovery of reverse transcriptase by Howard Temin and David Baltimore. A major reason for me to focus on exogenous viruses was the influence of people like Arsene Burny and his studies of bovine leukemia, William Jarrett on feline leukemia, and later those of Max Essex. These researchers, doing veterinary biology-virology, argued that naturally occurring leukemias and lymphomas in animals are apparently often due to exogenous retroviruses. At that time the concept of any cancer being infectious was thought to be naive at the very best. Subsequently, we learned that investigators (again, usually veterinary biologists) working in the avian systems had shown even earlier that an exogenous infecting retrovirus, known as avian leukosis virus, was a major cause of leukemia and lymphoma in chickens. Moreover, a closer examination of the murine leukemia virus literature suggested that mouse viruses may infect the developing offspring in utero or shortly after birth and enhance the probability of leukemia. Although a vertical transmission, this was, according to Gross, still an infection and not the simple gene transmission of unaltered endogenous retroviruses.

In the 1970s we obtained our first primate model. A Japanese-American, T. Kowakami, discovered the gibbon ape leukemia virus (GaLV); he showed that this retrovirus caused chronic myeloid leukemia in gibbons and that a variant of it causes T-cell acute lymphocytic leukemia. My coworkers and I isolated still another major variant of GaLV and we had the opportunity to study gibbon leukemic animals in detail, demonstrating the exogenous nature of GaLV and determining the presence of provirus in the tumor, and analyzing the GaLV genome. Dr. Flossie Wong-Staal in our group also showed that another newly isolated simian retrovirus, known as simian sarcoma virus (SSV), or woolly monkey virus, had viral sequences essentially identical to GaLV but contained additional sequences specifically homologous to cell sequences of the normal (uninfected) woolly monkey DNA. Moreover, Wong-Staal et al. and others showed that GaLV had homologous sequences in the DNA of normal mice, particularly in that of some Asian mice. From all these results we concluded that GaLV was an old infection of gibbons (many gibbons are infected in the wild), and that it entered these animals by way of an interspecies transmission of one of the Asian mouse endogenous retroviruses, perhaps by some intermediary vector, we also concluded that the woolly monkey virus (SSV) was derived by an interspecies transmission of GaLV from a pet gibbon to a pet woolly monkey housed in the same cage. (This history was verified by the owner of these animals and by studies which showed that woolly monkeys in the wild are not infected.) This resulted in a recombination of the viral sequences with cell sequences of the woolly monkey. These cellular sequences were later shown to be genetic sequences of platelet-derived growth factor (PDGF) as discussed by Aaronson and coworkers, Westermark and coworkers, and others.

These results influenced our thinking and the direction of our research. From this point, we considered the notion that a human retrovirus may have little or no homology to human DNA. With rare exception, this was a concept hitherto not even considered by the field. Animal retroviruses, including the disease-causing exogenous FeLV and avian leukosis virus (ALV), although clearly not endogenous, genetically transmitted elements clearly were substantially homologous to DNA sequences of the infected host cell in cat and chicken respectively. The results with GaLV showed little or no uninfected gibbon apes or woolly monkeys. All of these concepts and results have been detailed at previous Wilsede meetings. While we were still considering the possibility (in our view, probability) that human retroviruses would be found, we were, nevertheless, concerned that in these animal models (FeLV, ALV, MuLV, and GaLV) of retrovirus leukemias, virus was so readily found as to require no special techniques or efforts. In fact, viremia preceded leukemia, and it was frequently argued that extensive viremia is a prerequisite for viral leukemia. These facts had been presented as strong arguments against the existence of a human retrovirus and against the need for any special sensitive techniques to find them. Moreover, it was during the period of the first few Wilsede meetings that a few candidate human retroviruses turned out to be false leads, such as the RD114 virus and the virus called ESP-1, which were shown to be a new endogenous feline virus and mouse leukemia virus respectively. Both were contaminants of human cells.

Two model systems developed in work with animals – FeLV and BLV – helped sustain the thinking that human retroviruses probably do exist. Although FeLV was known to replicate extensively in most cat leukemias/lymphomas (see above), many of these cases were virus negative, as William Hardy and Max Essex emphasized at early Wilsede meetings. The epidemiology of these cats strongly implied that FeLV was involved. In addition, although virus could not be found in the tumor cells, it was often found at low levels in a few cells of the bone marrow. Therefore, Veffa Franchini, S. Josephs, R. Koshy and Flossie Wong-Staal in our group, pursued molecular biological studies of these tumors in collaboration with Essex and Hardy. We suspected that defective (partial) proviruses might explain the phenomenon. However, we were not able to prove this, and these interesting findings – as detailed at previous meetings – still lack an explanation. Presumably FeLV is involved in these leukemias by an indirect mechanism and not by a provirus integration into the cell destined to be the tumor.

The second example of an animal model system which became extremely important for human retroviruses is that of the bovine leukemia virus (BLV). This too was discovered at the beginning of the 1970's when Wilsede meetings were just getting underway. Since its discovery in Iowa by Van der Maartin and coworkers, much of the work on BLV biology was studied by Ferver et al. in Philadelphia and by Arsene Burny and his group in Brussels. It was also Burny et al. who carried out virtually all the BLV molecular biology. At the very first Wilsede meetings Arsene emphasized the minimal replication of BLV, the lack of viremia in infected animals, and the rare expression of virus in the tumor despite the presence of an integrated provirus. This was, of course, precisely the situation with HTLV-I and -II. Ironically, several features found for HTLV-I were later then found applicable to BLV.

There may be a lesson for us in this brief history: if our interest is a human disease, we should not allow ourselves to be trapped into focusing upon only one animal model but rather look more broadly at cell models.

During the mid 1970's and using the available monkey and ape viruses to make immunological and molecular probes, numerous groups including ours, reported finding virus-related molecules in some human cells, especially leukemias (our laboratory, Fersten group and Peter Bentvelyen and colleagues). The viruses were subsequently shown to be extremely closely related to the simian sarcoma virus (SSV) and GaLV or identical to them. Again, these studies were detailed in Wilsede meetings. Since there has been no further progress with these categories of virus, we must at least tentatively believe they were laboratory contaminants. Nonetheless, there are many indications that lead me to think that it will be interesting in the future to re-evaluate the question of retroviruses related to GaLV and SSV in humans.

In the remaining part of this presentation I will summarize our information on the known existing human retroviruses and highlight a few of the events that eventually led to their discovery.

When we began a search for human retroviruses beginning and reported at this first meeting it was in parallel with the late Sol Spiegelman and his colleagues, such as Arsene Burny and Rüdiger Hehlmann. Three approaches were used. As mentioned above, both Spiegelman's laboratory and ours exploited reverse transcriptase (RT) as a possible sensitive assay for discovering these viruses. Perhaps we could detect low levels of virus. Between 1970–

1975 the methods were made more sensitive and specific. The latter was necessary in order to distinguish viral RT from normal cellular DNA polymerases. These techniques, including the development and use of new synthetic homopolymeric template primers has been detailed in several reports. We were able intermittently to detect an enzyme which looked just like the viral RT, and we believed it might be a marker for an exogenous infecting retrovirus.

Spiegelman's group also used another approach that gave tantalizing results that most people couldn't quite accept, but I know of no one who has taken the trouble to re-evaluate these experiments. This approach made use of cDNA copies of messenger RNA transcripts from leukemic cells and showed some to be leukemia-specific, i.e., extra to the leukemic cells not present in normal cellular DNA. In at least a few cases Spiegelman and his colleagues could argue that these sequences were partly homologous to sequences present in some animal leukemia viruses. Thus, these experiments suggested that human leukemic cells contained *added* and probably virus-derived sequences. No one has yet pursued these studies further. The key criticism has always been that the amount of difference between the hybridization to leukemic cell DNA versus normal cell DNA was very extremely slight.

The second approach mentioned above, and one that we were lucky to take, was based on our attempts to define various growth factors for human blood cells, partly to help in our pursuit of a human retrovirus and partly because of our interests in blood cell biology. Initially we were looking specifically for a granulopoietic factor to grow granulocytic precursors. Our view for using a growth factor to help find virus was the belief that if a virus was present in low amounts, we could amplify it in this way, and if a viral gene was not expressed, we might induce its expression by growing the cells for a long period of time.

Thus, we were looking in any event for a growth factor that would grow granulopoietic cells, not, as Metcalf and Sachs had done, for colonies, but in mass amounts in liquid suspension. We had some temporary success in this. In these efforts we included conditional media from PHA-stimulated human lymphocytes, because in 1971–1972 we and others had discovered that stimulated lymphocytes released growth factors for some cell types. It was while looking for the granulocytic growth factor that we discovered IL-2, or T-cell growth factor, critical to our work. This discovery was made by Frank Ruscetti, the late Alan Wu and especially Doris Morgan. We also learned that activated but not "resting" T cells developed receptors for this growth factor. Peter Nowell had shown in the 1960s that after PHA lymphocytes live and grow for approximately two weeks, they tend to be lost and die out. We used the media, fractionated it, and added fractions back to the same stimulated cells. As long as we kept adding growth factor, the normal T cells continued to grow for considerable periods of time. We then approached studies of leukemic T cells; with one type of leukemia, the T cells grew as soon as we put them in culture and added IL-2. We did not need to activate them. They grew directly and they gave rise to the viruses that we have called HTLV-I.

The first human being from whom a retrovirus was isolated lived near Mobile, Alabama, in the south east of the United States. This man had no medical, personal, or social history when he developed a very aggressive T-cell malignancy. This was late 1978 when I called Arsene Burny for BLV reagents which, as Arsene likes to remind me, was on Christmas Eve. By that time we knew that the virus from this man behaved somewhat similar to bovine leukemia virus: it replicated poorly, seemed to cross-react slightly with BLV, and morphologically looked more like BLV than like other retroviruses. We thought, however, that we must rule out a bovine leukemia virus contaminant in the calf serum used in culturing human T cells. With the reagents to BLV provided by Arsene Burny this was done and soon we were able to characterize HTLV-I and to report on it at the beginning of 1979. We then published a series of papers on this in 1980 and early 1981. The clinicians called the malignancy an aggressive variant of mycosis fungoides (MF). Also known as cutaneous T-cell lymphoma, this is a T4 malignancy with skin manifestations, lymphoma cells infiltrating the skin, and usually a prolonged course.

We obtained a second isolate within a few months; this was from a young black woman in New York City who had come there from the Caribbean Islands. As in the case of the first patient, her illness resembled MF. It now seems, however, that MF may represent more than one disease (all with similar clinical manifestations), and that several forms of T-cell malignancies that are not MF may mimic that disease. By early 1981 the several sporadic cases which we had studied showed the presence of HTLV-I, all involved T4 cells, and all had an acute clinical course, often with hypercalcemia.

Tom Waldmann of NCI told me at that time of studies which had been conducted in Japan and published by Takatsuki, Yodoi, and Uchiyama. In 1977, they described a disease cases of which clustered in southern Japan. Although T4 cells and often accompanied by skin abnormalities, this disease seemed to differ from typical mycosis fungoides. They believed it to be a distinct disease, distinguished by its aggressiveness and, more importantly, by its geographical clustering. To my knowledge, this was the first time a reproducible clustering of human leukemia had been shown. They developed this lead by reexamining the epidemiology of lymphoid leukemia in Japan. Originally there were no leads, only that the relative incidence of B-cell leukemia in Japan was less than in the West. With availability of monoclonal antibodies, the cell surface molecules, they repeated the epidemiology studies with subtyping, i.e., B- versus T-cell leukemias. They found an increase in T-cell leukemias, particularly in the southwestern islands. However, they had no clues as to the cause. The prevailing causal suggestion at the time was that of parasitic infection.

Meanwhile our next HTLV-I isolate (the third) was obtained from a white, male, middle-aged merchant marine. When I learned of the evolving clinical-epidemiology story in Japan, we asked this patient social questions. As a merchant marine he had traveled extensively, including to the southern islands of Japan and to the Caribbean Islands. This fact and certain other aspects of his personal history allowed us to begin making a connection. In the meantime Bart Haynes, Dani Bolognesi, and their colleagues at Duke University were the first in the United States outside of our group to confirm an HTLV isolate, and this was followed by several more isolates from us. The Duke case was also of an aggressive T-cell leukemia, in this case in a Japanese-American woman who had come from the southern part of Japan to the Durham, North Carolina area. Otherwise only sporadic cases were identified in the United States.

By this time we had made contact with the late Professor Yohei Ito of Kyoto University. We received serum from him and his colleague Dr. Nakao, as well as from Tad Aoki in Niisita. Each of eight adult T-cell leukemias were positive, and their cultured cells also scored positive with our monoclonal antibodies to proteins of the virus. We were convinced that we had found the cause of that cluster. In the U.S., only sporadic cases were found. On March 1, 1981 at a workshop in Kyoto called by Prof. Ito for us to inform Japanese investigators of these results we reported on these isolates, the characterization of the virus, and the positive results on the Japanese ATL cases. Y. Hinuma, collaborating with Myoshi and working with Myoshi's cell line, presented the information that they too had identified a retrovirus but had not yet published their results. He furthermore suggested that the retrovirus was specific to this disease and referred to it as ATLV. Although confident that it would prove the same virus, we collaborated with Yoshida and Myoshi to demonstrate the identity of HTLV (now HTLV-I) and ATLV. Later Yoshida conducted the definite work of sequencing these viruses which ended this discussion and this phase of the work.

But how do these results help to explain the greater frequency of HTLV-I among black Americans? Sir John Dacie organized a small impromptu workshop in London attended by Bill Jarrett, Mel Greaves, Daniel Catovsky, Robin Weiss, and Bill Blattner (a key epidemiology collaborator in much of our work), and myself. At this session Catovsky reported a cluster of eight leukemias of very similar pattern, all similar to the Japanese disease, but all in black West Indians. In a collaborative study with Catovsky we showed all to be HTLV-I positive. The epidemiology of HTLV-I and its geographic prevalence is now fairly well known. It is present in the southeastern United States (especially among rural black populations), parts of Central America, the northern part of South America, Southern Japan and the Caribbean Islands. Half the lymphoid leukemias of adults in Jamaica (and presumably in many other Caribbean Islands) have been associated with HTLV-I. Unlike EBV, however, HTLV-I is far from ubiauitous and is totally absent from many areas of the world. In Europe, in addition to a cluster located in England, independent work in Amsterdam has led to the identification of a cluster among West Indian immigrants. A few areas of Europe have been found in which HTLV-I is endemic in a small proportion of the population; these include certain areas of Spain and a small region in southeastern Italy.

HTLV-I may have originated in Africa, arriving in the Americas via the slave trade. It may have been brought to Japan in the sixteenth century by Europeans who specifically entered the southern islands, bringing with them blacks and African monkeys. While this hypothesis may account for several aspects of the epidemiology, it cannot explain recent findings that the Ainu on the northern Japanese island of Hokaido also have a high prevalence of infection. Other studies have shown retroviruses very closely related to HTLV-I to be present in several African monkey and chimpanzees. Other studies have indicated that HTLV-I is transmitted only by intimate contact or by blood. Included in the latter, are the very disturbing arguments presented this year in Wilsede by Mel Greaves which suggest that HTLV-I may also be transmitted by the household mosquito, *Aedes egypti*. A similar conclusion has been drawn by Courtney Bartholomew from epidemiological studies done independently in Trinidad, West Indies.

The histological manifestations of leukemia/lymphoma associated with HTLV-I show variation in the histopathological pattern in the case of medium-sized lymphoma, mixed-cell lymphoma, large cell histiocytic lymphoma, and pleomorphic lymphoma, as well as in that of ATL. If it were not for the T4 and HTLV-markers, probably these would have been called four different diseases. The evidence that HTLV-I is the cause of a human cancer comes from several lines of evidence, not the least of which is the observation that many animal retroviruses can cause leukemia in various systems. Direct evidence for HTLV-I in ATL includes the clonal integration of HTLV-I provirus in the DNA of tumor cells, in vitro transformation of the right target cell (T_4 cells), and relatively straightforward epidemiology. It is important to note that the HTLV-I positive malignancies do not always show the clinical and histological pattern typical of ATL. There are some HTLV-I positive T-cell CLL, some HTLV-I positive apparently true mycosis fungoides, and some non-Hodgkins T-cell lymphomas. Careful clinical histological diagnosis is a two-edged sword. On the one hand, without greater precision of cell type Takatsuki et al. could not have described a cluster of ATL. On the other hand, too refined and we diagnose "a different disease" when it isn't.

Also, at Wilsede some have made the argument that we should throw away histology and clinical aspects and diagnose that leukemia solely by chromosomal changes. What happens when we do this with the T cell leukemias that are HTLV-I positive, i.e., where we have a cause? The result presents the problem that no consistent chromosomal change has been found in HTLV-I and leukemias, although a 14q abnormality has been found in about 40% of cases. These studies are hindered by lack of cell proliferation. However, in culture tumor cells more often than not release virus which infects the accompanying normal cells, and the normal cells outgrow the tumor cells. In 90% of cases the result is a diploid in vitro HTLV-I transformed cell line. Thus, more often than not, we cannot do the cytogenetics of the tumor.

Studies into the mechanism of HTLV-I transformation are among the most interesting features of this virus. Whereas the vast majority of animal retroviruses (excluding the usually defective transforming *onc* gene containing animal retroviruses which do not generally play a role in naturally occurring leukemias/lymphomas) do not have in vitro effects. In vitro HTLV-I mimics its in vivo effect, i.e., it chiefly infects T cells, particularly T4 cells, and induces immortalized growth in some. Perhaps the study of in vitro transformation of primary human T4 cells is akin to the study of initiation of T4 leukemia in vivo. Moreover, the molecular changes induced in vitro resemble the phenotypic characteristics of ATL cells. The major features in the mechanism of transformation are as follows:

1. ATL cells constitutively express IL-2 receptors (IL-2R) and in relatively large numbers. Normal T cells express IL-2R only transiently after immune activation and in an order of magnitude less than ATL cells. This is simulated by HTLV-I transformed T cells in vitro.

2. The integrated provirus is clonal and although each cell of the tumor have the provirus in the same location different tumors have different integration sites. These results obtained by Flossie Wong-Staal and coworkers in our group and by Yoshida and Seiki in Tokyo suggest that HTLV-I transforms its target T cell not by an activation of an adjacent or nearby cell gene, as suggested for some animal retroviruses, but by means of a *trans* mechanism.

3. Sequencing of the HTLV-I provirus has shown the presence of a new sequence not previously known in animal retroviruses. F. Wong-Staal and coworkers have demonstrated some of these sequences to be highly conserved and present in all biologically active HTLV-I isolates as well as in HTLV-II. Subsequently Haseltine has reported that these sequences encode a *trans*-acting protein known as the *trans*-acting transcriptional activator, or *tat*.

4. Transfection studies by Tanaguchi and by Warner Greene et al. have shown that *tat* not only induces more virus expression but also the expression of at least three types of cellular genes: IL-2, IL-2R, and HLA class II antigens. Thus, the first stage of transformation appears to be autocrine,

that is, each cell produces and responds to its own growth factor. There is reason to believe that secondary genetic events may be required for full malignant transformation, but these have not yet been defined. Finally, although one or more genetic changes in addition to HTLV-I may be required for development of leukemia, these probably need not be environmental in nature, since epidemiological studies only point to HTLV-I as the causative agent. In this sense HTLV-I leukemia differs from EBV and from Burkitt lymphoma.

Infection with HTLV-I may also lead to an increased incidence of B-cell CLL. This possibility has been raised by results of epidemiological studies in HTLV-I endemic areas. The mechanism here would have to be indirect however, because the viral sequences are not found in DNA of the B-cell tumor but in that of normal T cells. Some results suggest that this may be due to a chronic antigenic stimulation of B-cell proliferation, coupled with defective T4-cell function (due to HTLV-I infection) and spontaneous chance mutations in the hyperproliferating B cells.

Finally, HTLV-I has recently been linked to some CNS disease. The data are strictly epidemiological, and much work remains to be done with this interesting new opening.

HTLV-II, the second known human retrovirus, was isolated in my laboratory in 1981 in collaboration with D. Goldie at UCLA. The first isolate was from a young white male with hairy cell leukemia of T-cell type. There have only been few additional isolates. This is also T4-tropic, approximately 40% homologous to HTLV-I, shares some antigenic cross-reactivity, but shows certain morphological differences. The leukemias in which HTLV-II has thus far been found are few in number and have followed a fairly chronic course. As is the case with HTLV-I and HTLV-III, HTLV-II is apparently spreading among heroin addicts.

We began to think about a retrovirus cause of AIDS in late 1981. Beginning in 1982 we proposed that the likely cause of this disease was a retrovirus, a new one infecting T4 cells. I strongly suspected that it would be related to HTLV-I or -II. We knew from discussions with Max Essex and William Jarrett that feline leukemia virus (FeLV) can cause T-cell leukemia, and that a minor variant can cause AIDS or an AIDS-like disease. Recent studies by J. Mullins et al. indicate that this variation in FeLV may lie in the envelope. This observation plus the observations of the T4 tropism of HTLV-I, the mode of transmission of HTLV-I (sex, blood, congenital infection), seemed to fit what might be expected of an AIDS virus. We predicted that the difference in an AIDS virus from HTLV-I or HTLV-II would be in the envelope and/or in the *tat* gene. This prediction was not exactly right, for as we all know, the virus that causes AIDS posseses several additional features.

What do we know at present about the cytopathogenic effect of HTLV-III (HIV) and its mechanism? Studies by Peter Biberfeld at the Karolinska Institute and by Carlo Baroni in Rome indicate that the early sites of active infection may involve the follicular dendritic cells of the lymph nodes. Over time these cells degrade; first, lymphocytic hyperplasia develops and, later, there is an involution of the lymph nodes. The infected cells are those which enter germinal follicles. Those destined to be memory cells give rise to few progeny because upon T-cell immune activation they express virus and die; the population of memory T cells is therefore being destroyed regularly. The number of infected peripheral blood cells is only about 1% or less (as calculated by Southern blot hybridization). The number of cells expressing viral genes at any given time is in the range of only one in 10 000 to one in 100 000 (by RNA hybridization in situ). Examining these cells by electron microscopy, we see them bursting with virus release and dying. But why does this happen? Evidence from Zagury's laboratory at the University of Paris and from our own suggests that virus expression occurs specifically and only when T cells are immunologically activated, and that this is when the cell dies.

There is also strong evidence that T4 is required for cell killing, for when we transfect certain other cell types (T4−), thus producing virus, the cell does not die. Under certain conditions we can also transform T8 cells with HTLV-I; infected with HTLV-III, these cells produce virus but are not killed. Resting T4 cells can also be infected – without virus production but with immune activation. IL-2 receptor, IL-2, and gamma interferon genes are activated here, as in the case of normal T cells. Soon thereafter, however, viral genes are expressed, leading to the death of the cell. There has been much discussion of multi-nucleated giant formation as a mechanism of T4-cell killing by HTLV-III, but we now believe that this can be ruled out as a major contributing factor. Mandy Fisher, Flossie Wong-Staal, and others in our group have mutants of HTLV-III that replicate, show giant cell formation, but have very little T4-cell killing effect. Also, for this combination of diminished virus killing and maintained induction of giant cell formation Zagury has defined the conditions as decreased O_2 and/or temperature.

The genome of HTLV-III (HIV) reveals at least five extra genes. In addition to gag, pol, and env, this has a tat gene, a gene in the middle which we call sor, and a gene at the 3′ end called 3′ orf. It also shows a different splice which gives a different reading frame and different protein in the tat region, known as art or trs. Tat is involved in the transcriptional as well as post-transcriptional regulation of viral gene expression (T. Okamoto, F. Wong-Staal et al., and J. Sodrowski, C. Rosen, W. Haseltine et al., and P. Luciw et al.). The trs product determines whether viral env and gag genes will be expressed. The mechanism here is not yet understood, and we do not know the function of sor and orf. F. Wong-Staal and J. Ghrayeb have recently discovered a new gene known as the R gene, the function of which is also unknown.

Our general approach in studying the genes of HTLV-III and their function is to make deletion mutants or to perform site-directed mutations. This has been coupled with DNA transfection experiments in which human T cells have been transfected with various altered genes by the technique of protoplast fusion. Several coworkers and collaborators have contributed to this work. Notably, Amanda Fisher and Lee Ratner, Flossie Wong-Staal of our group, and Steve Pettaway at Dupont. Some of these studies show that tat and trs are essential for virus replication (not merely enhancement), that sor enhances replication, and that 3′-orf may repress virus production. Why HTLV-III should have so many regulatory genes is unknown.

Similar approaches have been used to determine which if any viral genes are involved in T4-cell killing. Is the mechanism indirect (e.g., analogous to tat of HTLV-I, activating a cellular gene) or direct? We have shown that a deletion in a few amino acids at the COOH terminus of the envelope leads to a mutant virus which can still replicate but does not kill. We therefore consider interaction of T4 and the envelope has a critical factor in virus killing. Nucleotide sequence data have now been obtained in our laboratory on many independent isolates of HTLV-III which have been published. These data show substantial heterogeneity regarding the envelope. How do these variations occur? We do not know the molecular mechanism here; however, most instances involve point mutations, perhaps due to error proneness of reverse transcriptase. One of our earliest virus isolates, called the HAT or

RF strain of HTLV-III (HTLV-III$_{RF}$) and mapped over two different time periods, showed no change in culture over many months. However other isolates obtained from patients showed significant changes over an 8-month period; these isolates were prepared by Wade Parks from Miami and analyzed by Beatrice Hahn, George Shaw, and Flossie Wong-Staal. This latter finding may be due to progressive mutation of the virus in vivo. Although a patient shows only one major virus type at any given time, minor variants of this virus emerge over time. Virus types found early on may nevertheless return at a later stage. These data can therefore not be solely explained by progressive mutation but probably by immune selection of different minor variants of a population of a number of variants which probably entered together at the time of infection.

Regarding vaccine, these analyses have good and bad news. The bad news, of course, the wide heterogeneity of viruses. The good, on the other hand is that we have not seen a patient infected with more than one strain of virus. In patients infected with a given type we have found only variants of that type, regardless of exposures. This may indicate that patients infected with one strain are protected against other strains.

The nucleotide sequence heterogeneity is reflected in biological variation. M. Popovic and S. Gartner in our group have shown that virus from the thymus is solely T4 tropic, that from the brain chiefly monocyte-macrophage tropic, and that from blood both T4 and macrophage tropic. Eva-Marie Fenyoe and Brigitta Anyos have reported at Wilsede their observation that virus isolated late in a disease can be biologically significantly different from isolates obtained earlier in the disease.

Infection with HTLV-III is associated with an increased incidence of malignancies, yet the sequences of the virus are not found in any of the major tumor types (Kaposi's sarcoma, B-cell lymphomas, and certain squamous cell carcinomas). It is therefore often assumed that these tumors develop chiefly because of immune suppression. I would suggest that these will be shown at least in part to involve other viruses, some of which are yet to be discovered.

The most astonishing thing about viruses and leukemia/lymphoma I have learned since the Wilsede meetings began some 15 years ago is the multiplicity of ways in which viruses can produce these malignancies. We know, for instance, of insertional mutagenesis (the apparent mechanism for avian leukemia virus and probably several other *gag-pol-env* retroviruses), which apparently operates by LTR activation of nearby cell genes important to growth. We also know of the infection of an *onc* gene containing retroviruses (only in animals and admittedly very rare). We have heard that FeLV may regularly recombine with cat cell sequences and acquire *onc* genes within the life of the infected cat and reinserting these genes may result in leukemia. We know, furthermore, that the mechanism for HTLV-I, and -II and BLV differs and involves a *trans*-acting mechanism; and there is evidence for some of these viruses as well as for others influencing the development of leukemia/lymphoma by indirect mechanisms. So, in this field, you do not have to go to California, like Hans Eidig, to find gold. I wish to thank Rolf Neth, his family, and his friends in this region for inviting me for this lecture and for enriching my life with the friendships made in Wilsede.

Reference

Modern Trends in Human Leukemia II – VI (1976–1985). Springer, Berlin Heidelberg New York Tokyo

Frederick Stohlman Jr. Memorial Lecture

Wilsede, June 21, 1978

Memorial Tribute to Dr. Frederick Stohl-man Presented by William C. Moloney

Gallo, Robert C.: Cellular and Virological Studies Directed to the Pathogenesis of the Human Myelogenous Leukemias

Pinkel, Donald: Treatment of Childhood Acute Lymphocytic Leukemia

Wilsede, June 18, 1980

Klein, George: The Relative Role of Viral Transformation and Specific Cytogenetic Changes in the Development of Murine and Human Lymphomas

Kaplan, Henry S.: On the Biology and Immunology of Hodgkin's Disease

Wilsede, June 21, 1982

Greaves, Melvyn F.: Immunobiology of Lymphoid Malignancy

Thomas, E. Donnall: Bone Marrow Transplantation in Leukemia

Wilsede, June 17, 1984

Klein, Jan: Introduction for N. Avrion Mitchison

Mitchison, N. Avrion: Repertoire purging by medium-concentration self-macromole-cules is the major factor determining helper and suppressor repertoire differences

June 18, 1984

Gallo, Robert C.: Introduction for Peter H. Duesberg

Duesberg, Peter H.: Are Activated Proto-*Onc* Genes Cancer Genes?

Wilsede, June 22, 1986

Vogt, Peter K.: Introduction for Harald zur Hausen

Harald zur Hausen: Viruses in Human Tumors

Malcolm A.S. Moore: Introduction for Donald Metcalf

Donald Metcalf: Hemopoietic Growth Factors and Oncogenes in Myeloid Leukemia Development

Haematology and Blood Transfusion   Vol. 31
Modern Trends in Human Leukemia VII
Edited by Neth, Gallo, Greaves, and Kabisch
© Springer-Verlag Berlin Heidelberg 1987

Introduction for Harald zur Hausen

P. K. Vogt [1]

Ladies and Gentlemen:

Tonight I have the pleasure to introduce the first speaker for the Frederick Stohlman Jr. Memorial Lectures, Harald zur Hausen.

Let me begin with some biographical data. Harald zur Hausen attended the medical schools of Bonn, Hamburg, and Düsseldorf and received his M.D. in 1960. This was followed by 2 years of internship and 4 years of postdoctoral research at the Institute of Microbiology of the University of Düsseldorf, where zur Hausen worked with Professor Kikuth. In 1966 Harald zur Hausen went to the United States to the Children's Hospital of Philadelphia, joining the laboratory of Werner and Gertrude Henle. He was appointed Assistant Professor of Virology at the University of Pennsylvania in 1968.

I think I am not taking excessive liberties in stating that the training with Werner and Gertrude Henle was the most decisive in Harald zur Hausen's research career. The period in the Henles' laboratory formed him. It was there that Harald zur Hausen acquired the basic tools and the broad intellectual outlook for his research. Harald zur Hausen has carried on the tradition of the Henles as great innovators in medical virology; through his work he has augmented and enriched it, becoming himself an eminent representative of this tradition.

Harald zur Hausen returned to Germany in 1969, first going to the institute of another ex-Philadelphian, Eberhard Wecker, in Würzburg. In 1972, Harald zur Hausen ac-

cepted the offer to head an independent institute of medical virology as Professor and Chairman at the University of Erlangen. From 1977 to 1983 he was Professor and Chairman of the Institute of Virology at the University of Freiburg, and in 1983 he accepted the challenging position of Scientific Director of the German Cancer Center at Heidelberg.

Zur Hausen has received numerous awards and prizes: the Richtzenhain Prize of the University of Heidelberg, the Warner Prize of the University of Hamburg, the Schaudinn Medal of the German Dermatological Society, and an Honorary Doctor of Science degree from the University of Chicago. He has been visiting professor at the university of Belo Horizonte in Brazil and the universities of Brisbane and Perth in Australia. Just 2 weeks ago, Harald zur Hausen received one of the most prestigious awards in cancer research, the Charles S. Mott Prize, presented by the General Motors Cancer Research Foundation for the most outstanding recent contribution to our knowledge about the causes and hence to the ultimate prevention of cancer.

Harald zur Hausen is a pioneer of medical virology. His work concentrated early on persistent infections with DNA viruses. This focus of interest quite naturally led him to a study of herpesviruses. He was the first to demonstrate the DNA of Epstein-Barr virus in Burkitt's lymphoma cells that do not produce the complete infectious virus. He showed that Epstein-Barr virus DNA was present in Burkitt tumor tissue and in the tissue of another tumor, nasopharyngeal carcinoma, in multiple genome equivalents per

[1] Dept. of Microbiology, 2025 Zonal Avenue, Los Angeles, California 90033, USA

cell. His observations indicate an important role of the Epstein-Barr virus in the genesis of Burkitt's lymphoma and of nasopharyngeal carcinoma.

Harald zur Hausen's recent work deals with human papillomaviruses. There are numerous, distinct types of these viruses. None of the them can be grown in tissue culture, so their study relies heavily on molecular biology techniques. Harald zur Hausen has demonstrated that papillomavirus sequences are present in most human genital tumors, that there is a correlation between the specific type of papillomavirus and the benign or malignant nature of the tumor, and that papillomavirus sequences are expressed in tumor tissue. All this together strongly indicates that papillomaviruses play an important role in the initiation and possibly the maintenance of these human tumors.

In his work on herpesviruses Harald zur Hausen was at the forefront of a large group of scientists who had been drawn to this field by the initial discovery that linked Epstein-Barr virus to Burkitt's lymphoma. The study of papillomaviruses has gained far fewer adherents, and here Harald zur Hausen has always been and remains the prime and dominant advocate for the oncogenic importance of these viruses.

If I mentioned only herpesviruses and papillomaviruses, I would ignore one of Harald zur Hausen's greatest accomplishments: the current healthy state of the German Cancer Center in Heidelberg. When Harald zur Hausen took over as the scientific director a mere 3 years ago, that institution had fallen on hard times. It was torn by internal strife and dissent, and much of its research program was widely perceived by the international scientific community as being in need of improvement. Within a remarkably short time Harald zur Hausen has restored peace, lifted scientific standards, attracted first-rate research talent, and created a modern scientific institution that has become worthy of the national effort devoted to its maintenance. This almost miraculous turnaround did not come about by a revolution or by confrontations but through Harald zur Hausen's determined, firm and persuasive leadership, his vision, his high ideals, and his diplomatic skill. The Federal Republic owes Harald zur Hausen its Cancer Center; he has revived it.

Ladies and gentlemen,

I introduce to you Harald zur Hausen, distinguished scholar, accomplished leader, and seasoned diplomat.

Haematology and Blood Transfusion Vol. 31
Modern Trends in Human Leukemia VII
Edited by Neth, Gallo, Greaves, and Kabisch
© Springer-Verlag Berlin Heidelberg 1987

Viruses in Human Tumors

H. zur Hausen [1]

Table 1 lists possible interactions of viruses in oncogenesis and emphasizes the role of human pathogenic viruses. The majority of tumor viruses known today insert their genetic material into the host cell nucleus, where it persists. The expression of at least one viral function appears to be a prerequisite for the maintenance of the transformed state.

An interesting difference in interactions in oncogenesis is noted in infections by herpes simplex viruses. Abortive infection by these viruses modifies the host cell DNA [30, 31]. Transformation of rodent cells by these infections does not require persistence of viral DNA, but selective DNA amplification induced by these agents may play a crucial role in transformation [15]. Recently, it has been noted that besides herpes simplex viruses other members of the herpesvirus group, such as the pseudorabies virus (B. Matz, per-

sonal communication) and murine cytomegaloviruses (R. Heilbronn, unpublished data) share this property. Even a member of the poxvirus group, vaccinia, is able to induce selective DNA amplification [32]. It remains to be seen whether this property is consistently linked to transforming functions.

A third group of agents is represented by viruses causing the acquired immunodeficiency syndrome (AIDS). In this condition, specific types of tumors develop as a consequence of the depressed immune function without being directly related to the AIDS virus infection.

The fourth rather interesting group is represented by agents suppressing oncogenicity. This property has thus far been observed exclusively in infections with autonomous or helper-dependent parvoviruses. Their mode of interaction with infected host cells may provide some clues on early events in carcinogenesis. Available evidence suggests an interference of these viruses with early events,

[1] Deutsches Krebsforschungszentrum, Im Neuenheimer Feld 280, 6900 Heidelberg, FRG

Table 1. Interactions of viruses with hosts and host cells in oncogenesis

Interaction	Example
Integration of the viral genome into host cell chromosomes, or episomal persistence of viral DNA	Hepatitis B, papillomaviruses, EBV, HTLV-I
Induction of changes analogous to chemical and physical carcinogens without persistence of viral DNA in modified cells	Herpes simplex virus; cytomegalovirus (?)
Induction of immunodeficiencies; secondary development of lymphomas and Kaposi sarcomas	HIV (AIDS)
Inhibition of oncogenesis	Parvoviruses

Table 2. Viruses involved in human oncogenesis

Virus	Related cancer(s)
Epstein-Barr viruses	Burkitt's lymphoma; nasopharyngeal cancer; lymphomas in immuno-suppressed individuals
Hepatitis-B virus	Primary hepatocellular carcinoma
HTLV-I	Adult T-cell leukemia
Human papillomaviruses types 5, 8, 14, 17	Squamous cell carcinomas in patients with epidermodysplasia verruciformis
Human papillomaviruses types 16, 18, 31, 33, 35	Cervical cancer, vulvar cancer, penile cancer, perianal and anal cancer

Table 3. Approximate latency periods for virus-associated human cancers

Virus	Cancer	Latency period (years)
Hepatitis B	Primary hepato-cellular carcinoma	30–50
HTLV-I	T-cell leukemia	30–50
Epstein-Barr	Burkitt's lymphoma	3–12
Epstein-Barr	Nasopharyngeal cancer	30–50
HPV 5, 8, 14, 17	Skin cancer in epidermodysplasia verruciformis	3–12
HPV 16, 18, 31, 33, 35	Cervical cancer, vulvar cancer, penile cancer, perianal and anal cancer	20–50

possibly related to initiation, in oncogenesis [15].

The following contribution concentrates on viruses in human tumors inserting their genetic material within the host nucleus. Members of four groups of viruses have thus far been identified as playing a role in human tumors. These viruses and the respective human tumors are listed in Table 2.

The percentage of human tumors which can be linked to these infections on a worldwide scale is remarkably high, at present approximately 15% for both sexes [41]. In females close to 20% of all cancers can be linked to viral infections, most notably cervical cancer, amounting to almost 16%. In males slightly less than 10% are virally linked; 6.2% represent primary hepatocellular carcinomas.

All cancers developing as a consequence of these viral infections share some characteristics:

1. They are monoclonal.
2. They develop only after long latency periods (in most instances after several decades; see Table 3).
3. Only a small percentage of infected individuals eventually develop cancer.
4. Expression of the persisting viral genome is the rule but appears to be restricted to a specific set of genes.

Attempts to clarify the role of viruses in human tumors will have to take into account these observations.

During the past few years a remarkable role of viruses of the papillomavirus group in human cancer has become evident. Particularly human anogenital cancer (including cervical, vulvar, penile, and perianal cancer) and specific rare forms of human skin cancer have been linked to these infections [43]. The mechanism of cancer induction following some of these infections may provide clues for the understanding of virus-linked oncogenesis in man and will be discussed in more detail subsequently.

Observations made by Rigoni-Stern (published in 1842) on a vastly different incidence of cervical cancer in prostitutes as compared with nuns mark the first important contribution to etiological factors in human genital cancer [27]. These studies, confirmed by many subsequent analyses, stimulated research on the role of sexually transmitted agents in the genesis of this neoplasia. Up to the end of the 1960s speculations were made concerning a possible role of gonorrhea, syphilis, and trichomoniasis in the induction of genital cancer, without there being any really supportive epidemiological evidence [28].

At the end of the 1960s a significant change occurred: two groups almost simultaneously reported seroepidemiological data implying an involvement of herpes simplex virus (HSV) type-2 infections in the etiology of cervical cancer [23, 26]. During the following 10 years a surprising number of confirmatory manuscripts were published, including experimental data on viral reactivation from tumor tissue, on the presence of a variety of HSV-specific antigens, on viral ribonucleic acid, and (much more scarce) on fragments of viral DNA within premalignant and malignant tissue (reviewed in zur Hausen [40]). Since partially inactivated HSV was also shown to induce transformation of rodent cells [9], by the end of the 1970s HSV appeared to be a strong candidate for a role in the induction of cervical cancer.

In 1969 my group in Würzburg attempted to demonstrate Epstein-Barr virus DNA in Burkitt's lymphomas and nasopharyngeal cancer. After succeeding in the purification of EBV DNA, it was readily possible to find genomes of this herpes-group virus regularly in Burkitt's lymphomas and nasopharyngeal cancer biopsies by DNA-DNA or DNA-RNA hybridizations [42, 44]. Therefore, it was an obvious task to use the same technology in attempts to find HSV DNA in anogenital cancer. Somewhat unexpectedly, we encountered difficulties. The analysis of a large number of biopsies provided exclusively negative results [45]. In early 1972 I became convinced that HSV, if at all involved in genital cancer, could not interact with host cells analogous to other tumor virus systems known at that time by leaving persisting viral DNA with partial gene expression in the transformed cell. Since another mode of interaction appeared to be unlikely at this period, and cervical cancer nevertheless remained a strong candidate for a viral etiology, during 1972 we started looking for a role of other viruses in human genital cancer.

There were good reasons for selecting human papillomavirus (HPV) for the subsequent study: a virus had been known since 1907 [4] to be the causative factor of human warts. Genital warts, a particularly unpleasant infection characterized by exuberant exophytic growth, had been shown electron microscopically to contain viral particles morphologically identical to those in common warts [1]. More importantly, there existed a substantial number of anecdotal reports, published over almost a whole century, on malignant conversion of genital warts (condylomata acuminata), usually after long duration and therapy resistance (reviewed in zur Hausen [37]).

Wart viruses had barely been characterized at this period: this was mainly due to the lack of in vitro systems for viral propagation and to a remarkable host specificity of these viruses [29]. Studies depended entirely on the availability of biopsy materials containing large quantities of viral particles. Our initial studies were performed with cRNA preparations obtained from an individual plantar wart. The first hybridization data published in 1974 [45] showed that many, but by far not all, DNAs from common warts hybridized with the radioactive probe. None of the genital warts and none of the cervical cancer biopsies showed a positive reaction. Since some of the genital warts analyzed contained electron microscopically visible viral particles, this was a clearcut suggestion that, most likely, different types of HPV are causative agents of condylomata acuminata. This result prompted a period of analyses of individual virus particle-containing papillomas for a genetic heterogeneity of papillomas; this was established in 1976 [10] and led to the identification of individual types 1 year later [12, 25].

The identification of genital papillomavirus infections turned out to be difficult

7

because of low particle production in genital warts. HPV 6 was identified in 1980 [11] from a rare condyloma with a high particle yield. Two new methodological approaches were of major importance for the subsequent developments: the introduction of gene cloning techniques into the papillomavirus field and the application of hybridization procedures at lowered stringency revealing the relatedness of distinct papillomavirus types, both first used in Peter Howley's laboratory [18]. The use of these methods led to a rapid expansion of identified types of HPVs: today 42 types have been established, and this number will most likely increase further.

Gerard Orth in Paris, Stephania Jablonska in Warsaw, and their colleagues identified a large number of HPV types from a rare human condition, epidermodysplasia verruciformis [25]. This syndrome is characterized by an extensive verrucosis and a remarkably high rate of malignant conversions of specific types of papillomas at sunexposed sites. It was of particular interest to demonstrate specific types of HPV, preferentially HPV 5, but also HPV 8 and – rarely – others, within the carcinomas, although patients with epidermodysplasia verruciformis commonly reveal infections with up to 15 additional types of papillomaviruses. Cancers in this condition therefore appear to represent a particularly interesting example of interactions between a specific virus infection and physical carcinogens such as the ultraviolet part of sunlight.

Returning to genital papillomavirus infections, cloning of HPV 6 DNA [6] permitted the identification of a closely related HPV DNA, HPV 11, in genital warts and laryngeal papillomas [13, 14, 22]. Applying conditions of low-stringency hybridization our group identified two additional types of genital papillomavirus infections, HPV 16 and HPV 18, by cloning their DNA directly from cervical cancer biopsies [3, 7]. Subsequently, additional types have been identified, most notably HPV 31 [19] and HPV 33 [2], both somewhat related to HPV 16. The total number of virus types found in the genital tract to date is 14. It appears at present that HPV 6 and 11 are the most prevalent virus types in genital warts, accounting for approximately 90% of all condylomata

acuminata and for about one third of all oral papillomas. In contrast, HPV 16 and probably also HPV 18 are found at external genital sites, most commonly in very different lesions, characterized as Bowenoid papulosis or Bowen's disease [16]. The histology reveals marked nuclear atypia and shows characteristics of a carcinoma in situ.

All four types of HPV also infect cervical tissue. Typical papillomatous proliferations at the cervix are rare. The most common colposcopically visible lesion is the "flat condyloma" [20].

Although ardently disputed at gynecological and cytological meetings, it is likely that the histology of HPV 6 and 11 lesions differs from that of HPV 16 and 18 [5]. The former viruses induce lesions characterized by a high degree of koilocytosis as a pathognomonic marker for this type of infection. HPV 16 and 18 viruses appear to preferentially induce lesions with marked nuclear atypia, a low degree of koilocytosis, or absence of visible koilocytosis. It is likely that some of the rather confusing data on the histopathology of HPV types result from infections with more than one type of HPV. Probably the majority of histopathologists would not have difficulties in discriminating a Bowenoid lesion from a koilocytotic condyloma at an external genital site. It would be rather surprising if the same type found in both of these lesions induced a uniform histopathological pattern at cervical sites.

Kreider and his colleagues [17] recently demonstrated that HPV 11 infections induce changes characteristic of koilocytotic dysplasia upon infection of human cervical tissue heterografted beneath the renal capsule of nude mice. It is anticipated that this technique will establish the causative role of HPVs in cervical dysplasias and therefore point to an etiological role of these agents in a clearly premalignant condition. Since HPV 16 and 18 have been directly isolated from cervical carcinoma biopsies, it is of course important to clarify their role in this type of cancer.

HPV 16 DNA is present in approximately 50% of biopsies from cervical, vulvar, and penile cancer. It is also found in some perianal and anal cancers and in a small percentage of oral, tongue, laryngeal, and lung carcinomas. HPV 18 DNA has so far been detected only in anogenital cancer, occurring in about 20% of the biopsies tested. Approximately an additional 10% of these biopsies contain HPV 33, 31, or 11 DNA, bringing the total percentage of biopsies with identifiable HPV types to about 80%. It is likely that the majority of additional genital tumors also contain HPV DNA of yet undefined types since bands become visible in blot hybridizations under conditions of lowered stringency. Therefore, it appears justified to summarize this part by stating that the majority of, if not all cervical, vulvar, and penile cancers contain HPV DNA.

Similar to cancer biopsies, the majority of cervical cancer-derived cell lines tested so far contain HPV 16 or HPV 18 DNA, among them the well-known HeLa line [3, 34]. The availability of these lines and of primary cervical cancer biopsies permitted an analysis of the state of the viral DNA within the tumor cells. From the results it became evident that cell lines contain exclusively integrated viral DNA; in primary tumors integration is also regularly noted, revealing a monoclonal pattern. Some of the primary tumors contain in addition episomal viral DNA [7]. Precursor lesions, Bowenoid papulosis, and cervical dysplasias appear to contain preferentially nonintegrated viral DNA [8].

The integrational pattern reveals some specificity on the viral side, opening the viral ring molecules most frequently within the E1–E2 open reading frames and thus disrupting the early region [34]. No preferential chromosomal sites have been noted for integration [21]. One line, Caski, contains at least 12 different integration sites in 11 distinct chromosomes.

In all cell lines analyzed thus far and in a number of primary tumors, transcription of the persisting HPV DNA has been noted. Commonly, transcripts covering the E6–E7 open reading frames are present [34]. Some of the transcripts are fused to adjacent host cell sequences. It is not clear whether these fusion transcripts play any functional role.

Sequencing of cDNA clones of HPV 18 transcripts in three cervical cancer lines revealed the existence of a small intron within the E6 open reading frame [33]. The second E6 exon is read in a different reading frame, resulting in a putative protein which shows some distant relationship to epidermal growth factor. It is interesting to note that the same splice donor and acceptor sites also exist in HPV 16 and 33 DNA, but are absent in HPV 6 and 11 DNA. It remains to be seen whether this has any functional significance.

The regularity of transcription in HPV-positive cervical cancer cells and the consistent expression of the E6–E7 open reading frames suggest a role of this genetic activity in the maintenance of the transformed state. Integration of viral DNA within E1–E2 with a likely disruption of an intragenomic regulation may represent another event important for malignant conversion. Several recent, still somewhat preliminary studies further emphasize the role of HPV expression in the maintenance of the malignant phenotype. Stanbridge and his co-workers [35] demonstrated that fusion of HeLa cells to normal human fibroblasts or keratinocytes results in a suppression of the malignant phenotype. Loss of chromosomes from the nontransformed donor, apparently in particular that of chromosome no. 11, leads to a reacquisition of malignant growth upon heterotransplantation into nude mice. Since HeLa cells express HPV 18 RNA, it was of obvious interest to analyze HPV 18 expression in the nonmalignant HeLa hybrids as well as in their malignant revertants.

The data obtained thus far (E. Schwarz et al., in preparation) indicate that no difference in HPV 18 expression occurs in HeLa cells, in their hybrids with normal cells, or in malignant revertants upon cultivation of these cells in tissue culture. Also under these conditions, no differences are noted in clonability and growth in soft agar. Whereas HeLa cells and malignant revertants continue to express HPV 18 DNA after transplantation into nude mice, initial experiments suggested a complete block of HPV 18 expression in the nonmalignant hybrid lines. Although these data were difficult to interpret due to the invasion of murine cells into the chamber, these and more recent studies using differentiation-inducing chemicals in vitro suggest a control of HPV expression at the transcriptional level in nontumorigenic hybrid cells.

The interpretation of these data is schematically outlined in Fig. 1. The data point to an intracellular control of HPV ex-

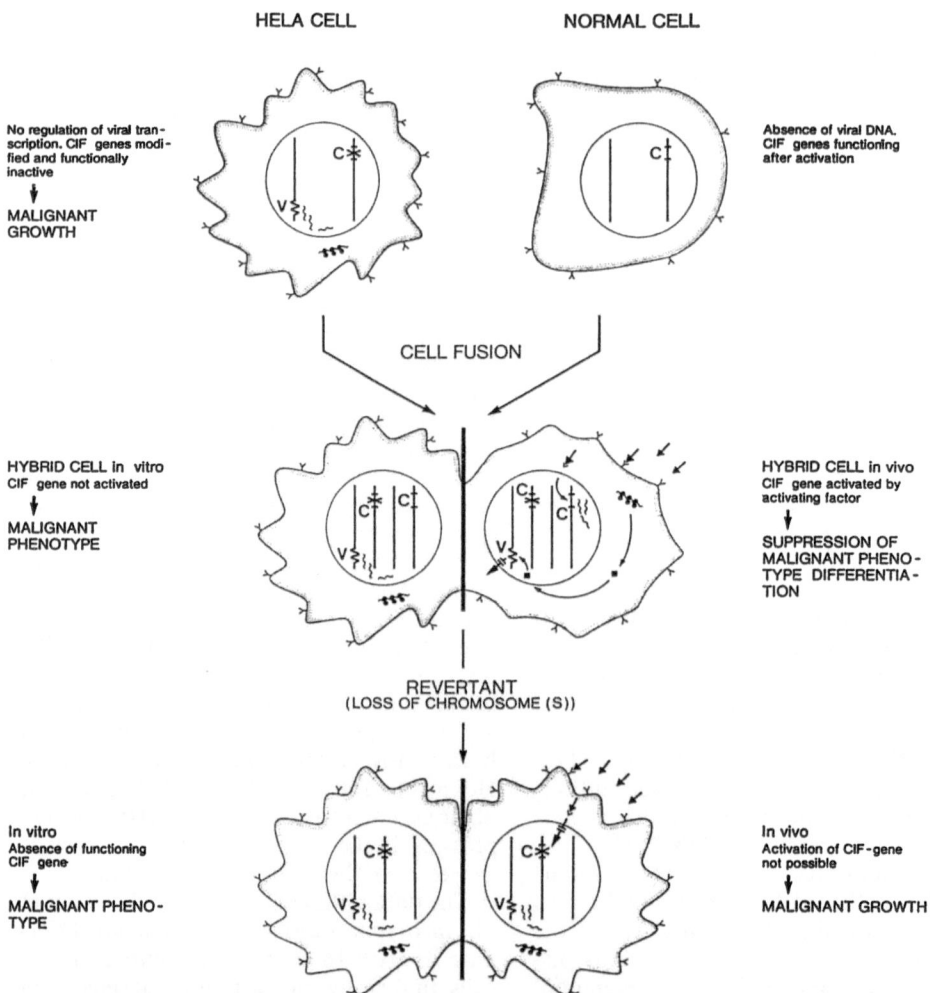

HELA CELL   NORMAL CELL

No regulation of viral transcription. CIF genes modified and functionally
inactive   Absence of viral DNA.
                                                                CIF genes functioning
                                                                after activation

MALIGNANT
GROWTH

CELL FUSION

HYBRID CELL in vitro
CIF gene not activated   HYBRID CELL in vivo
                                                                CIF gene activated by
MALIGNANT   activating factor
PHENOTYPE
                                                                SUPPRESSION OF
                                                                MALIGNANT PHENO-
                                                                TYPE DIFFERENTIA-
                                                                TION

REVERTANT
(LOSS OF CHROMOSOME (S))

In vitro
Absence of functioning
CIF gene   In vivo
                                                                Activation of CIF-gene
MALIGNANT PHENO-   not possible
TYPE
                                                                MALIGNANT GROWTH

Fig. 1. Interpretation of data on HPV 18 expression

pression by cellular genes. These genes are most likely modified and functionally inactive in HeLa cells but are contributed to the hybrids by the normal donor. Obviously, they are not expressed in tissue culture, but they seem to require activation by a putative humoral factor. This occurs upon hetero-transplantation to the nude mouse.

These data, if confirmed for other human tumor cell lines, support a concept viewing the development of human cancer as a failing host-cell control of persisting viral genes [36–38, 41]. The model derived there from can readily explain the frequently observed synergism between papillomavirus infec-

tions and initiating events [40]. Initiators should interact by modifying cellular control functions or the binding sites recognized by the cellular suppressing factor within the viral genome.

Factors modifying cellular genes in the development of genital cancer are presently poorly defined. Smoking, viral infections with initiating properties (e.g., herpes simplex virus and cytomegalovirus), and potentially mutagenic metabolites in chronic inflammations should be of particular risk for cervical sites and are probably much less active at external genital sites [40]. This could account for the much higher risk of cervical cancer in comparison with vulvar and penile cancer and for a different age distribution of the latter compared with cancer of the cervix.

The data suggest the existence of an intracellular surveillance mechanism which controls papillomavirus infections. It may have far-reaching implications for other human tumor virus infections as well, possibly controlled by a similar mechanism. This could represent an ancestral defense mechanism, preceding immunological control functions, that protects the host at the cellular level against potentially lethal functions of coevolving viruses. The expression of these viral functions in differentiating cells which are unable to proliferate, permitting replication and maturation of the respective papillomaviruses, points to a fine tuning of host-virus and virus-host adaptations.

Cancer as a result of a failing host-cell control of persisting viral genes could readily explain long latency periods between primary infections of cancer-linked viruses and tumor appearance. It also provides a convenient explanation for the fact that only a small number of infected individuals develop the respective cancer type. Since, in addition to a persisting viral genome, modifications in both alleles of suppressing genes are required, monoclonality of the arising tumor can be predicted.

The concept developed here offers a new approach to understanding the etiology of smoking-related cancers. Increasingly, HPV genomes have been demonstrated in some of them [41]. If such tumors arise from a similar interaction between persisting viral infections and smoking-related chemical carcinogens, new strategies may be developed for the control and therapy of these common human cancers.

References

1. Almeida JD, Oricl JD, Stannard LM (1969) Characterization of the virus found in human genital warts. Microbios 3:225–229
2. Beaudenon S, Kremsdorf D, Croissant O, Jablonska S, Wain-Hobson S, Orth G (1986) A novel type of human papillomavirus associated with genital neoplasias. Nature 321:246–249
3. Boshart M, Gissmann L, Ikenberg H, Keinheinz A, Scheurlen W, zur Hausen H (1984) A new type of papillomavirus DNA, its presence in genital cancer biopsies and in cell lines derived from cervical cancer. EMBO J 3:1151–1157
4. Ciuffo G (1907) Innesto positivo con filtrato di verruca vulgare. Giorn Ital Mal Venereol 48:12–17
5. Crum CP, Mitao M, Levine RU, Silverstein S (1985) Cervical papillomaviruses segregate within morphologically distinct precancerous lesions. J Virol 54:675–681
6. de Villiers E-M, Gissmann L, zur Hausen H (1981) Molecular cloning of viral DNA from human genital warts. J Virol 40:932–935
7. Dürst M, Gissmann L, Ikenberg H, zur Hausen H (1983) A papillomavirus DNA from a cervical carcinoma and its prevalence in cancer biopsy samples from different geographic regions. Proc Natl Acad Sci USA 80:3812–3815
8. Dürst M, Kleinheinz A, Hotz M, Gissmann L (1985) The physical state of human papillomavirus type 16 DNA in benign and malignant genital tumors. J Gen Virol 66:1515–1522
9. Duff R, Rapp F (1973) Oncogenic transformation of hamster embryo cells after exposure to inactivated herpes simplex virus type I. J Virol 12:209–217
10. Gissmann L, zur Hausen H (1976) Human papilloma viruses: physical mapping and genetic heterogeneity. Proc Natl Acad Sci USA 73:1310–1313
11. Gissmann L, zur Hausen H (1980) Partial characterization of viral DNA from human genital warts (condylomata acuminata). Int J Cancer 25:605–609
12. Gissmann L, Pfister H, zur Hausen H (1977) Human papilloma viruses (HPV): characterization of four different isolates. Virology 76:569–580
13. Gissmann L, Diehl V, Schulz-Coulon H, zur Hausen H (1982) Molecular cloning and characterization of human papillomavirus DNA from a laryngeal papilloma. J Virol 44:393–400
14. Gissmann L, Wolnik H, Ikenberg H, Koldovsky U, Schnürch HG, zur Hausen H (1983) Human papillomavirus type 6 and 11 sequences in genital and laryngeal papillomas and in some cervical cancer biopsies. Proc Natl Acad Sci USA 80:560–563
15. Heilbronn R, Schlehofer JR, Yalkinoglu AÖ, zur Hausen H (1985) Selective DNA amplification induced by carcinogenes (initiators): evidence for a role of proteases and DNA polymerase alpha. Int J Cancer 36:85–91

16. Ikenberg H, Gissmann L, Gross G, Grussendorf-Conen E-I, zur Hausen H (1983) Human papillomavirus type 16-related DNA in genital Bowen's disease and in Bowenoid papulosis. Int J Cancer 32:563–565
17. Kreider JW, Howett MK, Wolfe SA, Bartlett GL, Zaino RJ, Sedlacek TV, Mortel L (1985) Morphological transformation in vivo of human uterine cervix with papillomavirus from condylomata acuminata. Nature 317:639–641
18. Law MF, Lancaster WD, Howley PM (1979) Conserved polynucleotide sequences among the genomes of papilloma viruses. J Virol 32:199–211
19. Lorincz AT, Lancaster WD, Temple GF (1985) Detection and characterization of a new type of human papilloma virus. J Cell Biochem [Suppl 9c] 75
20. Meisels A, Roy M, Fortier M, Morin C, Casas-Cordero M, Shah KV, Turgeon H (1981) Human papilloma virus infection of the cervix: the atypical condyloma. Acta Cytol 25:7–16
21. Mincheva A, Gissmann L, zur Hausen H (1987) Chromosomal integration sites of human papillomavirus DNA in three cervical cancer cell lines mapped by in situ hybridization. Med. Microbiol. Immunol. 176:245–256, 1987
22. Mounts P, Shah KV, Kashima H (1982) Viral etiology of juvenile – and adult – onset squamous papilloma of the larynx. Proc Natl Acad Sci USA 79:5425–5429
23. Nahmias AJ, Josey WE, Naib ZM, Luce CF, Guest BA (1970) Antibodies to herpes virus hominis types I and II in humans. II. Women with cervical cancer. Am J Epidemiol 91:547–552
24. Orth G, Favre M, Croissant O (1977) Characterization of a new type of human papillomavirus that causes skin warts. J Virol 24:108–120
25. Orth G, Favre M, Breitburd F, Croissant O, Jablonska S, Obalek S, Jarzabek-Chorzelska M, Rzesa G (1980) Epidermodysplasia verruciformis: a model for the role of papillomaviruses in human cancer. In: Essex M, Todaro G, zur Hausen H (eds) Viruses in naturally occurring cancers. Cold Spring Harbor, N.Y. pp 259–282
26. Rawls WE, Tompkins WAF, Figueroa ME, Melnick JL (1968) Herpes simplex virus type 2: association with carcinoma of the cervix. Science 161:1255–1256
27. Rigoni-Stern D (1842) Fatti statistici relativi alle malattie cancrose. Giornale Service Progr Pathol Terap Ser 2:507–517
28. Rotkin ID (1973) A comparison review of key epidemiological studies in cervical cancer related to curent searches for transmissible agents. Cancer Res 33:1353–1367
29. Rowson KEK, Mahy BWJ (1967) Human papova (wart) virus. Bacteriol Rev 31:110–131
30. Schlehofer JR, zur Hausen H (1982) Induction of mutations within the host cell genome by partially inactivated herpes simplex virus type 1. Virology 122:471–475
31. Schlehofer JR, Gissmann L, Matz B, zur Hausen H (1983) Herpes simplex virus induced amplification of SV 40 sequences in transformed Chinese hamster cells. Int J Cancer 32:99–103
32. Schlehofer JR, Ehrbar M, zur Hausen H (1986) Vaccinia virus, herpes simplex virus and carcinogens induce DNA amplification in a human cell line and support replication of a helper-dependent parvovirus. Virology 152:110–117
33. Schneider-Gaedicke A, Schwarz E (1986) Different human cervical carcinoma cell lines show similar transcription patterns of human papillomavirus type 18 genes. EMBO J 5:2285–2292
34. Schwarz E, Freese UK, Gissmann L, Mayer W, Roggenbuck B, zur Hausen H (1985) Structure and transcription of human papillomavirus sequences in cervical carcinoma cells. Nature 314:111–114
35. Stanbridge EJ, Der CJ, Doersen C-J, Nishimi RY, Peehl DM, Weissman BE, Wilkinson JE (1982) Human cell hybrids: analysis of transformation and tumorigenicity. Science 215:252–259
36. zur Hausen H (1977) Human papillomaviruses and their possible role in squamous cell carcinomas. Curr Top Microbiol Immunol 78:1–30
37. zur Hausen H (1977) Cell-virus gene balance hypothesis of carcinogenesis. Behring Institute Mitt 61:23–30
38. zur Hausen H (1980) The role of viruses in human tumors. Adv Cancer Res 33:77–107
39. zur Hausen H (1982) Human genital cancer: synergism between two virus infections or synergism between a virus infection and initiating events. Lancet 2:1370–1373
40. zur Hausen H (1983) Herpes simplex virus in human genital cancer. Int Rev Exp Pathol 25:307–326
41. zur Hausen H (1986) Intracellular surveillance of persisting viral infections: human genital cancer resulting from a failing cellular control of papilloma-virus gene expression. Lancet 2:489–491
42. zur Hausen H, Schulte-Holthausen H (1970) Presence of EB virus nucleic acid homology in a "virus-free" line of Burkitt tumor cells. Nature 227:245–248

43. zur Hausen H, Schneider A (1986) The role of papillomaviruses in human anogenital cancer. In: Howley PM, Salzman NP (eds) The pepovaviridae, the papillomaviruses. Plenum Press, New York (in press)

44. zur Hausen H, Schulte-Holthausen H, Klein G, Henle W, Henle G, Chifford P, Santesson L (1970) EBV DNA in Burkitt tumours and anaplastic carcinomas of the nasopharynx. Nature 228:1056–1058

45. zur Hausen H, Meinhof W, Scheiber W, Bornkamm GW (1974) Attempts to detect virus-specific DNA sequences in human tumors. I. Nucleic acid hybridizations with complementary RNA of human wart virus. Int J Cancer 13:650–656

Haematology and Blood Transfusion   Vol. 31
Modern Trends in Human Leukemia VII
Edited by Neth, Gallo, Greaves, and Kabisch
© Springer-Verlag Berlin Heidelberg 1987

Introduction for Donald Metcalf

M. Moore [1]

It is a personal pleasure to introduce my friend and former colleague, Donald Metcalf. He is best recognized as one of the founding fathers of modern experimental hematology, but we should not forget his pioneering work on the thymus. From 1956 and the decade thereafter, Don undertook a series of elegant studies on thymic cell kinetics and was one of the first to analyze the impact of thymectomy and thymic grafting on lymphopoiesis. Indeed, he should be considered the first to demonstrate the effects of thymectomy on lymphoid tissue and the autonomous control of lymphocyte proliferation within the thymus. In addition, his analysis of leukemogenesis in AKR mice is still considered definitive, revealing his ability to compare and contrast the cellular biology of the normal and neoplastic to gain insight into the etiology and pathogenesis of leukemia. The same consummate skills as an experimentalist, and the same insight and interest, were to mark his subsequent investigations into myelopoiesis and myeloid leukemia that have occupied the last two decades.

I had known and admired Don's work during his "thymic phase," since I also began my research career on thymic development, and it was this area that led me to move from England to Australia in 1967 to begin what was to be a 7-year collaboration with Don. Why, you may ask, did Don move out of the thymus area at the very time that it became a major preoccupation of immunologists? To understand this you must understand the environment, the man, and the interplay of chance and the prepared mind. In 1965 the Nobel Laureate, Sir Macfarlane Burnet, retired as Director of the Walter and Eliza Hall Institute for Medical Research (WEHI), appointing as his successors his two protégés, Gus Nossal as Director and Don Metcalf as Assistant Director and Head of the Cancer Research Unit. This was a wise decision, since Don remained relatively unburdened by administrative responsibilities, which he naturally finds irksome, and was able to pursue his scientific interests. The "golden age of immunology" can be considered to have begun in the mid-1960s and the Hall Institute was very much at the forefront. Don has always disliked the "bandwagon" concept of research, choosing instead to move in his own directions and as much as possible into uncharted territory.

At this time, experimental hematology was emerging from its lowly status as a descriptive morphological discipline, helped by radioisotope labeling kinetics and the first stem cell assay (CFU-S), as well as some knowledge about erythropoietin and regulation of erythropoiesis. While vision and concepts are necessary to move a field, there is a third essential, the catalyst of methodology. Hematology lacked in vitro systems for quantitation of hematopoietic cell proliferation and differentiation, and so an important milestone was reached in 1965 when Don, with Dr. Ray Bradley, developed a semisolid culture technique, permitting the clonal growth and maturation of granulocytes and macrophages, from committed precursors in the bone marrow. This tech-

[1] Memorial Sloan-Kettering Cancer Center, 1275 York Avenue, New York, N.Y. 10021, USA

nique was subsequently modified by him and his colleagues to permit the clonal culture of eosinophils, megakaryocytes, B-lymphocytes and multipotential cells. With the use of these clonal culture techniques and cell separation procedures, he and his collaborators succeeded in characterizing hematopoietic stem cells and progenitor cells. His analysis of the growth requirements of granulocytes and macrophages led to the discovery of a group of specific glycoprotein regulators, the colony stimulating factors (CSFs). All four murine CSFs have been purified by his group, and work by his group and others has now led to the cloning of cDNAs for all four murine and human CSFs. His recent work, using bacterially synthesized recombinant CSFs, has shown that the CSFs' function in vivo is to control the production and function of granulocytes, monocytes, and related blood cells. In this era of megabuck science, it is instructive to remember that much of the pioneering work and the seminal observations were made in agar cultures using tools no more sophisticated than a microscope, a handheld micropipette, glass slides, and orcein stain.

To the requirements of vision, technical expertise, and powers of observation, there must be added "Chance, Fortune, Luck, Destiny, Fate, Providence which determine whether you walk to the right or left of a particular tree ..." I think this is best illustrated by recalling the circumstances surrounding the murine myelomonocytic leukemia WEHI-3. This tumor arose very early in a very large experiment on mineral oil induction of plasmacytomas in BALB/c mice, being carried out by Noel Warner and myself. Not only was this tumor unique among all the hundreds of tumors that subsequently developed, it was exactly the right tumor (myelomonocytic leukemia), with the right properties (responded to CSFs by proliferation or differentiation, produced CSFs, cloned in agar), in the right place (Cancer Research Unit, WEHI), at the right time (1968–1969), when our interests were extending from the role of growth factors in normal myelopoiesis to regulatory aberrations in myeloid leukemia.

Studies on WEHI-3 led to subsequent studies in which human myeloid leukemic populations were shown to remain CSF-dependent for cell proliferation, but one CSF, G-CSF, also had the property of suppressing myeloid leukemic cells by enforced differentiation. While showing that myeloid leukemia development need not involve autocrine mechanisms, Don and his group have recently shown that the genes for GM-CSF and interleukin-3 (IL-3) can function as proto-oncogenes. It is exceedingly unlikely that WEHI-3 would have been analyzed to the extent it was if it had developed elsewhere and one wonders without it how long it would have taken to "discover," purify, and clone IL-3 and G-CSF, since both growth factors were discovered as a direct result of the use of the WEHI-3 cell lines as constitutive sources of IL-3 and as specific responders to G-CSF.

Early in 1986 I had the pleasure of attending a Birthday Party Symposium at the Hall Institute to celebrate the 21st anniversary of the discovery of the in vitro hematopoietic colony assay. It was very much a coming-of-age party for experimental hematology, heralding its own golden age, which Don was so instrumental in creating. For those who attended the final party, the image of Don Metcalf, Ray Bradley, Leo Sachs, and Bun McCulloch, festooned with colored balloons of varying sizes representing the cellular and regulatory aspects of their respective contributions to hematology, was a vision better seen than described. What was also evident was the contribution that Don has made in inspiring the second, and what is now the third generation of "new wave" experimental hematologists.

Don's contributions were recognized by his recent award of the Wellcome Prize of the Royal Society which is, I am sure, just the beginning of a succession of recognitions for his pioneering role in the modern era of hematology and leukemia research. Your work has not only led to the discovery and characterization of hematopoietic growth factors, but as a former clinician (1953, Royal Prince Alfred Hospital, Sydney), the initiation of clinical trials with recombinant growth factors must be a source of satisfaction to you – ("Only if they are done right," I hear you say). With these words, ladies and gentlemen, it is my distinct personal pleasure to present to you an extraordinary scientist, Dr. Donald Metcalf.

Haematology and Blood Transfusion   Vol. 31
Modern Trends in Human Leukemia VII
Edited by Neth, Gallo, Greaves, and Kabisch
© Springer-Verlag Berlin Heidelberg 1987

Hemopoietic Growth Factors and Oncogenes in Myeloid Leukemia Development *

D. Metcalf [1]

A. Introduction

Understanding of the abnormal nature of cancer cells has advanced rapidly in the past decade because of work in two apparently separate fields – those of oncogenes and specific growth-regulatory factors. What has intrigued workers in both fields has been the recognition that, in a number of instances, the products of oncogenes or proto-oncogenes have been shown to be related either to growth factors themselves or to the receptors for such growth factors. The reported examples of this association are already numerous enough to make a chance association improbable – c-sis and PDGF [1], c-erb-B and the EGF receptor [2], c-fms and the CSF-1 receptor [3]. When this association is considered in the light of the numerous documented examples, particularly in the leukemias and lymphomas, of non-random chromosomal translocations that involve proto-oncogenes [4], a strong case exists for formalizing earlier notions of cancer into a concept that neoplastic change results from aberrant or aberrantly expressed genes that code for growth factors or growth factor receptors.

Where this concept of cancer becomes less than adequate is in its extension to two more

specific proposals: (a) that cancer is the simple consequence of over-stimulation (either excessive or inappropriate persistence) of the proliferation of the cells involved, or (b) that this over-stimulation has an origin within the cell itself – the autocrine hypothesis of cancer. At first sight, these extensions seem reasonable, both on grounds of simplicity and because experimental cancers can often be transplanted to syngeneic recipients using a single cancer cell, with the resulting transplanted cancer being documentable as being derived from the transplanted cell.

There are three types of evidence indicating that these more extreme views of cancer formation are likely to be naive and incorrect:

1. Neoplastic change is not simply a question of stimulation of cell division but depends on incorrect responses to proliferative stimulation with the occurrence of an abnormally high proportion of self-replicative versus differentiative divisions. Rapid cell division in excess of that shown by any cancer population is exhibited by many normal tissues. Rates of cell division are therefore not the key feature distinguishing the behavior of normal from neoplastic cells, the latter depending on intrinsic defects in the qualitative nature of the daughter cells being produced. At the very least, therefore, the concept of cancer, whether initiated by proto-oncogenes or by some other mechanism, requires the existence of a crucial heritable abnormality in the genetic programming of the cell that determines its abnormal pattern of response to proliferative signals.

[1] Cancer Research Unit, Walter and Eliza Hall Institute, P.O. Royal Melbourne Hospital, 3050, Victoria, Australia
* The work from the author's laboratory was supported by the Carden Fellowship Fund of the Anti-Cancer Council of Victoria, The National Health and Medical Research Council, Canberra and The National Institutes of Health, Bethesda, Grant Nos. CA-22556 and CA-25972.

2. For many growth factors it is known that multiple tissues produce the factor in question, and the ability or otherwise of the first emerging cancer cell to produce the same factor is likely to be a trivial influence in determining the concentration of the factor impinging on the receptors of the cell.

3. Many, perhaps all growth factors have actions on responding cells that are not simply proliferative in nature. Some of these effects are indeed quite opposed to extended cell division, e.g. the induction of differentiation commitment, and this complex situation can in fact result in cancer cell suppression by a growth factor. This again indicates that the critical abnormality in cancer cell lies in its response pattern to signalling rather than to the signal itself.

Because information on the molecular control of hemopoietic cells is now quite extensive, the complex issues involved in the development of leukemia are at present better recognized than those for other cancers. These questions will therefore be reviewed in the special context of the development of myeloid leukemia.

Both normal and leukemic granulocyte-macrophage precursor cells can be grown clonally in vitro, and the specific regulatory molecules controlling these events are well characterized [5]. In the case of murine myeloid leukemia cells, individual colonies grown in vitro can be shown to be able to induce transplanted leukemia in recipients, and by this means the clonogenic cells can be shown to be stem cells of the leukemic population. We can be somewhat confident, therefore, that our knowledge of the behavior of murine clonogenic myeloid leukemic cells in vitro does encompass the factors likely to have controlled the emergence of the first leukemic cells in vivo. The situation is less favorable for human myeloid leukemic cells, because in chronic myeloid leukemia and in some cases of acute myeloid leukemia the originating leukemic cell lies in the multipotential stem cell compartment of the hemopoietic population. Information on the mechanisms controlling the behavior of hemopoietic stem cells is much less complete, as these involve – in part at least – control by stromal cells, and the nature of these control systems has been documented only in qualitative but not yet in molecular terms. Studies on human myeloid leukemic cells that have entered the granulocyte-monocyte lineage and are clonogenic in vitro have been extensive and can be discussed at the molecular level but it must be kept in mind that for many human myeloid leukemias, there remains an important black box that prevents us from being certain regarding the controls operating during the emergence of the first clonogenic leukemic cell in the stem cell compartment.

B. Control of Normal Granulocyte-Macrophage Populations

Analysis of the factors controlling the proliferation of murine granulocyte-macrophage populations has shown that the glycoprotein colony-stimulating factors (CSFs) are the only known molecules in biological materials that are able by direct action to stimulate cell proliferation in these populations. Four such murine CSFs have been identified, purified and sequenced, and cDNAs for three have been isolated and expressed in mammalian and bacterial expression systems (Table 1). Several features of these CSFs have become evident: (a) All are glycoproteins, but the extensive carbohydrate portion of each molecule seems not to be needed for the biological actions of the molecule on responding cells either in vitro or in vivo. (b) Three are monomers with mandatory disulfide bridges, while one (M-CSF) is a dimer, also with some form of necessary disulfide bridging. (c) No sequence homology exists between the CSFs or between the CSFs and known oncogene products or growth factors for other tissues. (d) Each CSF has a corresponding specific membrane receptor, one of which (for M-CSF) is, or is closely related to, the *c-fms* proto-oncogene product [3]. (e) Responding granulocyte-macrophage progenitor cells simultaneously co-express receptors for more than one CSF and cross-down modulation of these receptors can occur following the occupancy of one type of receptor by its specific CSF [13].

Table 1. The granulocyte-macrophage colony-stimulating factors

Species	Type	Alternative acronyms	Approximate mol. wt.[a]	cDNAs cloned
Mouse	GM-CSF	MGI-1 GM	23 000	Yes [6]
	G-CSF	MGI-1G	25 000	Yes (S. Nagata, personal communication)
	M-CSF	CSF-1, MGI-1M	35 000–70 000	?
	Multi-CSF	IL-3, PSF	23 000–28 000	Yes [7, 8]
Man	GM-CSF	CSFα Pluripoietin α	22 000	Yes [9]
	G-CSF	CSF β Pluripoietin	19 000	Yes [10, 11]
	M-CSF	CSF-1	45 000	Yes [12]

[a] Observed molecular weights of purified native CSFs vary according to degree of glycosylation.

To date, only three corresponding human CSFs have been identified, so others may well exist. The three known human CSFs have also been purified and sequenced and cDNAs isolated and expressed. Significant sequence homology exists between corresponding murine and human CSFs. Despite this, there is not necessarily species cross-reactivity. For example, human and murine GM-CSFs do not cross-stimulate cells from the other species, whereas the G-CSFs are fully cross-reactive [14].

Two of the functional activities of the CSFs have particular relevance for leukemogenesis: (a) the CSF's are mandatory for all cell divisions in granulocyte-macrophage precursor cells, the concentration determining the length of the cell cycle, and (b) the CSFs can irreversibly induce differentiation commitment in granulocyte-macrophage progenitors, a process requiring the presence of the committing CSF for one to three cell divisions and being asymmetrical in pattern [15].

C. Responsiveness of Myeloid Leukemia Cells to CSFs

Murine myeloid leukemic cells from primary tumors or recently isolated cell lines display a similar dependency on CSF for proliferation to that of normal cells, although on continued culture in vitro, such cell lines eventually lose most or all of their CSF dependency.

Conversely, CSFs can inhibit the proliferation of leukemic cells. In one extensively studied murine myeloid leukemia (WEHI-3B D$^+$) the commitment action of the CSFs was demonstrated to have profound effects on the behavior of the leukemic population. Culture of these cells in vitro in the presence of M-CSF (or multi-CSF) did not influence their pattern of differentiation or proliferation [16]. However, culture in the presence of purified GM-CSF or G-CSF led to the production of differentiating granulocytic and monocytic cells [17, 18]. Of the latter two, the action of G-CSF was by far the more striking, and culture for two to six cycles in the presence of G-CSF led to suppression of stem cell self-generation, with complete extinction of these leukemic cell populations in vitro and demonstrable loss of leukemogenicity on transplantation [19, 16]. Single-cell analysis of this process indicated that the irreversible commitment process closely resembled the commitment action of the CSFs on normal granulocyte-macrophage progenitors [20]. A differentiation-unresponsive subline of WEHI-3B cells (D$^-$ cells) was shown to be unresponsive because of failure to express membrane receptors for G-CSF [21], although other abnormalities could have co-existed in such cells, preventing their responsiveness.

It is of interest that even with responsive but autonomously growing WEHI-3H D$^+$ cells, culture in the presence of G-CSF did result in initial growth stimulation of the leukemic cells [20], suppression of the population commencing only following the induction of significant levels of differentiation commitment. Thus, even in this otherwise optimal system for demonstrating CSF-induced suppression, the opposing actions of the CSFs were clearly evident.

This work with WEHI-3B cells has been criticized as dealing only with a single cell line and therefore possibly not being of general relevance for other myeloid leukemias. However, in current experiments a similar differentiation induction has been observed with other murine myeloid or myelomonocytic leukemias, suggesting that the effects of G-CSF are not restricted to this one model system.

D. Role of CSFs in Leukemia Induction

Three sets of observations have recently been reported on the question of whether autocrine production of CSF by emerging leukemic cells is necessary for leukemic transformation.

Two groups have noted that when continuous hemopoietic cell lines that are not leukemogenic by transplantation tests subsequently acquire the ability to produce transplanted leukemias, this is associated with the production of detectable amounts of CSF [22, 23]. The possibility raised by these observations is that autocrine production of CSF, by providing an internal, nonregulatable source of the appropriate growth factor, is the final step in the multistage leukemogenic process.

A somewhat similar conclusion can be reached from experiments in which cells of the non-leukemic FD-CP1 cell line were transformed to leukemogenic cells by the insertion of a retroviral construct containing GM-CSF cDNA [24]. The resulting constitutive production of GM-CSF on which the FD cells are dependent for survival and proliferation was the only obvious effect of the experimental procedure that resulted in leukemic transformation.

A quite different conclusion was reached from studies in which continuous hemopoietic cell lines were transformed to autonomous, leukemogenic cells by infection with the Abelson virus [25, 26]. In this case, no transcription of mRNA for either GM-CSF or multi-CSF was detected, nor was there detectable synthesis of either CSF or the occurrence of abnormal expression of membrane receptors for either CSF. It is evident from these latter experiments that leukemogenic transformation does not of necessity require either the autocrine production of growth factors or the expression of abnormal numbers of growth factor receptors.

Although FD-CP1 cells are non-leukemic and absolutely CSF dependent, they are highly abnormal, being immortalized, incapable of differentiation, possessing eight metacentric marker chromosomes, and exhibiting a very high capacity (greater than 90%) for clonogenic self-renewal. The high self-renewal capacity of FD-CP1 cells (Table 2) despite their inability to produce transplanted tumors suggests that high self-renewal is necessary, but not in itself sufficient, for a cell to behave as a leukemic cell. Because of their properties, FD-CP1 cells could quite properly be regarded as already having passed through one or more preleukemic changes, so none of the above observations really addresses in totality the ques-

Table 2. Self-generation by clonogenic FD-CP1 cells compared with self-generation by leukemic FD-CP1 cells transformed by GM-CSF cDNA

Colony type	No. of colonies recloned	Mean no. of cells per colony	Mean no. of clonogenic cells per colony	Percent of clonogenic cells
FD-CP1	20	3630	3220 ± 2680	89
GMV FD 1.	10	1770	2080 ± 980	118
2.	10	4380	3220 ± 1000	74

FD-CP1 colony formation was stimulated by purified recombinant GM-CSF; GMV FD colony formation was unstimulated. Colonies were recloned after 6 days of culture.

tion of what transforms a normal into a leukemic cell.

Granted their abnormal state, the question remains as to what final step was required for the transformation of FD-CP1 cells into leukemic cells. One proposal that would resolve the apparent contradiction arising from these leukemogenicity studies is that the Abelson virus product may be able to activate the terminal stages of the signalling cascade induced by binding of CSF to its receptor. This would bypass the necessity of involving CSF, yet result in a common sequence of end-stage changes. There is in fact evidence that when the CSFs act on responding normal granulocyte-macrophage cells, marked changes can occur in transcription rates of known proto-oncogenes [27; C. Willman, personal communication], so it is not improbable that the dysregulated expression of a viral oncogene could result in activation of signalling pathways normally involved in CSF-initiated signalling. If these common pathways are indeed of significance, then the role of CSF as a mandatory proliferative stimulus for both normal and emerging leukemic cells acquires extra significance in the leukemogenic process.

Despite these emerging links, it is necessary to repeat that the crucial abnormality required for an emerging leukemic cell is its abnormal response pattern to such signalling, and when this is considered in the light of the clonal nature of the resulting leukemia it is still necessary to propose that other heritable abnormalities must exist in the responding cell that determine its abnormal response pattern to the signalling cascade, whether CSF induced or oncogene initiated. What the G-CSF experiments discussed earlier indicate, however, is that for at least some myeloid leukemias, the abnormal gene programming in the cells is able to be corrected or reversed by G-CSF action.

Do the experiments in which CSF in a retroviral construct induces leukemia indicate that the CSF genes can be added to the list of proto-oncogenes? The answer is probably affirmative, since the evidence is of a similar nature to that establishing a number of other genes as proto-oncogenes [28].

An intriguing story is emerging concerning the chromosomal location of the CSF genes in human cells; it has obvious parallels with the involvement of *c-myc* in Burkitt's lymphoma and *c-abl* in chronic myeloid leukemia. The genes for GM-CSF, M-CSF and the M-CSF receptor have all been localized in a tight cluster on the 5q chromosome at the site of the breakpoint in the 5q deletion syndrome [29, 30]. In its simplest clinical form, this syndrome involves the dominant clonal proliferation of a granulocyte, monocyte and erythroid population resulting in refractory anemia with excess blast cells, typically in elderly women, and sometimes classified as smouldering leukemia. In association with other chromosomal abnormalities, the 5q deletion is also a characteristic feature of secondary acute myeloid leukemias occurring following chemotherapy. The deleted portion of the 5q chromosome appears not to be translocated to another chromosome, and it remains to be determined how such a deletion might result in the evolution of a CSF-responsive dominant clone.

E. Other Biological Agents Suppressing Myeloid Leukemia

While the CSFs are the only known proliferative agents for granulocyte-macrophage cells, it is important to recognize that CSFs are not the only biological agents able to induce differentiation in myeloid leukemia cells with subsequent loss of leukemogenicity. Extensive studies have documented the presence in various conditioned media of differentiation-inducing factors (DF, DIF or MGI-2) that do not appear to be proliferative agents but are able to induce similar suppressive effects to G-CSF on a variety of murine and human leukemic cell lines, the most extensively studied being the murine M1 model [31–33]. In vivo evidence indicates that production of the murine factor can be T-cell-dependent [34], unlike the situation with G-CSF, and biochemical purification studies have indicated that DF is separable and distinct from G-CSF [33, 35]. Injection of crude material containing MGI-2 inhibited the growth of transplanted myeloid leukemic cells in SL and SJL/J mice [36], and it will be of interest to determine the structure and actions of this factor in vivo when cDNA clones and recombinant material can be obtained. Certainly, if DF or related factors lack proliferative effects on responding leukemic cells but exhibit strong differentiating effects, such factors would be quite clearly superior to the CSFs as antileukemic agents.

It is quite conceivable that the production of molecules such as DF (MGI-2) could be elicited within a cell in response to CSF signalling and account for the observed differentiation occurring in both normal and leukemic cells following exposure to G-CSF [37, 38]. Any explanation of the differentiation-inducing action of CSFs on leukemic cells requires the production of some type of signalling molecule to mediate the observed effects, and such a molecule would need to achieve an irreversible alteration in the genome of the cell, since the effects are known to be irreversible following CSF removal. What seems improbable is that the DF would need to be secreted by the responding cells and to activate the cells by binding to membrane receptors. This proposal encounters the same types of difficulties as the autocrine hypothesis of leukemia with respect to the CSFs, namely that DF and the CSFs are also produced by other tissues. Significant actions of these molecules might be achieved by remaining within the cell producing them, but the minute amounts secreted by individual leukemic cells are unlikely to be of significance in the context of cells residing in fluid containing the same molecules produced by vastly more numerous cells in other tissues. It is also improbable that secreted DF could be responsible for the differentiation that can be induced by G-CSF in cultures of a single normal cell or leukemic cell in 1-ml volumes, since it is unlikely that any one cell could synthesize sufficiently high concentrations to achieve any significant binding to membrane receptors.

Thus, even though differentiating normal and some leukemic cells have been shown to generate DF or comparable material able to induce differentiation in other leukemic cells [37, 39], the single-cell experiments suggest that if these molecules are critical in differentiation induction, they are likely to act while still within the responding cell and could equally well be regarded as mediator molecules of CSF-induced events.

F. Human Myeloid Leukemia

Turning to the situation with human myeloid leukemia, the most striking observation has been that the clonogenic proliferation in vitro of cells from most patients with both chronic and acute myeloid leukemia is absolutely dependent on stimulation by extrinsically added CSF or by CSF produced by other cells in the culture [15]. More recently, some examples of apparently autonomous growth by acute myeloid leukemia cells have been encountered (C. G. Begley, D. Metcalf, N. A. Nicola: unpublished data), but these are a minority of cases and the CSF dependency of these cells earlier in their evolution cannot be determined. For the large majority of primary human leukemias, therefore, the clonogenic GM cells exhibit no capacity for autonomous proliferation in dispersed suspension cultures, a situation which appears to effectively eliminate an autocrine basis for their neoplastic behavior. The differentiating cells (monocytes) in many populations of CML, AMML and AMonoL have a clear capacity to produce CSF, but this capacity is no higher than that of corresponding normal cells and it occurs in vivo in the context of widespread tissue production of significant concentrations of CSF [40].

From the viewpoint of leukemia development, the above in vitro data would indicate that the CSFs must play a mandatory role in myeloid leukemia development in most patients since the leukemia clone is CSF dependent. However, based on the general comments made earlier, CSF stimulation cannot be the sole leukemogenic event, since this fails to account for the clonal nature of the disease or for the abnormal pattern of self-generation following CSF stimulation. These latter two facts require the presence of intrinsic abnormalities in the initiating cell, quite possibly involving the signalling events following CSF stimulation.

Different AML populations vary in their pattern of expression of CSF receptors and in their quantitative responsiveness to CSF stimulation. However, in neither case is the variation in these phenotypic characteristics outside the wide range observable in normal progenitors, and such differences between myeloid leukemic populations can be expected since each is clonally derived from a heterogeneous population. For the two human CSFs (GM-CSF and G-CSF) with proliferative effects on human cells the responsiveness of individual AML populations is quite similar, and there has been no evidence that a particular AML population might be uniquely responsive to only a single CSF. To date, leukemic populations from all patients examined with acute and chronic myeloid leukemia have exhibited G-CSF receptors and no examples of the WEHI-3B D⁻ situation have been encountered [14].

Suppression of clonogenic self-renewal in cultures of primary human myeloid leukemia has been difficult to monitor since the clones in conventional CSF-stimulated cultures uniformly lack clonogenic cells. This may indicate an extremely strong commitment action of the CSFs, or it may merely indicate that the clonogenic cells grown in such cultures are already committed and have lost their self-generative capacity. Studies using an alternate culture system for AML blast cells do indicate a capacity for self-generation by clonogenic cells [41]. While this process remains CSF dependent, the regulation of the behavior of true leukemic stem cells in AML populations has not yet been fully characterized [42].

Established human leukemic cell lines can be subjected to the same types of study outlined above for WEHI-3B cells. Like the mouse cell lines, the human HL60 cell line has now become autonomous with respect to dependency on extrinsic CSF, but it remains capable of chemically induced differentiation [43] and can therefore be used to determine the ability of human CSFs also to induce differentiation commitment.

The behavior of HL60 cells in clonal culture appears to have been variable in different laboratories, either because of subclone differences or because the fetal calf serum used in such cultures seems to have an influence on the observed effects. Culture in the presence of either GM-CSF or G-CSF does not induce obvious morphological differentiation in these cells but does lead to expression on the membranes of lineage-specific markers associated with maturing cells [44; C. G. Begley, D. Metcalf, N. A. Nicola: unpublished data]. Of more importance, both GM-CSF and G-CSF have an ability to suppress clonogenic self-renewal as assessed by recloning of treated HL60 cells (Table 3). This raises the interesting possibility that suppression of self-renewal need not be accompanied by morphological differentiation and that use of the latter criterion may lead to a serious underestimation of the ability of the CSFs to induce differentiation.

Given that the proliferation of human myeloid leukemic cells is usually CSF dependent but that the CSFs can exhibit a capacity to extinguish such a population by differentiation commitment, a dilemma is presented in assessing whether their use would represent a useful procedure in the treatment of myeloid leukemia. Use of the CSFs to accelerate the regeneration of surviving normal clones during remission presents less of a problem unless significant numbers of clonogenic leukemic cells persist during such a remission.

These questions have some immediacy, since mass-produced recombinant human GM-CSF and G-CSF will shortly be avail-

Table 3. Action of GM-CSF and G-CSF on differentiation and clonogenic content of HL60 cells

Incubated with	CSF concentration (Units/ml)	Total cells ($\times 10^{-5}$)	Total clonogenic cells ($\times 10^{-5}$)	Percent of cells				
				Blasts	Promyelocytes	Myelocytes	Metamyelocytes	Monocytes
–	0	66.0	56.2	2.5	94.0	3.0	0	0.5
GM-CSF	400	23.6	4.1	0.5	95.5	4.0	0	0
G-CSF	150	38.1	5.4	1.5	96.5	1.0	0	1.0

Cells cultured for 2 weeks in the presence of purified recombinant human GM-CSF or purified cross-reacting murine G-CSF (C. G. Begley, D. Metcalf, N. A. Nicola, unpublished data).

able for clinical trials. On the balance of existing evidence, G-CSF may have a better prospect of being a useful antileukemic agent, but such trials will need to be undertaken with circumspection and careful monitoring of leukemic cell levels prior to and following the administration of this agent. The results with clinical trials of conventional cytotoxic agents have emphasized the complexities involved in the accurate assessment of patients with a heterogeneous clinical course and, as a consequence, the need for collaborative studies following an agreed clinical protocol. It can only be hoped that clinical trials on the CSFs will benefit from the experience with the introduction of interferons and will be carried out from the outset with meticulous attention to objective assessment of the effects induced by the CSFs.

G. Summary

Most primary myeloid leukemias are dependent for proliferative stimulation on the glycoprotein colony-stimulating factors. These agents are therefore mandatory co-factors in the development of myeloid leukemia. The CSFs also modify oncogene transcription, and in model leukemogenesis experiments GM-CSF has been shown to be a proto-oncogene. However, most evidence is against an autocrine hypothesis of myeloid leukemia based solely on CSF production by emerging leukemic cells. Because the CSFs also have differentiation commitment actions, they can induce differentiation in myeloid leukemic cells, and G-CSF in particular has an impressive capacity to suppress myeloid leukemic populations by this action. The antagonistic actions of the CSFs on myeloid leukemic cells make it difficult to predict whether they will prove to be useful agents in the management of myeloid leukemias.

References

1. Johnson A, Heldin C-H, Wasteson A, Westermark B, Deuel TF, Huang JS, Seeburg PH, Gray A, Ullrich A, Scrace G, Stroobant P, Waterfield MD (1984) The *c-sis* gene encodes a precursor of the B chain of platelet-derived growth factor. EMBO J 3:921–928

2. Ullrich A, Coussens L, Hayflick JS, Dull TJ, Gray A, Tam AW, Lee J, Yarden Y, Liebermann TA, Schlessinger J, Downward J, Mayes ELV, Whittle N, Waterfield MD, Seeburg PH (1984) Human epidermal growth factor receptor cDNA sequence and aberrant expression in the amplified gene in A431 epidermal carcinoma cells. Nature 309:418–425

3. Sherr CJ, Rettenmier CW, Sacca R, Roussel MF, Look AT, Stanley ER (1985) The *c-fms* proto-oncogene product is related to the receptor for the mononuclear phagocytic growth factor CSF-1. Cell 41:665–676

4. Cory S (1986) Activation of cellular oncogenes in hemopoietic cells by chromosome translocation. Adv Cancer Res 47:189–234

5. Metcalf D (1986) The molecular biology and functions of the granulocyte-macrophage colony-stimulating factors. Blood 67:257–267

6. Gough NM, Gough J, Metcalf D, Kelso A, Grail D, Nicola NA, Burgess AW, Dunn AR (1984) Molecular cloning of cDNA encoding a murine haemopoietic growth regulator, granulocyte-macrophage colony-stimulating factor. Nature 309:763–767

7. Fung MC, Hapel AJ, Ymer S, Cohen DR, Johnson RN, Campbell HD, Young IG (1984) Molecular cloning of cDNA for mouse interleukin-3. Nature 307:233–237

8. Yokota T, Lee F, Rennick D, Hall C, Arai N, Mosmann T, Nabel G, Cantor H, Arai K (1984) Isolation and characterization of a mouse cDNA clone that expresses mast cell growth factor in monkey cells. Proc Natl Acad Sci (USA) 81:1070–1074

9. Wong GG, Witek J, Temple PA, Wilkens KM, Leary AC, Luxenberg DF, Jones SS, Brown EC, Kay RM, Orr EC, Shoemaker C, Golde DW, Kaufman RJ, Hewick RM, Wang EA, Clark SC (1985) Human GM-CSF: molecular cloning of the complementary DNA and purification of the natural and recombinant proteins. Science 228:810–815

10. Nagata S, Tsuchiya A, Asano S, Kaziro Y, Yamazaki T, Yamamoto O, Hirata Y, Kubota N, Oheda M, Nomura H, Ono M (1986) Molecular cloning and expression of cDNA for human granulocyte colony-stimulating factor. Nature 319:415–418

11. Souza LM, Boone TC, Gabrilove J, Lai PH, Zsebo KM, Murdock DC, Chazin VR, Braszewski J, Lu H, Chen KK, et al. (1986) Recombinant human granulocyte colony-stimulating factor: Effects on normal and leukemic myeloid cells. Science 232:61–65

12. Kawasaki ES, Ladner MB, Wang AM, Arsdell J Van, Warren MK, Coyne MY, Schweickart VL, Lee M-T, Wilson KJ, Boos-

man A, Stanley ER, Ralph P, Mark DF (1985) Molecular cloning of a complementary DNA encoding human macrophage-specific colony-stimulating factor (CSF-1). Science 230:291–296

13. Walker F, Nicola NA, Metcalf D, Burgess AW (1985) Hierarchical down-modulation of hemopoietic growth factor receptors. Cell 43:269–276

14. Nicola NA, Begley CG, Metcalf D (1985) Identification of the human analogue of a regulator that induces differentiation in murine leukaemic cells. Nature 314:625–628

15. Metcalf D (1984) The hemopoietic colony-stimulating factors. Elsevier, Amsterdam

16. Metcalf D (1982) Regulatory control of the proliferation and differentiation of normal and leukemia cells. Natl Cancer Inst Monogr 60:123–131

17. Metcalf D (1979) Clonal analysis of the action of GM-CSF on the proliferation and differentiation of myelomonocytic leukemic cells. Int J Cancer 24:616–623

18. Metcalf D, Nicola NA (1982) Autoinduction of differentiation in WEHI-3B leukemia cells. Int J Cancer 30:773–780

19. Metcalf D (1980) Clonal extinction of myelomonocytic leukemic cells by serum from mice injected with endotoxin. Int J Cancer 25:225–233

20. Metcalf D (1982) Regulator-induced suppression of myelomonocytic leukemic cells: clonal analysis of early cellular events. Int J Cancer 30:203–210

21. Nicola NA, Metcalf D (1984) Binding of the differentiation-inducer, granulocyte colony-stimulating factor to responsive but not unresponsive leukemic cell lines. Proc Natl Acad Sci USA 81:3765–3769

22. Hapel AJ, Lee JC, Farrar WC, Ihle JN (1981) Establishment of continuous cultures of Thy 1.2$^+$ Ly1$^+$2$^-$ T cells with purified interleukin-3. Cell 25:179–186

23. Schrader JW, Crapper RM (1983) Autogenous production of a hemopoietic growth factor "P-cell-stimulating factor" as a mechanism for transformation of bone marrow-derived cells. Proc Natl Acad Sci USA 80:6892–6896

24. Lang RA, Metcalf D, Gough NM, Dunn AR, Gonda TJ (1985) Expression of a hematopoietic growth factor cDNA in a factor-dependent cell line results in autonomous growth and tumorigenicity. Cell 43:531–542

25. Cook WD, Metcalf D, Nicola NA, Burgess AW, Walker F (1985) Malignant transformation of a growth factor-dependent myeloid cell line by Abelson virus without evidence of an autocrine mechanism. Cell 41:677–683

26. Pierce JH, Di Fiore PP, Aaronson SA, Potter M, Pumphrey J, Scott A, Ihle JN (1985) Neoplastic transformation of mast cells by Abelson MuLV: abrogation of IL-3 dependence of a nonautocrine mechanism. Cell 41:685–693

27. Muller R, Curren T, Muller D, Guilbert L (1985) Induction of c-fos during myelomonocytic differentiation and macrophage proliferation. Nature 314:546–548

28. Weinberg RA (1985) The action of oncogenes in the cytoplasm and nucleus. Science 230:770–776

29. Heubner K, Isobe M, Croce CM, Golde DW, Kaufman SE, Gasson JC (1985) The human gene encoding GM-CSF is at 5q 21-q32 the chromosome region deleted in the 5q$^-$ anomaly. Science 230:1282–1285

30. Le Beau MM, Westbrook CA, Diaz MO, Larson RA, Rowley JD, Gasson JL, Golde DW, Sherr CJ (1986) Evidence for the involvement of GM-CSF and FMS in the deletion (5q) in myeloid disorders. Science 231:984–987

31. Lotem J, Lipton JH, Sachs L (1980) Separation of different molecular forms of macrophage- and granulocyte-inducing proteins for normal and leukemic myeloid cells. Int J Cancer 25:763–771

32. Yamamoto Y, Tomida M, Hozumi M (1980) Production by spleen cells of factors stimulating differentiation of mouse myeloid leukemic cells that differ from colony-stimulating factor. Cancer Res 40:4804–4809

33. Olssen I, Sarngadharan MG, Breitman TR, Gallo RC (1984) Isolation and characterization of a T-lymphocyte-derived differentiation-inducing factor for the myeloid leukemic cell line HL-60. Blood 63:510–517

34. Lotem J, Sachs L (1985) Control of in vivo differentiation of myeloid leukemia cells. V. Regulation by response to antigen. Leuk Res 9:1479–1486

35. Tomida M, Yamamoto-Yamiguchi Y, Hozumi M (1984) Purification of a factor inducing differentiation of mouse myeloid leukemic M1 cells from conditioned medium of mouse fibroblast L929 cells. J Biol Chem 259:10978–10982

36. Lotem J, Sachs L (1984) Control of in vivo differentiation of myeloid leukemic cells. IV. Inhibition of leukemia development by myeloid differentiation-inducing protein. Int J Cancer 33:147–154

37. Lotem J, Sachs L (1983) Coupling of growth and differentiation in normal myeloid precursors and the breakdown of this coupling in leukemia. Int J Cancer 32:127–134

38. Nicola NA, Metcalf D, Matsumoto M, Johnson GR (1983) Purification of a factor

inducing differentiation in murine myelomonocytic leukemia cells. Identification as granulocyte colony-stimulating factor (G-CSF).
J Biol Chem 258:9017–9023

39. Symonds G, Sachs L (1982) Autoinduction of
    differentiation in myeloid leukemic cells: res-
    toration of normal coupling between growth
    and differentiation in leukemia cells that con-
    stitutively produce their own growth-induc-
    ing protein. EMBO J 1:1343–1346

40. Metcalf D, Nicola NA (1985) Role of the
    colony-stimulating factors in the emergence
    and suppression of myeloid leukemia popula-
    tions. In: Wahren B et al. (eds) Molecular bi-
    ology of tumor cells. Raven, New York, pp
    215–232

41. Buick RN, Minden MD, McCulloch EA
    (1979) Self-renewal in culture of proliferative
    blast progenitor cells in acute myeloblastic
    leukemia. Blood 54:95–104

42. Nara N, McCulloch EA (1986) A comparison
    of the growth-supporting capacities of fresh
    and cultured leukemic blast cells. Leuk Res
    10:273–277

43. Abraham J, Rovera G (1981) Inducers and in-
    hibitors of leukemic cell differentiation in cul-
    ture. In: Baserga R (ed) Tissue growth fac-
    tors. Springer-Verlag, Berlin Heidelberg New
    York, pp 405–425

44. Boyd AW, Metcalf D (1984) Induction of dif-
    ferentiation in HL60 cells: a cell cycle-depen-
    dent all-or-none effect. Leuk Res 8:27–43

25

New Strategies in Leukemia Diagnostic and Therapy

Haematology and Blood Transfusion Vol. 31
Modern Trends in Human Leukemia VII
Edited by Neth, Gallo, Greaves, and Kabisch
© Springer-Verlag Berlin Heidelberg 1987

Poster Award for U. Creutzig

E. Henderson[1]

Through the years considerable advances have been made, and have been highly publicized in developing curative regimens for acute lymphocytic leukemia. For most large series the probability of a long-term continuous complete remission exceeds 0.5. Equally well publicized have been the less dramatic, but steady advances in the management of adult nonlymphocytic acute leukemias where long-term survivals are reported in 10%–30% of cases, depending both on the rigorousness of treatment and the constraints of eligibility to the study. Surprisingly, relatively little attention has been afforded the good news in the treatment of acute myelocytic leukemias occurring in pediatric patients during this same period.

Clearly a child with AML has a harder row to hoe than does his counterpart with ALL. At the same time a few single-institution studies have achieved strikingly good results with these patients (Weinstein, Leventhal) using aggressive chemotherapy, and a not inconsiderable proportion of the successes of allogeneic bone marrow trans-

plantation have depended upon HLA-matched siblings of this younger age group. However, only recently have large controlled trials been conducted and analyzed which employed intensive chemotherapy in childhood AML. The studies presented by Creutzig and her coworkers within the Berlin-Frankfurt-Münster group are notable examples of the signal advances in pediatric patient management and the outstanding contributions made by West German clinical investigators during the past decade.

All students of leukemia have been inspired by the early studies of the treatment of childhood ALL, conducted by pathologists, internists, and even pediatricians in those happy times when an ecumenical spirit of achievement held sway. Today we continue to turn to advanced studies in childhood cancers for those leads which may be used in hematological malignancies of all age groups.

For these several reasons the poster presentation by Creutzig et al. was chosen not only "best of class" but "best of show."

[1] Roswell Park Memorial Institute, Medical Oncology, 666 elm Street, Buffalo, New York 14263, USA

Edward Henderson
T. A. Lister, K. A. McCreche
The poster awards selection committee

Haematology and Blood Transfusion   Vol. 31
Modern Trends in Human Leukemia VII
Edited by Neth, Gallo, Greaves, and Kabisch
© Springer-Verlag Berlin Heidelberg 1987

Treatment Results in Childhood AML, with Special Reference to the German Studies BFM-78 and BFM-83 *

U. Creutzig[1], J. Ritter[1], M. Budde[2], H. Jürgens[3], H. Riehm[2], and G. Schellong[1]

A. Introduction

The number of children with acute myelogenous leukemia (AML) who achieve remission and the number of long-term survivors have increased in the last 10 years owing to intensified chemotherapy and better supportive care. This report reviews nine pediatric studies, particularly the German AML studies BFM-78 and BFM-83.

A total of 294 children with AML under 17 years of age entered the AML studies BFM-78 ($n = 151$) and BFM-83 ($n = 143$) between December 1978 and January 1986. The second study is still open for patient entry. The treatment in the first study consisted of a seven-drug regimen over a period of 8–10 weeks, together with prophylactic cranial irradiation, and was followed by maintenance therapy with 6-thioguanine and cytosine arabinoside (Ara-C) for 2 years and additional Adriamycin during the 1st year [1]. In the BFM-83 study an 8-day induction with Ara-C, daunorubicin, and VP-16 precedes the BFM-78 protocol.

The initial patient data of the two studies are in general comparable – age: median 9.11 and 9.3 years; sex: boys 54% and 52%; WBC: median ($\times 10^3/\mu$l) 24.0 and 28.5; initial CNS involvement: 9% and 7%, respectively. Extramedullary organ involvement (excluding liver and spleen enlargement) was seen more often in the BFM-83 study (32%);

it accounted for only 18% of patients in the BFM-78 study. But the involvement of bone, orbits, and kidney (7% in the BFM-83 study) was not evaluated in the BFM-78 study. The distribution of the FAB subtypes [2] shows a higher proportion of the FAB M5 type (28%) in the BFM-83 study (only 21% in BFM-78). In both studies the myeloblastic subtypes M1 and M2 account for 20%–24% of patients, whereas the M3 and the M6 subtypes were rarely seen (2%–4%).

The overall results are presented in Table 1. In the BFM-78 study, 54 relapses (8 with CNS involvement) occurred after a median follow-up time of 5.3 years (range 3.3–7.0 years). The life table estimations for an event-free survival (EFS, total group) and an event-free interval (EFI, remission group) after 7.0 years are 38% (SD 4%) and 47% (SD 5%), respectively (Fig. 1). In the BFM-83 study, 25 relapses occurred (4 with CNS involvement) after a median follow-up of 1.8 years (range 0.2–3.0 years). The life table estimations are EFS 48% (SD 5%) and EFI 62% (SD 6%) (Fig. 1).

Risk factor analysis shows that hyperleukocytosis (WBC $\geq 100 \times 10^3/\mu$l) is the main risk factor for early hemorrhage and/or leukostasis ($p < 0.001$, X^2 test), for nonresponse ($p < 0.05$, X^2 test), and also for relapse ($p = 0.08$, log rank test). In addition, in the monocytic subtypes M4 and M5, extramedullary organ involvement was a risk factor for early hemorrhage and/or leukostasis ($p < 0.001$) and also for relapse ($p = 0.07$, log rank test). The M1 subtype has the best prognosis: EFS 55% (SD 7%) and EFI 66% (SD 7%) after 7 years.

* Supported by the Bundesminister für Forschung und Technologie, FRG.
Universitäts-Kinderklinik Münster [1], Hannover [2], and Düsseldorf [3], FRG.

Table 1. Results of the AML studies BFM-78 and BFM-83, January 1986

	BFM-78	BMF-83
Patients	151	143
Death before onset of therapy	2	9
Death during induction		
Hemorrhage/leukostasis	12	7
Other complications	5	2
Partial/nonresponder	13	21
Complete remission achieved	119 (80%)	104 (78%)
Death in remission	6	4
Withdrawals (BMT)	5 (2)	6 (6)
Relapses (with CNS involvement)	54 (8)	25 (4)
In continuous complete remission	54	69
Alive	66	88
Event free survival (%)[a]	38 (SD 4)	48 (SD 5)
Event free interval (%)[a]	47 (SD 5)	62 (SD 6)

BMT, bone marrow transplantation.
[a] Kaplan-Meier estimated after 7.0 years in BMF-78 and 3.1 years in BFM-83.

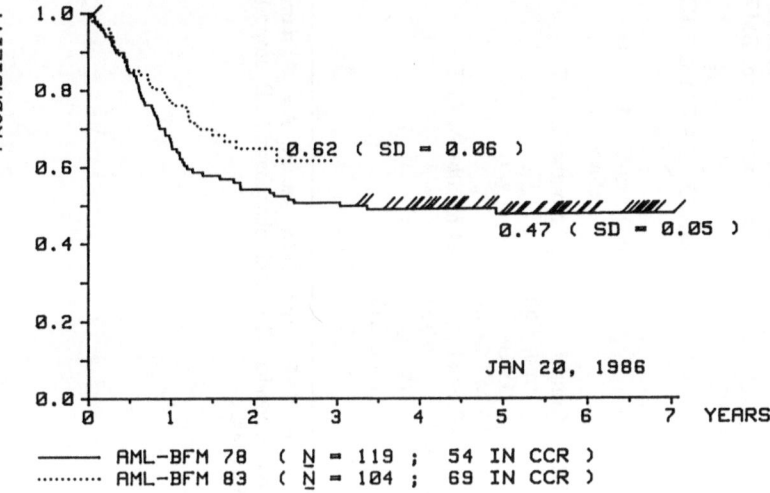

Fig. 1. Probability of event-free interval in AML studies BFM-78, and BFM-83. /, patients in CCR (all patients of BFM-78 study, last patient entered the BFM-83 study group). *CCR,* continuous complete remission

B. Discussion

In most pediatric trials starting before 1976, the median duration of complete remission was short – less than 12 months; after 3 or 4 years, life table estimation for EFI was about 30% and for survival 20% in the best studies [3].

Eight recent pediatric chemotherapy protocols with high remission rates and good results are presented in Table 2, together with one bone marrow transplantation (BMT) trial. Even though the induction/consolidation regimens with two to seven drugs differ considerably, they all include one of the anthracyclines and Ara-C. Vincristine and

Table 2. Design and results of nine AML trials in patients <20 years of age

Study institute	Start of trial	Induction/consolidation	CNS prophylaxis	Intensification/maintenance	No. patients	No. in CR	No. relapses	No. CNS relapses	EFI[a] %
VAPA 80-035 (4)	1976 1980	VAPA 1–7, 1–5 DA 3+7, 2+5	– Ara-C i. th.	12 months, intensive sequential chemotherapy	61 64	45 (74%) 45 (70%)	22 20	8 3	48 ⎱ 5 years 40 ⎰ >5 years
St. Jude's (5)	1976 1980	D, V, AZA, A×2–5 DA 3+7, 2+5	MTX i. th. –	30 months maintenance 12 months intensive sequential chemotherapy (or BMT)	95 87	68 (72%) 65 (75%) (15)	50 33 (7)	6 5	29 ⎱ 35 ⎰ 3 years (53)
UK–MRC (6)	1982	DAT 3+10×2	–	MAZE ⎨ melphalan, DAT/MAZE/HD-Ara-C (BMT)	66	60 (91%) (15)			35 ⎱ 2.5 years (70) ⎰
Norway (7)	1981	DAT (modified)	–	HD-Ara-C 2–4 courses + retinol	12	12	1		70 – 3 years
BFM (1)	1978	V, P, A, A, T, CTX (8 weeks)	Cranial irradiation (18 Gy) MTX i. th.	24 months A, A, T	149	119 (80%)	54	8	47 – 7 years
BFM	1983	ADE 8+3+3 followed by 8 weeks induction/consolidation	Cranial irradiation (18 Gy) Ara-C i. th.	24 months A, A, T	134	104 (78%)	25	4	62 – 3 years
Seattle (8)	1978			BMT		23	7		70 – 6 years

V, vincristine; P, prednisone; A, Ara-C (in VAPA and BFM, second A = Adriamycin); AZA, azauridine; D, daunorubicin; MTX, methotrexate; T, thioguanine; MAZE, amsacrine; AZA, etoposide; CTX, cyclophosphamide; E, etoposide; BMT, bone marrow transplantation.
[a] Event-free interval, Kaplan-Maier estimation.

prednisone were also administered in the VAPA [4] and BFM [1] studies. The first St. Jude's study [5] combined Ara-C with 6-aza-uridine. In consolidation of the BFM studies, cyclophosphamide was given at least twice.

In most studies, remission was induced by relatively short and intensive therapy with a seven-plus-three regimen (Ara-C plus daunorubicin), with or without thioguanine, which induced a complete myelosuppression and was followed by a therapy pause of approximately 3 weeks. In contrast, the BFM-78 study used a prolonged induction/consolidation regimen for 8 weeks, which also caused severe bone marrow hypoplasia, but in most cases the necessary therapy pauses were short.

A new strategy in intensive post-remission therapy – called intensification – was initiated with the VAPA-10 protocol [4] and is now part of most of the new studies presented in Table 2. Lie et al. [7] reported excellent results with high-dose Ara-C as postremission therapy in a small group of children. The results of BMT, which is another way of intensification in remission, are very encouraging, especially in young patients [8].

In conclusion, new therapy strategies including intensive induction regimens together with consolidation and intensification or intensive maintenance with noncross-resistant drugs will improve the treatment results in childhood AML and increase the proportion of patients in long-term remission to 50%. The low incidence of CNS relapses in the BFM studies indicates that prophylactic CNS treatment early in remission can prevent CNS disease, and the increasing number of long-term survivors emphasizes the need for effective prevention of CNS relapse in pediatric patients. It still remains to be seen whether prophylactic cranial irradiation together with intrathecal methotrexate or Ara-C is necessary or whether systemic treatment with Ara-C infusion or especially HD-Ara-C would produce an effective liquor level.

Although some results favor BMT, this therapy is currently limited to patients with HLA-compatible donors, and the long-term effects are unknown. Prospective comparisons of BMT with chemotherapy intensification or maintenance are necessary.

References

1. Creutzig U, Ritter J, Riehm H-J, et al. (1985) Improved treatment results in childhood acute myelogenous leukemia: a report of the German cooperative study AML-BFM 78. Blood 65:298–304
2. Bennett JM, Catovsky D, Daniel MT, et al. (1976) Proposals for the classification of the acute leukaemias. Br J Haematol 33:451–458
3. Ritter J, Creutzig U, Riehm H, et al. (1984) Acute myelogenous leukemia: current status of therapy in children. In: Thiel E, Thierfelder S (eds) Recent results in cancer research, vol 93. Springer, Berlin Heidelberg New York, pp 204–215
4. Weinstein H, Grier H, Gelber R, et al. (1987) Post remission induction intensive sequential chemotherapy for children with AML – treatment results and prognostic factors. In: Büchner T, Schellong G, Hiddemann W et al. (eds) Haematology and blood transfusion, vol 30. Acute leukemias. Springer, Berlin Heidelberg New York, pp 88–92
5. Dahl GV, Kalwinsky DK, Mirro J, et al. (1987) A comparison of cytokinetically based versus intensive chemotherapy for childhood acute myelogenous leukemia. In: Büchner T, Schellong G, Hiddemann W et al. (eds) Haematology and blood transfusion, vol 30. Acute leukemias. Springer, Berlin Heidelberg New York, pp 83–87
6. Marcus RE, Catovsky D, Prentice HG, et al. (1987) Intensive induction and consolidation chemotherapy for adults and children with acute myeloid leukaemia – Joint AML trial 1982–1985. In: Büchner T, Schellong G, Hiddemann W et al. (eds) Haematology and blood transfusion, vol 30. Acute leukemia. Springer, Berlin Heidelberg New York, pp 346–351
7. Lie SO, Slørdahl SH (1987) High-dose cytosine-arabinoside and retinol in the treatment of acute myelogenous leukemia in childhood. In: Büchner T, Schellong G, Hiddemann W et al. (eds) Haematology and blood transfusion, vol 30. Acute leukemias. Springer, Berlin Heidelberg New York, pp 399–402
8. Appelbaum FR, Thomas ED (1985) The role of marrow transplantation in the treatment of leukemia. In: Bloomfield CD (ed) Chronic and acute leukemias in adults. Nijhoff, Boston, pp 229–262

Additional participating members of the BFM-AML-Study Group M. Neidhardt (Augsburg); G. Henze (Berlin); H.-J. Spaar (Bremen); M. Jacobi (Celle); W. Andler (Datteln); J.-D. Beck (Erlangen); B. Stollmann (Essen); B. Kornhuber (Frankfurt);

A. Jobke (Freiburg); G. Prindull (Göttingen); F. Lampert (Gießen); W. Brandeis (Heidelberg); N. Graf (Homburg/Saar); H. Kabisch (Hamburg); G. Nessler (Karlsruhe); H. Wehinger (Kassel); M. Rister (Kiel); F. Berthold (Köln-Univ.); W. Sternschulte (Köln); O. Sauer (Mannheim); C. Eschenbach (Marburg); P. Gutjahr (Mainz); K.-D. Tympner (München-Harlaching); Ch. Bender-Götze (München-Univ.); St. Müller-Weihrich (München-Schwabing); R. J. Haas (München v. Haunersches Spital); A. Reiter (Nürnberg); W. Ertelt (Stuttgart); D. Niethammer (Tübingen); G. Gaedicke (Ulm); Th. Luthardt (Worms)

Haematology and Blood Transfusion Vol. 31
Modern Trends in Human Leukemia VII
Edited by Neth, Gallo, Greaves, and Kabisch
© Springer-Verlag Berlin Heidelberg 1987

The Treatment of Acute Myelogenous Leukemia

R. Bassan, A. Z. S. Rohatiner, W. Gregory, J. Amess, R. Biruls, M. J. Barnett, and T. A. Lister

A. Introduction

It has recently been suggested that it is possible to cure at least 25% of younger adults who have acute myelogenous leukaemia [1]. The results achieved at St. Bartholomew's Hospital, London, demonstrate this and may be used to illustrate the still outstanding problems.

B. Patients and Methods

One hundred and eighty-five consecutive, previously untreated patients, aged 15–59 years, commenced short-term chemotherapy between 1978 and 1986, some as part of three sequential open studies and some in a randomised clinical trial. The majority (106), who received BX therapy comprising an intended six cycles of adriamycin (25 mg/m^2 days 1, 2, and 3), cytosine arabinoside by i.v. bolus (100 mg/m^2 twice daily) and 6-thioguanine orally (200 mg daily), each of the last two for 7 days, form the basis of this analysis. The intercycle (day 1–day 1) time was proposed to be 21 days but ranged from 18 to 66 days, depending on the clinical state of the patient and the morphological appearance of the bone marrow.

Patients were cared for in an open ward. Bowel decontamination was attempted with non-absorbable antibiotics; fever was assumed to be due to bacterial infection and was treated with appropriate antibiotic combinations, and prophylactic platelet transfusions were given to maintain the platelet count above $20 \times 10^9/l$.

C. Results

Complete remission was achieved in 64 of 106 patients; the reasons for failure are shown in Table 1. Of these 64, 34 patients continue in unmaintained complete remission with a median follow-up of 1 year (four proceeded to allogenic or syngeneic bone marrow transplantation, and have been "censured" since that time). Thirty-seven others are alive, five in second or subsequent complete remission. All deaths were attributable to leukaemia (at presentation or relapse) or its therapy (Fig. 1). Multivariate analysis demonstrated that the only factor to correlate either with prolonged freedom from leukaemia or with survival was the interval between cycles 1 and 2. The other factors considered were:

- Age
- FAB classification
- Blast count
- Serum albumin

Table 1. Responses to BX therapy among 106 patients

Complete remission	64 (60%)
Resistant leukaemia	11
Supportive-care failure	30
Other cause	1
Total	106

ICRF Department of Medical Oncology, St. Bartholomew's Hospital, London, England

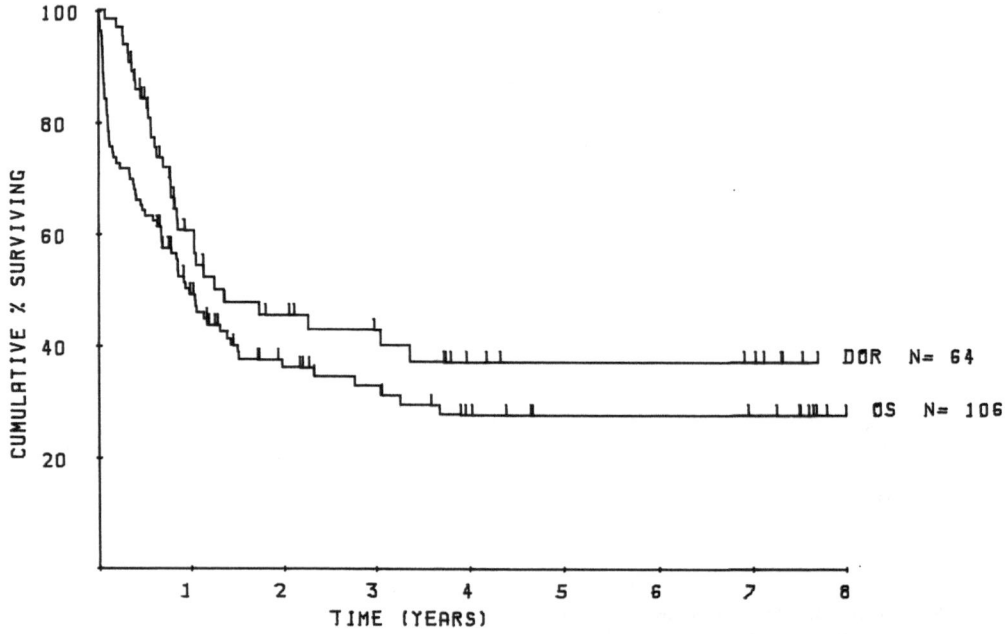

Fig. 1. Overall survival (*OS*) and duration of remission (*DOR*) in patients aged 15–59 years

- Hepatosplenomegaly
- Total no. of treatment cycles
- Cycles of treatment to achieve CR
- Cycles of consolidation after CR

There was *no* correlation between the number of cycles of therapy received (beyond a minimum of three) and duration of remission.

D. Discussion

These results clearly demonstrate that cure is possible for at least 25% of younger patients with acute myelogenous leukaemia. They identify failure to eradicate leukaemia as by far the greatest problem, 11 patients having died of resistant disease and 30 having had a recurrence within 3 years. Previous results from St. Bartholomew's Hospital suggest that the likelihood of many recurrences after the 3-year point is small, although it does exist. It may be inferred that further attention must be given to very early treatment if the results are to be improved, and that prolonging therapy is unlikely to have a major effect. It may even be possible to reduce the duration of treatment and obtain equally good results, provided the intensity is maintained. Whether or not improvements will be achieved by increasing the number of drugs, altering the scheduling, or incorporating either allogeneic or autologous transplantation remains to be demonstrated.

It is probable, regardless of which approach is investigated, that prospective analyses of patient variables, particularly in cytogenetics, may identify those patients for whom the current strategy already carries a high probability of success, those for whom an alternative must be found if cure is to be achieved, and those who, no matter what the nature of the bone marrow defect, cannot tolerate the treatment and for whom it should not be prescribed.

Reference

1. Weinstein HJ, Mayer RJ, Rosenthal DS, Coral FS, Camitta BM, Gelber RD (1983) Chemotherapy for acute myelogenous leukemia in children and adults: VAPA update. Blood 62:315–319

Haematology and Blood Transfusion   Vol. 31
Modern Trends in Human Leukemia VII
Edited by Neth, Gallo, Greaves, and Kabisch
© Springer-Verlag Berlin Heidelberg 1987

Long-Term Follow-up After Therapy Cessation in Childhood Acute Lymphoblastic Leukemia

R. Rokicka-Milewska, D. Derulska, J. Armata, W. Balwierz, J. Bogusławska-Jaworska,
R. Cyklis, B. Duczmal, D. Michalewska, T. Newecka, M. Ochocka, U. Radwańska,
B. Rodziewicz, and D. Sońta-Jakimczuk

A. Introduction

The duration of complete remission (CR) after cessation of treatment is regarded as the only criterion of cure in ALL patients. Most authors agree that patients with stable remission 4 years after termination of therapy can be regarded as cured. Relapses after 4 years are extremely rare [1–5].

B. Patients and Methods

The subject of the present analysis was a group of children with ALL in whom complete remission had persisted for over 4 years after therapy cessation. The follow-up ended on Dec. 31, 1984.

Among 1230 children with ALL treated by the Polish Children's Leukemia/Lym-

Dept. of Pediatric Oncology and Hemorrhagic Diatheses, Institute of Pediatrics, Medical Academy, Warsaw

phoma Study Group, treatment was withdrawn for 371 after long-standing CR. For 111 children from this group CR persisted for more than 4 years after therapy withdrawal. This group consisted of 62 boys and 49 girls. The age of the children at the time of ALL diagnosis ranged from 6 months to 15 years. At the time of diagnosis risk factors were found in 53 of the 111 children.

Treatment methods varied, depending on the time of the diagnosis and the therapy routinely used at that time [6, 7]. Treatment was stopped for 103 children during the first long CR. Eight children had extramedullary relapses before the therapy was stopped. In two patients relapses involved the testes, while six had CNS relapses.

C. Results

When therapy methods were intensified the percentage of children achieving long-term remission increased. It rose from 2.1% at the

Table 1. Methods of treatment for ALL in children

Methods of therapy	Number of patients	Patients with over 4 years' remission after therapy cessation	
		Number	Percent
Zuelzer's	522	11	2,1
Varied, gradually intensified	349	21	6
Intensive chemotherapy + irradiation	359	79	22
Total	1 230	111	

time of monotherapy to 22% when poly-chemotherapy with CNS irradiation was introduced (Table 1).

In the group of 111 children remaining in remission for over 4 years after treatment cessation, the period of follow-up measured from the time of diagnosis ranged from 6 to 26 years. The follow-up from the moment of treatment cessation varied from 4 to 18 years (Fig. 1).

In only one case, 54 months after treatment had been stopped, was testicular infiltration observed. The other 110 children are disease-free long-term survivors.

Height retardation was recognized in only two children. The long-living ALL patients lead normal lives. The children of school age are continuing their education. The adults are either working or still studying. Twenty children had learning difficulties connected with mathematical thinking or memory retention.

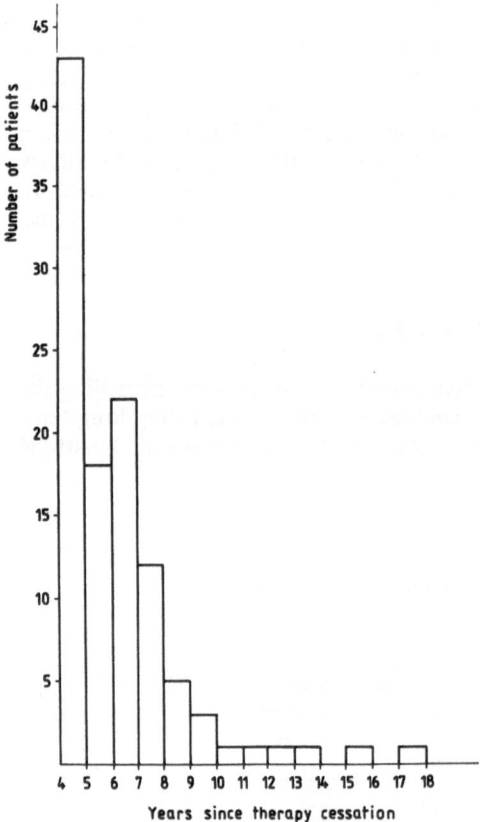

Fig. 1. Duration of follow-up after cessation of therapy in 111 children with ALL

In a majority of the patients no permanent internal organ damage has been noticed. In one case hepatic cirrhosis was discovered and in another schizophrenia.

Menstruation in all the women is normal. Seven persons, three male and four female, have healthy children who were born between 3 and 16 years after termination of ALL treatment.

We observed no secondary neoplasm in any case.

D. Conclusions

1. Intensive polychemotherapy combined with CNS irradiation resulted in a considerable increase in the percentage of cured ALL patients.
2. Long-lasting remission after treatment cessation was possible, not only in children in the first remission but also in those who suffered an extramedullary ALL relapse.
3. Risk factors lose their prognostic value in long-lasting survival for female patients but not for male patients.
4. Patients with ALL who underwent long treatment had no visible deviations in physical development and no permanent internal organ lesions.
5. ALL patients are able to have progeny and lead normal lives.

Acknowledgement. This work was supported by a grant from the Governmental Program for Cancer Control.

References

1. Derulska D, Rokicka-Milewska R, Ochocka M, Newecka T (1985) Acta Haematol Pol 16:7–13
2. Ekert H, Balderas A, Waters D, Mathews RV (1981) Med J Aust 1:523–525
3. Jacquillat Cl, Weil M, Auclerc MF, Schaison G, Bernard J (1981) Nouv Presse Med 10:1903–1908
4. Mauer AM (1980) Blood 56:1–10
5. Moe PJ (1984) Eur Pediatr Haematol Oncol 1:119–126
6. Pinkel D, Simone J, Hustu HO, Aur RJA (1972) Pediatrics 50:246–251
7. Zuelzer W (1964) Blood 24:477–494

Haematology and Blood Transfusion   Vol. 31
Modern Trends in Human Leukemia VII
Edited by Neth, Gallo, Greaves, and Kabisch
© Springer-Verlag Berlin Heidelberg 1987

Progress in Treatment of Advanced Non-Hodgkin's Lymphoma in Children – Report on Behalf of the Polish Children's Leukemia/ Lymphoma Study Group

J. Bogusławska-Jaworska, B. Rodziewicz, B. Kazanowska, J. Armata, R. Cyklis, P. Daszkiewicz, A. Dłużniewska, M. Matysiak, M. Ochocka, U. Radwańska, R. Rokicka-Milewska, M. Sroczyńska, Z. Wójcik, and I. Żmudzka

A. Introduction

It is well known that children with non-Hodgkin's lymphoma (NHL) are highly curable by modern treatment schedules [3]. As has been reported, with the LSA_2L_2 protocol the Polish Children's Leukemia/Lymphoma Study Group was able to cure about 90% of NHL children in stages I and II [2]. However, the outcome of disseminated NHL, particularly with initial central nervous system (CNS) or bone marrow (BM) involvement and B-cell histology remained unsatisfactory [2]. Therefore, between 1983 and 1986 two other therapy modalities, COAMP [1] and the Murphy [3] protocols were applied for children with nonlocalized NHL.

B. Material and Methods

Two hundred and four children with highly malignant NHL entered this multicenter study. The Kiel histologic classification scheme was used. The clinical staging was done according to the criteria of Murphy et

Departments of Pediatric Hematology and Medical Schools of Wrocław, Kraków, Poznań, Warszawa, and Zabrze, Poland

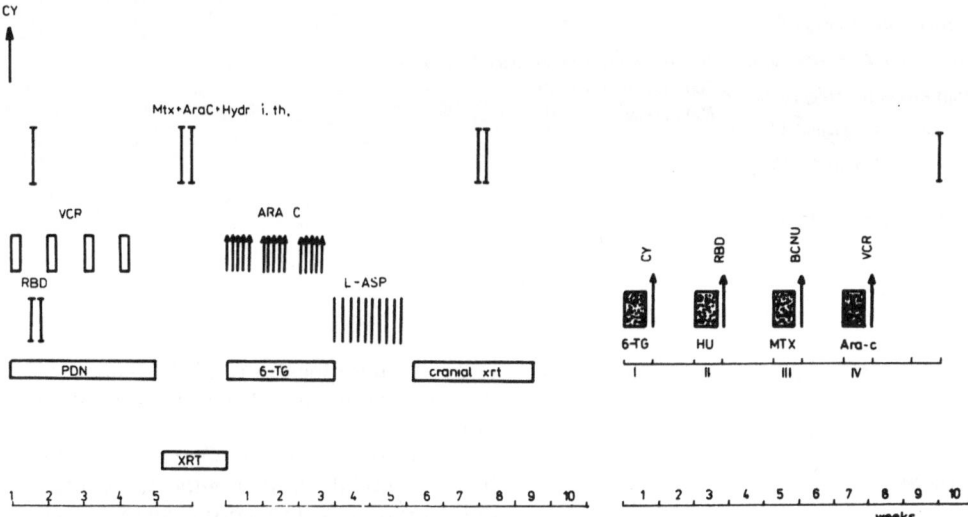

Fig. 1. Modified LSA_2L_2 protocol. *CY,* Cyclophosphamide 1200 mg/m³ i.v. *VCR,* Vincristine 1.5 mg/m² i.v. *RBD,* Rubidomycin 60 mg/m² i.v. *L-ASP,* Asparaginase 10 000 µ/m² i.v. *6-Tg,* Tioguanine 75 mg/m² o. *BCNU,* Belustine 60 mg/m² o. *Mtx,* Methotrexate 10 mg/m² o. Mtx, 6,25 mg i.th. Ara-C, 30 mg i.th.; hydrocortisone i.th. 30 mg; cranial *xrt,* cranial Cobalt

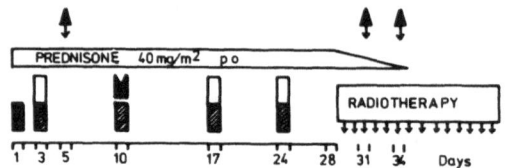

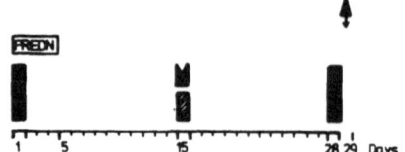

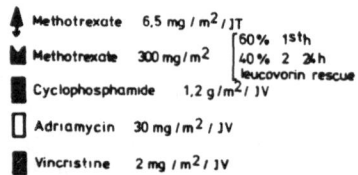

Fig. 2. The COAMP protocol

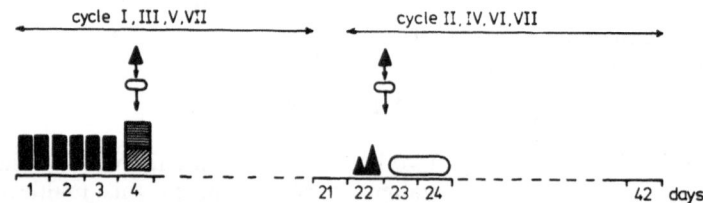

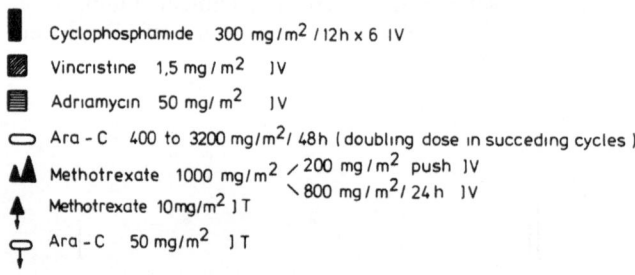

Fig. 3. The Murphy-Bowman protocol

al. [3]. The therapy protocols are outlined in Figs. 1–3.

C. Results

The comparison of actuarially estimated event-free survival rates in children with stages III or IV treated according to the three different regimens and the influence of primary tumor location and B cell immunology on the outcome of treatment are shown in Figs. 4–8.

A comparison of the effects of the three therapy modalities in nonlocalized disease indicates that the most promising results are achieved with the COAMP program in stage III, including NHL with a mainly abdominal location and B-cell histology. It is evident, however, that the treatment results in

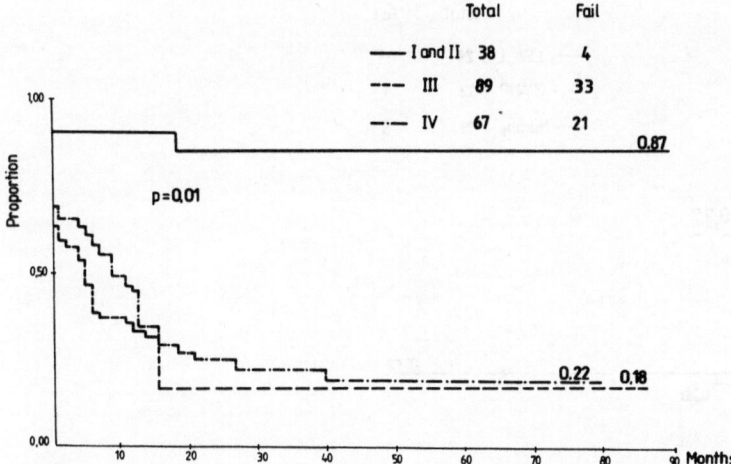

Fig. 4. Probability of event-free survival of children with NHL stages I–IV treated with the LSA_2L_2 regimen

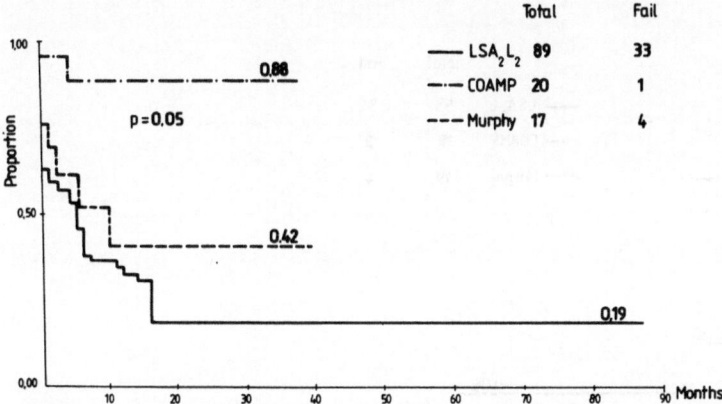

Fig. 5. Comparison of event-free survival of children with stage-III NHL using three different regimens

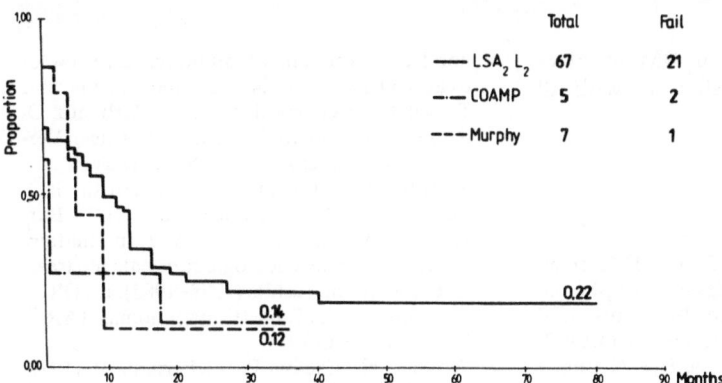

Fig. 6. Comparison of event-free survival of children with stage-IV NHL using three different regimens

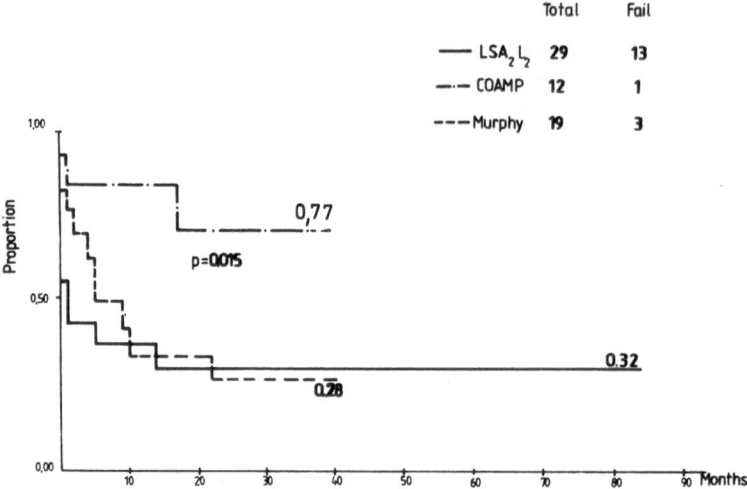

Fig. 7. Comparison of event-free survival of children with stage-III and -IV NHL using three different regimens

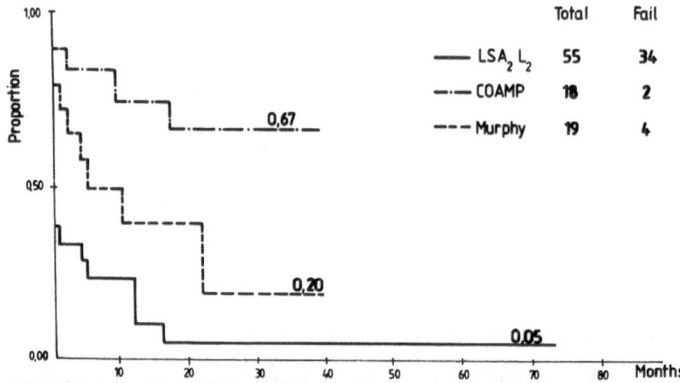

Fig. 8. Comparison of event-free survival of children with stage-III and -IV NHL with a mainly abdominal location using three different regimens

children with initial CNS or BM involvement remain highly unsatisfactory with all the protocols used.

References

1. Anderson JR, Wilson JS, Jenkin DT, et al. (1983) Childhood non-Hodgkin's lymphoma. The results of a randomized therapeutic trial comparing a four-drug regimen (COAMP) with a ten-drug regimen (LSA₂L₂). N Engl J Med 308:559–565

2. Bogusławska-Jaworska J, Rodziewicz B, Kazanowska B, Armata J, et al. (1986) Childhood non-Hodgkin's lymphoma: a review of treatment results in 243 children. In: Büchner T, Schellong G, Hiddemann W, Urbanitz D, Ritter J (eds) Acute leukemias. Springer-Verlag, Berlin Heidelberg New York Tokyo

3. Murphy SB, Bowmann WP, Hustu HO, Berard CW (1984) Advanced stage III–IV Burkitt's lymphoma and B-cell ALL in children. Kinetic and pharmacologic rationale for treatment and recent results (1979–1983). In: O'Conor, Lenoir (eds) Burkitt's lymphomas. IARC-WHO Publications

4. Wollner N, Exelby P, Lieberman P (1979) Non-Hodgkin's lymphoma in children. A progress report on the original patients treated with the LSA₂L₂ protocol. Cancer 44:1990

Haematology and Blood Transfusion   Vol. 31
Modern Trends in Human Leukemia VII
Edited by Neth, Gallo, Greaves, and Kabisch
© Springer-Verlag Berlin Heidelberg 1987

Strategies for the Future Chemotherapy of Human Immunodeficiency Virus (HIV)

S. Broder [1]

Acquired immune deficiency syndrome (AIDS) is caused by the third known human T-lymphotropic virus [1, 2]. One designation for the virus is HIV. In order to develop therapeutic strategies for the treatment of AIDS and related disorders, one must first consider the life cycle of the etiologic agent. As we review this life cycle, we will touch upon certain stages of particular interest for the development of new therapies. HIV (also called HTLV-III, LAV and ARV) belongs to the family of RNA viruses known as retroviruses [3–6] which must replicate through a DNA intermediate (i.e., at one step in their cycle of replication, genetic information flows from RNA and DNA, a reverse or "retro" direction).

The first step in infection of a cell by HIV is the binding to the target cell receptor. In the case of helper-inducer cells, this receptor is thought to be on or near the CD4 antigen [7–9], but other receptors may possibly be used by HIV in infecting different cell types. This binding step may be vulnerable to attack by antibodies either to the virus or to the receptor, and one can speculate that in the future, certain defined substances could be designed to occupy the receptor and accomplish the same thing.

It is conceivable that an experimental agent could alter the properties of the viral surface itself (e.g., by altering the lipid composition), and this might be one mechanism by which a new lipid agent could act [10]. It

is known that there is some variation in the surface envelope from one viral isolate to another [1]. The range of possible alterations in the envelope binding site is, however, most likely limited by the need to bind to CD4 (which is relatively constant), and antibody directed against this site would probably bind to (and neutralize) most strains of HIV.

Thus, monoclonal antibodies to HIV may have a therapeutic role in patients with AIDS or related diseases. A potential difficulty of this approach, however, is that virally infected cells could make infectious cell-to-cell contacts. In this regard, the recognition that macrophages can harbor the virus and can infect T cells through cell-to-cell contacts makes it important to include assays of infectivity that test this route of transmission in testing new agents in vitro. It is also worth testing whether antibodies can gain access to relevant epitopes under such circumstances. Also, it has been shown that AIDS can occur in the face of neutralizing antibodies to HIV. Whether this occurs because the titers of such antibodies are low is a topic for ongoing research [11, 12]. After binding to a cell, HIV enters the target cell by a poorly defined mechanism, perhaps by a fusion process. It is conceivable that drugs which block this step could be developed.

After it enters a target cell, the virus loses its envelope coat and RNA is released into the cytoplasm. (Pharmacologic agents which block this "uncoating" might be developed in future strategies for the experimental treatment of AIDS.) HIV uses a lysine transfer RNA as a primer and its special DNA polymerase, i.e., the reverse transcrip-

---

[1] Associate Director, Clinical Oncology Program, National Cancer Institute, Bethesda, Maryland 20892, USA

tase (RT), to copy itself, employing the viral RNA as a template. The viral DNA polymerase is encoded in a genetic region denoted as the *pol* gene. Eventually, the genetic information encoded by the virus as a single strand of RNA is transcribed into a double-stranded DNA form. RT is the enzyme that characterizes the entire family of retroviruses. Because of its unique role in retroviral replication and because a great deal is known about it [13], RT is a high-priority target for antiviral therapy, and, as noted below, a number of drugs which inhibit RT have been shown to block infection of cells with HIV in vitro. Recently we have been particularly intrigued by the capacity of oligonucleotides (which are linked by phosphorothioate esters) to inhibit retroviral replication, perhaps by serving as competitive inhibitors of primer for reverse transcription (Matsukura et al., unpublished).

The DNA copy of the virus is circularized soon after its formation, and it can either remain in an unintegrated form or become integrated into the host cell genome. It is not known whether the circularized form of the virus is biologically important. It is possible that chemicals could be developed to interfere with the viral "integrase" (thought to be a function of the *pol* segment) which mediates this integration step.

At some later time, perhaps after activation of the infected cell, the DNA is transcribed to messenger RNA using host RNA polymerases, and this RNA is then translated to form viral proteins, again using the biochemical apparatus of the host cell. However, within any given cell, the retrovirus could either remain latent (perhaps for the life of the cell) or begin another cycle of replication, sometimes in response to T-cell activating stimuli. It has recently been shown that HIV has a transcriptional and/or translational activating gene which makes a product (called the *tat*-III protein) that markedly enhances the production of viral proteins. All of the known pathogenic human retroviruses have special transcriptional or translational activating (*tat*) genes; but there are significant differences [1, 14–18], and certain ideas about these *tat* genes are still evolving.

The *tat*-III protein is thought to increase both translation of the viral RNA and its transcription, although this point requires further research. It is also thought to provide the virus with a positive-feedback loop in infected cells in which a viral product can in turn increase production of new virions. One of the hallmarks of HIV is its capacity to replicate within and destroy target T cells. This capacity seems to require a functional *tat*-III gene, although it is likely that genes outside the *tat*-III region will also be found to play a role in the cytopathic effect.

The *tat*-III protein is small (86 amino acids), with a cluster of positively charged amino acids, and it is thought the *tat*-III gene product influences the translation of other proteins by binding to critical regulatory sequences at the 5′-end of messenger RNA. It is possible that drugs or other agents may be found which inhibit either the *tat*-III product itself, a crucial nucleic acid binding site for this protein, or both.

Recently, Sodroski et al. have provided data for the existence of a seventh gene in the genome of HIV [19]. The data suggest that a product of this gene provides a *second* post-transcriptional kind of *trans*-regulatory function for the efficient synthesis of HIV *gag* and *env*, but not *tat*-III proteins. The segment of DNA required for this novel second *trans* function partly overlaps the *tat*-III and *env* genes in an alternate reading frame. It is apparent that this new gene could also be an important target for new therapies.

It is conceivable that a class of agents which interfere with the structure and function of retroviral messenger RNA in infected cells could have a role in AIDS. One drug, ribavirin, is believed to act as a guanosine analogue that interferes with the 5′-capping of viral messenger RNA in other viral systems, and perhaps this activity could be useful in retrovirally induced disorders [19, 20]. To date, ribavirin has not been shown to exert an in vivo effect against the AIDS virus.

One novel approach that may conceivably inhibit the translation (or transcription) of viral products would be the use of "antisense" oligodeoxynucleotides. Basically, these could be short sequences of DNA (or DNA which is chemically modified to enable better cell penetration and resistance to enzymatic degradation) whose base pairs are complementary to a vital segment of the viral genome [21–25]; by binding to this segment, such oligonucleotides could theoretically block expression of the viral genome through a kind of hybridization arrest or possibly by interfering with the binding of a regulatory protein such as *tat*-III or the second *trans*-regulatory gene already discussed, or with both. In principle, it might be possible to achieve the same goal by constructing an "anti-sense" virus (i.e., a retrovirus which has been genetically engineered to produce a stretch of messenger RNA that will bind to the messenger made by the wild-type virus).

The final stages in the replicative cycle of HIV involve the secondary processing of viral proteins by cleavage and glycosylation, assembly of the virus, and finally viral budding. Interferons may act to interfere with this stage of HIV replication. Other strategies for interfering with retroviral proteases and glycosylation could be explored in the future experimental treatment of AIDS.

While we have focused the discussion on how to suppress HIV, it might be worth noting that the virus could theoretically set off a chain of secondary events in vivo (autoimmune reaction, toxic lymphokine production, etc.) that is necessary for the expression of clinical disease. However, we will not be able in this article to discuss strategies for intervening against potential secondary events.

I would now like to turn to a discussion of a broad family of 2′, 3′-dideoxynucleoside analogues that can be potent inhibitors of the RT of HIV. From one perspective, these are certainly not new chemicals, and in several cases pioneering studies have been accomplished over the past 20 years or so [26–32]. However, their application as potential antiretroviral chemotherapeutic agents in human beings will require an expansion of how these agents might have previously been categorized. It is worth stressing that work with animal viruses often fails to provide a good model for how these drugs act against human viruses. Moreover, these drugs illustrate the need to combine virologic, immunologic, and pharmacologic perspectives in AIDS drug development. They are of special interest because they underscore the fact that a simple chemical modification of the sugar moiety can predictably convert a normal substrate for nucleic acid synthesis into a potent compound with the capacity to inhibit the replication and cytopathic effect of HIV, at least in vitro.

Certain relationships between the structure and activity of these nucleoside analogues have been explored in previous work [33]. It can be shown that a simple reduction (removal of the hydroxyl group) at the 3′-carbon of the sugar can convert a normal nucleoside into a potent agent against HIV in this system. A further reduction at the 5′-carbon, creating 2′,3′,5′-trideoxynucleoside, nullifies the antiretroviral effect. However, not all dideoxynucleosides have an antiretroviral effect, and a putative effect needs to be established on a case by case basis.

The National Institutes of Health, through the Developmental Therapeutics Program of the National Cancer Institute, is developing 2′,3′-dideoxycytidine and 2′,3′-dideoxyadenosine as possible experimental agents for HIV infections. Interestingly, deoxycytidine kinase can phosphorylate both drugs. The dideoxycytidine derivative is farthest along in its preclinical development, and preliminary studies in mice and dogs suggest that it will prove to have good oral bioavailability and to be comparatively nontoxic (Grieshaber, unpublished observations). This drug is now in phase I clinical trials. The dose-limiting toxicity appears to be a peripheral neuropathy, in the phase I study.

While there are several issues related to the antiviral effects of dideoxynucleosides which are as yet not resolved, it would appear that as 2′,3′-dideoxynucleosides are successively phosphorylated inside a target cell to yield 2′,3′-dideoxynucleoside-5-triphosphates, they become analogues of the 2′-deoxynucleosides that are the natural substrates for cellular DNA polymerase *and* viral DNA polymerase (RT). It is important to stress that the crucial phosphorylation reactions are catalyzed by host cellular kinases; the retrovirus does not provide these enzymes and, therefore, it (unlike *herpes* versus certain antiviral drugs) cannot adopt a simple strategy of mutating a kinase gene to develop drug resistance, although drug resistance (e.g., a mutation in the viral DNA polymerase) must always be among the reasons why an experimental agent could fail. Similar considerations apply to 3′-azido-3′-deoxythymidine (AZT) [34], a compound which we will discuss in more detail below. In this context, the lack of activity against HIV that was observed using 2′,3′,5′-trideoxyadenosine probably related to the unavailability of the 5′-site to undergo phosphorylation. It is also worth noting that cells with different histologic or species origins may show different profiles of phosphorylating activity. Therefore, in testing these drugs in animals it is important to determine such phosphorylating profiles in advance.

We are now focusing our research efforts on various 2′,3′-dideoxynucleosides. There are data to suggest that the DNA polymerase (RT) of HIV is much more susceptible to the inhibitory effects of these drugs as triphosphates than is mammalian DNA polymerase alpha (Mitsuya and Broder, unpublished work), an enzyme which has key DNA synthesis and repair functions in the life of a cell. This parallels what has been learned in animal retroviral systems (see discussion in [33]). *One* explanation for the activity of these drugs is that following anabolism to nucleotides (triphosphates), they bring about a selective chain termination as the RNA form of the virus attempts to make DNA copies of itself, because normal 5′→3′ phosphodiester linkages cannot be completed. Thus, one model for the activity of these compounds is that the viral DNA polymerase is more easily fooled into accepting the dideoxynucleotide than is the mammalian enzyme counterpart, or that the viral DNA polymerase has less capacity to repair the incorporation of the false nucleotide, or both.

We have found that with the sugar in a 2′,3′-dideoxy configuration, almost every purine and pyrimidine tested suppresses HIV replication in vitro; however, dideoxythymidine had substantially less activity than the others [33]. This represents a drastic departure from what we had expected on the basis of observations in certain animal retroviral systems with this drug, and is another warning that one cannot extrapolate from animal models in developing drugs against pathogenic human retroviruses. Interestingly, the substitution of an azido group at the 3′-carbon of the sugar in place of a hydrogen (AZT) significantly restored the antiviral effect of the 2′,3′-dideoxythymidine

against HIV [35]. This azido substitution yields AZT.

In the remaining portion of this article, I would like to summarize some of our preliminary clinical observations made when using AZT in patients with AIDS and related disorders [35]. This drug is an interesting compound that was synthesized over 20 years ago [27] and shown by Ostertag et al. more than 12 years ago [34] to inhibit C-type murine retrovirus replication in vitro; however, no application of the agent was found for the practice of medicine. It was recently developed as an experimental agent against HIV in a clinical collaboration between the Clinical Oncology Program of the National Cancer Institute, and Duke University. The drug is manufactured by the Burroughs-Wellcome company under the tradename Retrovir™. It was found to have in vitro activity against HIV as part of the Clinical Oncology Program's screening effort in February 1985, after it had been shown to have potent in vitro activity in a murine retroviral system at the Wellcome Research Laboratories. At that time, it had not been used as a drug in human beings. We gave the first patient the drug as part of a phase I AIDS therapy protocol in July 1985, at the Clinical Center of the National Institutes of Health [36].

Initially, the patients received AZT intravenously. It was subsequently shown that the drug was well absorbed when given orally (60% bioavailability), and each patient was then switched to receive oral AZT after an initial 2-week administration of AZT intravenously. Pharmacokinetic studies showed that peak levels of 1.5–2 μM were attained following a 1-h infusion of 1 mg/kg or oral administration of 2 mg/kg, and that the drug has a half-life of approximately 1 h. Increased doses of the drug yielded proportionally increased peak levels; for example, 5 mg/kg given intravenously over 1 h yielded a peak level of 6–10 μM and a concentration of 0.6 μM 4 h after the start of the infusion. In addition, sampling of the cerebral spinal fluid (CSF) showed penetration of AZT; CSF levels have ranged from 15% to >100% of simultaneously measured plasma levels ([36], and Klecker et al., unpublished observation). The excellent capacity of this drug to cross the blood-brain barrier is a noteworthy feature, given the propensity of HIV to replicate within the central nervous system [37].

More than twenty-five patients have so far been studied in this phase I trial. This was an escalating-dose trial, and patients received 3, 7.5, 15, 30, or 45 mg/kg per day intravenously for 2 weeks, followed by twice that dose given orally for 4 weeks. The first four-dose regimens have previously been described [36]. For the first two-dose schedules, the drug was administered three times a day, and for the last three-dose schedules, it was divided into six doses spaced 4 h apart. This scheduling modification was made because of the relatively short half-life of AZT. Bone marrow suppression was observed in half the patients on the two highest doses, suggesting that these doses might not be suitable for prolonged therapy in most patients; however, this issue is still under study. Even at lower doses, certain side effects (especially anemia) occurred under conditions of long-term administration, and this will be discussed later.

While the primary purpose of this phase I study was to determine whether AZT could be tolerated over 6 weeks in patients with AIDS or AIDS-related complex, the results might indicate in addition that at least partial immunologic and/or clinical responses occurred in some of the patients during this short-term administration. In particular, a majority of the patients had increases in the absolute number of circulating helper-inducer T-lymphocytes, 6 of the 16 patients who were anergic at entry developed positive skin tests while on AZT, and the one patient who was serially studied had the restoration of an in vitro cytotoxic response to influenza virus-infected autologous cells. (This test requires an intact collaboration between helper cells and cytotoxic cells, and is almost always depressed in patients with AIDS). At least some immunologic improvement seemed to occur in patients receiving 7.5 or 15 mg/kg per day intravenously (followed by twice that dose given orally), and in fact, each of the 11 patients at these doses had an increase in their absolute number of helper-inducer (CD4+) cells ($p < 0.001$). At the highest dose tested (45 mg/kg on day IV), the data suggest that drug-induced bone marrow toxicity represented a significant side effect (Yarchoan and Broder, unpublished observations). However, some patients with fulminant AIDS have bone suppression even before experimental therapy is initiated. One must keep open the possibility that patients with early HIV infections will tolerate drugs better than patients with advanced disease.

In addition to the partial immunologic reconstitution observed in these patients, some short-term clinical improvement may have been seen in some. Two patients who had chronic nail-plate fungal infections at entry experienced clearing of these infections without specific antifungal therapy. In addition, 1 patient who had debilitating aphthous stomatitis before therapy had healing of the lesions, a majority of patients had weight gains of 2 kg or greater (not explainable by fluid retention and associated with an increase in appetite), and 6 patients noted that their fevers stopped or that they had an improved sense of well-being. One patient had lower extremity weakness and dysesthesia accompanied by electromyelogram abnormalities which were attributed to HIV infection. After receiving AZT, his symptoms resolved, and a repeat electromyelogram was normal. Finally, one patient with an expressive aphasia and one patient with severe impairment of cognitive functions improved on AZT therapy. It is worth emphasizing that phase I studies by definition do not have a special control arm, and in the absence of a control arm (see discussion later in this presentation), no definitive conclusions can be drawn from these results. This is because AIDS is an inherently variable disease, and for certain parameters (e.g., weight gain), it is virtually impossible to rule out the power of a placebo effect.

Four of the patients developed non-life-threatening infections (localized herpes zoster, sinusitis, pneumonia, and *Pneumocystis carinii* pneumonia, respectively) during the 6-week period of the initial protocol; each of these infections responded to appropriate therapy. The patient with *Pneumocystis carinii* pneumonia developed clinical evidence of infection 5 days after starting on the highest dose of AZT, and it is likely that this infection was present even before he started on therapy.

In spite of the possible clinical and immunologic improvements, HIV could be identified in several of the patients on the lower dose regimens by using the technique of phytohemagglutinin-stimulated lymphocyte culture to detect the virus. At the higher doses (e.g., $\geqq 30$ mg/kg per day intravenously followed by $\geqq 60$ mg/kg per day orally), however, the virus was generally not detected in the patients on therapy, in whom such an evaluation could be made, thus suggesting that a virustatic effect might have been attained with high-dose AZT.

One of the fundamental problems of clinical research involving HIV is that a reliable and quantitative assay for viral load is still not available. Most of the techniques in use were designed to detect and isolate HIV in experiments where the object was to *find* virus, however little there might be. At the beginning of such research, it was a technical breakthrough just to identify and propagate the retrovirus on a wide scale [38, 39]; quantifying the amount of virus present in vivo was never a primary goal. The current techniques usually depend on detecting RT or a structural protein of the virus in cultures of peripheral blood lymphocytes that have been activated by a polyclonal T-cell mitogen. It is difficult to distinguish de novo activation of viral replication in vitro (i.e., unmasking a previously latent state) from a previously established chain of viral replication which had been underway in the patient and is permitted to continue in tissue culture. Physicians should take these factors into consideration as they evaluate reports summarizing HIV-related treatment protocols, and it is especially important to recognize the pitfalls of relying on viral cultures alone as an end point. More recent techniques such as measuring p24 expression in the circulating plasma might be very useful.

The earliest patients entered on this trial were taken off AZT for about 1 month and then restarted on the drug. As more experience was gained, patients who were enrolled into the later phases of the study were sometimes continued on the drug after the initial 6-week course of treatment, and in several cases an escalating-dose regimen was used. At the National Cancer Institute, we are currently following 12 patients on extended AZT therapy. While it is too early to draw conclusions, preliminary results suggest that in patients with fulminant AIDS the number of helper-inducer T cells may reach a plateau after 6 weeks of therapy using the current regimens, and in some patients (particularly at higher doses), the number of helper-inducer T cells may show a decline. Such patients appear to remain at some risk for developing opportunistic infections. Seven of the patients being followed have Kaposi's sarcoma; of these, one has had a complete remission of his Kaposi's sarcoma, and three have had some clearing of their lesions (Yarchoan and Broder, unpublished observations). Interestingly, the patient with complete clearing had worsening of his lesions during the early part of the AZT regimen but had clearing starting in the 8th week of experimental therapy. At this time, we cannot say whether these changes are due to the antiviral effects of the drug or to an unanticipated antitumor effect. At the least, it would appear from the preliminary results that if one is following a response to an antiviral drug by monitoring the Kaposi's sarcoma lesions as an end point in patients with HIV infection, one should be prepared to wait at least 3 months before making a definitive assessment about a response.

Thus, experimental treatment with AZT was associated with objective responses of the Kaposi's sarcoma in certain patients on a short-term basis. However, the number of helper-inducer lymphocytes reached a plateau after an initial rise and often fell in patients whose daily dose was escalated. At the same time, as doses were increased, some patients developed megaloblastic changes in their bone marrows (not explainable by folate or vitamin B12 deficiencies which do, in fact, occur in this patient population), accompanied by falls in the total white blood cell counts. Some patients develop red-cell hypoplasia on long-term treatment. (Interestingly, in our studies, AZT seemed to spare platelets, and, indeed, some patients seemed to have significant increases in platelet counts. Therefore, perhaps patients with idiopathic thrombocytopenic purpura in the setting of HIV infection would be particularly interesting to study with this drug.)

Recent data suggest that certain changes in bone marrow function, including the late depression of white blood cells, are related to a drug-induced depletion of normal pyrimidine pools. We have recently shown that T cells exposed to high concentrations of AZT in vitro have decreased levels of thymidine triphosphate, and AZT-induced pyrimidine starvation, due in part to an inhibition of thymidylate kinase, may be one factor responsible for this late toxicity (Balzarini et al., unpublished results). Therefore, one of the important challenges for future clinical investigation will be to develop approaches that minimize this depletion of normal pyrimidines, which if successful, might permit long-term administration without unacceptable toxicity. In patients known not to have other explanations such as folate or vitamin B12 deficiencies, it may also be possible to monitor the increase in the mean corpuscular volume of circulating red blood cells (a peripheral reflection of the megaloblastic changes in the bone marrow, which in turn appears to be a function of pyrimidine starvation) as an index of impending drug toxicity (Yarchoan and Broder, unpublished observations).

We are currently trying to explore regimens which take the above observations into consideration. In collaboration with the Wellcome Research Laboratories, we are exploring how to clinically modify hepatic glucuronidation since this is a major route of AZT elimination, particularly when the drug is given orally. (It is interesting to note that in preclinical testing, dideoxycytidine, the nucleoside analogue discussed earlier, is excreted into the urine essentially unchanged.) We are also planning regimens which might be able to test combinations of antiviral modalities in the future. An alternating regimen of AZT and dideoxycytidine may offer several pharmacologic advantages, and preliminary results are encouraging.

These initial results with AZT suggest that this drug can be administered with potentially interesting effects in patients in a short-term regimen. A randomized, double-blind/placebo-controlled trial of orally administered AZT was recently conducted. This was a multi-center study that involved approximately 280 patients. Roughly equal numbers of patients received drug and placebo. The study was initiated (using the pharmacokinetic and dosing data observed in our phase I study) in February of 1986, and patients were accrued over a four month period of time. By September of 1986, there were 19 deaths in the placebo arm and one death in the drug arm. There were a number of immunologic and clinical parameters that provided additional data that patients were deriving at least a short-term benefit from the administration of AZT, and accordingly on September 19, 1986, an independent data-safety monitoring board recommended that patients in the placebo arm begin to receive drug. AZT has now been approved as a prescription drug for the therapy of certain patients with AIDS and its related disorders in the United States and in several European countries.

More recent studies (Yarchoan and Broder, unpublished) suggest that AZT may have the capacity to at least temporarily reverse some of the dementias that are associated with AIDS. From a clinical point of view, some of the neurologic improvements may sometimes be more evident than other features of AZT therapy. From one point of view, the capacity of the drug to improve the neurologic function of certain patients is unexpected and should be the topic of continued basic and clinical research.

AZT is certainly not a final answer, and in some patients the drug may exhibit prominent bone-marrow suppressive effects. Nevertheless, the studies involving AZT have confirmed in a general way the hypothesis that an antiretroviral intervention can provide a clinical benefit to patients suffering from pathogenic retroviral infections, even in advanced disease.

References

1. Wong-Staal F, Gallo RC (1985) Human T-lymphotropic retroviruses. Nature 317:395–403
2. Wayne-Hobson S, Montagnier L (1986) Genetic structure of the lymphadenopathy-AIDS virus. Cancer Rev 1:18–34
3. Baltimore D (1970) RNA-dependent DNA polymerase in virions of RNA tumor viruses. Nature 226:1209–1211
4. Temin MH, Mizutani S (1970) RNA-directed DNA polymerase in virions in Rous sarcoma virus. Nature 226:1211–1213

5. Poiesz BJ, Ruscetti FW, Gazdar AF, Bunn PA, Minna JD, Gallo RC (1980) Detection and isolation of type C retrovirus particles from fresh and cultured lymphocytes of a patient with cutaneous T-cell lymphoma. Proc Natl Acad Sci USA 77:7415–7419

6. Gallo RC (1984) Isolation and characterization of human T-cell leukemia/lymphoma virus. In: Broder S (ed) T-cell lymphoproliferative syndrome associated with human T-cell leukemia/lymphoma virus. Ann Intern Med 100:543–557

7. Dalgleish AG, Beverly PCL, Clapham PR, et al. (1984) The CD4 (T4) antigen is an essential component of the receptor for the AIDS retrovirus. Nature 312:763–767

8. Klatzmann D, Champagne E, Chamerat S, et al. (1984) T-lymphocyte T4 molecule behaves as the receptor for human retrovirus LAV. Nature 312:767–768

9. Popovic M, Gallo RC, Mann DL (1984) OKT-4 antigen bearing molecule is a receptor for the human retrovirus HTLV-III. Clin Res 33:560A

10. Sarin PS, Gallo RC, Scheer DI, et al. (1985) Effects of a novel compound (AL 721) on HTLV-III infectivity in vitro. N Engl J Med 313:1289–1290

11. Weiss RA, Clapham PR, Cheingsong-Popov R, et al. (1985) Neutralization of human T-lymphotropic virus type III by sera of AIDS and AIDS-risk patients. Nature 316:69–72

12. Robert-Guroff M, Brown M, Gallo RC (1985) HTLV-III-neutralizing antibodies in patients with AIDS and AIDS-related complex. Nature 316:72–74

13. Veronese FD, Copeland TD, DeVico AL, Rahman R, Oroszlan S, Gallo RC, Sarngadharan MG (1986) Characterization of highly immunogenic p66/p51 as the reverse transcriptase of HTLV-III/LAV. Science 231:1289–1291

14. Sodroski JG, Rosen CA, Haseltine WA (1984) Trans-acting transcriptional activation of the long terinal repeat of human T lymphotropic viruses in infected cells. Science 225:381–385

15. Rosen CA, Sodroski JG, Haseltine WA (1985) The location of the cis-acting regulatory sequences in the human T cell lymphotopic virus type III (HTLV-III/LAV) long terminal repeat. Cell 41:813–823

16. Rosen CA, Sodroski JG, Goh WC, et al. (1986) Post-transcriptional regulation accounts for the trans-activation of the human T-lymphotropic virus type III. Nature 319:555–559

17. Fisher AG, Feinberg MB, Josephs SF, et al. (1986) The trans-activator gene of HTLV-III is essential for firus replication. Nature 320:367–371

18. Dayton AI, Sodroski JG, Rosen CA, Goh WC, Haseltine WA (1986) The trans-activator gene of the human T-cell lymphotropic virus type III is required for replication. Cell 44:941–947

19. Sodroski J, Goh WC, Rosen C, Dayton A, Terwilliger E, Haseltine W (1986) A second posttranscriptional trans-activator gene required for HTLV-III replication. Nature (to be published)

20. McCormick JB, Getchell JP, Mitchell SW, Hicks DR (1984) Ribavirin suppresses replication of lymphadenopathy-associated virus in cultures of human adult T lymphocytes. Lancet 2:1367–1369

21. Stephenson ML, Zamecnik PC (1978) Inhibition of Rous sarcoma viral RNA translation by a specific oligodeoxyribonucleotide. Proc Natl Acad Sci USA 75:285–288

22. Izant JG, Weintraub H (1984) Inhibition of thymidine kinase gene expression by antisense RNA: a molecular approach to genetic analysis. Cell 36:1007–1015

23. Pestka S, Daugherty BL, Jung V, et al. (1984) Anti-mRNA: specific inhibition of translation of single mRNA molecules. Proc Natl Acad Sci USA 81:7525–7528

24. Murikami A, Blake KR, Miller PS (1985) Characterization of sequence-specific oligodeoxyribonucleoside methylphosphonates and their interaction with rabbit globin mRNA. Biochemistry 24:4041–4046

25. Wickstrom E, Simonet WS, Medlock K, Ruiz-Robles I (1986) Complementary oligonucleotide probe of vescular stomatitis virus matrix protein mRNA translation. Biophys J 49:15–17

26. Robins MJ, Robins RK (1964) The synthesis of 2′,3′-dideoxyadenosine from 2′-deoxyadenosine. J Am Chem Soc 86:3585–3586

27. Horwitz JP, Chua J, Noel M (1964) Nucleosides. V. The Monomesylates of 1-(2′-deoxy-beta-D-Lyxofuranosyl) thymine. J Organ Chem 29:2076–2078

28. Robins MJ, McCarthy JR, Robins RK (1966) Purine nucleosides. XII. The preparation of 2′,3′-dideoxyadenosine, 2′,5′-dideoxyadenosine, and 2′,3′,5′-trideoxy-adenosine from 2′-deoxyadenosine. Biochemistry 5:224–231

29. Horwitz JP, Chua J, Noel M, Donatti JT (1967) Nucleosides. XI. 2′,3′-dideoxycytidine. J Organ Chem 32:817–818

30. Doering AM, Jansen M, Cohen SS (1966) Polymer synthesis in killed bacteria: Lethality of 2′,3′-dideoxyadenosine. J Bacteriol 92:565–574

31. Toji L, Cohen SS (1970) Termination of deoxyribonucleic acid in *Escherichia coli* by 2′,3′-dideoxyadenosine. J Bacteriol 103:323–328

32. Lin TS, Prusoff WH (1978) Synthesis and biological activity of several amino acid analogues of thymidine. J Med Chem 21:109–112

33. Mitsuya H, Broder S (1986) Inhibition of the in vitro infectivity and cytopathic effect of human T-lymphotropic virus type III/lymphadenopathyassociated virus (HTLV-III/LAV) by 2′,3′-dideoxynucleosides. Proc Natl Acad Sci USA 83:1911–1915

34. Ostertag W, Roesler G, Krieg CJ, Kind J, Cole T, Crozier T, Gaedicke G, Steinheider G, Kluge N, Dube S (1974) Induction of endogenous virus and of thymidine kinase by bromodeoxyuridine in cell cultures transformed by friend virus. Proc Natl Acad Sci USA 71:4980–4985

35. Mitsuya H, Weinhold KJ, Furman PA, et al. (1985) 3′-azido-3′-deoxythymidine (BWA 509U): an antiviral agent that inhibits the infectivity and cytopathic effect of human T-lymphotropic virus type III/lymphadenopathy-associated virus in vitro. Proc Natl Acad Sci USA 82:7096–7100

36. Yarchoan R, Klecker RW, Weinhold JR, et al. (1986) Administration of 3′-azido-3′-deoxythymidine,an inhibitor of HTLV-III/LAV replication, to patients with AIDS or AIDS-related complex. Lancet I:575–580

37. Shaw G, Hahn BH, Arya SK, et al. (1984) Molecular characterization of human T cell leukemia (lymphotropic) virus type III in the acquired immunodeficiency syndrome. Science 226:1165–1171

38. Popovic M, Sarngadharan MG, Reed E, Gallo RC (1984) Detection, isolation, and continuous production of cytopathic retroviruses (HTLV-III) from patients with AIDS and pre-AIDS. Science 224:497–500

39. Gallo RC, Salahuddin SZ, Popovic M, et al. (1984) Frequent detection and isolation of cytopathic retroviruses (HTLV-III) from patients with AIDS and at risk for AIDS. Science 224:500–503

Haematology and Blood Transfusion   Vol. 31
Modern Trends in Human Leukemia VII
Edited by Neth, Gallo, Greaves, and Kabisch
© Springer-Verlag Berlin Heidelberg 1987

Intra-arterial *Cis*-platinum in Osteosarcoma

C. H. Carrasco, C. Charnsangavej, W. J. Richli, and S. Wallace

Conventional radiography continues to be the most important imaging modality in the initial diagnosis and assessment of skeletal neoplasms. However, this technique is usually inadequate to determine the local extent of the tumor, particularly in malignancies. Angiography also fails to define accurately the local extent of most skeletal neoplasms. Computed tomography, however, demonstrates the intramedullary and extraosseous extent of skeletal neoplasms much more accurately and is currently the modality most frequently used for this purpose.

The use of angiography in skeletal neoplasms is now almost completely limited to those that are managed with intra-arterial therapy, either infusion chemotherapy or embolization, including osteosarcomas, nonresectable giant cell tumors, and metastases. Angiography is employed to define the vascular anatomy for optimal catheter placement and also to assess the therapeutic response, including detection of residual or recurrent tumor. In addition, demonstration of abnormal vascularity is employed in the planning of the biopsy with some neoplasms.

A. Osteosarcoma

Osteosarcoma comprises a variety of neoplasms capable of osteoid matrix pro-

1515 Holcombe BLVD., Department of Diagnostic Radiology, The University of Texas M.D. Anderson Hospital and Tumor Institute at Houston, Houston, Texas 77030 USA. Phone (713) 792–8295

duction in at least a small focus. These tumors vary in their biological behavior from the relative indolence of the parosteal osteosarcoma to the extreme aggressiveness of the telangiectatic type. The etiology of osteosarcoma is unknown; however, Paget's disease, radiation, and osteogenesis imperfecta are known precursors in some instances. Osteosarcoma is the most frequent primary malignant neoplasm of bone after myeloma, and its peak incidence is in the second decade of life. Males are more frequently affected than females.

The site of predilection for osteosarcoma is the metaphyseal portion of the long bones, with the distal femur, the proximal tibia, and the proximal humerus accounting for the majority of the cases. Conventional radiographs usually suggest the diagnosis, but the relative nonspecificity of the radiographic signs makes a tissue diagnosis mandatory prior to the initiation of therapy. Osteosarcoma may be completely lytic or predominantly sclerotic, but it usually exhibits a combination of these features. The hallmark of the roentgenologic diagnosis of osteosarcoma is given by mineralized tumor osteoid matrix, which characteristically presents as nests of cloud-like to ivory-like density.

B. Therapy

For many years, radical surgery was the principal mode of therapy for primary osteosarcoma and yielded an overall survival rate of approximately 20% [1]. Radiologic evidence of pulmonary metastases was seen at a median of 8.5 months following potentially curative surgery [2, 3], and patients usually died within 6 months after detection of pulmonary metastases.

The fatal outcome of most osteosarcoma patients following surgery led to the use of radiation therapy for local control [4–6] in an effort to spare patients likely to develop pulmonary metastases from unnecessary mutilation. Preoperative radiation therapy was also employed with the hope of changing tumor cell viability and to prevent implantation of cells dislodged during surgery. However, this approach yielded survival rates comparable to those achieved by surgery alone [1], so radiation therapy was discarded as a primary treatment modality.

Subsequently, various chemotherapeutic agents were shown to be active against established metastases and the primary tumor, resulting in prolongation of survival. The fact that osteosarcoma is microscopically disseminated at the time of diagnosis in the vast majority of patients, as evidenced by the rapid onset of clinically evident pulmonary metastases soon after amputation, has led to the administration of adjuvant chemotherapy following surgery [7, 8].

Advances achieved with chemotherapy led to the search for alternative methods to treat the primary tumor short of amputation, the most significant of which has been limb salvage [9–11]. Preoperative chemotherapy was initially used to control the primary tumor while awaiting the production of a customized endoprosthesis for limb salvage surgery [12]. Subsequently, preoperative chemotherapy was employed with the intent to treat the primary tumor and identify an effective chemotherapeutic agent for adjuvant therapy based on the degree of tumor necrosis [10, 13]. Using a combination of various chemotherapeutic agents, Rosen et al. [14] reported a 92% continuous disease-free survival for a median of 2 years in a group of 79 patients.

C. Intra-arterial Chemotherapy

Since the therapeutic activity of most antineoplastic agents is related to their concentration at the site of the tumor, several authors administered them intra-arterially in an attempt to improve on the results achieved with intravenous administration. Cis-platinum has been demonstrated to be an active agent against osteosarcoma [15], yielding a response rate of 67% in 17 patients in whom it was administered via the intra-arterial route [16]. There were nine complete and two partial responses as determined by clinical, angiographic, and pathological parameters. The local concentrations of cis-platinum in the vein draining the region of the neoplasm were higher than those of a peripheral vein, reflecting the systemic concentration of the drug. It was also noted that increased tumor destruction was a function of the number of infusions, high cis-platinum concentration within the tumor, and the tumor subtype. In another report, Benjamin et al. [17] noted ten responses in 18 adult patients treated with intra-arterial cis-platinum and systemic adriamycin.

Preoperative intra-arterial cis-platinum 120–200 mg/m^2 is currently being administered to patients with localized osteosarcomas at UT M.D. Anderson Hospital and Tumor Institute in order to treat the primary tumor and determine the efficacy of this agent for adjuvant therapy. Patients who are 16 years of age or older also receive systemic adriamycin 90 mg/m^2.

D. Technical Considerations

In pediatric patients, the procedure is performed under general anesthesia. In older patients, mild sedation and local anesthesia suffice. The usual access route for the arterial catheterization is the contralateral femoral artery for patients with lower extremity and pelvic neoplasms, while either femoral artery can be used for tumors located elsewhere. Catheterization is performed employing the Seldinger technique. The patients are anticoagulated with 50 U/kg heparin as soon as the catheter is in the arterial system, and an equal dose is administered during the course of the infusion of cis-platinum.

Since thrombotic complications are related in part to the caliber of the catheters employed, these should be of the smallest caliber that will allow for a safe and atraumatic catheterization. We prefer to use 3.5-F catheters in the pediatric age-group and 5-F catheters for older patients. Straight guide wires will decrease the likelihood of producing vascular spasm in younger patients.

Although curved catheters facilitate catheterization, their tip will often rest on the vessel wall, thus exposing a localized area of endothelium to a greater concentration of the chemotherapeutic agent; this can be avoided with the use of straight catheters. A deflector wire is employed to advance the straight catheter over the aortic bifurcation to the contralateral extremity. For upper-extremity neoplasms, the catheter tip is preshaped to facilitate engagement of the brachiocephalic vessels, and it should conform to the anatomy of the catheterized vessel to provide greater stability and decrease endothelial trauma.

Since the majority of osteosarcomas are located about the knee, the vessels most frequently catheterized for their infusion are the superficial femoral and popliteal arteries. Neoplasms in this region are frequently supplied by multiple vessels consisting of the geniculate arteries and hypertrophied periosteal-cortical arteries. The catheter tip should be placed proximally to the branches supplying the tumor, bypassing as many musculocutaneous branches as possible. Laminar flow within the infused vessel may prevent adequate mixing of the chemotherapeutic agent and result in streaming of the infusion for variable distances from the catheter tip. This phenomenon may cause large amounts of the chemotherapeutic agent to bypass some of the branches supplying the tumor, to flow into a branch supplying only part of the tumor, or to flow into a musculocutaneous branch that does not supply the tumor at all. In the latter instance, necrosis of normal tissues and subsequent scarring may occur. Streaming of the infusion can be disrupted by the use of a pulsatile pump (Gianturco; Cook, Inc.) which delivers the infusion in one to three short pulses per second, creating turbulence, better mixing, and a more homogeneous distribution of the infusion chemotherapy.

Rarely, a tumor will have a single branch providing most of its blood flow, and at least one of the chemotherapy infusions is then delivered selectively into this vessel. In this manner, a greater cytotoxic effect related to the greater drug concentration is achieved.

The main blood supply to proximal femoral osteosarcomas is provided by the femoral circumflex artery, which arises from the deep femoral artery, frequently just beyond its origin, providing an extremely short segment in which to place the tip of the infusion catheter. A catheter in this position is unstable and may dislodge into the superficial femoral artery, whose contribution to proximal femoral neoplasms is negligible. When this situation is encountered, the catheter tip is placed within the common femoral artery.

Osteosarcomas of the femoral diaphysis may receive their blood supply from branches of both the superficial and deep femoral arteries. When the contribution by the superficial femoral artery is provided by only a few vessels, redistribution of the blood supply may be performed by occluding these branches with segments of Gelfoam. The blood supply to the tumor will then be provided solely by the deep femoral artery, the infusion of which will cover the entire neoplasm. When flow redistribution is impractical, the infusions should be alternated between the deep and the superficial femoral arteries or should be performed in the common femoral artery.

Osteosarcomas located in the proximal humerus usually receive a major portion of their blood supply from the circumflex humeral artery, which should be selectively infused for at least one of the courses of preoperative chemotherapy.

Angiography in the frontal and lateral planes is performed at the time of each catheterization. Photographic subtraction of the arteriograms allows assessment of the degree of vascularity of the neoplasm.

E. Determination of Response

A cytotoxic effect may be apparent on the plain radiographs of the tumor by the appearance of reactive calcification and a decrease in the size of the soft tissue mass. The margins of the neoplasm may become better defined, and varying degrees of cortical remodeling occur. Computed tomography will demonstrate similar findings in cross section. An increase in the size of the soft tissue mass or in the area of osteolysis usually indicates progression of the disease. However, the conventional determination of response, where a complete response is indicated by total disappearance of the tumor and a partial response represents at least a 50% decrease in the size of the tumor, cannot be employed in skeletal neoplasms since they frequently do not decrease in size as they respond to therapy.

In a group of 37 patients treated prior to 1983, we observed that those with 90% or more histologic tumor necrosis had a 95% disease-free survival at 2 years, compared with 21% for those with lesser degrees of necrosis. Therefore, a clinical test that correlates with the degree of histologic tumor necrosis would be useful in devising the therapeutic strategy prior to resection. The features of healing noted by conventional radiography and computed tomography are variable and not predictive of the degree of tumor necrosis. However, the tumor vascularity as noted on subtraction arteriograms correlates reasonably well with the histologic tumor necrosis. In a group of 79 patients with osteosarcoma, we observed that a complete or near-complete disappearance of the tumor vascularity had a sensitivity of 95% and a specificity of 58% in predicting 90% or more histologic tumor necrosis in the resected specimen. The presence of residual tumor vascularity almost always indicates the presence of significant viable tumor.

Following several courses of preoperative chemotherapy, the neoplasm is resected as part of a limb salvage procedure or an amputation, depending on the response. The neoplasm is sectioned longitudinally, and a slice through the center of the tumor or through the region where residual vascularity was noted in the last arteriogram is mapped out in multiple sections. The percentages of viable and necrotic tumor within each section are estimated, averaged for all sections, and expressed as an overall percentage of tumor necrosis.

F. Results

A group of 65 patients 16 years of age or older with extremity osteosarcomas were evaluated. These patients were treated pre-operatively with systemic adriamycin and intra-arterial *cis*-platinum for a total of three to six courses. Adjuvant chemotherapy of adriamycin and *cis*-platinum was continued until cumulative *cis*-platinum toxicity and then changed to adriamycin and dacarbazine. Since 1983, patients with less than 90% tumor necrosis have been treated with an alternating program adding high-dose methotrexate and bleomycin, cyclophosphamide, and dactinomycin. The overall 3-year disease-free survival is 65%, which is superior to our historical control of 20%. The 28 patients treated since 1983 have a 75% disease-free survival at 2 years, compared with 62% for those treated from 1979–1982 [18].

Downstaging the tumor with preoperative chemotherapy increased the number of patients who were considered for limb salvage procedures. Only 8% of the patients fulfilled the criteria for limb salvage procedures prior to chemotherapy, but 60% underwent limb salvage following chemotherapy [19].

Two groups of patients with favorable prognosis were identified, those with osteosarcomas in the humerus and those with the telangiectatic type. All six patients with humeral osteosarcomas underwent limb salvage and are alive and free of disease. Six of the seven patients with telangiectatic osteosarcomas are alive and free of disease; the seventh died of treatment-related complications.

References

1. Friedman MA, Carter SK (1972) The therapy of osteogenic sarcoma: Current status and thoughts for the future. J Surg Oncol 4:482–510
2. Marcove RC, Mike V, Hajek JV, et al. (1971) Osteogenic sarcoma in childhood. NY State J Med 71:855–859
3. Jeffree CM, Price CHG, Sessons HA (1975) The metastatic patterns of osteosarcoma. Br J Cancer 32:87–107
4. Cade S (1955) Osteogenic sarcoma: a study based on 113 pts. J R Coll Surg Edinb 1:79–111
5. Lee ES, Mackenzie DH (1964) Osteosarcoma: a study of the value of preoperative megavoltage radiotherapy. Br J Surg 51:252–274

6. Jenkin RDT, Allt WEC, Fitzpatrick PJ (1972) Osteosarcoma: an assessment of management with particular reference to primary irradiation and selective delayed amputation. Cancer 30:393–400

7. Cortes EP, Necheles TF, Holland JF, Glidewell O (1979) Adriamycin (ADR) alone versus ADR and high-dose methotrexate–citrovorum factor rescue (HDM-CFR) as adjuvant to operable primary osteosarcoma. A randomized study by Cancer and Leukemic group B (CALGB). Proc Am Assoc Cancer Res 20:412

8. Sutow WW, Sullivan MP, Wilbur JR, Cangir A (1975) A study of adjuvant chemotherapy in osteogenic sarcoma. J Clin Pharmacol 7:530–533

9. Jaffe N, Watts H, Fellows KE, Vawter C (1978) Local en bloc resection for limb preservation. Cancer Treat Rep 62:217–223

10. Rosen G, Marcove RC, Caparros B, Nirenberg A, Kosloff C, Huvos AG (1979) Primary osteogenic sarcoma. The rationale for preoperative chemotherapy and delayed surgery. Cancer 43:2163–2177

11. Morton DL, Eilber FR, Townsend CN Jr, Grant TT, Mirra J, Weisenburger TH (1976) Limb salvage from a multidisciplinary treatment approach for skeletal and soft tissue sarcomas of the extremity. Ann Surg 184:268–278

12. Rosen G, Murphy ML, Huvos AG, et al. (1976) Chemotherapy, en bloc resection and prosthetic bone replacement in the treatment of osteogenic sarcoma. Cancer 37:1–11

13. Rosen G, Caparros B, Huvos A, et al. (1982) Preoperative chemotherapy for osteogenic osteosarcoma: selection of postoperative adjuvant chemotherapy based on the response of the primary tumor to preoperative chemotherapy. Cancer 49:1221–1230

14. Rosen G, Marcove RC, Huvos AG, et al. (1983) Primary osteogenic sarcoma: eight-year experience with adjuvant chemotherapy. J Cancer Res Clin Oncol 106[Suppl]:55–67

15. Ochs JJ, Freeman AI, Douglass HO, Hibgy DJ, Mindell R, Sinks T (1978) Cis-dichlorodiammineplatinum (II) in advanced osteogenic sarcoma. Cancer Treat Rep 62:239–245

16. Jaffe N, Bowman R, Wang Y-M, et al. (1984) Chemotherapy for primary osteosarcoma by intra-arterial infusion. Review of the literature and comparison with results achieved by the intravenous route. Cancer Bull 36:37–42

17. Benjamin RS, Chuang VP, Wallace S, et al. (1982) Preoperative chemotherapy for osteosarcoma (abstract C-675) ASCO 1:174

18. Benjamin RS, Chawla SP, Carrasco CH, et al. (1986) Primary chemotherapy of patients with extremity osteosarcoma. (abstract C-) ASCO

19. Benjamin RS, Murray JA, Wallace S, et al. (1984) Intra-arterial preoperative chemotherapy for osteosarcoma – a judicious approach to limb salvage. Cancer Bull 36:32–36

Haematology and Blood Transfusion   Vol. 31
Modern Trends in Human Leukemia VII
Edited by Neth, Gallo, Greaves, and Kabisch
© Springer-Verlag Berlin Heidelberg 1987

In Vitro Treatment of Bone Marrow from Patients with T-Cell Acute Lymphoblastic Leukemia and Non-Hodgkin's Lymphoma Using the Immunotoxin WT1-Ricin A

M. J. Barnett[1], A. Z. S. Rohatiner[1], J. E. Kingston[1], K. E. Adams[1], E. L. Batten[1], R. Bassan[2], P. E. Thorpe[3], M. A. Horton[1], J. S. Malpas[1], and T. A. Lister[1]

A. Introduction

The murine monoclonal antibody WT1 [1] identifies a glycoprotein of molecular weight 40000 present on normal thymocytes and blasts from patients with T-cell acute lymphoblastic leukaemia (T-ALL) [2]. The antibody may be linked by a disulphide bond to the A chain of ricin [3] to form an immunotoxin (WT1-ricin A) which kills cells that express the WT1 antigen but does not have an inhibitory effect on haematopoietic precursors [4].

WT1-ricin A has been used to treat bone marrow from patients in remission of T-ALL and non-Hodgkin's lymphoma (NHL), in an attempt to eradicate occult neoplastic cells. The study was conducted with the intention of then using such cryopreserved marrow to support the treatment of these patients with intensive chemoradiotherapy in second remission.

B. Materials and Methods

I. Patients

Clinical details are shown in Table 1.

[1] ICRF Department of Medical Oncology, St. artholomew's Hospital, London EC1A 7BE, UK
[2] Ospedali Ruiniti, Bergamo, Italy
[3] ICRF Drug Targeting Laboratory

Table 1. Results obtained in patients studied

Pa-tient	Age	Sex	Diag-nosis	Pre WT1-ricin A				Post WT1-ricin A		
				BM vol. (ml)	MNC ($\times 10^9$)	WT1 (%)	CFU-GM on day 12 (per 10^5 MNC)	MNC ($\times 10^9$)	WT1 (%)	CFU-GM on day 12 (per 10^5 MNC)
1	33	M	ALL[a]	1420	2.2	5	50	1.7	<1	36
2	41	M	NHL[a]	1437	2.7	5	45	1.7	<1	51
3	49	M	ALL	1376	2.3	8	36	1.8	<1	27
4	13	M	ALL	1239	2.0	10	157[b]	1.1	<1	183[b]
5	26	M	ALL	1736	2.5	13	28	1.6	<1	3
6	9	M	ALL	579	0.7	20	72	0.6	<1	36
7	12	M	ALL	740	1.4	27	49	1.2	<1	147
8	14	F	NHL	578	1.4	22	26	0.6	<1	80

BM, bone marrow.
[a] Second remission, all others first remission.

57

II. Methods

In Vitro Treatment of Marrow

Bone marrow was harvested during morphological and immunological remission (no detectable WT1+/TdT+ cells), and the mononuclear cell (MNC) fraction was isolated. Half the cells were cryopreserved untreated and half were treated with WT1-ricin A. The cells were transferred to tissue culture flasks at a concentration of 5×10^6 cells/ml in incubation medium (RPM1 1640 + 15% autologous serum + penicillin and streptomycin). Ammonium chloride and WT1-ricin A were then added to a final concentration of 6 M ammonium chloride and 0.25 µg ricin A/ml. The flasks were incubated for 20 h at 37 °C in a 5% CO_2-humidified incubator. The cells were then resuspended and washed twice prior to cryopreservation.

C. Results

In all cases, the percentage of WT1+ cells decreased from between 5% and 27% to less than 1% after incubation with the immunotoxin. In four of eight cases, this was accompanied by a decrease in colony-forming unit–granulocyte macrophage (CFU-GM) numbers.

D. Discussion

The method described is practical and, as far as can be deduced from this study, effective.

Experience needs to be gained with the reinfusion of such marrow and the monitoring of subsequent haematological and immunological reconstitution. Furthermore, the interest in such in vitro methods of treating the autograft should not eclipse the major issue of disease eradication in the patient.

Acknowledgments. The contribution of the medical and nursing staff of Duty Theatre, Kenton and Dalziel Wards at St. Bartholomew's Hospital is gratefully acknowledged. We thank Angie Mehta for typing this manuscript.

References

1. Tax WJM, Willems HW, Kibbelaar MDA, De Groot J, Capel PJA, Waal RMW De, Reekers P, Koene RAP (1982) Monoclonal antibodies against human thymocytes and T lymphocytes. In: Peeters H (ed) Protides of the biological fluids, vol 29. Pergamon, Oxford, pp 701–704
2. Vodinelich L, Tax WJM, Bai Y, Pegram S, Capel P, Greaves MF (1983) A monoclonal antibody (WT1) for detecting leukaemias of T-cell precursors (T-ALL). Blood 62:1108–1113
3. Thorpe PE, Ross WCJ (1982) The preparation and cytotoxic properties of antibody-toxin conjugates. Immunol Rev 62:119–158
4. Myers CD, Thorpe PE, Ross WCJ, Cumber AJ, Katz FE, Tax WJM, Greaves MF (1984) An immunotoxin with therapeutic potential in T-cell leukaemia: WT1-ricin A. Blood 63:1178–1185
5. Gilmore MJML, Prentice HG, Blacklock HA, Ma DDF, Janossy G, Hoffbrand AV (1982) A technique for rapid isolation of bone marrow mononuclear cells using ficoll-metrizoate and the IBM 2991 blood cell processor. Br J Haematol 50:619–626

Haematology and Blood Transfusion Vol. 31
Modern Trends in Human Leukemia VII
Edited by Neth, Gallo, Greaves, and Kabisch
© Springer-Verlag Berlin Heidelberg 1987

Ablative Therapy Supported by Autologous Bone Marrow Transplantation with In Vitro Treatment of Marrow in Patients with B-Cell Malignancy

A. Z. S. Rohatiner, M. J. Barnett, S. Arnott, N. Plowman, F. Cotter, K. Adams,
E. L. Batten, S. Outram, J. A. L. Amess, M. A. Horton, and T. A. Lister

A. Introduction

Patients with non-Hodgkin's lymphoma who relapse almost invariably die as a consequence of the disease regardless of histological subtype [1–4]. Ablative therapy supported by autologous bone marrow transplantation (BMT) may result in durable remissions in a proportion of such patients [5–8] although this approach is limited by the high frequency of bone marrow (BM) infiltration. Nadler et al. [9] have used the B-cell-specific monoclonal antibody anti-B1 [10] and rabbit complement to deplete autologous marrow of residual, morphologically

ICRF Department of Medical Oncology, St. Bartholomew's Hospital, London EC1A, UK

undetectable lymphoma. A study is in progress at St. Bartholomew's Hospital to evaluate the use of ablative therapy supported by such in vitro-treated autologous BM as consolidation of second or subsequent remission in patients with B-cell malignancy.

B. Patients and Methods

I. Patients

Thirteen patients have been treated since June 1985. Clinical characteristics are shown in Table 1. Patient 6 had minimal splenomegaly at the time of treatment, the remainder had no evidence of disease by computerized tomography (CT) scan criteria and on the basis of BM morphology and phenotyping.

Table 1. Clinical characteristics

Patient	Age	Histology	Stage at presentation	Site	Remission status
1	38	Follicular	IIIA	Lymph node	3rd
2	44	Follicular	IVB	Lymph node, liver, spleen, BM	2nd
3	42	Follicular	IVB	Lymph node, pl. effn., ascites, BM	2nd
4	55	Follicular	IVB	Lymph node, lung, pl. effn., BM	2nd
5	36	Follicular	IIIB	Lymph node	2nd
6	29	Follicular	IVB	Lymph node, liver, spleen, BM	3rd
7	39	Follicular	IIA	Lymph node	2nd
8	61	Follicular	IVA	Lymph node, BM	3rd
9	26	Burkitt	IVB	Lymph node, CNS, kidney, BM	1st
10	56	Centroblastic	IVB	Lymph node, liver, spleen	2nd
11	49	Centroblastic	IVB	Lymph node, bowel	3rd
12	50	Follicular	IVA	Lymph node, BM	2nd
13	38	Follicular	IIIA	Lymph node	3rd

II. In Vitro Treatment of BM

BM was aspirated from the anterior and posterior iliac crests under general anaesthetic. The mononuclear cell fraction was treated with three cycles of anti-B1 and rabbit complement (Pel-Freez) [9] and the cells cryopreserved.

III. Therapy

Patients received cyclophosphamide, 60 mg/kg IV on days 1 and 2, followed by total body irradiation, 200 cGy bd on days 3, 4 and 5 (except for the first four patients, who received a single dose of 900 cGy on day 3). Marrow was reinfused within 24 h of completion of radiotherapy.

C. Results

I. Haemopoietic and Immunological Reconstitution

Neutrophil recovery ($>0.5 \times 10^9$/l) occurred after 25 days (mean) with a range of 15–45 days. Platelet recovery ($>20 \times 10^9$/l) occurred after 28 days (mean) with a range of 15–

54 days, except in one patient with follicular lymphoma with a persistently hypocellular bone marrow who continues to require platelet transfusions at 5-month intervals. Normal numbers of B cells were detectable in the peripheral blood at 3 months. Circulating immunoglobulin M and G (IgM and IgG) levels fell to <25% of normal 2–3 months after transplantation, returning towards normal at 6 months. The ratio of T8+ve (cytotoxic/suppressor) to T4+ve (helper/inducer) cells has reversed in all patients and this abnormality has persisted for over 6 months. (Data not shown.)

II. Toxicity

Twelve patients were discharged from hospital 15–42 days after reinfusion of marrow, one died of bronchopneumonia on day 9 (Table 2).

III. Survival

Eleven patients are well without evidence of disease; the patient with B-cell acute lymphoblastic leukaemia (B-ALL) has relapsed and died.

Table 2. Haematological reconstitution

Patient	N. of cells reinfused ($\times 10^9$/l)	Days to		Complications
		Neutrophils ($=0.5 \times 10^9$/l)	Platelets ($>20 \times 10^9$/l)	
1	3.6	21	23	Fever, no organism[a]
2	0.98	28	29	Pneumonia $\times 2$[a]
3	1.7	18	25	Fever, no organism[a]
4	1.6	16	13	Fever, no organism
5	2.2	23	23	Septicaemia
6	1.3	45	45	Septicaemia[a]
7	1.9	15	15	Herpes simplex
8	0.99	42	>5m	Fever, no organism[a]
9	2.3	20	54	Fever, no organism
10	1.6	Patient died on day 9		Bronchopneumonia
11	1.3	25	35	Fever, no organism
12	1.4	25	25	Fever, no organism[a]
13	1.9	25	25	Fever, no organism

All patients lost up to10% of their body weight.
[a] Oral ulceration.

D. Conclusions

The experience to date confirms the feasibility of this approach. It remains to be established whether such intensive therapy given as consolidation prolongs remission duration.

Acknowledgements. We thank the medical and nursing staff of Annie Zunz and Dalziel Wards for their expert care and Angie Mehta for typing the manuscript. Anti-B1 was kindly supplied by Dr. Lee Nadler and subsequently by Coulter Immunology.

References

1. Sweet DL, Golomb HM, Ultmann JE, et al. (1980) Cyclophosphamide, vincristine, methotraxate with leucovorin rescue, and cytarabine (COMLA) combination sequential chemotherapy for advanced diffuse histiocytic lymphoma. Ann Intern Med 92:785
2. Skarin AT, Canellos GP, Rosenthal DS, et al. (1983) Improved prognosis of diffuse histiocytic and undifferentiated lymphoma by use of high dose methotraxate alternating with standard agents (M-BACOD). J Clin Oncol 1:91
3. Fisher RI, De Vita VT Jr, Hubbard SM, et al. (1983) Diffuse aggressive lymphomas: increased survival after alternating flexible sequences of ProMACE and MOPP chemotherapy. Ann Intern Med 98:304
4. Gallagher CJ, Gregory WM, Jones AE, et al. (1986) Follicular lymphoma: prognostic factors for response and survival. J Clin Oncol (in press)
5. Appelbaum FR, Herzig GP, Ziegler JC, et al. (1978) Successful engraftment of cryopreserved autologous bone marrow in patients with malignant lymphoma. Blood 52:85
6. Appelbaum FR, Thomas ED (1983) Review of the use of marrow transplantation in the treatment of non-Hodgkin's lymphoma. J Clin Oncol 1:440
7. Philip T, Biron P, Maraninchi D, et al. (1984) Role of massive chemotherapy and autologous bone marrow transplantation in non-Hodgkin's malignant lymphoma. Lancet I:391
8. Carella AM, et al. (1984) High-dose chemotherapy and nonfrozen autologous bone marrow transplantation in relapsed advanced lymphomas or those resistant to conventional chemotherapy. Cancer 33:1382
9. Nadler LM, Botnick L, Canellos GP, et al. (1984) Anti-B1 monoclonal antibody and complement treatment in autologous bone marrow transplantation for relapsed B-cell non-Hodgkin's lymphoma. Lancet
10. Stashenko P, et al. (1980) Characterization of a human B-lymphocyte-specific antigen. J Immunol 125:1678

Haematology and Blood Transfusion   Vol. 31
Modern Trends in Human Leukemia VII
Edited by Neth, Gallo, Greaves, and Kabisch
© Springer-Verlag Berlin Heidelberg 1987

Use of Autologous Bone Marrow Transplantation in Acute Myeloid Leukemia

A. K. Burnett [1]

A. Introduction

Progress in achieving initial remission of disease in acute myeloblastic leukaemia (AML) has taken place in recent years, with rates of 70%–80% being reported [1–3]. This has been effected by different scheduling of drugs rather than by the introduction of new chemotherapeutic agents. The ability of chemotherapy protocols to maintain remission is less easy to demonstrate. Unlike remission maintenance chemotherapy in acute lymphoblastic leukaemia (ALL), there is little evidence to suggest that continuous chemotherapy has prevented subsequent relapse for the majority of patients. Some improvements have been claimed for very intensive protocols, with better results being achieved in children [4, 5]. However, since the majority of patients with the disease are adults, alternative approaches are required.

Allogeneic bone marrow transplantation (BMT) has proved to be an effective remission maintenance strategy, with approximately 50% of patients becoming long-term survivors [6–8]. This approach, however, is not without its limitations. When the procedure goes well, it is probably much less toxic than conventional intensive chemotherapy, but in a proportion of patients who do become long-term survivors, morbidity can be significant and there are important late consequences. Procedure-related deaths due to the immunobiological problems of allograft represent a risk. About 30%–40% of

patients transplanted succumb to problems such as pneumonitis, graft-versus-host disease (GVHD) or the consequences of immunosuppression. A crucial point is that the actuarial risk of relapse following allograft appears to be 15%–30%, which represents a substantially better antileukaemic effect than that achieved by any other approach. Such results are only achieved in first remission. When allografts are attempted at later stages of the disease, results are worse primarily owing to a higher rate of relapse. An important limitation of allograft with regard to the problem of cure in AML is that it is only applicable to younger patients (conventionally under 40 years of age) with a fully HLA-matched donor, thus restricting the technique to 10%–15% of those with the disease. The prospects for younger patients (under 20 years of age) are good, with 70% –80% surviving; but conventional chemotherapy is also offering improved results in these cases. It can be anticipated that morbidity and mortality of allograft patients will be reduced by such measures as T-cell depletion to abrogate GVHD [9], and cytomegalovirus-negative blood product support for seronegative recipients [10, 11].

The mechanism involved in the cures obtained by allograft may be complex. Two major factors may operate. Allografted marrow rescue has permitted the administration of ablative doses of cyclophosphamide and total body irradiation (TBI) to the patient's marrow, which may alone be capable of eradicating leukaemia. There may in addition be an antileukaemic effect exerted by the graft on any residual leukaemia [graft-versus-leukaemia (GVL) effect]. Such an ef-

[1] Glasgow Royal Infirmary, Castle Street, Glasgow G4 OSF, UK

fect has been shown to operate in lymphoid leukaemia models in mice [12, 13] and was part of the rationale behind introducing BMT into clinical practice.

Autologous remission bone marrow represents a source of replacement haemopoietic stem cells following ablative chemotherapy or chemoradiotherapy. Potential advantages offered by autologous BMT (ABMT) are: (a) there would be an additional option available to patients who lack a donor; (b) procedural morbidity and mortality may be less; not only would GVHD be eliminated as a complication but syngeneic data suggest that pneumonitis and immunosuppression would be less; (c) if toxicity was limited, this approach could be offered to older patients and would thus represent an option for more patients with the disease. Theoretical objections must also be recognised, the first of which relates to loss of the GVL effect. This mechanism may operate in AML in remission in man, but such evidence is indirect and the effect may not be great. It should be borne in mind that the often-quoted experimental data refer to lymphoid models usually involved in transplantation across histocompatibility boundaries. An association of an antileukaemic effect of acute GVHD, based on statistical prediction, in man is not significant for AML in remission, although there is apparent an effect of AML in relapse and ALL in remission and relapse [14]. Perhaps the most useful parallel is the relapse rate in twin transplants for AML in first remission, where half of a relatively small number of patients with various preparative protocols developed recurrent disease usually within the first 12 months after transplant [15].

The second objection is that orthodox assumptions about the nature of remission suggest that the inevitability of relapse indicates that while the patient may fulfil the clinical criteria of remission, residual cells remain which are responsible for relapse. Remission marrow therefore will contain some residual leukaemic cells, and relapse is therefore probable. This raises the important issue of the importance of cleansing (or "purging") the bone marrow.

If the twin data are accepted at face value, they have three important implications for autograft: (a) there will predictably be a higher relapse rate, perhaps at least 50% in autograft, owing to lack of a GVL effect; (b) further risk of relapse may occur if contamination of the autologous marrow is relevant; and (c) morbidity and procedural mortality will be low.

Purging of residual leukaemia in vitro in the context of AML presents special problems. There is little evidence to suggest that density separation is of value. Specific monoclonal-antibody-based techniques are not available at present, and most attention currently centres around pharmacological treatment in vitro [16]. This originated from experimental data in a rat myeloid leukaemia model of efficacy which used a cyclophosphamide metabolite (4-hydroperoxy-cyclophosphamide) because the tumour was very sensitive in vivo to cyclophosphamide [17]. An unsatisfactory aspect of such an approach is that there is no way of assessing effectiveness in vitro in any individual case.

B. Choice of Ablative Protocol

On the basis of allogeneic experience, the timing of the autograft is predictably going to influence outcome. In relapsed disease and second remission allograft, even with the advantages of an uncontaminated graft and the postulated GVL effect, relapse rates are high; consequently, autograft is unlikely to be of benefit. Subsequent clinical studies confirm such an impression. For optimum results, use in first remission is logical.

Cyclophosphamide and TBI constitute the standard preparative protocol for allograft and represent a useful benchmark. There is some evidence to suggest that substitution of cyclophosphamide by melphalan may have enhanced antileukaemic effect [18]. Although increased TBI has little effect on reducing the relapse rate in allograft of relapsed disease, it may offer some advantage if used in remission. Chemotherapy can be an effective alternative preparative regime for allograft.

A number of studies involving chemotherapy-based protocols with ABMT are currently under way, but there is insufficient follow-up at present to indicate whether a TBI or chemotherapy protocol is superior. An interesting approach is that of double autograft, whereby chemotherapy with ABMT is given on two occasions. A possible advantage of this approach, apart from the fact that it intensifies treatment, is that a degree of "in vitro purging" may be achieved [19].

C. Results of Autograft in First Remission

In our own experience in Glasgow, with the use of unpurged marrow, 22 patients have received an autograft in first remission.

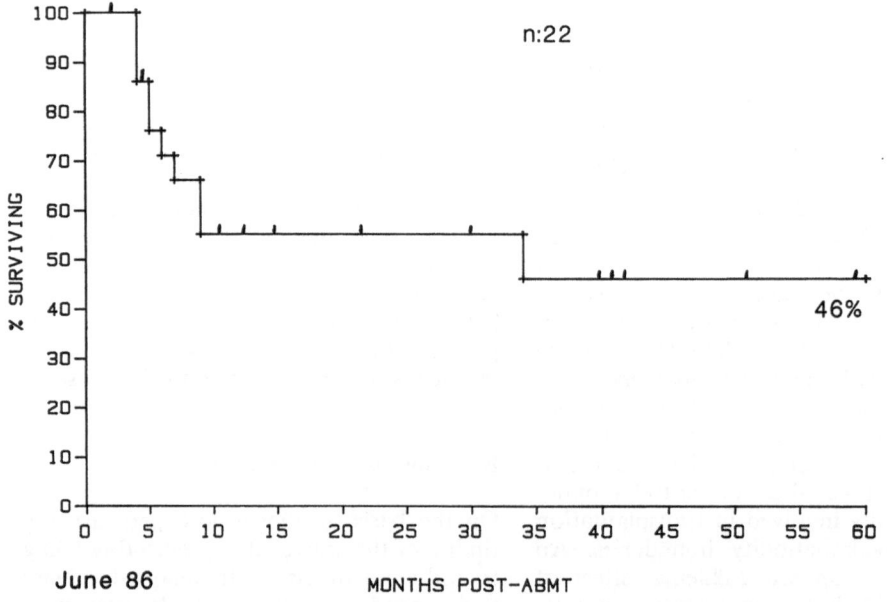

Fig. 1. Survival of patients receiving ABMT for AML in first remission (Glasgow)

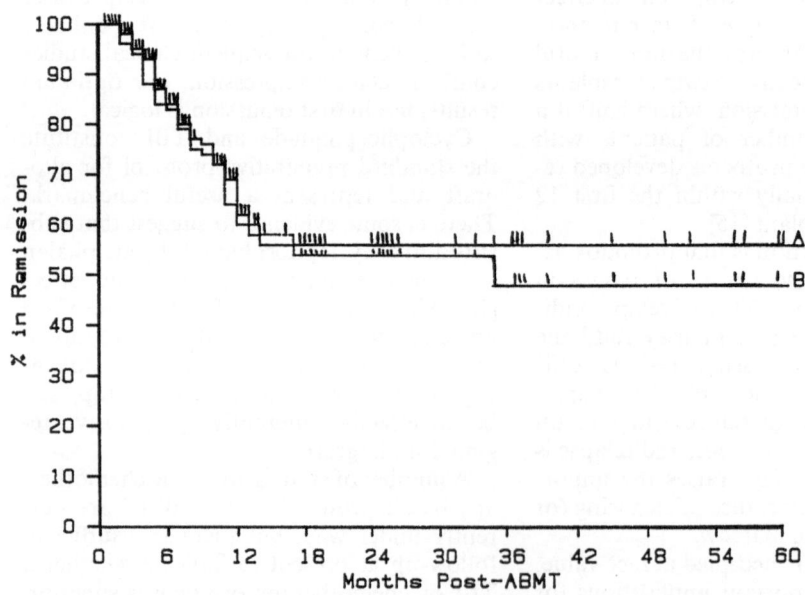

Fig. 2. Multi-centre study [20] of ABMT in first remission. *A*, leukaemia-free survival; *B,* overall survival

64

These patients ranged in age from 13 to 53 years (median 36). The first 13 patients received cyclophosphamide and single fraction TBI (950 cGy) and autologous marrow stored at 4 °C for 54 h. The next 9 patients received melphalan (110 mg/m²) and fractionated TBI (6 × 200 cGy) with cryopreserved marrow. Nine patients have relapsed, all within 12 months of transplant, 12 continue in remission and 8 have been in remission for over 2 years. There was no procedural mortality, and morbidity was acceptable. One patient died of a cerebral haemorrhage in complete remission 35 months after ABMT. The actuarial survival at 4 years is 46% and leukaemia-free survival 57% (Fig. 1).

In a review of data from other European centres using unpurged bone marrow, 90 cases were assessed [20]. Of these cases, 5 died of non-leukaemic, usually infective causes, 3 within 3 months of autograft. The age range of patients was 10–57, but 33 patients were over 35 years old and may therefore be considered outside the acceptable age range for allograft. A variety of cytoreductive protocols were used: single-pulse high-dose chemotherapy, double autograft, and cyclophosphamide and TBI; 53 patients received TBI, and 37 a chemotherapy protocol (including 14 as double autografts). Twenty-seven patients relapsed, all but 2 within 1 year of autograft. The leukaemia-free survival at 3 years after ABMT was 56% (Fig. 2).

Relatively few data are available to assess whether purging confers additional benefit. Such comparisons as have been made show no advantage.

D. Conclusions

Available studies suggest autologous transplantation may have a contribution to make to remission maintenance in AML in first remission. Prolonged follow-up of more patients is awaited with interest, but in the meantime it is important to be aware of possible selection bias in these patients. In particular, they were in remission for variable periods prior to autograft and may have selected themselves as having more responsive disease; similarly, patients who relapsed

prior to autograft would be excluded from the protocol. In the multi-centre study [20], when leukaemia-free survival was stratified according to time elapsed prior to autograft, there were improved prospects for those autografted at 4–8 months (58%) compared with those at < 4 months (38%). This could obviously be due to the selection bias referred to above, but it may also indicate that chemotherapy prior to autograft plays an important role.

These results are of importance in the future evaluation of purging techniques, since the leukaemia-free survival is similar to that observed in syngeneic transplants. This may suggest that the question of residual leukaemia in the graft is unimportant. It will also be difficult to demonstrate, at least in first remission, significant benefit from purging.

References

1. Rees JKH, Gray R, Hayhoe FGJ (1985) Late intensification therapy in the treatment of acute myeloid leukaemia. (abstract). Proc Am Soc Clin Oncol C621
2. Preisler HD, Rustum Y, Henderson ES et al. (1979) Treatment of acute non-lymphocytic leukaemia: use of anthracyclin – cytosine arabinoside induction therapy and comparison of two maintenance regimens. Blood 53:455–464
3. Gale RF, Foon KA, Cline MJ et al. (1981) Intensive chemotherapy for acute myelogenous leukaemia. Ann Intern Med 94:753–757
4. Weinstein HJ, Mayer RJ, Rosenthal DS et al. (1983) Chemotherapy for acute myelogenous leukaemia in children and adults: VAPA Update. Blood 62:315–319
5. Creutzig U, Riefim RH, Langermann HJ (1985) Improved treatment results in childhood acute myelogenous leukaemia: a report of the German Co-operative Study AML-BRM-78. Blood 65:298–304
6. Thomas ED, Buckner CD, Clift RA (1979) Marrow transplantation for acute non-lymphoblastic leukaemia in first remission. N Engl J Med 301:597–599
7. Powles RL, Morgenstern G, Clink HM et al. (1980) The place of bone marrow transplantation in acute myelogenous leukaemia. Lancet 1:1047–1050
8. Zwaan FE, Hermans J, Barrett AJ et al. (1984) Bone marrow transplantation for

acute non-lymphoblastic leukaemia: a survey of the European group for bone marrow transplantation. Br J Haem 56:645–653

9. Prentice HG, Blacklock HA, Janossy G et al. (1984) Depletion of T lymphocytes in donor marrow prevents significant graft-versus-host disease in matched allogeneic leukaemics marrow transplant recipient. Lancet I:472–476

10. Bowden RA,Sayers M, Flournoy N et al. (1986) Cytomegalovirus Immune Globulin and Seronegative Blood Products to Prevent Primary Cytolomegalovirus Infection after Bone Marrow Transplantation. N Engl J Med 314:1006–1010

11. McKinnon S, Burnett AK, Crawford RG et al. (1986) Prevention of CMV infection in allogeneic bone marrow transplant recipients by using CMv-negative blood products. Bone Marrow Transplantation 1:67(Suppl)

12. Barnes DWH, Loutit JF (1975) Treatment of murine leukaemia with x-rays and homologous bone marrow. Br J Haem 3:241–252

13. Boranic M (1971) Time pattern of anti-leukaemic effect of graft-versus-host reaction in mice. J Natl Cancer Inst 4:421–432

14. Weiden PL, Flournoy N, Thomas ED et al. (1979) Anti-leukaemia effect of graft-versus-host disease in recipients of allogeneic marrow grafts. N Engl J Med 300:1068–1073

15. Gale RP, Champlin RE (1984) How does bone marrow transplantation cure leukaemia? Lancet II:28–30

16. Santos GW, Colvin OM (1986) Pharmacological Purging of Bone Marrow with Reference to Autografting. Clin Haematol 15; 1:67–83

17. Sharkis SJ, Santos GW, Colvin M (1980) Elimination of acute myelogenous leukemic cells from marrow and tumor suspensions in the rate with 4-hydroperoxycyclophosphamide. Blood 55:521–523

18. Goss GD, Powles RL, Barrett A et al. (1985) Melphalan and total body irradiation (TBI) versus Cyclophosphamide plus TBI prior to bone marrow transplantation in acute myeloid leukaemia in first remission. Exp Haematol 13; 12–13 (Suppl 17)

19. Anderson CC, Linch DC, Goldstone AH (1986) Double autografting: a potential curative regimen for acute leukaemia. Minimal residual disease in acute leukaemia 1986. Hagenbeck B, Lowenberg A (eds) Martinus Nijhoff, Amsterdam, pp 221–233

20. Burnett AK, McKinnon S (1986) Autologous bone marrow transplantation in first remission AML using non-purged marrow – update. Minimal residual disease in acute leukaemia 1986. Hagenbeck B, Lowenberg A (eds). Martinus Nijhoff, Amsterdam, pp 211–220

Haematology and Blood Transfusion   Vol. 31
Modern Trends in Human Leukemia VII
Edited by Neth, Gallo, Greaves, and Kabisch
© Springer-Verlag Berlin Heidelberg 1987

Monoclonal-Antibody-Purged Autologous Bone Marrow Transplantation for Relapsed Non-T-Cell Acute Lymphoblastic Leukemia in Childhood

C. M. Niemeyer, J. Ritz, K. Donahue, and S. E. Sallan

A. Introduction

Acute lymphoblastic leukemia (ALL) in childhood is a curable disease for the majority of patients [1]. Most children who relapse, however, have a poor prognosis. Although second complete remission can usually be obtained, the long-term disease-free survival in most series is less than 10% [2, 3]. Therefore, allogeneic bone marrow transplantation has been considered the treatment of choice for children with ALL in second hematologic remission who have an HLA-identical mixed leukocyte culture (MLC) nonreactive sibling donor. An alternative approach has been autologous bone marrow transplantation.

Since leukemic cells almost certainly contaminate remission bone marrow, methods to eradicate leukemic cells in vitro have been developed. The essential elements of in vitro purging are removal of leukemic cells and in vivo hematopoietic reconstitution by the treated bone marrow. The two strategies for in vitro removal of contaminating leukemic cells include the use of pharmacologic agents, mainly the cyclophosphamide derivatives ASTA Z 7557 [4] and 4-hydroperoxycyclophosphamide [5], and the use of heteroantisera [6] or monoclonal antibodies directed against cell surface antigens of leu-

kemic cells. Monoclonal antibodies are utilized with exogenous complement [7, 8] or immunotoxins [9, 10] or immunophysical methods [11]. In a model system that utilizes leukemic cell lines, one can demonstrate that monoclonal antibodies, complement, and drugs have a higher efficacy in the selective elimination of clonogenic cells than either modality alone [12, 13].

There are a number of practical and theoretical obstacles to overcome. Chemotherapeutic agents might have excessive toxicity to stem cells, and, thus, hematopoietic recovery would be impossible. The antigenic heterogeneity of malignant cells in the individual patient might mitigate against in vitro cytolysis of all blast cells. Furthermore, antibodies may cross-react with normal cells, especially progenitors or stem cells. The phenotype of a small population of progenitor cells for leukemic blasts may not be the same as the phenotype for the majority of blast cells [14]. It would be more important to purge these malignant progenitor cells and perhaps their precursors. Finally, none of the clinical studies that apply one or the other method of in vitro purging of remission bone marrow has been done in a setting where the efficacy of the in vitro manipulation could be compared to the use of nonpurged bone marrow.

In this report, we provide an update and critical evaluation of our clinical experience in autologous bone marrow transplantation for children with ALL in second and subsequent remissions. Moreover, we will compare these results with our concurrent allogeneic transplant experience.

Dana Farber Cancer Institute, Division of Medical and Pediatric Oncology, Dana Farber Cancer Institute, Childrens' Hospital, Boston, MA, USA, 02115, 44 Binney Street

B. Methods and Materials

Between November 1980 and June 1986 we transplanted 31 children under the age of 18 for non-T-cell ALL.

I. Elimination of Leukemic Cells from Remission Bone Marrow In Vitro

Two murine monoclonal antibodies, J5 [15] and J2 [16, 17], were utilized with rabbit complement. The J5 antibody reacts with the common acute lymphoblastic leukemia antigen (CALLA), a 100-kd glycoprotein expressed on leukemic cells of approximately 80% of patients with non-T-cell ALL. J2 recognizes an associated 26-kd glycoprotein (gp26). Although in the majority of cases of non-T-cell ALL leukemic cells express both CALLA and gp26 antigen, there are instances when only one of these antigens is present [18]. In over 90% of cases, leukemic cells will express at least one of these antigens, which independently might serve as a target for monoclonal antibody binding and complement lysis. The generation, characterization, and utilization of the monoclonal antibodies in the in vitro elimination of leukemic cells have been described previously [7, 19, 20]. The first 13 patients had marrow treated with only one antibody: J5 in 12 patients and J2 in 1 patient. After an experimental in vitro system indicated that two antibodies resulted in higher cell kill [21], the next 18 patients had their marrow treated with both antibodies.

II. Cytoreductive Chemotherapeutic Treatment and Radiation Therapy In Vivo

Patients with relapsed ALL were eligible if their leukemic cells expressed CALLA or gp26. Patients with HLA-compatible donors, as well as those in whom a complete remission could not be induced with chemotherapy alone, were excluded. After remission induction (usually with vincristine, prednisone, and asparaginase), all children received at least one course of intensification therapy consisting of VM-26, cytosine arabinoside (ara-C), and asparaginase, together with intrathecal hydrocortisone and ara-C (Table 1). Patients who had not previously

Table 1. Intensification therapy

		Day			
		1	3	7	10
Vm-26	200 mg/m² i.v.	×	×	×	×
Ara-C	300 mg/m² i.v.	×	×	×	×
Aspara-ginase	25 000 IU/m² i.m.	×		×	
Ara-C	40 mg i.t.	×	×	×	×
Hydro-cortisone	15 mg i.t	×	×	×	×

Table 2. Ablation therapy

			Pretransplant day									
			−9	−8	−7	−6	−5	−4	−3	−2	−1	0
Vm-26	200 mg/m²		×				×					
Ara-C	500 mg/m² × 5	n = 22										
	500 mg/m² × 7	n = 6										
	3 g/m² × 6	n = 3										
Cyclophosphamide	60 mg/kg						×	×				
TBI 850 cGy		n = 12										
1200 cGy	(200 cGy × 6)	n = 16							×	× × ×	× ×	
1300 cGy	(216 cGy × 6)	n = 3										
Bone marrow reinfusion												×

N: number of patients treated;
TBI: total body irradiation.

received intensive treatment with an anthra-cycline were also given a single dose of dox-orubicin. After recovery from intensification therapy, bone marrow was harvested and ablation initiated (Table 2). During the study period, several dose adjustments were implemented. All patients received cyclo-phosphamide (60 mg/kg) in the days im-mediately preceding radiation therapy. They also received ara-C during the days preced-ing cyclophosphamide treatment. Twenty-two patients were given ara-C (500 mg/m^2) per day for 5 days by continuous infusion. In an effort to improve antileukemic efficacy, six children were given the same daily dose for 7 days. This schedule was abandoned be-cause of concern about increased morbidity secondary to prolonged marrow aplasia. The most recently treated patients were given 3 gm/m^2 for six doses. VM-26 was ad-ministered on the first and last day of the ara-C infusion. Additionally, eight patients were treated with asparaginase at the time of the first VM-26 dose. All patients received total body irradiation at 5 cGy per minute. During the trial the total dose was increased and fractionated. The first 12 patients re-ceived 850 cGy in a single fraction, and the following 16 patients received 1200 cGy fraction in six 200 cGy doses delivered twice daily. Most recently, the total dose was fur-ther increased to 1300 cGy with 216 cGy fraction twice daily. Small lead shields were used to attentuate the pulmonary dose by 15%. Following the last dose of total body irradiation, the antibody-treated autologous bone marrow was thawed and directly in-fused by rapid intravenous bolus. No che-motherapy was administered after trans-plantation.

III. Study Population

Of the 31 patients, 21 were transplanted in second remission, 8 in third remission, and 1 child in fourth remission. The analysis also includes one child transplanted in first re-mission. This child had required more than 100 days to enter remission. Thirteen of the children had experienced an initial relapse while receiving therapy, and 17 had relapsed after stopping treatment. The median dura-tion of first remission was 24 months (range

2–84), and the median duration of the sec-ond remission for the nine children trans-planted in subsequent remissions was 8 months (range 2–54). The last remission prior to transplant had a median duration of 2 months (range 1–7).

Analysis of the sites of relapse prior to transplantation showed that 18 patients had bone marrow (BM) relapse, 2 had central nervous system (CNS) disease, and 2 had isolated testicular relapses only. Either con-secutively or simultaneously, five children had recurrent BM and CNS disease, two had BM and testicular disease, and one had in-volvement of BM, CNS, and testis. The me-dian age at the time of transplantation was 7.4 years (range 3.2–15.7). There were 24 males and 7 females.

Beginning in 1979, we adopted a treat-ment policy of allogeneic bone marrow transplantation for all patients with relapsed ALL who had histocompatible donors. This policy was modified in 1981 to exclude indi-viduals whose relapse occurred more than 1 year after stopping chemotherapy. Twenty-two patients received an allogeneic bone marrow transplant at our own center, the Memorial Sloan-Kettering Cancer Center, the Seattle Bone Marrow Transplantation Center, the University of Kentucky, or the University of Iowa. The autologous and al-logeneic transplant populations were com-parable with respect to age and white blood count at diagnosis, as well as to the duration of the initial complete remission. There were two major differences between the groups. Most patients in the allogeneic group had re-lapsed after intensive chemotherapy, whereas the majority of patients in the autol-ogous group had relapsed after more con-ventional chemotherapy. Ablative therapy for the allogeneic patients included only cyclophosphamide and total body irradi-ation, as compared to the more intensive preparative regimen for the autologous pa-tients.

IV. Statistical Methods

For analysis of event-free survival, events were defined as relapses or remission deaths. Times were calculated from the day of bone marrow transplantation. The Kaplan-Meier method was used to estimate survival distributions for event-free survival [33]. The two-sided log-rank procedure was utilized to assess the statistical significance of treatment differences between time distributions [34]. The Fisher exact test was used to compare outcome with respect to prognostic features which were categorized [34].

C. Results

After autologous bone marrow transplantation, the probability of event-free survival at 5 years was $27\% \pm 16\%$ (Fig. 1). Of the 31 patients, 21 had an event and 10 remained in continuous complete remission. There was a high incidence of remission deaths (9 patients), with all deaths secondary to toxicity occurring within 3 months of transplantation. Four patients died of aspergillosis, three of hemorrhage, and two of interstitial pneumonitis of unknown etiology. The majority of transplants were performed in single isolation rooms without high-energy particulate filtration. Hematologic recovery was noted in all patients who survived more than 20 days.

Twelve patients relapsed between 2 and 14 months (median 4.5 months) after transplantation. Nine of them relapsed in the BM only, two simultaneously in the BM and an extramedullary site, and one in the retro-orbital space. The three patients with recurrent extramedullary disease were all individuals who had previously relapsed in only extramedullary sites prior to the procedure. Of the five patients with only extramedullary disease prior to transplantation, one is in continuous complete remission at 53 months, one died of toxicity, and three relapsed, all within the BM and an extramedullary site.

The occurrence of an isolated or combined extramedullary relapse prior to transplantation was not a prognostic factor, nor was the initial presenting white blood count. The duration of the initial remission, however, was prognostically highly significant ($p = 0.0028$) for event-free survival post-transplantation (Fig. 2). Of the 14 patients with an initial remission of more than 24 months, 3 died secondary to toxicity, 2 relapsed, and 9 remained in continuous complete remission. Of the 17 children whose initial remission was shorter than 24 months, 6 died

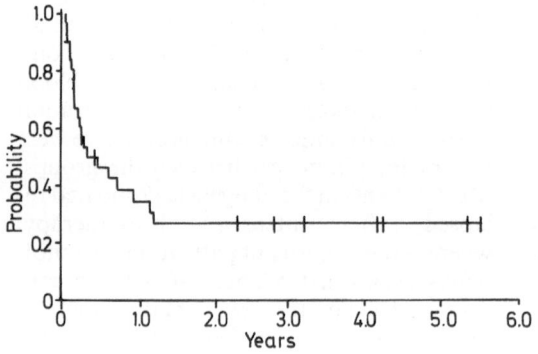

Fig. 1. Probability of event-free survival after autologous bone marrow transplantation

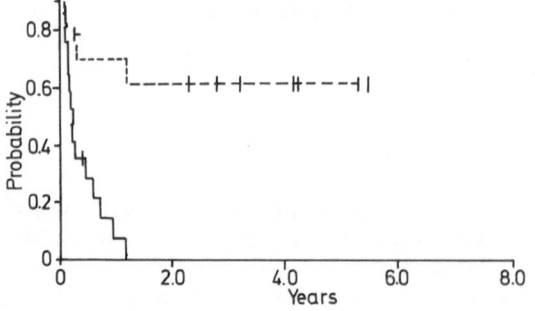

Fig. 2. Probability of event-free survival as a function of duration of longest remission prior to transplantation.
(——— less than 24 months; – – – more than 24 months)

70

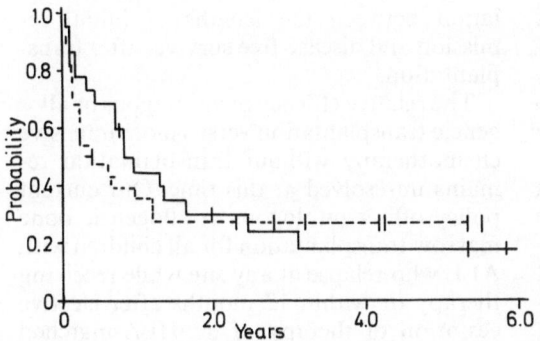

Fig. 3. Probability of event-free survival of allogeneic (——) versus autologous (– – –) bone marrow transplantation

from toxicity, 10 relapsed, and 1 is in continuous complete remission 3 months after transplantation. None of the children transplanted after a remission of 30 months or longer has relapsed.

When the outcome of the 31 autologous transplant patients was compared with that of the 22 allogeneic patients, the probability of event-free survival at 5 years was seen to be very similar, with $27 \pm 16\%$ for the autologous patients and $18\% \pm 18\%$ for the allogeneic transplant patients (Fig. 3) [25]. The median time to failure was shorter for the autologous group owing to acute toxicity and relapse.

D. Discussion

Thirty-one children received an autologous bone marrow transplant for treatment of ALL in second or subsequent remission. Event-free survival at 5 years was $27\% \pm 16\%$. Toxicity rate was high, with 9 out of 31 children suffering a remission death. Duration of initial remission prior to transplantation was prognostically highly significant for long-term event-free survival after transplantation. The outcome of autologous transplantation compared favorably with that of our allogeneic transplant experience.

At the University of Minnesota, two consecutive studies of autologous bone marrow transplantation for recurrent ALL have been conducted since 1982 [8, 22]. Both studies utilized the same monoclonal antibodies, BA-1 (pan B cell), BA-2 (anti-gp26), BA-3 (anti-CALLA), and complement for in vitro purging of the harvested bone marrow. The

preparative regimen differed in the sequential studies.

In the first study, 23 children and 5 adults were treated with two doses of cyclophosphamide (60 mg/kg) and total body irradiation (1320 cGy) delivered twice daily in 165 cGy fractions. The second study utilized a single fraction irradiation dose of 850 cGy followed by ara-C to a total dose of 38 gm/m^2. Thirteen patients were enrolled on this study prior to December 1985. Toxicity in both studies was low, with three toxic deaths from infection: one in Study One and two in Study Two [22]. Twenty-one of the 28 patients in the first study relapsed 1–9 months after transplantation, with a median time to relapse of 3.3 months. Seven of the 13 patients in the second study relapsed. The relapse-free survivals at 1 year are 22% and 30%, respectively. The duration of longest remission prior to transplantation was not of prognostic significance for post-transplant event-free survival [22].

In contrast to our study, all the Minnesota patients' initial relapses occurred while they were receiving treatment. Furthermore, a higher percentage of patients were transplanted in third or fourth remission, and the median duration of the longest remission prior to transplantation was 14 months [23], as opposed to 24 months in our study.

The high relapse rate after autologous bone marrow transplantation for ALL could be due to an insufficient conditioning regimen or to inadequate removal of leukemic cells during the in vitro treatment. At the University of Minnesota, the same conditioning regimen was used for allogeneic and autologous transplants. A review of 121 patients transplanted between 1978 and

1985 showed that patients with autografts and allografts had a similar event-free survival at 2 years of 28% ± 14% and 34% ± 16%, respectively [24]. Patients with autografts relapsed earlier and more frequently than patients with allografts. However, patients who received allogeneic transplants and did not have graft-versus-host disease had the same relapse rate as those who received autologous grafts. This suggests that the relapses in autologous transplant patients were due to refractory disease in vivo, and possibly the lack of graft-versus-leukemia effect, rather than to reinfused leukemic cells.

The Seattle transplant group reported similar survival rates for allogeneic transplantation of children with ALL in second or subsequent remission, with 13 out of 15 patients in long-term remission [26]. Better results for allogeneic transplantation have been reported by the Memorial Sloan-Kettering Cancer Center, with a projected 2-year disease-free survival for 22 patients in second remission of 67% ± 10% [27].

In our study, two out of ten patients in continuous complete remission after autologous bone marrow transplantation had experienced an initial relapse more than 1 year off therapy. It could be argued that those children could have been treated as effectively with an intensive chemotherapy regimen without total body irradiation and transplantation. Johnson and coworkers compared the outcome of 24 children who received allogeneic transplants in second or subsequent remission to that of 21 children treated with conventional chemotherapy [28]. A follow-up of that study showed that all 21 children treated with chemotherapy died within 3.5 years of entering the study, whereas 6 out of 21 children who were transplanted remained leukemia-free from 4.5–8 years after transplantation [29]. That study, however, was hampered by the fact that the median duration of initial remission was only 13 months for the chemotherapy group, as compared to 25 months for the transplant group. A report from the Hospital for Sick Children in London found no advantage for 15 children treated with allogeneic transplantation, compared to 40 children treated with chemotherapy only [30]. In both groups, there was a highly significant correlation between the lengths of initial remission and disease-free survival after transplantation.

The relative efficacy of autologous or allogeneic transplantation versus more intensive chemotherapy without transplantation remains unresolved at this time. Our current policy offers autologous or allogeneic bone marrow transplantation for all children with ALL who relapse at any site while receiving therapy or within 12 months after elective cessation of therapy. If an HLA-matched donor is available, an allogeneic transplant is recommended; if not, the child who is CALLA-positive is eligible for an autologous marrow transplant. Children who relapse more than 12 months after elective cessation of therapy are treated with only intensive chemotherapy.

Children with relapsed ALL have a dismal prognosis. Recent reports [31, 32] suggest that for a selected group of patients the outcome of intensive chemotherapy might be as good as that reported with bone marrow transplantation. For some time to come, we will continue to be confronted by the problem of optimal therapy for treatment of children with relapsed ALL.

References

1. Niemeyer CM, Hitchcock-Bryan S, Sallan SE (1985) Comparative analysis of treatment programs for childhood acute lymphoblastic leukemia. Semin Oncol 12:122–130
2. Sallan SE, Hitchcock-Bryan S (1981) Relapse in childhood acute lymphoblastic leukemia after elective cessation of initial treatment: Failure of subsequent treatment with cyclophosphamide, cytosine arabinoside, vincristine and prednisolone (COAP). Med Pediatr Oncol 9:455–462
3. Chessels J, Leiper A, Rogers D (1984) Outcome following late marrow relapse in childhood acute lymphoblastic leukemia. J Clin Oncol 10:1088–1091
4. Gorin NC, Douay L, Laporte JP, Lopez M, Mary JY, Najman A, Salmon C, Aegerter P, Stachowiak J, David R, Pene F, Kantor G, Deloux J, Duhamel E, van den Akker J, Gerota J, Parlier Y, Duhamel G (1986) Autologous bone marrow transplantation using marrow incubated with ASTA Z 7557 in adult acute leukemia. Blood 67:1367–1376

5. Kaizer H, Stuart RK, Brookmeyer R, Beschorner WE, Braine HG, Burns WH, Fuller DJ, Korbling M, Mangan KF, Saral R, Sensenbrenner L, Shadduck RK, Shende AG, Tutschka PJ, Yeager AM, Zinkham WH, Calvin OM, Santos GW (1985) Autologous bone marrow transplantation in acute leukemia: a phase I study of in vitro treatment of marrow with 4-hydroperoxycyclophosphamide to purge tumor cells. Blood 65:1504–1510

6. Thierfelder S, Netzel B, Hoffmann-Fezer G, Kranz B, Haas J (1984) Treatment of autologous bone marrow grafts with antibodies against ALL cells. In: Lowenberg B, Hagenbeek A (eds) Minimal residual disease in leukemia. Nijhoff, Amsterdam, pp 241–253

7. Ritz J, Sallan SE, Bast R, Lipton J, Clavell L, Feeney M, Hercend T, Nathan DG, Schlossman S (1982) Autologous bone marrow transplantation in CALLA-positive acute lymphoblastic leukemia after in vitro treatment with J5 monoclonal antibody and complement. Lancet 2:60–63

8. Ramsey N, LeBien T, Nesbit M, McGlave P, Weisdorf D, Kenyon P, Hurd D, Goldman A, Kim T, Kersey J (1985) Autologous bone marrow transplantation for patients with acute lymphoblastic leukemia in second or subsequent remission: results of bone marrow treated with monoclonal antibodies BA-1, BA-2, and BA-3 plus complement. Blood 66:508–513

9. Gorin NC, Donay L, Laporte JP, Lopez M, Zittoun R, Rio B, Stachowski J, Jansen J, Cazallas P, Poncelet P, Liance MC, Viosin GA, Salmon C, LeBlanc G, Deloux J, Najman A, Duhanell G (1985) Autologous bone marrow transplantation with marrow decontaminated by immunotoxin T101 in the treatment of leukemia and lymphoma: first clinical observations. Cancer Treat Rep 69:953–959

10. Kersey JH (1986) Autologous bone marrow transplantation in B and T cell lineage ALL: The Minnesota experience. (Abstract) J Cell Biochem 10D:91

11. Dicke KA, Poyntou CH, Reading CL (1984) Elimination of leukemic cells from remission marrow suspensions by an immunomagnetic procedure. In: Lowenberg B, Hagenbeek A (eds) Minimal residual disease in leukemia. Nijhoff, Amsterdam, pp 209–211

12. LeBien TW, Anderson JM, Vallera DA, Uckun FM (1986) Increased efficacy in selective elimination of leukemic cell line clonogenic cells by a combination of monoclonal antibodies BA-1, BA-2, BA-3 and complement and Mafosfamide (ASTA Z 7557). Leuk Res 10:139–143

13. DeFabritiis P, Bregni M, Lipton J, Greenberger J, Nadler L, Rothstein L, Korbling M, Ritz J, Bast RC (1985) Elimination of clonogenic Burkitt's lymphoma cells from human bone marrow using 4-hydroxycyclophosphamide in combination with monoclonal antibodies and complement. Blood 65:1064–1070

14. Griffin JD, Larcoin P, Schlossman SF (1983) Use of surface markers to identify subset of acute myelomonocyte leukemia cells with progenitor cell properties. Blood 62:1300–1303

15. Ritz J, Pesando JM, Notis-McContary J, Lazarus H, Schlossman SF (1980) A monoclonal antibody to human acute lymphoblastic leukemia antigen. Nature 283:583–585

16. Kersey JH, LeBien TW, Abramson CS (1981) A human hemopoietic progenitor and acute lymphoblastic leukemia-associated cell surface structure identified with a monoclonal antibody. J Exp Med 153:726

17. Hercend T, Nadler LM, Pesando JM (1981) Expression of a 26,000 dalton glycoprotein on activated human T-cells. Cell Immunol 64:192

18. Ritz J, Sallan SE, Bast R, Takvorian T, Schlossman S (1985) Serotherapy and bone marrow transplantation. In: Springer TA (ed) Hybridoma technology in the biosciences and medicine. Plenum, New York, pp 493–504

19. Ritz J, Bast RC, Takvorian T, Sallan SE (1985) Clinical application of monoclonal antibodies in acute leukemia. Technology Impact. Potential Directions for Laboratory Medicine. The New York Academy of Sciences. 428:308–317

20. Bast R, Ritz J, Lipton JM, Feeney M, Sallan SE, Nathan DG, Schlossman S (1983) Elimination of leukemic cells from human bone marrow using monoclonal antibody and complement. Cancer Res 43:1389–1394

21. Bast R, Defabritiis, Mayer C (1983) Elimination of malignant clonogenic cells from human bone marrow using multiple monoclonal antibodies and complement (C). Am Assoc Cancer Res 24:223

22. Ramsey NR, Nesbit M, McGlave P, Weisdorf D, Hurd D, Goldman A, Kim T, Kersey J, Woods W, LeBien T (1986) Autologous bone marrow transplantation (BMT) for patients with acute lymphoblastic leukemia (ALL) in second or subsequent remission: results of bone marrow treated with monoclonal antibodies BA-1, BA-2, BA-3 and complement using two sequential preparative regimens. In: Gale RP, Champlin R (eds) Recent advances in bone marrow transplantation. UCLA symposia on molecular and cellular biology, new series, vol 53. Liss, New York

23. Ramsey N (Personal communication)
24. Kersey J, Weisdorf D, Nesbit N, Woods W, LeBien T, McGlave P, Kim T, Tiliporid A, Vallera D, Haahe R, Bostrom B, Hurd D, Kvirit W, Goldmann A, Ramsey N (1986) Allogeneic and autologous bone marrow transplantation for acute lymphoblastic leukemia (ALL) (abstract). J Cell Biochem 10D:207
25. Niemeyer (Unpublished data)
26. Sanders JE, Flourney N, Thomas D, Buckner CD, Lum LG, et al. (1985) Marrow transplant experience in children with acute lymphoblastic leukemia. An analysis of factors associated with survival, relapse, and graft versus host disease. Med Pediatr Oncol 13:165–172
27. Dinsmore R, Kirkpatrick D, Flomenberg N, Gulati S, Kapoor N, Shank B, Reid A, Groshen S, O'Reilly RJ (1983) Allogeneic bone marrow transplantation for patients with acute lymphoblastic leukemia. Blood 62:381–388
28. Johnson FL, Thomas ED, Clark B, Chard R, Hartmann JR, Storb R (1981) A comparison of marrow transplantation with chemotherapy for children with acute lymphoblastic leukemia in second or subsequent remission. N Engl J Med 305:846–851
29. Storb R (1985) Marrow grafting for leukemia. Exp Hematol 13:6–8
30. Chessells JM, Rogers DW, Leiper AD, Blacklock H, Plowman PN, Richards S, Levinsky R, Festenstein H (1986) Bone marrow transplantation has a limited role in prolonging second marrow remission in childhood lymphoblastic leukemia. Lancet 1:1239–1241
31. Rivera GK, Buchanan G, Boyett JM, Camitta B, Ochs J, Kalwinsky D, Amylon M, Vietti TJ, Crist WM (1986) Intensive retreatment of childhood acute lymphoblastic leukemia in first bone marrow relapse. A Pediatric Oncology Group Study. N Engl J Med 315:273–278
32. Henze G, Buchanan S, Fengler R (1976) The BFM-relapse studies in childhood ALL: concepts of 2 multicentric trials and results after 2½ years. (Abstract) International symposium: acute leukemias, prognostic factors and treatment strategies. Münster, West Germany, March 1986
33. Kaplan EL, Meier P (1958) Non parametric estimation from incomplete observation. J Am Statist Assoc 53:457–481
34. Gelber RD, Zelen M (1985) Planning and reporting of clinical trials. In: Calabresi P, Schein PS, Rosenberg SA (eds) Medical oncology. Basic principles and clinical management of cancer. Macmillan, New York, pp 406–425

Haematology and Blood Transfusion   Vol. 31
Modern Trends in Human Leukemia VII
Edited by Neth, Gallo, Greaves, and Kabisch
© Springer-Verlag Berlin Heidelberg 1987

The Use of Cultured Bone Marrow Cells for Autologous Transplantation in Patients with Acute Myeloblastic Leukemia

N. G. Testa[1], L. Coutinho[1], J. Chang[2], G. Morgenstern[2], J. H. Scarffe[3], and T. M. Dexter[1]

A. Introduction

The permissive or inductive environment provided by bone marrow stromal cells in long-term cultures allows the persistent proliferation and differentiation of haemopoietic stem and progenitor cells [1]. Cells harvested from cultures of murine bone marrow can reconstitute the haemopoietic system when transplanted into lethally irradiated mice [2]. If bone marrow heavily infiltrated with leukaemic cells is cultured using similar conditions, the leukaemic blast cells become undetectable within 1 week, and the cultured marrow can then be used to rescue

[1] Department of Experimental Haematology, Paterson Laboratories
[2] Department of Haematology
[3] Department of Medical Oncology, Christie Hospital and Holt Radium Institute, Manchester M20 9BX, England

lethally irradiated mice [3]. In cultures of bone marrow cells from untreated patients with chronic granulocytic leukaemia (CML), the Philadelphia chromosome decreased, after being present in over 95% of mitoses, to almost undetectable levels. In the same cultures, Ph-negative cells became the predominant mitotic population [4]. Similarly, in some cultures established from bone marrow from patients with newly diagnosed acute myeloblastic leukaemia (AML), the size of the leukaemic clone (assessed either by chromosome markers or by a characteristic abnormal growth pattern in colony assays) diminished to undetectable levels, while normal haemopoiesis became dominant ([5, 6] and our unpublished results). A similar pattern may also be seen in cultures established from bone marrow in relapse.

From these experimental data, summarized in Table 1, it would appear that the conditions prevailing in vitro may both suppress the growth of leukaemic cells and fa-

Table 1. Emergence of normal cells in long-term cultures of leukaemic bone marrow

Bone marrow	Diagnosis	Parameters measured	Reference
Murine	Disseminated thymoma	Disappearance of blast cells Ability to reconstitute the haemopoietic system upon transplant	[3]
Human	CML	Disappearance of Ph chromosome Reappearance of Ph-negative (normal?) mitosis	[4]
	AML	Disappearance of chromosome markers Disappearance of leukaemic colony growth pattern Appearance of normal colony growth pattern Appearance of normal chromosome pattern	[5, 6]

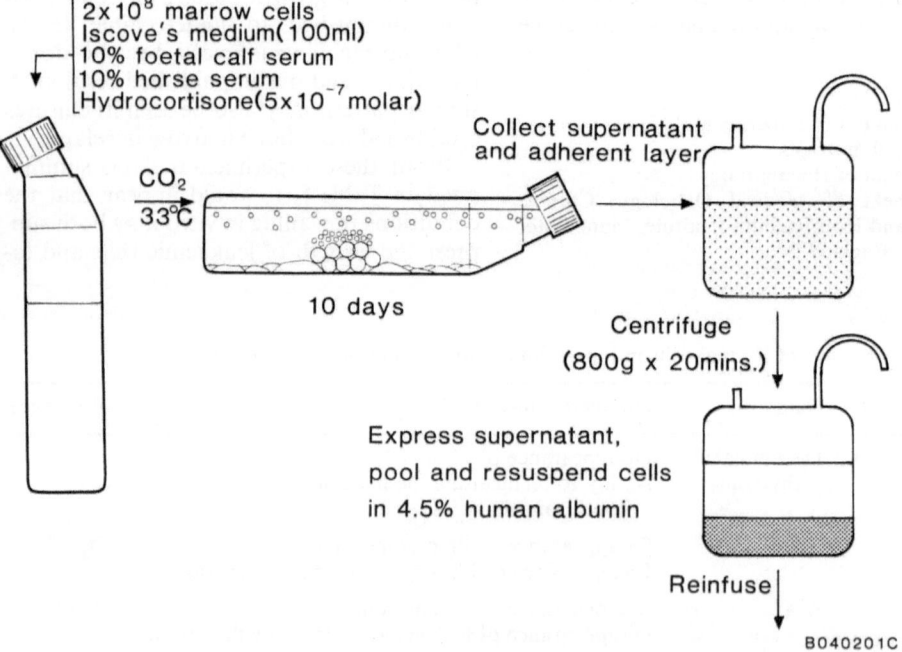

2×10^{8} marrow cells
Iscove's medium(100ml)
10% foetal calf serum
10% horse serum
Hydrocortisone(5×10^{-7}molar)

CO_2
$33^{\circ}C$

10 days

Collect supernatant
and adherent layer

Centrifuge
(800g x 20mins.)

Express supernatant,
pool and resuspend cells
in 4.5% human albumin

Reinfuse

B040201C

Table 3. Patients who received autologous transplant of cultured bone marrow cells

Patient (FAB)	Age	Status at marrow harvest	Interval – end of chemotherapy to BMT (weeks)	Total nucleated cells infused ($\times 10^8$/kg)	GM-CFC infused ($\times 10^3$/kg)	Survival from BMT (weeks)	Current status
MC (M4)	15	First relapse (40% blasts in bone marrow)	15	1.3	16.2	62+	Relapse (week 30); receiving chemotherapy
TC (M2)	39	First relapse (60% blasts in bone marrow)	13	1.2	10.7	16+	Relapse (week 12); receiving chemotherapy
FB (MDS)	35	First remission (but myelodysplastic bone marrow)	32	1.0	27.0	42	Died infection/myelodysplasia
TB (M4)	19	First remission	25	2.3	98.0	58+	Complete remission; well
JW (M1)	16	First remission	27	1.7	107.1	30+	Complete remission; well

diated red-cell transfusions and systemic antimicrobials, as indicated.

C. Results

Details of BMT, haematological recovery and outcome are shown in Tables 3 and 4. The first patient was in early relapse at the time of marrow harvest. Serial cytogenetic studies performed during the preceding clinical remission had shown that the 16q abnormality which characterised his leukaemic clone had persisted in about one-fifth of the mitoses from the bone marrow. However, only normal mitoses were detected after the bone marrow had been in culture for 7–14 days [6]. Following transplantation, full reconstitution was achieved, the 16q marker became undetectable (for the first time since diagnosis) and the patient entered a full remission. The second patient transplanted in relapse (without a chromosomal marker) regenerated leukaemia 12 weeks after BMT. He continue sin good clinical condition, leading an active life on haematological support.

One patient transplanted in remission following chemotherapy for transformation of a myelodysplastic syndrome reverted not to normal haemopoiesis, but to myelodysplasia after the transplant. She required support transfusions until she died. Two patients transplanted in first remission are in complete remission after 58 and 30 weeks, respectively.

Table 4. Haematological reconstitution

Parameter	
Engraftment	5/5
Discharge from hospital after BMT	4.5– 9 weeks
Time of last red-cell transfusion[a]	10 –13 weeks
Time of last platelet transfusion[a]	8 –12 weeks
Time to reach $> 0.5 \times 10^9$/1 neutrophils[a]	7 – 8 weeks

[a] Excluding relapse and patient FB; the latter reverted to myelodysplasia and had low platelet counts that required transfusions until her death.

D. Discussion

The haematological recovery and lack of procedural mortality in the five patients transplanted strongly suggest that the cultured cells engrafted and that this technique can be reliably used for autologous BMT. The recovery of peripheral blood cells, and especially of platelets, was slower than after allogeneic transplantation, but prolonged thrombocytopenia has been observed after conventional autologous transplantation [7]. In this context, as one of the patients in this series shows, a history of myelodysplasia may be a contraindication for autologous transplant.

The altered balance between the leukaemic and normal populations in culture is likely to be responsible for the remission achieved in the first patient. However, the high leukaemic load existing in the patient at the time of the ablative therapy, prior to transplantation, made the eventual relapse not unexpected. It is probable that relapses after autologous and allogeneic BMT are usually due to leukaemic cells which remain in the host after the conditioning treatment preceding the transplant. Because of this, relapses are to be expected with the present conditioning regimes in at least 25% of patients transplanted in first remission of AML.

The results, although preliminary, are encouraging and allow us to consider the possibility of manipulating the cultures by regulatory molecules (colony-stimulating factors, interferons and others) which may induce differentiation of leukaemic cells [8] and favour the growth of normal haemopoietic progenitors. Experiments along these lines are in progress. In addition, the use of cultured bone marrow for autologous transplants in CML, poor-prognosis acute lymphoblastic leukaemia or in some patients with solid tumors are possible developments for the future.

Acknowledgements. This work is supported by the Cancer Research Campaign (CRC) and the Leukaemia Research Fund. T. M. Dexter is a Fellow of the CRC.

References

1. Dexter TM, Spooncer E, Simmons P, Allen TD (1984) Long-term marrow cultures: an overview of techniques and experience. In: Wright DG, Greenberger JJ (eds) Long-term bone marrow culture. Liss, New York, p 57
2. Spooncer E, Dexter TM (1983) Transplantation of long-term cultured bone marrow cells. Transplantation 35:624
3. Hays EF, Hale L (1982) Growth of normal hemopoietic cells in cultures of bone marrow from leukaemic mice. Eur J Cancer Clin Oncol 18:413
4. Coulumbel L, Kalousek DK, Eaves CS, Gupta CM, Eaves AC (1983) Long-term marrow culture reveals chromosomally normal hemopoietic progenitor cells in patients with Ph-positive chronic myelogenous leukemia. N Engl J Med 306:1493
5. Eaves C, Coulumbel L, Duke I, Kalousek J, Cashman J, Eaves AC (1985) Maintenance of normal and abnormal hemopoietic cell populations in long-term cultures of CML and AML marrow cells. In: Cronkite EP, Dainiak N, McCaffrey RP, Palek J, Quesenberry PJ (eds) Hematopoietic stem cell physiology. Liss, New York, p 403
6. Chang J, Coutinho L, Morgenstern G, Scarffe JH, Deakin D, Harrison C, Testa NG, Dexter TM (1986) Reconstitution of haemopoietic system with autologous marrow taken during relapse of acute myeloblastic leukaemia and grown in long-term culture. Lancet I:294
7. Burnett AK, Tansey I, Watkins R, Alcorn M, Maharaj D, Singer CRJ, McKinnon S, McDonald GA (1984) Transplantation of unpurged autologous bone marrow in acute myeloid leukaemia in first remission. Lancet II:1068
8. Nicola NA, Metcalf D (1985) Binding of the differentiation – inducer GM-CSF to responsive, but not unresponsive leukaemia cell lines. Proc Natl Acad Sci USA 81:3765

Haematology and Blood Transfusion Vol. 31
Modern Trends in Human Leukemia VII
Edited by Neth, Gallo, Greaves, and Kabisch
© Springer-Verlag Berlin Heidelberg 1987

Bone Marrow Transplantation in Leukemia in the Absence of an HLA-Identical Sibling Donor

R. Dopfer[1], G. Ehninger[2], and D. Niethammer[1]

A. Introduction

Bone marrow transplantation is a potentially curative treatment for patients with leukemia, aplastic anemia, metabolic disorders, and immunodeficiency. One of the main problems of this procedure is the graft-versus-host reaction induced in the recipient by the immune function of the transplanted marrow. In order to minimize the risks of graft rejection and graft-versus-host disease (GVHD), marrow transplantation has in general been limited to patients with HLA-identical sibling donors. The majority of patients, however, will not have such a family member available. To cope with such patients, several alternative approaches have been investigated. One of them is autologous bone marrow transplantation (with or without antileukemic treatment of the marrow); another is transplantation of haploidentical marrow after T-cell depletion by separation with lectins, E rosetting, or monoclonal antibodies. Most experience in this field has been gained in patients with severe combined immunodeficiency. Another alternative for these patients is bone marrow transplantation with the marrow of an unrelated but matched or partially matched donor, or even a mismatched family donor. Only few clinical data are available to assess the latest acceptable limits for HLA incompatibility in human bone marrow transplantations with

a mismatched related or unrelated donor. Such transplantations have been performed to explore the limitations of this procedure, mainly in the United Kingdom and the United States. The results of these transplantations are described in this short overview.

B. Mismatched Unrelated Donors

It is evident that there are major logistic problems in identifying suitable unrelated donors quickly enough and in sufficient numbers to make an impact on the management of leukemia or aplastic anemia. Table 1 describes the probability for a given antigen system that the donor pool will include at least one person phenotypically identical to a random recipient [1]. Values are applied to Caucasian donors and recipients, and are based on haplotype frequency estimates published in *Histocompatibility Testing 1980*, with the exception of HLA-A,B, for which haplotype frequencies from the Terasaki laboratory were used. As one can imagine, the donor pool has to be very large (for some rare haplotypes, over 1 million) to find a suitable donor. However, for selecting donors who are only partially identical, the pool needed is significantly smaller. Experience with matched and mismatched bone marrow transplantations has been gained in several centers. In Tables 2–5, the results from the United Kingdom (Hammersmith and Westminster Hospitals) and the United States (Seattle and Iowa City) are summarized [2–5].

[1] Department of Pediatric Hematology and Oncology, University Children's Hospital, Ruemelinstrasse 21–26, Tuebingen, FRG
[2] Department of Internal Medicine, University of Tuebingen, Otfried-Müller-Strasse 23

Table 1. Pool size calculations for the search for HLA-identical bone marrow donors. (After [1])

Pool Size	A	B	DR	A, B	A, DR	B, DR	A, B, DR
1	3.08	0.807	3.29	0.097	0.166	0.085	0.013
5	13.4	3.9	14.9				
10	23.7	7.5	27.1				
20	38.1	14.1	45.6	1.86	4.0	3.6	
40	54.5	29.9	73.4	3.6	6.9	5.2	
80	70.0	40.1	86.3	6.7	11.9	8.0	
500	94.8	81.9	99.3	25.9	39.3	26.3	
1 000	97.9	90.7	99.8	37.2	53.3	37.6	
5 000	99.7	98.8	100.0	65.3	81.4	66.5	
10 000				75.5	89.2	77.3	29.1
50 000				91.1	97.9	93.3	55.5
100 000							66.6
500 000							86.4

Table 2. Seattle experience with BMT from phenotypically identical unrelated donors (After [2])

BMT with phenotypically
identical donors

	n	Survival	GVHD, acute	Causes of death
ALL II. rem.	1	711	0	relapse
AML I. rem.	1	288 +	II	
AA	3	224, 161, 29	II, II, I	Asp., no graft, bleeding
CML-CP	6	61, 101, 47, 31, 56, 40 +	III, IV, III, II, IV, I	CMV, GVHD, VOD, I.P.
CML-AP	1	139	IV	GVHD
CML-BC-CP	1	349 +	I	

Table 3. Westminster experience with BMT from unrelated donors. (After [3])

Age	Disease	HLA				GVHD prophylaxis	Take	GVHD	Outcome
		A	B	DR	MLC				
19	ALL 2. CR	=	=	ND	=	CyA	Early	No	Hemorrhage + 15
18	ALL 3. CR	=	=	ND	=	CyA	Full	III	+ 45
39	AML 1. CR	=	=	=	=	CyA	Full	Chronic	Well > 1 500 days
9	ALL 3. CR	=	=	ND	=	T-Dep CyA	Full	II	Aspergillus + 55
4	ALL 1. CR	=	=	=	=	T-Dep CyA	Full	No	Metabolic + 27
9	ALL 1. CR	=	=	=	=	T-Dep CyA	Full	No	Aspergillus + 27
22	PreAML	=	=	=	=	T-Dep CyA	Full, Rej	No	Aspergillus + 66

Table 4. Hammersmith experience with BMT of unrelated donors. (After [4])

Disease	Engraftment	GVHD	Survival
SAA 8			
CGL – CP 2			4/14 (120–1 599 days)
CGL – AP 1	8/14	6/9	
		Grade 3–4	
Fanconi 3			

SAA, severe aplastic anemia.

Table 5. Outcome of BMT with unrelated DR,D-matched donors in Iowa City (After [5])

Disease		n	Survival: Continuous and/or > 1 yr.	Causes of Death
ANLL	2nd CR	3	3	
	3rd CR	0		
	4th CR	1	0	HSV/CMV
	Relap	7	0	ARDS, Asp., Leg, GVHD/HSV, Mucor, Gm-, Gm-,
ALL	2nd CR	2	0	Gm-/CDS, GVHD
	3rd CR	4	1	CMV, Crypto, P. carinii*
	Relap	2	0	Asp., HSV
AUL	2nd CR	1	0	GVHD/Asp
CML	SP	4	1	GHVD/Gm-, P. carinii*
	AP	9	4	GVHD/HSV, GVHD, Asp., Can., Gm-
	BC SP	2	0	GVHD, Gm-
RAEB			1	
SAA		4	1	NE/Asp, Asp, NE/VOD
Total		39	11	

* TMP-SM allergy
HSV, herpes simplex virus infection; CMV, cytomegalovirus infection; GVHD, graft-versus-host disease; ASP, aspergillus infection; ARDS, acute respiratory distress syndrome; LEG, legionella infection; Gm-, gram-negative sepsis; VOD, veno-occlusive disease; Crypto, cryptococcus infection; Can, candida infection; Ne, engraftment failure.

Table 6. Correlation of GVHD with HLA class I match[a]. (From [5])

		Grade aGVHD[b]				
		0	I	II	III	IV
Number of	0	–	–	–	1	1
HLA A & B	1	–	3	1	1	–
Matches	2	–	3	2	1	–
	3	2	3	–	1	2
	4	2	2	–	1	1
Totals:		4	+11	+3	+5	+4=27

[a] All patients matched at HLA class II antigens.　　[b] Median time of onset GVHD, day 22 (12–40)

Table 7. Clinical status of survivors. (From [5])

UPN	Age	Disease	Match, HLA A,B[a]	(mos.)	Status	cGVHD[b]	Karnofsky
94	18	CML-AP	1A, 1B	28+	Bronchitis	L	90
101	39	CML-AP	1A	24+	Sinusitis, bronchitis	S, L	90
108	32	ANLL 2nd CR	2A	25+	Well	–	100
127	12	SAA	1A, 1B	18+		S	100
131	5	CML	1B	15+	Bronchitis	S	80
150	32	ANLL 1st CR	1A, 2B	9+		G	80
151	38	CML-AP	1A, 2B	8.8+	Bronchitis	S	90
159	28	RAEB	2A, 2B	6+	CMV enteritis	–	90

[a] all patients HLA D/DR matched
[b] S = skin, L = Liver, G = gut
RAEB, refractory anemia with excess of blasts.

Because the GVHD prophylaxis, state of disease, and degree of HLA identity vary, comparison of the results is difficult. However, it is possible to draw the conclusion that bone marrow transplantation with phenotypically identical or partially matched marrow from unrelated donors is a feasible method for patients lacking an HLA-identical sibling donor. Fatal septic complications would seem to be a major problem. GVHD occurs more frequently than with identical sibling donor transplants and contributes to the cause of death in some patients. But the frequency of severe GVHD is not correlated with the degree of mismatch in DR-matched patients (Table 6). The infections which occur are probably due to the higher incidence of GVHD. The long-term outcome is doubtful, however, with regard to the clinical status of the patients in Iowa City (Table 7). More than half of the survivors suffer from chronic bronchitis, which is well known as a GVHD equivalent. These patients with GVHD of the lung have clinical problems with the trapped-air phenomenon and restrictive bronchitis.

It is not known whether in transplants from fully HLA-matched (A, B, D, DR) unrelated donors the possibility of graft failure or GVHD is due to undetermined histocompatibility antigens outside the major locus, or whether different DP and DQ antigens are responsible for these reactions. Basic research in HLA typing requires intensification to illuminate the correlations between different HLA antigens or minor antigens and graft failure or GVHD.

C. Mismatched Family Donors

Bone marrow transplantation from related phenotypically identical or related mismatched donors has been performed in greater number in Seattle than elsewhere [6]. A total of 105 patients have been grafted: 41 with acute leukemia in remission, 51 with acute leukemia in relapse, 5 with chronic granulocytic leukemia (CGL) in chronic phase, and 8 with CGL in blast crisis. Engraftment was delayed in a significant number of patients, thus resulting in persistent granulocytopenia. The risk of GVHD was higher in mismatched transplantation than in the control group, and this risk increased with the degree of HLA disparity (Fig. 1). The survival of patients with one unshared antigen was the same as in the control group (Fig. 2). These data clearly demonstrate that bone marrow transplantation with mismatched family donors is feasible, that results with one antigen mismatch are good, but that engraftment and GVHD problems have to be considered.

D. Strategies of Bone Marrow Transplantation in Childhood

Data concerning bone marrow transplantation with unrelated donors and partially

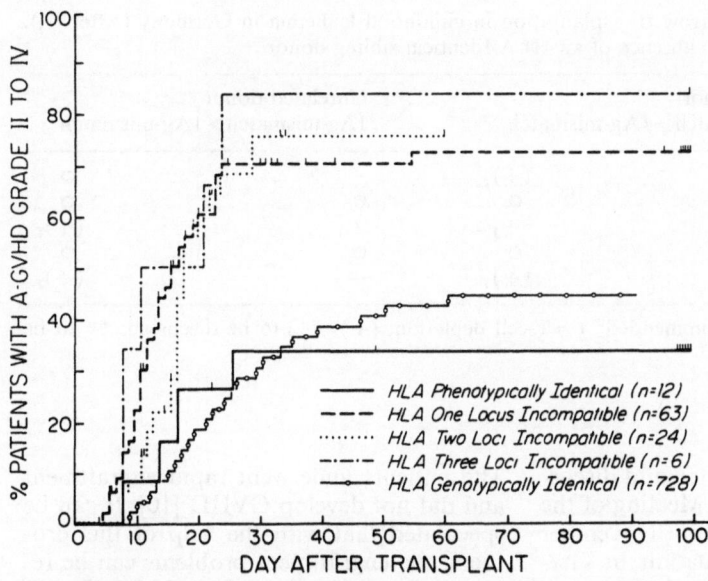

Fig. 1. GVHD incidence in 105 patients after BMT with phenotypically identical or mismatched family donors. (After [6])

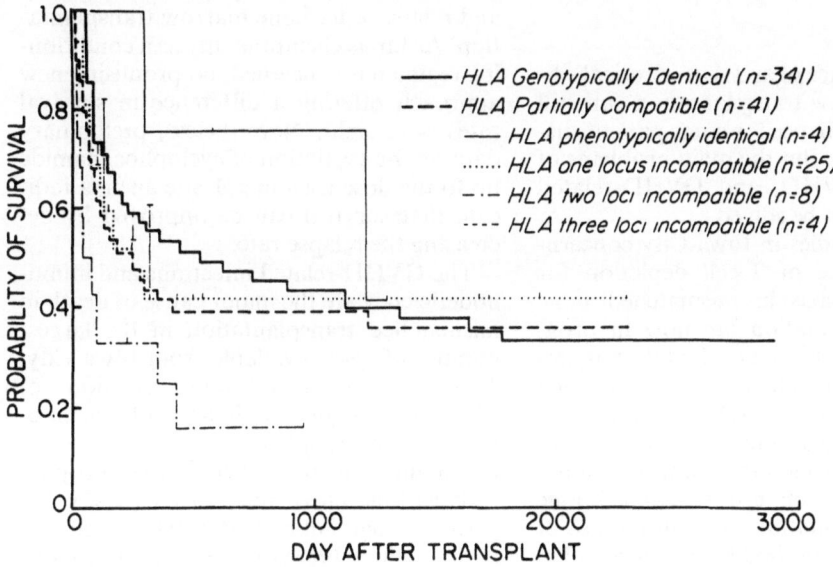

Fig. 2. Survival of 105 patients grafted from phenotypically matched or mismatched family donors. (After [6])

Table 8. Strategies for bone marrow transplantation in childhood leukemia in Germany (After [7]). Mismatch transplantation in the absence of an HLA-Identical sibling donor

	Sibling donor 1Ag-mismatch > 1Ag-mismatch		Unrelated donor 1Ag-mismatch > 1Ag-mismatch	
CML	+	$(+)_T$	+	o
ALL 1.CR	o*	o	o	o
ALL 2.CR	+	$+_T$	$+_T$	$(+)_T$
AML 1.CR	$(+)_{(T)}$	o	o	o
AML 2.CR	$+_{(T)}$	$(+)_T$	$+_T$	$(+)_T$

o = not recommended; + = recommended; T = T-cell depletion; (+) = (T) to be discussed; * = to be discussed for high-risk patients

matched donors were presented and discussed in part at the 4th Expert Meeting of the Kind-Philipp Foundation in November 1985. For the pediatric situation in Germany, we have drawn the conclusions presented in Table 8 [7].

E. New Developments to Prevent GVHD, Engraftment Failure, and Relapse of Leukemia

Even in the absence of an HLA-identical sibling, bone marrow transplantation can still offer a curative chance for some patients using other donors. But the main problems of engraftment, GVHD, and GVHD-related infections have to be solved.

Controlled studies in Iowa City concerning the relevance of T-cell depletion for GVHD prophylaxis in mismatched bone marrow transplantation are now in progress. For mismatched transplantation in immunodeficient patients, it can be concluded [8] that significant GVHD does not occur but that engraftment failure can be a problem with T-cell depletion. Promising initial results have been obtained in matched bone marrow transplantation through the use of such monoclonal antibodies as Campath I in vitro for T-cell depletion and in vivo, after bone marrow transplantation, for GVHD prophylaxis [9]. The combination of T-cell depletion in vitro and use of LFA1 monoclonal antibody in vivo after bone marrow transplantation has been successfully employed in Paris in two patients with osteopetrosis and the Wiskott-Aldrich syndrome.

The patients underwent rapid engraftment and did not develop GVHD [10]. It can be speculated that with the help of this protocol, the engraftment problems can be resolved. Intensification of total body irradiation (TBI) and chemoconditioning have been associated with a significant increase in toxicity, but there are some interesting data on the combination of TBI and total nodal irradiation to prevent engraftment failure and relapse after bone marrow transplantation. As far as chemotherapy as a conditioning regimen is concerned, no promising new approach offering a difference in survival rates is in sight. Nevertheless, preliminary data on the escalation of cyclophosphamide up to the dose used in aplastic anemia indicate that survival can be improved by decreasing the relapse rate.

The GVHD-related infections and immunodeficiency are the major cause of death in mismatched transplantation in the largest number of cases available from Iowa City. Through consequent administration of trimethoprim for prophylaxis of pneumocystis carinii, prophylactic use of 7S immunoglobulins, adequate herpes virus prophylaxis with acyclovir and perhaps CMV hyperimmunoglobulin, and total decontamination with elimination of gram-negative bacteria, the problems with infections may prove to be of minor importance.

Both improvement in the prophylactic treatment of graft failure and GVHD and improvement in the prophylaxis of GVHD-related infections may lead to increased survival rates in mismatched bone marrow transplantation.

84

References

1. Mickey MR (1985) Donor pools size for bone marrow transplantation. NIH technology assessment meetings, May 13–15, 1985
2. Personal communication: Deeg, Seattle
3. Hows JM, Yin J, Jones L, Apperley J, Econimou K, James DCO, Batchelor J, Goldman JM, Gordon-Smith EC (1986) Allogeneic bone marrow transplantation with volunteer unrelated donors. Bone Marrow Transpl 1, suppl 1:125 (Abstract)
4. Barrett AJ, Beard J, McCarthy D, Shaw PJ, Hugh-Jones K, Hobbs JR, James DOC (1986) Bone marrow transplant for leukemia with matched unrelated donors. Bone Marrow Transpl 1, suppl 1:127 (Abstract)
5. Personal communication: Gingrich, Iowa City
6. Beatty PG, Clift PhD, Mickelson EM, Nisperos BB, Flournoy A, Martin PJ, Sanders JE, Stewart P, Buckner CD, Storb R, Thomas ED, Hansen JA (1985) Marrow transplantation from related donors other than HLA-identical siblings. N Engl J Med 313, 13:765–771
7. Niethammer D, Ostendorf P, Dopfer R, Klingebiel Th (1986) Knochenmarktransplantation bei Leukämien in Abwesenheit von HLA-identischen Geschwistern. Ergeb Pädiatr Onkol 10:155–170
8. O'Reilly R, Brochstein J, Dinsmore R, Kirkpatrick D (1984) Marrow transplantation for congenital disorders. Semin Hematol 21, 3:188–220
9. Hale G, Waldmann H (1986) Depletion of T-cells with Campath 1 and human complement. Analysis of GVHD and graft failure in a multi-centre study. Bone Marrow Transpl 1, suppl 1, 93:(Abstract)
10. Personal communication, Griscelli, Paris

Haematology and Blood Transfusion   Vol. 31
Modern Trends in Human Leukemia VII
Edited by Neth, Gallo, Greaves, and Kabisch
© Springer-Verlag Berlin Heidelberg 1987

Bone-Marrow Purging with Monoclonal Antibodies and Human Complement in ALL and AML

O. Majdic [1], K. Sugita [1], I. Touw [2], U. Köller [1], H. Stockinger [1], R. Delwel [2], B. Löwenberg [2], and W. Knapp [1]

High-dose treatment followed by infusion of histocompatible allogeneic bone marrow has been shown to be curative in many patients with acute leukemia. Inherent in this treatment modality are a number of problems, however. Most prominent among them: graft versus host disease or, when using T cell-depleted marrow, graft failure. In addition, age restriction, conventionally applied to minimize morbidity and mortality, reduces the application of allogeneic bone marrowtransplantation to, on the average, about one third of those with the disease, and of these only about one in three will have a suitable donor.

Autologous bone marrow support may circumvent some of these problems and restrictions and, under certain conditions, be more effective than currently available conventional treatment protocols. In autologous bone marrow transplantation one of the major problems is the danger of reinfusing residual clonogenic leukemia cells. Remission is usually conceived to be a situation where bone marrow function is apparently normal but there is residual disease undetectable by conventional techniques. It is therefore probable that at least a few leukemic cells will be included in the bone marrow autograft from the remission patient. The numbers reinfused will nevertheless be relatively low, and with the currently used therapeutic modalities it would seem that the observed relapses after ABMT are not infrequently due to endogenous recurrence rather than to proliferation of reinfused tumor cells. It is therefore difficult to clearly prove the additional beneficial effect of bone marrow purging in autologous transplantation.

For this reason the safety requirements for any purging protocol must be particularly stringent. The cytotoxic effects have to be reproducibly selective and the procedural handling as simple as possible. The easiest way to achieve this is incubation with specific monoclonal antibodies which have the capacity to lyse their respective target cells, together with autologous serum as a complement source.

Lysis with MoAbs and human serum makes the purging extremely easy and reproducible and eliminates any foreseeable risks otherwise potentially introduced by the use of heterologous sera as a complement source. It can also be better controlled than more drastic and less specific procedures such as purging with pharmacologic agents. We therefore have concentrated our efforts on finding monoclonal antibodies or mixtures thereof which have that capacity.

Among acute leukemias, purging with monoclonal antibodies has so far been restricted to ALL. For AML no immunology-based techniques were available because of the lack of a suitable specific monoclonal antibody.

In our laboratory as well, the first protocol developed for the elimination of leukemic cells with monoclonal antibodies and human complement was a purging protocol for ALL cells [1]. In this protocol lysis of ALL blasts is induced with a cocktail of

[1] Institute of Immunology, University of Vienna, A-1090 Vienna, Austria
[2] Dr. Daniel Den Hoed Cancer Center, Rotterdam, Netherlands

Table 1. VIM2-reactivity of AML-CFU in AML patients

Patient no.	FAB classification	VIM2 reactivity[a]
1	M2	−
2	M4	+
3	M4	+
4	M4	+
5	M4	+ +
6	M1	+ +
7	M1	+ +
8	M1	+ +
9	M1	+ +
10	M2	+ +
11	M5	+ +
12	M2	+ +
13	M1	+
14	M4	+
15	M1	−
16	M2	−
17	M2	−
Normal CFU-GM		−

[a] Bone marrow cells from AML patients and healthy controls were stained with VIM2 antibody in indirect immunofluorescence and then sorted with a fluorescence-activated cell sorter into three fractions of relative fluorescence intensity, i. e., negative (−) weakly positive (+), and intensely positive (+ +) cells. These separated fractions were inoculated in colony culture to determine the distribution of AML-CFU as a function of antigen density expression in each of the cases.

three IgM-type monoclonal antibodies (termed VIB-pool). These are directed against the CALLA (CD10) antigen (VILA1 antibody) and against two different epitopes of the CD24 surface structure (VIBC5 and VIBE3 antibodies). The purging efficiency was evaluated with leukemic cell lines of the common ALL types (Reh6 and Nalm6) and with blast cells from common ALL patients. Optimal lysis was obtained with antibody and human serum concentrations as low as 1 µg/ml and 7% respectively. As a standard purging protocol we proposed one 20-min incubation at room temperature with antibody, followed by two 30-min incubations at 37 °C with 25% human complement. In dye-exclusion tests 99% purging efficiency and in clonogenic assays detecting elimination of up to 5 logs of clonogenic tumor cells 99.99% (= 4 logs) purging efficiency was achieved. Treatment with VIB-pool and human complement had no negative effect on the growth of normal hemopoietic progenitor cells CFU-GM, CFU-E, and BFU-E.

Based on these encouraging results we next screened all our monoclonal anti-leukocyte antibodies for lytic efficiency with human complement [2]. It turned out that some anti-myeloid antibodies also had the capacity to lyse their respective target cells in the presence of human complement.

The most interesting of these antibodies is certainly the broadly reactive anti-myeloid antibody VIM2 [3]. This antibody reacts in >90% of acute myeloid leukemias with a considerable proportion of blast cells. It is not expressed on day-14 CFU-GM cells [4], but the clonogenic leukemia cells (AML-CFU) seem to be VIM2 positive in a considerable proportion of AML patients [5] (Table 1).

Also cytolytic with human complement are the anti-myeloid antibodies VIMD5 [6] and VIM8 [7]. Like VIM2, they are not reactive with day-14 CFU-GM or with CFU-E or BFU-E cells [4] and can, although not as frequently, be found on AML blast cells [6, 7]. We therefore prepared a cocktail of these

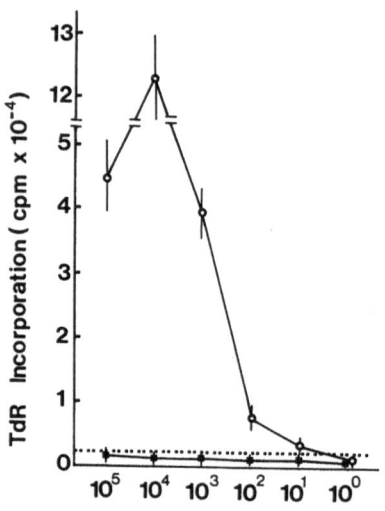

Number of HL 60 cells

Fig. 1. Proliferation of malignant myeloid cells (HL-60 cells) after treatment with a cocktail of three anti-myeloid monoclonal antibodies (VIM2, VIMD5, VIM8 ■——■) and control antibody (VILA1 o——o) respectively, in the presence of human complement. Cell suspensions were first incubated for 20 min at room temperature with monoclonal antibody. After that, two rounds of complement treatment for 30 min each were performed. The cells were then washed, resuspended in the original volume, and seeded in 96 well microplates at different cell concentrations ($1-10^5$ leukemic cells/well). Plates were cultured for 4 days and proliferation was measured by ^{3}H-thymidine uptake

three antibodies (VIM2, VIMD5, and VIM8) and tested the lytic efficiency of this cocktail in a model system using HL-60 cells as target cells (Fig. 1). As can be seen, the purging efficiency in the model system is quite impressive. More relevant experiments to evaluate the effect of this treatment on clonogenic tumor cells (AML-CFU) in individual AML patients must still be done, however.

Acknowledgement. This study was supported by the *Mediz. wissensch. Fonds des Bürgermeisters der Bundeshauptstadt Wien.*

References

1. Sugita K, Majdic O, Stockinger H, Holter W, Köller U, Peschel C, Knapp W (1986) Int J Cancer 37:351–357
2. Sugita K, Majdic O, Stockinger H, Holter W, Burger R, Knapp W (1987) Transplantation 43:570–574
3. Majdic O, Bettelheim P, Stockinger H, Aberer W, Liszka K, Lutz D, Knapp W (1984) Int J Cancer 33:617–623
4. Peschel C, Konwalinka G, Geissler D, Majdic O, Stockinger H, Braunsteiner H, Knapp W (1985) Exp Hematol 13/11:1211–1216
5. Delwel R, Touw I, Löwenberg B (1986) In: Hagenbeek A, Löwenberg B (eds) Minimal residual disease in acute leukemia. Nijhoff, Dordrecht, pp 68–75
6. Majdic O, Liszka K, Lutz D, Knapp W (1981) Blood 58:1127–1133
7. Knapp W, Majdic O, Stockinger H, Bettelheim P, Liszka K, Köller U, Peschel C (1984) Med Oncol Tumor Pharmacother 4:257–262

Haematology and Blood Transfusion   Vol. 31
Modern Trends in Human Leukemia VII
Edited by Neth, Gallo, Greaves, and Kabisch
© Springer-Verlag Berlin Heidelberg 1987

Purging of Bone Marrow with a Cocktail of Monoclonal Antibodies (VIB-pool) for Autologous Transplantation *

F. Zintl, B. Reiners, H. Thränhardt, J. Hermann, D. Fuchs, and J. Prager

A. Introduction

Children with relapsed common acute lymphoblastic leukemia (ALL), B-non-Hodgkin lymphoma (B-NHL), and B-acute lymphocytic leukemia (B-ALL) have a very poor prognosis. If there is no HLA-identical donor, the patient should be considered for autologous bone marrow transplantation. Collected autologous marrow should be cleansed of contaminating tumor cells without destroying hemopoietic stem cells. We report here the results of our investigations with a cocktail of three monoclonal antibodies (VIL-A 1, VIB-C 5, and VIB-E 3 – the VIB pool – kindly given to us by Dr. Knapp of Vienna) concerning in vitro cytotoxicity against ALL blast cells and leukemic cells lines, lytic capacity with rabbit and human complement, and stem cell toxicity, together with our findings concerning the ex vivo purging of the marrow of four children. The antibodies have the particular advantage of being able to lyse blast cells of common ALL-type and B cells very effectively with human complement [5].

B. Material and Methods

I. Antibodies

The VIB pool used is a cocktail consisting of three monoclonal antibodies of the IgM type

* This investigation was supported by the Internationale Gesellschaft für Chemo- und Immunotherapie, Vienna
Department of Pediatrics, University Hospital of Jena, GDR

(VIL-A 1, VIB-C 5, and VIB-E 3) and reacts with the common ALL antigen (CALLA) – VIL-A 1 – and with two different epitopes of the CD 24 surface structure – VIB-C 5 and VIB-E 3.

II. Complement

We used as complement human AB serum and selected rabbit serum batches not toxic against human hemopoietic stem cells, and autologous serum for the ex vivo purging.

III. Cells

Target cells were fresh or cryopreserved leukemic cells from children with ALL, hemopoietic cell lines Reh and Nalm, and mononucleated bone marrow cells from healthy adult volunteers.

IV. Treatment of Cell Mixtures

The cotoxicity of the antibodies for the target cells was tested by using the trypan blue exclusion test and the specific ^{51}Cr-release.

V. Purging Protocol

Bone marrow cells from four children (three Burkitt-type NHL, stage III, and one common ALL) were harvested from the anterior and posterior iliac crest, and anticoagulated with preservative-free heparin. Mononuclear cells were isolated on Ficoll-Amidotrizoate gradients and resuspended at a concentration of $1-2 \times 10^7$ cells/ml. They were incubated with the antibody cocktail (30 μg/ml) at room temperature for 20 min. This procedure was followed by a twice-repeated 30-min treatment with autologous serum (final concentration 50%). The cells were cryopreserved in RPMI medium containing 5% dimethyl sulfoxide, 20% human albumin, and 20% autologous serum.

VI. Colony-Forming Assay

The enumeration of CFU-GM by a modified technique of Irvine et al. (1984) [2] was done in all patients at each stage of the investigation: (a) on the fresh marrow; (b) after incubation before freezing; and (c) after thawing.

C. Results and Discussion

1. It was possible to demonstrate a high lytic capacity of the antibody cocktail (VIB pool) with complement against CALLA-positive leukemic cells, blast cells of a child with B-ALL, and Nalm and Reh cells. There was no difference in the lytic capacity, whether rabbit serum or human AB serum was used as complement source (Fig. 1).
2. Lysis of CALLA-positive leukemic cells was detectable at antibody concentrations of as low as 0.08 μg/ml. The per-

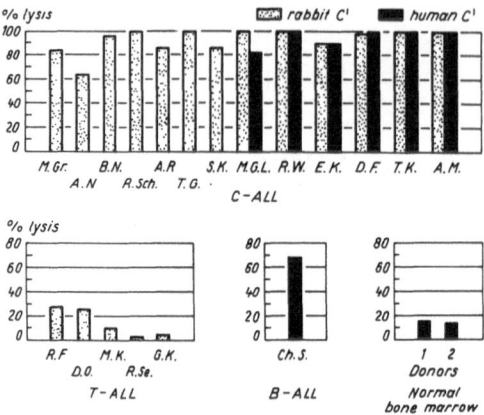

Fig. 2. Reactivity of the VIB antibody cocktail with CALLA $^+$ ALL cells

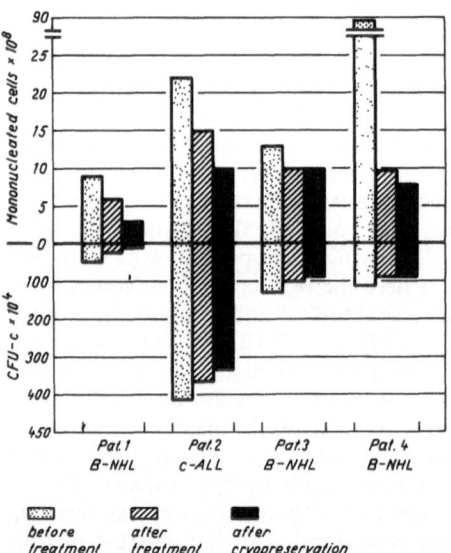

Fig. 3. Mononucleated cells and CFU-GM in bone marrow of four patients after in vitro purging with VIB pool and human complement

centage of lysed cells ranged from 82% to 100% with leukemic cells and amounted to 100% with Reh cells (Fig. 2).
3. Treatment with the VIB pool and rabbit or human complement did not cause a significant loss of CFU-GM. The loss of CFU-GM due to cryopreservation amounted to $15 \pm 9\%$ (Fig. 3).
4. After the ex vivo purging of remission marrow of four children (3 B-NHL, 1 common ALL) with the VIB pool and human complement for autologous

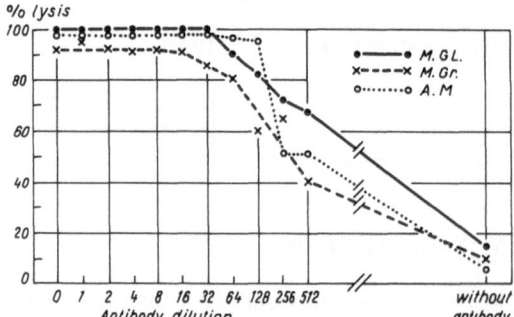

The single samples contained 20 μl of cell suspension (5 × 10⁶ c/ml), 20 μl antibody dilution (6-0,005 μg), and 40 μl human complement

Fig. 1. Reactivity of the VIB pool against different target cells

90

transplantation, there was a sufficient recovery of CFU-GM for cryopreservation ($2.2–10 \times 10^4$ CFU-GM/kg).

According to different investigations, an in vitro purging procedure with a combination of several monoclonal antibodies is more effective than with only one antibody [1]. All three components of the VIB pool are able to lyse leukemic cells of the common ALL type. The VIB-C 5 and VIB-E 3 components react with leukemic cells of the B-ALL type [3]. All three components are able to lyse CALLA ALL cells with human complement, as was shown by Sugita et al. (1986) [5] and ourselves. Compared to other monoclonal antibodies used for purging bone marrow [4, 1], which, as a rule, react with heterologous complement only, the VIB pool has the advantage of binding the rabbit and human complement. This results in a number of advantages for clinical application.

References

1. Bast RC Jr, Fabritiis P De, Lipton J et al. (1985) Elimination of malignant clonogenic cells from human bone marrow using multiple monoclonal antibodies and complement. Cancer Res 45:499–503
2. Irvine AE, Morris TCM, Kennedy H et al. (1984) Human umbical cord contitioned medium: stimulation for human CFU-G. Exp Hematol 12:19–24
3. Knapp W, Majdic O, Bettelheim P et al. (1983) Typing of leukemic cells with monoclonal antibodies. Ann NY Acad Sci 420:250–260
4. Ritz J, Bast RC Jr, Clavell L et al. (1982) Autologous bone marrow transplantation in CALLA positive acute lymphoblastic leukemia after in vitro treatment with J 5 monoclonal antibody and complement. Lancet 2:60–63
5. Sugita K, Majdic O, Stockinger H et al. (1986) Use of a cocktail of monoclonal antibodies and human complement in selective killing of acute lymphocytic leukemia. Int J Cancer 37:351–357

Haematology and Blood Transfusion   Vol. 31
Modern Trends in Human Leukemia VII
Edited by Neth, Gallo, Greaves, and Kabisch
© Springer-Verlag Berlin Heidelberg 1987

Autologous Bone Marrow Transplantation in Paediatric Solid Tumours

R. Pinkerton, T. Philip

A. Introduction

In leukaemia allogeneic bone marrow transplantation is a method by which high-dose, often curative therapy can be given without regard to marrow toxicity. Applying the same principle to paediatric solid tumours should allow selection of the most active agents for use in combinations, at doses limited only by extramedullary toxicity. The availability of HLA- and DR-matched allografts is very limited, however, restricting this type of marrow transplant to less than one in five children with malignancy. Other options are to use either autologous grafts or mismatched allografts, and at present, autologous bone marrow transplantation (ABMT) is the alternative of choice. ABMT is used either to shorten the period of aplasia after non-ablative high-dose chemotherapy such as melphalan [8] or as a rescue after massive myeloablative chemotherapy, often with total-body irradiation (TBI).

The use of high-dose melphalan in childhood solid tumours was pioneered by the Royal Marsden Group [9], and subsequently a wide variety of multiagent "massive therapy" regimens have been developed. High-dose TBI was introduced by a number of American groups [4, 11] and is now also widely used in European centres. In this review, we consider the application of massive therapy and ABMT to paediatric tumours, with particular reference to the three in which it has been most widely used, namely neuroblastoma (6.2 children/10^6 popula-

tion), rhabdomyosarcoma ($3.7/10^6$) and Ewing's sarcoma ($2.0/10^6$).

B. Chemo-Radiotherapy Regimens

There are several issues still to be resolved in devising massive therapy protocols. These include determining the effects of extending the time of exposure to a given drug after increasing its absolute concentration and investigating the possible interaction of drugs and irradiation. The choice of agents at high dose has been based either on the known responsiveness of particular tumours at conventional dosage or on theoretical considerations.

Extramedullary toxicity must be balanced against the possible benefits of dose escalation. High-dose therapy inevitably produces toxicity in other organs, particularly the oral mucosa and gastrointestinal tract, which share with the bone marrow a rapid cellular proliferative rate. Also of note are pneumonitis; hepatotoxicity – predominantly veno-occlusive disease; urological toxicity – acute renal failure, haemorrhagic cystitis; neurological complications – leukoencephalopathy, seizures, and cardiomyopathy.

The problems of age and other pre-existing disease encountered in adults are obviously not applicable to paediatric practice, but the extent of initial disease and the nature and complications of previous chemotherapy must be taken into account in anticipating treatment-related complications.

The radiosensitivity of most paediatric tumours is taken advantage of in many conventional treatment regimens, and it is a

Department of Paediatric Oncology, Centre Léon Berard, Lyon, France

logical step, therefore, to study the efficacy of this treatment modality in high dose. There is an understandable reluctance to use TBI in young children because of the early and, as yet ill-defined, long-term toxicity. Similarly, the advantages of fractionated TBI remain controversial. Although pulmonary toxicity is reduced, the relative cytotoxic effect in tumours with "shouldered" response curves remains to be clarified.

Alternative strategies to TBI are the further intensification of multiple chemotherapy and the use of double autografts [6], but the long-term consequences of high-dose alkylating agents must also be taken into account if these procedures are introduced for other than very poor prognosis patients.

C. Autologous Bone Marrow

One of the major problems associated with autologous transplantation is to ensure that the marrow is free from tumour cells. As many "small round cell tumours" appear similar to normal haemopoietic progenitors on conventional histological and cytological examination, new approaches to the detection of malignant cells in bone marrow have been sought. The ability to produce monoclonal antibodies has greatly enhanced the possibility of detecting tumour cells in bone marrow [7]. The conventional way to define bone marrow status at harvesting is by aspiration or biopsy. Experience in Lyon relating to neuroblastoma has confirmed that biopsies are more effective than aspirates for detecting tumour involvement. Moreover, increasing the number of sampled sites markedly increases the yield of positive results. Even in the absence of demonstrable tumour there may be residual disease, and this provides a rationale for attempting to "purge" the marrow.

Whilst the use of monoclonal antibodies and complement has found favour for purging leukaemic bone marrow, this is not the case for solid tumours. However, a recently reported anti-ganglioside antibody that fixes human complement may have a role here [18].

The drug 4-hydroperoxycyclophosphamide (4-HC) has been used extensively as an agent for destroying leukaemic cells in bone marrow in vitro and has been shown to be active in some human neuroblastoma cell lines. However, although 4-HC has been used in clinical practice, the effectiveness of this procedure still needs to be determined [6].

The most widely applied technique for removing neuroblasts from bone marrow is one employing a cocktail of monoclonal antibodies and magnetic microspheres coated with anti-mouse immunoglobulin. A panel of six anti-neuroblastoma antibodies are used in the procedure to maximize binding to tumour cells and attempt to overcome the problem of antigenic heterogeneity [20].

D. Clinical Results

Neuroblastoma is the most common solid malignancy in early childhood (up to 5 years age). Despite considerable progress in paediatric oncology, neuroblastoma is still a fatal disease for 90% of patients with stage-IV disease (which accounts for at least 70% of cases in children more than 1 year of age). Phase-II studies using high-dose melphalan or chemoradiotherapy followed by ABMT have shown promising response rates [1, 4–6, 15]. Several groups, including ours, have reported preliminary results in cases of stage-IV neuroblastoma using massive therapy and ABMT as an early consolidation procedure for children over 1 year of age, in either partial remission (PR) or complete remission (CR) [6, 13]. A study led by the European Neuroblastoma Study Group (ENSG) is one of the few in which a massive therapy regimen has been evaluated in a prospective randomized fashion. This has demonstrated that in patients with stage-III and -IV disease who received a common initial chemotherapy regimen "OPEC" [19], consolidation with high-dose melphalan increased the duration of relapse-free survival [16]. The southern French cooperative group (LMCE) is currently evaluating a regimen comprised of vincristine infusion, 4 mg/m^2, melphalan, 180 mg/m^2, and total-body irradiation with 12 Gy (1200 rads), fractionated at 6×2 Gy with lung shielding after 10 Gy. This is given to all stage-IV patients who are over 1 year old at diagnosis and who achieve at least partial remission within initial chemotherapy.

Of 38 such patients, seven died of toxicity (18%) and 13 relapsed; 18 are alive with NED, with a median observation time of 17 months post diagnosis. Our preliminary conclusions are that this massive therapy is effective in very poor prognosis neuroblastoma (76% response rate in evaluable patients), but that toxicity is high and may be related to the total-body irradiation. This unselected group of patients shows a clear improvement in duration of remission compared with the previous series without ABMT, although long-term survival cannot yet be assessed.

The Villejuif group have studied the use of combination regimens, excluding the use of TBI [6]. A double procedure was used, and autologous marrow was purged with Asta Z. The first regimen comprised carmustine (300 mg/m^2), viomycin 26 (1 g/m^2) and melphalan (180 mg/m^2), and this was repeated 3–4 months later. Of 14 patients thus treated, there were two early toxic deaths and one relapse, and 11 are alive in CR 4–20 months after ABMT (median 12 months). It should be emphasized that these patients were a highly selected subgroup who responded well to initial therapy and were grafted only after extensive staging confirmed CR.

Phase-II studies in children with relapsed or resistant rhabdomyosarcoma have demonstrated a high response rate to high-dose melphalan with autologous marrow rescue (greater than 90%). The duration of response was almost invariably brief, however, with few long-term survivors. As this is a radiosensitive tumour, it seemed appropriate to build on the basis of melphalan and study the value of TBI in such patients. In addition, because the long-term survival of children with stage-IV disease remains poor, massive therapy could be considered for consolidation treatment once CR had been achieved. To date, eight patients (median age 4 years) have been treated in our group: four received massive therapy in first CR, having presented with advanced disease involving metastases of bone in all cases, with or without metastases of marrow, lymph nodes or lungs; two were in second CR after responding to salvage therapy.

Massive therapy comprised vincristine infusion (4 mg/m^2 over 5 days), melphalan (140 mg/m^2), TBI (12 Gy in six fractions), followed by autologous bone marrow (purged with Asta Z in some patients), or melphalan (120–140 mg/m^2) and TBI (9 Gy in a single dose), followed by unpurged autologous marrow. Four patients remain disease free, all of whom were in CR at the time of massive therapy (three first CR and one second CR). Clearly, it is too early to make any firm conclusions about the value of such a procedure or the need to purge the marrow. However, it would appear that, as with most other tumours, one course of massive therapy, even including TBI, is unlikely to salvage patients with progressive or resistant disease.

The use of double procedures is also being studied in rhabdomyosarcoma. In the current International Society of Paediatric Oncology (SIOP) trial, stage-IV patients who achieve CR after chemotherapy alone are randomized (in certain major centres) to receive vincristine, carmustine and melphalan with ABMT (Asta-Z purged), followed after 3–4 months by procarbazine, VP16 and cyclophosphamide. A similar approach is taken for patients less than 5 years old with stage-II/III parameningeal disease who do not receive high-dose cranial irradiation.

In an American series of selected cases with very bad prognosis (relapses, initial stage IV), a combination of vincristine, actinomycin, cyclophosphamide and Doxyrubicin (adriamycin) (VACA) followed by TBI (8 Gy, 2 fractions) has produced 45% survivors (1 year median follow-up) [10].

In Ewing's sarcoma, promising preliminary results were obtained by Cornbleet et al. [3] using melphalan as a single agent. In a review of 35 cases in 1984, the European Bone Marrow Transplant (EBMT) Group similarly demonstrated a response rate of 66% in evaluable patients [12]. However, the general pattern of outcome of lymhoma patients after massive therapy is also observed with this solid tumour. The results are good for patients grafted in CR (80% survival at 12 months), reasonable for relapses still responding to rescue protocol (30%), and very poor despite a high response rate for patients grafted in progressive disease. In studies by the NCI of a group of 57 selected very bad prognosis patients [10] using the VACA massive therapy regimen and TBI (8 Gy, 2 fractions), 26 are survivors at 2 year's follow-up.

There are also several reports of the use of ABMT procedures with other tumours such as osteosarcoma [10], Wilms tumour [17], malignant germ cell tumours [2], and glioma [14]. However, the results are too preliminary to comment on the precise role of ABMT in these diseases.

In conclusion, therefore, massive therapy with ABMT is now an established treatment modality in paediatric oncology. The technical aspects and most treatment-related complications have been clarified, and many phase-II studies have shown encouraging results. In the future, management of poor-prognosis diseases such as neuroblastoma may involve the use of more intensive induction regimens to improve the quality of remission at the time of ABMT, which remains the single most important prognostic factor.

References

1. August CS, Serota FT, Koch PA, Burkey E, Schlesinger H, Elkins WL, Evans AE, D'Angio GJ (1984) Treatment of advanced neuroblastoma with supralethal chemotherapy, radiation, and allogeneic or autologous marrow reconstitution. J Clin Oncol 2:609–616
2. Biron P, Philip T, Maraninchi D, Pico JL, Cahn JY, Fumoleau P, Le Mevel A, Gastaut JL, Carcassonne JM, Kamioner D, Hervé P, Brunat-Mentigny M, Hayat M (1985) Massive chemotherapy and ABMT in progressive disease of non-seminomatous testicular cancer. In: Dicke K, Spitzer G, Zander AR (eds) Autologous bone marrow transplantation. University of Texas, Houston, pp 203–210
3. Cornbleet M, Corringham R, Prentice H, Boesen E, Mc Elwain TJ (1981) Treatment of Ewing sarcoma with high-dose melphalan and autologous bone marrow transplantation. Cancer Treat Rep 63:241–244
4. D'Angio GJ, August C, Elkins W, Evans AE, Seeger R, Lenarsky C, Feig S, Wells J, Ramsay N, Kim T, Woods W, Krivit W, Strandjord S, Coccio P, Novak L (1985) Metastatic neuroblastoma managed by supralethal therapy and bone marrow reconstitution (BMRc). Results of a four-institution children's cancer study group pilot study. In: Evans AE, D'Angio GJ, Seeger RC (eds) Advances in neuroblastoma research. Liss, New York, pp 557–563
5. Graham-Pole J, Lazarus HM, Herzig RH, Worthington D, Riley C (1984) High-dose melphalan therapy for the treatment of children with refractory neuroblastoma and Ewing sarcoma. Am J Pediatr Hematol Oncol 6:17–26
6. Hartmann O, Kalifa C, Beaujean F, Bayle C, Benhamou E, Lemerle J (1985) Treatment of advanced neuroblastoma with two consecutive high-dose chemotherapy regimens and ABMT. In: Evans AE, D'Angio GJ, Seeger RC (eds) Advances in neuroblastoma research. Liss, New York, pp 565–568
7. Kemshead JT, Goldman A, Fritschy J, Malpas JS, Pritchard J (1983) The use of monoclonal antibodies in the differential diagnosis of neuroblastoma and lymphoblastic disorders. Lancet I:12–15
8. Kingston JE, Malpas JS, Stiller CA, Pritchard J, Mc Elwain TJ (1984) Autologous bone marrow transplantation contributes to haemopoietic recovery in children with solid tumours treated with high-dose melphalan. Br J Haematol 58:589–595
9. Mc Elwain TJ, Hedley DW, Gordon MY, Jarman M, Millar JL, Pritchard J (1979) High-dose melphalan and non-cryopreserved autologous bone marrow treatment of malignant melanoma and neuroblastoma. Exp Hematol 7:[Suppl 5]360–371
10. Miser J (1986) High-dose therapy and ABMT in pediatric solid tumor. In: de Bernardi B (ed) Novel therapeutic approaches in pediatric oncology. Martinus Nijhoff, Boston (in press)
11. Munoz LL, Wharam MD, Kaizer H, Leventhal BG, Ruymann F (1983) Magna-field irradiation and autologous marrow rescue in the treatment of pediatric solid tumors. Int J Radiat Oncol Biol Phys 9:1951–1954
12. Philip T (1984) Status of the role of ABMT in solid tumors in Europe. Proc of European Bone Marrow Transplant Group, Granada
13. Philip T, Biron P, Philip I, Favrot M, Bernard JL, Zucker JM, Lutz B, Plouvier E, Rebattu P, Carton M, Chauvot P, Dutou L, Souillet G, Philippe N, Boridigoni P, Lacroze M, Clapisson G, Olive D, Trealaven J, Kemshead JT, Brunat-Mentigny M (1985) Autologous bone marrow transplantation for very bad prognosis neuroblastoma. In: Evans AE, D'Angio GJ, Seeger RC (eds) Advances in neuroblastoma research. Liss, New York, pp 568–586
14. Phillips GL, Fay JW, Herzig G, et al. (1983) Intensive 1,3-bis (2 chloroethyl)-1-ni-

trosourea (BCNU) and cryopreserved autologous marrow transplantation for refractory cancer. A phase I-II study. Cancer 52:1792–1802

15. Pritchard J, Mc Elwain TJ, Graham-Pole J (1982) High-dose melphalan with autologous bone marrow rescue for treatment of advanced neuroblastoma. Br J Cancer 48:86–92

16. Pritchard J, Germona S, Jones D, De Kraker J, Love S (1986) Is high-dose melphalan of value in treatment of advanced neuroblastoma? Proc ASCO, vol 5, A 805

17. Prats J, Toledo J, Payarols J, Gallego S, Macio J (1985) High-dose melphalan therapy for the treatment of children with refractory Wilms tumor. Proc SIOP, p 289

18. Saarinan UM, Coccia PF, Gerson SL, Pelley R, Cheung NKV (1985) Eradication of neuroblastoma cells in vitro by monoclonal antibody and human complement. Method for purging autologous bone marrow. Cancer Res 45:5969–5975

19. Shafford EA, Rogers DW, Pritchard J (1984) Advanced neuroblastoma: improved response rate using malignant regimen (OPEC) including sequential cis-platinum and VM26. J Clin Oncol 2:742–747

20. Treleaven JG, Gibson FM, Ugelstad J, Rembaum A, Philip T, Caine GD, Kemshead JT (1984) Removal of neuroblastoma cells from bone marrow with monoclonal antibodies conjugated to magnetic microspheres. Lancet I:70–73

Haematology and Blood Transfusion Vol. 31
Modern Trends in Human Leukemia VII
Edited by Neth, Gallo, Greaves, and Kabisch
© Springer-Verlag Berlin Heidelberg 1987

Cytokines with Possible Clinical Utility

R. Mertelsmann [1], J. Kolitz [2], K. Welte [2], and F. Herrmann [1]

A. Introduction

Biological response modifiers (BRM) are agents aimed at reducing tumor growth, not primarily by exerting direct cytotoxic effects but by modulation of tumor gene expression (e.g., induction of differentiation) or by enhancing host defense mechanisms directed against cancer cells. BRM as primary therapy or as adjuncts to cytotoxic agents in the treatment of cancers have attracted increasing interest in view of stagnating clinical results in many areas [1], and there is increasing evidence of in vitro and in vivo efficacy of these agents. Furthermore, advances in molecular biology suggesting that oncogenes and their products play a crucial role in oncogenesis support approaches to modulation of regulatory mechanisms as a means of controlling tumor cell growth.

Clinical trials of BRM are more complex than those evaluating cytotoxic agents which are generally given at maximum tolerated dosages. Maximum tolerated doses of BRM are not necessarily optimal for modifying biological response, nor are they always the most efficacious doses. A tentative classification for BRM with some representative agents is presented in Table 1.

Agents such as retinoic acid affect tumor cell proliferation and differentiation, apparently through modulation of tumor cell gene expression rather than through host mechanisms. It should be kept in mind, however, that tumor-host interactions are subject to an intricate regulatory network of cells and cytokines, similar to the endocrine system. Modulation of one parameter could have additional, indirect effects on the biological response network. Table 2 describes cytokines that have been cloned and have thus been identified as unique gene products.

It has now become increasingly clear that the original hypothesis of "one producer cell type – one cytokine – one target cell type" does not reflect the biological facts. Ample

[1] Department of Hematology, University of Mainz, Mainz, Federal Republic of Germany
[2] Laboratory of Cytokine Biology, Sloan-Kettering Institute, New York, NY, USA

Table 1. Biological response modifiers

Group	Examples
1. Monoclonal antibodies	Anti-melanoma, anti-T cell
2. Cytokines	IL 1, 2, 3; IFN α, β, γ; TNF α, β; G-, g/M 0-, M 0-CSF, EPO, EPA
3. Synthetic agents	retinoid acid, vitamin D3, HMBA
4. Immunoregulatory peptides	Tuftsin, endorphins

IL 1, 2, 3; Interleukin 1, 2, 3; *IFN α, β, γ,* interferon α, β, γ; *TNF α, β,* tumor necrosis factor α, β; *CSF for G, G/M0, M,* colony stimulating factors for granulocytes, granulocytes/macrophages, macrophages; *EPO,* erythropoietin; *EPA,* erythroid potentiating activity; *HMBA,* hexamethylene bisacetamide

Table 2. Recombinant human cytokines

Agent	Receptor	Hemopoietic producer cell	cDNA cloning reported by	Growth factor for	Activation factor for
IL1	–[a]	MO	March et al. (1985) Nature 315:641	T, B	T, B
IL2	Tac	T	Taniguchi et al. (1983) Nature 302:305	T, NK, B, MO[c]	T[c], NK[c], B, MO[c]
IL3	–	T	Not published	G/MO-PC, early RBC-PC	nd[d]
IFNα	–	B, MO, Nk	Goeddel et al. (1980) Nature 287:411	–	NK[c]
IFNβ	–	–	Derynck et al. (1980) Nature 285:542	–	–
IFNγ	–	T, NK	Gray et al. (1981) Nature 295:503	–	NK, MO[c]
TNFα	–	MO	Shirai et al. (1985) Nature 312:803	T (?)	MO[c]
TNFβ	–	T	Gray et al. (1984) Nature 312:721	nd	T
G-CSF	–	MO	Souza et al. (1986) Science 232:61	G-PC	G
GM-CSF	fes (?)[e]	T	Wong et al. (1985) Science 228:810	G/MO-PC, early RBC-PC	MO
M-CSF	fms	MO	Kawasaki et al. (1985) Science 230:291	–	MO
EPO	–	–	Lin et al. (1985) Proc Natl Acad Sci USA 82:7580	late RBC-PC[c]	–
EPA	–	T	Gasson et al. (1985) Nature 315:768	early and late RBC-PC	–

[a] Not cDNA cloned. *MO*, macrophages; *T*, T cells; *B*, B cells; *NK*, NK cells; *G*, granulocytes; *RBC*, red blood cells; *PC*, progenitor cells.
[b] Documented in clinical trials.
[c] Not determined.
[d] Related oncogene.

evidence has been accummulated demonstrating that a given cytokine can be produced by different cell types (e.g., IL1) and can exert effects on different cell types (e.g., IL2 on T cells, B cells, and monocytes). The biological effect appears to be dependent upon receptor density, receptor affinity, and ligand concentration, as well as on the functional state of the responder cell [2]. Since so far only one of these agents, IL2, has undergone more than preliminary clinical evaluation, the following brief review will focus on this agent.

B. Interleukin 2

The long-term proliferation of normal T-lymphocytes in suspension culture was first achieved by Morgan et al. [3], using the T-cell-derived cytokine intially designated "T-cell growth factor" (TCGF) and later renamed interleukin 2 (IL2).

The biochemical purification of IL2 and the molecular cloning and expression of its gene have led to a growing appreciation of the protean functional capabilities of this molecule. It supports the growth of human cytotoxic T cells (CTL) [4, 5] and natural killer (NK) cells [6], it enhances the functional capabilities of NK cells [1, 8], and it is the factor essential for the induction and growth of human lymphokine-activated killer (LAK) cells [9]. It induces antigen-specific T-cell lines to produce B-cell growth factor-I [10], and it is capable of enhancing gamma-interferon (gamma-IFN) production either alone [11] or in conjunction with mitogen [2]. An even broader immunoregulatory role for IL2 is suggested by its recently demonstrated ability to drive B cell proliferation and immunoglobulin production (13–16) and by the recent description of functionally active IL2 receptors on macrophages [12].

Not surprisingly, a number of human disease states have been found to be associated with varying defects in IL2 production and response. Among those affected are patients with primary and acquired immunodeficiency diseases, including common variable immunodeficiency (CVI) [18] and the acquired immunodeficiency syndrome (AIDS) [19, 20], bone marrow transplant recipients [21], and patients with severe burns and hemophilia [22] (K. Welte, unpublished observations). Furthermore, several immunosuppressive drugs appear to exert their effects by blocking IL2 gene expression [23, 24]. Defects in lectin- and mitogen-induced T-cell proliferation are frequently reversible in vitro by exogenous IL2. These observations, coupled with the demonstrated ability of IL2 to enhance the cytotoxicity of NK and LAK cells, have provided a rationale for clinical evaluation of IL2 in human malignancy and immunodeficiency.

The human IL2 gene has been cloned and sequenced [25], and its position on chromosome 4 has been determined by us and others [26, 27]. Several recombinant IL2 (rIL2) preparations (Cetus, Amgen, Biogen) have been compared in our laboratory with human purified IL2 (hpIL2) and, except for higher background mitogenic activity on the part of rIL2, no differences were detected in a variety of human in vitro and murine in vitro and in vivo systems (K. Welte, V. J. Merluzzi, unpublished observations).

C. IL2 in the Treatment of Cancer

The ability of IL2 to restore T cell functional defects in vivo and in vitro and to induce and enhance cytoxicity against fresh and cultured tumor targets led to early exploration of its potential as an agent in the treatment of cancer. The anti-tumor activity of IL2 has been most clearly demonstrated in conjunction with the infusion of specific immune cultured T cells or nonspecific LAK cells.

B6 mice with syngeneic Friend virus-induced FBL-3 leukemia are cured with the combination of noncurative doses of cyclophosphamide and administration of tumor-immune congeneic lymphocytes cultured in vitro and expanded in vivo with IL2 [28]. High doses of IL2 and infusions of autologous LAK cells cause major regressions of murine transplantable sarcomas and melanomas [29], with IL2 inducing in vivo proliferation of the adoptively transferred cells [30]. IL2 alone causes major regressions of murine sarcomas when given in extremely high doses (400 000 U intraperitoneally every 8 h) [31].

Following i.v. bolus administration of Jurkat hpIL2, the serum half-life of IL2 in man was 5–7 min, with a second component of clearance of 30–120 min [32]. Such a two-compartment model is compatible with our own observations following treatment of 30 patients with rIL2 (Cetus) given by 6 hour continuous i.v. infusion [35].

We completed an initial trial of hpIL2 in human malignancy and immunodeficiency at Memorial Hospital in 1983 [33]. The IL2 was purified from human PBL-conditioned medium in our laboratory [34]. The s.c. route of administration was chosen in order to achieve maximal lymphatic drainage. Escalating doses were given, to a maximum daily dose of 20000 U/m^2 and a maximum total dose of 855000 U/m^2, administered over 77 days.

Sixteen patients with malignancy and AIDS were treated. Except for occasional skin irritation at the injection site, no toxicity was observed. One patient, a child with probable Nezelof's syndrome who died of infectious complications after 5 days of therapy with IL2 and after an unsuccessful T-cell-depleted bone marrow graft from a haplotype-identical half brother, was found at autopsy to have all lymph nodes lymphocyte depleted, except for inguinal nodes proximal to s.c. IL2 injection sites, where lymphoid follicles were noted. This was an early suggestion of the in vivo biological activity of IL2.

While there was some suggestion of improved responsiveness to OKT3-inducible T-cell activation in the only two patients receiving treatment for at least 50 days, there was no clear evidence for significant biological response modification in this trial.

A trial of Jurkat hpIL2 in human malignancy has been completed at the National Cancer Institute [32]. Twelve patients with a range of solid tumors received IL2 at doses of up to 2000 µg by i.v. bolus or continuous infusion weekly for 4 weeks. Biological observations included an acute decrease in peripheral blood T cells, affecting all major T cell subsets, and an increase in circulating cells capable of responding to IL2 and expressing LAK activity. No clinical response was seen. Toxicity consisted primarily of fever, chills, malaise, and reversible hepatopathy.

In a recently completed clinical trial, we administered rIL2 (Cetus) as a continuous 6-h i.v. infusion to 17 patients with advanced malignancy and to 13 patients with AIDS [35]. The maximum tolerated dose was 1000000 U/m^2, with dose-limiting toxicity consisting of fever > 40 °C, thrombocytopenia, and diarrhea at the 2000000 U/m^2 dose level. Except for one patient with a myelodysplastic syndrome, who had a fall in marrow blasts from > 10% to 1% over a 2-month period, no significant clinical responses were seen. Dose-dependent biological response-modifying effects were observed, however.

At the higher dose levels a reproducible lymphocytosis occurred, peaking on day 15 of each treatment cycle, with an up to five-fold increase in the absolute lymphocyte count. The expansion consisted of a polyclonal increase in all T-cell subsets, with no substantive change observed in any T-cell marker or in the T4/T8 ratio.

Twenty patients with solid tumors were treated with rIL2 (Cetus) at the National Cancer Institute [36] using i.v. bolus administration. No clinical responses were seen, but a Tac+ lymphocytosis was also observed, along with induction of detectable gamma-interferon serum levels.

Much interest has recently been generated by the report of major tumor regressions in patients with solid tumors (primarily melanoma, colon carcinoma, and hypernephroma) treated with infusions of autologous LAK cells and high doses (100000 U/kg every 8 h i.v.) of rIL2 [37]. A major focus of research activity will be to reduce the considerable toxicity of this approach, which has included marked fluid retention, pulmonary edema, hypotension, and reversible renal dysfunction. Whether the therapeutic effect is due primarily to the infusions of LAK cells or to the high doses of rIL2 is also presently unclear.

Given the ability of IL2 to induce LAK cells with wide anti-tumor efficacy both in vivo and in vitro and the clear demonstration of potent biological effects achievable in treated patients, additional efforts will have to be made to translate the promise of this lymphokine into clinically meaningful results. Subcutaneous, i.p., (P. Chapman et al., submitted) and intralesional administration might achieve sufficiently high local concentration of IL2 to generate LAK cells in vivo with acceptable toxicity. The use of cyclo-phosphamide in low doses directed against suppressor T cells is a potential means of countering regulatory mechanisms limiting the efficacy of IL2 (J. Kolitz, manuscript in preparation). Defining the phenotype and optimizing the activation conditions for LAK cells may lead to therapies with re-duced toxicities. The use of monoclonal an-tibodies directed against tumor antigens might lead to local inflammatory infiltrates in tumor sites [38]. CTL numbers and NK/LAK cytotoxicity could then possibly be amplified in vivo by IL2. These approaches are being utilized in current or planned clini-cal trials at Memorial Hospital, New York, and at the Department of Hematology of the University of Mainz.

References

1. Bailar JC, Smith EM (1986) Progress against cancer? N Engl J Med 314:1226–1232
2. Herrmann F, Cannistra SA, Griffin JD (1986) T cell-monocyte interactions in the produc-tion of humoral factors regulating human granulopoiesis in vitro. J Immunol 136:2856–2862
3. Morgan DA, Ruscetti FW, Gallo RC (1976) Selective in vitro growth of T-lymphocytes from normal human bone marrows. Science 193:1007–1008
4. Gillis S, Smith KA (1977) Long-term culture of tumor-specific cytotoxic T cells. Nature 268:154–156
5. Gillis S, Baker PE, Ruscetti FW, et al. (1978) A long-term culture of human antigen-spe-cific cytotoxic T cell lines. J Exp Med 148:1093–1098
6. Flomenberg N, Welte K, Mertelsmann R, et al. (1983) Interleukin 2-dependent natural kil-ler (NK) cell lines from patients with primary T cell immunodeficiencies. J Immunol 130:2635–2643
7. Henney CS, Kuribayashi K, Kern DE, et al. (1981) Interleukin 2 augments natural killer cell activity. Nature 291:335–338
8. Trinchieri G, Matsumoto-Kobayshi M, Clark SC, et al. (1984) Response of resting pe-ripheral blood natural killer cells to interleu-kin 2. J Exp Med 160:1147–1169
9. Grimm EA, Mazumder A, Zhang HZ, et al. (1982) Lymphokine-activated killer cell phe-nomenon: lysis of natural killer-resistant fresh solid tumor cells by interleukin 2 activated au-tologous peripheral blood lymphocytes. J Exp Med 155:1823–1841
10. Howard M, Matis L, Malck TR, et al. (1983) Interleukin 2 induces antigen-reactive T cell lines to secrete BCGF-1. J Exp Med 158:2024–2039
11. Kasahara T, Hooks JJ, Dougherty SF, et al. (1983) Interleukin 2 mediated immune inter-feron (IFN-gamma) production by human T cells and T cell subsets. J Immunol 130:1789–1989
12. Pearlstein KT, Palladino MA, Welte K, et al. (1983) Purified human interleukin 2 enhanced induction of immune interferon. Cell Immu-nol 80:1–9
13. Zubler RH, Lowenthal JW, Erard F, et al. (1984) Activated B cells express receptor for, and proliferate in response to, pure interleu-kin 2. J Exp Med 160:1170–1183
14. Waldmann TA, Goldman CK, Robb RJ, et al. (1984) Expression of interleukin 2 recep-tors on activated human B cells. J Exp Med 160:1450–1466
15. Boyd AW, Fisher DC, Fox DA, et al. (1985) Structural and functional characterization of IL-2 receptors on activated human B cells. J Immunol 134:2387–2392
16. Ralph P, Jeong G, Welte K, et al. (1984) Stim-ulation of immunoglobulin secretion in hu-man B-lymphocytes as a direct effect of high concentrations of IL-2. J Immunol 133:2442–2445
17. Herrmann F, Cannistra SA, Levine H, et al. (1985) Expression of interleukin 2 receptors and binding of interleukin 2 by gamma inter-feron-induced human leukemic and normal monocytic cells. J Exp Med 162:1111–1116
18. Kruger G, Welte K, Ciobanu N, et al. (1984) Interleukin 2 correction of defective in vitro T cell mitogenesis in patients with common variable immunodeficiency. J Clin Immunol 4:295–303
19. Ciobanu N, Welte K, Kruger G, et al. (1983) Defective T cell response to PHA and mito-genic monoclonal antibodies in male homo-sexual with acquired immunodeficiency syn-drome and its in vitro correction by interleu-kin 2. J Clin Immunol 3:332–340
20. Murray HW, Welte K, Jacobs JL, et al. (1985) Production of and in vitro response to inter-leukin 2 in the acquired immunodeficiency syndrome. J Clin Invest 76:1959–1964
21. Welte K, Ciobanu N, Moore MAS, et al. (1984) Defective interleukin 2 production in patients after bone marrow transplantation and in vitro restoration of defective T-lym-phocyte proliferation by highly purified inter-leukin 2. Blood 64:380–385
22. Antonacci A, Calvano SE, Reaves A, et al. (1984) Autologous and allogeneic mixed lym-phocyte responses following thermal injury in man: the immunomodulatory effects of inter-

leukin 1, interleukin 2 and a prostaglandin inhibitor, WY-18251. Clin Immunol Immunopath 30:304–320

23. Kröncke M, Leonard WJ, Depper JM (1984) Cyclosporin A inhibits T-cell growth factor gene expression at the level of mRNA transcription. Proc Natl Acad Sci USA 81:5214–5218

24. Arya SK, Wong-Staal F, Gallo RC, et al. (1984) Dexamethasone-mediated inhibition of human T-cell growth factor and gamma-interferon messenger RNA. J Immunol 133:273–276

25. Holbrook NJ, Smith KA, Fornace AJ Jr, et al. (1984) T-cell growth factor: complete nucleotide sequence and organization of the gene in normal and malignant cells. Proc Natl Acad Sci USA 81:1634–1638

26. Siegal LJ, Harper ME, Wong-Staal F, et al. (1984) Gene for feline chromosome B1. Science 223:175–178

27. Sykora KW, Kolitz J, Szabo P, et al. (1984) The human IL2 gene is located on chromosome 4. Cancer Invest 2:261–265

28. Cheever MA, Greenberg PD, Fefer A (1982) Augmentation of the anti-tumor therapeutic efficacy of long-term cultured T-lymphocytes by in vivo administration of purified interleukin 2. J Exp Med 155:968–980

29. Mazumder A, Rosenberg SA (1984) Successful immunotherapy of natural killer-resistant established pulmonary melanoma metastases by the intravenous adoptive transfer of syngeneic lymphocytes activated in vitro by interleukin 2. J Exp Med 159:495–507

30. Ettinghausen SE, Lipford EH, Mule JJ, et al. (1985) Recombinant interleukin-2 stimulates in vivo proliferation of adoptively transferred lymphokine-activated killer (LAK) cells. J Immunol 135:3623–3635

31. Rosenberg SA, Mule JJ, Spiess PJ, et al. (1985) Regression of established pulmonary metastases and subcutaneous tumor mediated by the systemic administration of high-dose recombinant interleukin 2. J Exp Med 161:1169–1188

32. Lotze MT, Frana LW, Sharrow SO, et al. (1985) In vivo administration of purified human interleukin 2. Half-life and immunologic effects of the Jurkat cell line-derived interleukin 2. J Immunol 134:157–166

33. Mertelsmann R, Welte K, Sternber C, et al. (1984) Treatment of immunodeficiency with interleukin 2: initial exploration. Resp Modif 4:483–490

34. Welte K, Wang CY, Mertelsmann R, et al. (1982) Purification of human interleukin 2 to apparent homogeneity and its molecular heterogeneity. J Exp Med 156:454–464

35. Kolitz JE, Holloway K, Welte K, et al. (1985) A multiple-dose phase-I trial of recombinant interleukin 2 in advanced malignancy. Proc Am Soc Clin Oncol 135:2865–2875

36. Lotze MT, Frana LW, Sharrow SO, et al. (1985) In vivo administration of purified human interleukin 2. II. Half-life, immunologic effects, and expansion of peripheral lymphoid cells in vivo with recombinant interleukin 2. J Immunol 135:2865–2875

37. Rosenberg SA, Lotze MT, Muul LM, et al. (1987) A progress report on the treatment of 157 patients with advanced cancer using lymphokine-activated killer cells and Interleukin-2 or high-dose Interleukin-2 alone. N Engl J Med 316:889–897

38. Houghton AN, Mintzer D, Cordon-Cardo C (1985) Mouse monoclonal IgG 3 antibody-detecting GD3 ganglioside: a phase-I trial in patients with malignant melanoma. Proc Natl Acad Sci USA 82:1242–1246

Haematology and Blood Transfusion Vol. 31
Modern Trends in Human Leukemia VII
Edited by Neth, Gallo, Greaves, and Kabisch
© Springer-Verlag Berlin Heidelberg 1987

Biological Approaches to Cancer Therapy

K. A. Foon[1]

A. Introduction

Progress had been made over the past 5 years toward the development of specific biological approaches to the treatment of cancer. The techniques of genetic engineering and mass cell culture, and improved techniques in protein and nucleic acid sequencing have made available biologics as highly purified molecules. The most definitive investigations have been carried out with natural and cloned interferon-α preparations, and it is clear that the latter are capable of inducing responses primarily in patients with certain types of lymphomas and leukemias. Preliminary trials with murine monoclonal antibodies have demonstrated excellent in vivo tumor localization and transient clinical responses, but durable responses are rare events. Antibodies conjugated to drugs, toxins, and isotopes have greater antitumor activity in vitro and in animal models; clinical trials are currently under way.

B. Monoclonal Antibodies

Clinical trials with monoclonal antibodies in humans have been designed to approach preliminary questions with respect to the feasibility and toxicity of monoclonal antibody therapy and to the rationale for the use of these reagents. While most of these trials

---

[1] Division of Clinical Immunology, Roswell Park Memorial Institute, 666 Elmst, Buffalo NY 14263

have involved single patients or small series of patients, early indications are that an unlabeled monoclonal antibody alone may have some therapeutic effect, albeit rather limited.

Results of serotherapy trials in patients with a wide variety of hematologic malignancies and solid tumors are shown in Table 1 [1–18]. Transient reductions (24–48 h) in circulating leukemia cells were common, as were transient improvements in cutaneous lesions in patients with cutaneous T-cell lymphoma. At least 50% of patients with B-cell lymphomas/leukemias treated with anti-idiotype monoclonal antibodies had partial responses; one patient had a complete response (lasting over 4 years). Excellent targeting of antibody to tumor cells was reported in most of these studies.

Sears and coworkers [15, 16] treated 20 patients with gastrointestinal tumors with the 17-1A IgG_{2a} antibody, 3 of whom remained tumor-free 22, 13, and 10 months after therapy. Houghton and coworkers [18] reported 3 partial responses in 12 patients with melanoma treated with an IgG_3 antibody recognizing a ganglioside antigen (G_{D3}). Interestingly, this antibody is cytotoxic in vitro with human complement and human effector cells. Inflammatory reactions were observed around tumor sites in some of the patients treated with this antibody.

Toxicities associated with monoclonal antibody therapy are generally quite mild. Fevers, chills, and urticaria are quite common but are not treatment-limiting toxicities. Rare patients have developed shortness of breath associated with the rapid infusion

Table 1. Monoclonal antibody clinical trials

Disease	Antibody/class	Specificity	No. of patients	Toxicity	Effect	Institution	Reference
B-lymphoma	Ab89/IgG$_{2a}$	Lymphomas	1	Renal (transient)	Transient reduction in circulating cells	Dana-Farber	[1]
B-lymphoma	4D6/IgG$_{2b}$	Idiotype	1	None	Complete remission	Stanford	[2]
B-lymphoma	Anti-idiotype/ IgG$_1$ of IgG$_{2a}$ or IgG$_{2b}$	Idiotype	10	Fever, chills, nausea, vomiting, headache, diarrhea, transient dyspnea	5 objective responses	Stanford	[3]
B-CLL	Anti-idiotype/ IgG$_{2b}$ and IgG$_1$	Idiotype	1	Fever, urticaria	Transient reduction in circulating cells	NCI	[4]
B-CLL	T101/IgG$_{2a}$	T65	13	Dyspnea, hypotension, fever (101–102° F), urticaria	Transient reduction in circulating cells	NCI	[5]
B-CLL	T101/IgG$_{2a}$	T65	4	Dyspnea, hypotension, fever, malaise, urticaria	Transient reduction in circulating cells	U. Calif. San Diego	[6, 7]
ATL	L17F12 (anti-Leu-1)/IgG$_{2a}$	Leu-1	1	Renal, hepatic (transient)	Transient reduction in circulating cells	Stanford	[8]
CTCL	L17F12/IgG$_{2a}$	Leu-1	6	Dyspnea, hives, cutaneous pain	Minor remission in 5 out of 7 patients	Stanford	[9, 10]
CTCL	T101/IgG$_{2a}$	T65	12	Dyspnea, fever (101°–102° F)	Minor remission in 4 patients	NCI	[11]
CTCL	T101/IgG$_{2a}$	T65	4	Dyspnea, fever	Minor remissions	U. Calif. San Diego	[7]
T-ALL	L17F12/IgG$_{2a}$ 12E7/IgG$_1$ 4H9/IgG$_{2a}$	Leu-1 T & B cells T cells	8	Sporadic coagulopathy	Transient reduction in circulating cells	Stanford	[12]
cALL	J5/IgG$_{2a}$	CALLA	4	Fever (101°–102° F)	Transient reduction in circulating cells	Dana-Farber	[13]
AML	PM/81/IgM AML-2-23/ IgG$_{2b}$ PMN 29/IgM PMN 6/IgM	NR$^+$ NR NR NR	3	Fever, back pain, arthralgia, myalgia	Transient reduction in circulating cells	Dartmouth	[14]
Gastro-intestinal	17-1A/IgG$_{2a}$	NR	20	Urticaria, bronchospasm, mild hypotension	Limited response	Wistar/ Fox Chase	[15, 16]
Melanoma	9.2.27/IgG$_{2a}$	250K	20	Fever, serum sickness	None	NCI	[17]
Melanoma	R25/IgG$_3$	G$_{D3}$	12	Urticaria, pruritis, fever, wheezing, vomiting	Major tumor regressions in 3 patients	Memomrial Sloan-Kettering	[18]

cALL, common acute lymphoblastic leukemia; ATL, adult T-cell leukemia-lymphoma; CTCL, cutaneous T-cell lymphoma; B-CLL, B-chronic lymphocytic leukemia; AML, acute myelogenous leukemia. NR, not reported.

of monoclonal antibodies, and others have developed hypotension and tachycardia. A limited number of patients have developed transient reduction in their creatinine clearance and elevation of their liver enzymes, thought to be secondary to immune complexes. In conclusion, murine-derived monoclonal antibodies can be safely infused; although side effects can be expected, they are usually mild.

Another attractive therapeutic application of monoclonal antibodies is to "clean up" autologous bone marrow prior to bone marrow transplantation. Patients who are in clinical remission will often have morphologically undetectable tumor cells in their bone marrow which theoretically could be detected and destroyed with specific antibodies and complement (or antibodies conjugated to toxins). Most of the obstacles and toxicities with monoclonal antibody infusion would be eliminated by using this technology. Such an approach has been reported when using the B1 monoclonal antibody to clean up autologous bone marrow from patients with non-Hodgkin lymphoma [19] and a variety of antibodies to clean up bone marrow from patients with acute lymphoblastic leukemia [20, 21]. Early results have demonstrated that bone marrow reconstitution takes place in virtually every patient. Therapy is tolerated quite well, and most of the patients will enter a complete remission. However, for acute lymphoblastic leukemia only one-third of the patients have been maintained for more than 1 year in remission, and this is not different from what is seen in allogeneic bone marrow transplantation. The results for non-Hodgkin lymphoma are more promising, with over 50% of the patients remaining in remission with a median duration of 22 months. Long-term disease-free survival will be necessary before concluding that these therapies have been curative.

Antibodies conjugated to drugs, toxins, and radionuclides can be used for therapy and radioimaging. There is considerable evidence, at least in animal tumor models, suggesting that antibodies covalently linked to certain toxins such as ricin or diphtheria toxin have a greater antitumor effect both in vitro and in vivo than unconjugated free antibodies [22, 23]. A number of centers are currently studying monoclonal antibodies conjugated to radionuclides such as ^{111}In or ^{131}I to determine diagnostic efficacy in man.

C. Interferon

Interferons are a family of proteins produced by cells in response to virus, double-stranded ribonucleic acid, antigens, and mitogens. In addition to antiviral activity, the interferons have profound effects on a number of components of the immune system, including B cells, T cells, natural killer cells, and macrophages, and have antiproliferative activity. With respect to the interferons and cancer therapy, it is still unclear whether the interferons work primarily by their antiproliferative activity or through alterations of immune responses. It is clear, however, from both preclinical and clinical studies that interferons have antitumor activity in a number of tumor systems [29].

The most extensively studied interferons clinically are the natural and recombinant interferon-α preparations (Table 2). Antitumor activity for the alpha interferons has been quite limited in regard to solid tumors. The best results have been achieved in AIDS-related Kaposi's sarcoma, with approximately a 50% response rate [30, 31]. Results for breast cancer have been mixed, with 30%–40% responses reported in some studies and no responses in others [32–34]. Renal cell carcinoma is among the tumors most unresponsive to any known cytotoxic agents, and approximately a 15% partial response rate to interferon-α has been reported [35]. Partial response rates of around 10%–20% have been reported for patients with melanomas, similar to the chemotherapy response rates [36, 37]. Responses for other common solid tumors such as bronchogenic carcinoma and colon cancer have been negative. Preliminary trials with crude interferon-α preparations from Yugoslavia suggested some activity for head and neck cancers; however, these results have not been confirmed outside Yugoslavia.

The most impressive results for interferon-α have been obtained in the hematologic malignancies. Approximately 50% response rates for patients with low-grade

Table 2. Clinical trials with interferon-α[a]

Tumor	Number of evaluable patients	Response rates			Total response %
		CR[a]	PR[a]	MR[a]	
Hematologic malignances					
Hairy-cell leukemia	121	14[b]	69	35	95
Non-Hodgkin lymphoma (low-grade)	92	9	30	6	42
Non-Hodgkin lymphoma (intermediate- and high-grade)	36	1	4	2	14
Cutaneous T-cell lymphoma	20	2	7	2	45
Chronic lymphocytic leukemia	67	0	12		18
Multiple myeloma	177	3[b]	18		17
Chronic myelogenous leukemia	68	2	46	7	81
Essential thrombocythemia	4	3	0		75
Acute leukemia	62		19[c]		31
Solid Tumors					
Kaposi's sarcoma (AIDs-related)	44	9	12		48
Osteogenic sarcoma	15	0	1		7
Melanoma	167	6	13	2	11
Renal cell	252	6	37	28	17
Breast	187	0	14	10	7
Ovarian	42	5	3		19
Bladder (papillomatosis or superficial)	20	10	8		90
Colorectal	66	0	2		3
Carcinoid	9	0	6		67
Lung, small-cell	10	0	0		0
Lung, non-small-cell	70	0	1		1

[a] Special thanks to Dr. Mark Roth for compiling the data shown in this table. CR, complete response; PR, partial response; MR, minor response. Complete response means absence of hairy cells in the bone marrow (in most studies) and normalization of peripheral blood white cells, platelets, and erythrocytes. Partial response means a normalization of peripheral blood white cells, platelets, and erythrocyte counts, and > 50% reduction in hairy cells in the bone marrow. Minor response generally means improvement in hemoglobin to more than 10 g/dl or improvement in platelets to more than $100 \times 10^9/1$ or improvement in neutrophils to more than $1 \times 10^9/1$.
[b] Complete response and partial response not available from all trials; % total response includes all responses.
[c] Most responses were of short duration.

non-Hodgkin lymphoma and cutaneous T-cell lymphoma have been reported [38–41]. These responses have lasted from 6–10 months, and in many patients, responses have continued for a number of years. Patients with chronic lymphocytic leukemia have been reported to have approximately an 18% response rate, and in our trials at the National Cancer Institute (NCI) we reported only two brief responses among 18 evaluable patients [42].

We and other investigators have reported excellent responses for patients with hairy-cell leukemia treated with recombinant leukocyte A interferon [43–46]. Responses appear to be equivalent for patients who have not had prior splenectomy. Greater than 90% response rates have been widely reported. While complete responses are not common (careful evaluation of the bone marrow usually reveals residual hairy cells), partial responses and even minimum responses usually lead to a dramatic improvement in blood counts. We also reported immunologic improvement, with natural killer cell activity returning in most patients following therapy with interferon, as well as normalization of T-lymphocyte subpopulations.

Chronic myelogenous leukemia also appears to be responsive [47] to interferon-α, with hematologic remission reported in 55 out of 68 patients (81%). These patients have had improved hematologic parameters as well as reduction in size of enlarged spleens and suppression of the Ph^1 chromosome.

These studies have demonstrated that interferon-α has the highest reported response rate for any standard or experimental agent in advanced, previously treated cutaneous T-cell lymphoma patients. They also establish interferon-α as a new non-cross-resistant modality of therapy for low-grade- and possibly intermediate-grade-histology non-Hodgkin lymphoma. Interferon-α may be the most active single agent for hairy-cell leukemia and should be considered first for therapy when splenectomy is no longer effective in controlling the disease. Whether 2'-deoxycoformycin is more effective than interferon-α for hairy-cell leukemia remains to be determined. Phase III trials for previously untreated patients with non-Hodgkin lymphoma, cutaneous T-cell lymphoma, and hairy-cell leukemia, and chronic myelogenous leukemia patients are clear avenues of future investigation.

References

1. Nadler LM, Stashenko P, Hardy R, et al. (1980) Serotherapy of a patient with monoclonal antibody directed against a human lymphoma-associated antigen. Cancer Res 40:3147–3154
2. Miller RA, Maloney DG, Warnke R, Levy R (1982) Treatment of a B cell lymphoma with monoclonal anti-idiotype antibody. N Engl J Med 306:517–522
3. Meeker TC, Lowder J, Maloney DG, et al. (1985) A clinical trial of anti-idiotype therapy for B cell malignancy. Blood 65:1349–1363
4. Giardina SL, Schroff RW, Kipps TJ, et al. (1985) The generation of monoclonal anti-idiotype antibodies to human B cell-derived leukemias and lymphomas. J Immunol 135:653–658
5. Foon KA, Schroff RW, Bunn PA, et al. (1984) Effects of monoclonal antibody therapy in patients with chronic lymphocytic leukemia. Blood 64:1085–1094
6. Dillman RO, Shawler DL, Sobel RE, et al. (1982) Murine monoclonal antibody therapy in two patients with chronic lymphocytic leukemia. Blood 59:1036–1045
7. Dillman RO, Shawler DL, Dillman JB, Roystan I (1984) Therapy of chronic lymphocytic leukemia and cutaneous T cell lymphoma with T101 monoclonal antibody. J Clin Oncol 2:881–891
8. Miller RA, Maloney DG, McKillop J, Levy R (1981) In vivo effects of murine hybridoma monoclonal antibody in patient with T cell leukemia. Blood 58:78–86
9. Miller RA, Levy R (1981) Response of cutaneous T cell lymphoma to therapy of hybridoma monoclonal antibody. Lancet 2:225–230
10. Miller RA, Oseroff AR, Stratte PT, Levy R (1983) Monoclonal antibody therapeutic trials in seven patients with T cell lymphoma. Blood 62:988–995
11. Foon KA, Schroff RW, Sherwin SA, Oldham RK, Bunn PA, Hsu S-M (1983) Monoclonal antibody therapy of chronic lymphocytic leukemia and T cell lymphoma: preliminary observations. In: Boss BD, Langman RE, Towbridge IS, Dulbecco R (eds) Monoclonal antibodies and cancer. Academic, New York, pp 39–52
12. Levy R, Miller RA (1983) Tumor therapy with monoclonal antibodies. Fed Proc 42:2650–2656
13. Ritz J, Pesando JM, Sallan SE, et al. (1981) Serotherapy of acute lymphoblastic leukemia with monoclonal antibody. Blood 58:141–152
14. Ball ED, Bernier GM, Cornwell GG, McIntyre OR, O'Donnell Jr, Fanger MW (1983) Monoclonal antibodies to myeloid differentiation antigens: in vivo studies of three patients with acute myelogenous leukemia. Blood 62:1203–1210
15. Sears HF, Mattis J, Herlyn D, et al. (1982) Phase I clinical trial of monoclonal antibody in treatment of gastrointestinal tumors. Lancet 1:762–765
16. Sears HG, Herlyn D, Steplewski Z, Koprowski H (1984) Effects of monoclonal antibody immunotherapy in patients with gastrointestinal adenocarcinoma. J Biol Response Mod 3:138–150
17. Oldham RK, Foon KA, Morgan AC, et al. (1984) Monoclonal antibody therapy of malignant melanoma: in vivo localization in cutaneous metastasis after intravenous administration. J Clin Oncol 2:1235–1244

18. Houghton AN, Mintzer D, Cordon-Cardo C, et al. (1985) Mouse monoclonal IgG$_3$ antibody detecting GD3 ganglioside: a phase I trial in patients with malignant melanoma. Proc Natl Acad Sci USA 82:1242–1246

19. Nadler L, Takvorian T, Botnick L, et al. (1984) Anti-B1 monoclonal antibody and complement treatment in autologous bone marrow transplantation for relapsed B cell non-Hodgkin's lymphoma. Lancet 2:427–443

20. Ritz J, Bast RC, Clavell LA, et al. (1982) Autologous bonemarrow transplantation in CALLA-positive acute lymphoblastic leukemia after in vivo treatment with J5 monoclonal antibody and complement. Lancet 2:60–63

21. Ramsay N, LeBien T, Nesbit M, et al. (1985) Autologous bonemarrow transplantation for patients with acute lymphoblastic leukemia after in vitro treatment with monoclonal antibodies BA-1, BA-2, and BA-3 plus complement. Blood 66:508

22. Foon KA, Bernhard MI, Oldham RK (1982) Monoclonal antibody therapy: Assessment by animal tumor models. J Biol Response Mod 1:277–304

23. Hwang KM, Foon KA, Cheung PH, Pearson JW, Oldham RK (1984) Selective antitumor effect of a potent immunoconjugate composed of the A chain of abrin and monoclonal antibody to a hepatoma-associated antigen. Cancer Res 44:4478–4486

24. Order SE, Klein JL, Ettinger D, et al. (1980) Use of isotopic immunoglobulin in therapy. Cancer Res 40:3001–3007

25. Leichner PK, Klein JL, Garrison SB, et al. (1981) Dosimetry of ^{131}I labeled antiferritin in hepatoma: a model for radioimmunoglobulin dosimetry. Int J Radiat Oncol Biol Phys 7:323–333

26. Leichner PK, Klein JL, Siegelman SS, et al. (1983) Dosimetry of ^{131}I labeled antiferritin in hepatoma: specific activities in the tumor and liver. Cancer Treat Rep 67:647–657

27. Ettinger DS, Order SE, Sharam MD, et al. (1982) Phase I–II study of isotopic immunoglobulin therapy for primary liver cancer. Cancer Treat Rep 66:289–297

28. Lenhard RE, Order SE Jr, Spunberg JJ, Asbell SO, Leibel SA (1985) Isotopic immunoglobulin: a new systemic therapy for advanced Hodgkin's disease. J Clin Oncol 3:1296–1300

29. Kirkwood JM, Ernstoff M (1984) Interferons in the treatment of human cancer. J Clin Oncol 2:336–352

30. Krown SE, Real FX, Cunningham-Rundles S (1983) Preliminary observations on the effect of recombinant leukocyte A interferon in homosexual men with Kaposi's sarcoma. N Engl J Med 308:1071–1076

31. Groopmen JE, Gottlieb MS, Goodman J, et al. (1984) Recombinant alpha-2 interferon therapy for Kaposi's sarcoma associated with the acquired immunodeficiency syndrome. Ann Intern Med 100:671–676

32. Gutterman JU, Blumenschein GR, Alexanian R, et al. (1980) Leukocyte interferon-induced tumor regression in human metastatic breast cancer, multiple myeloma, and malignant lymphoma. Ann Intern Med 93:399–406

33. Bordon EC, Holland JF, Dao TL, et al. (1982) Leukocyte-derived interferon (alpha) in human breast carcinoma. The American Cancer Society Phase II Trial. Ann Intern Med 97:1–6

34. Sherwin SA, Mayer D, Ochs J, et al. (1983) Recombinant leukocyte A interferon in advanced breast cancer. Ann Intern Med 98:598–602

35. Quesada JR, Swanson DA, Trindade A, et al. (1983) Renal cell carcinoma: antitumor effects of leukocyte interferon. Cancer Res 43:940–947

36. Cregan ET, Ahmann DL, Green SJ, Long HJ, Frytak S, Itri LM (1985) Phase II study of recombinant leukocyte A interferon (IFN-rA) plus cimetidine in disseminated malignant melanoma. J Clin Oncol 3:977

37. Kirkwood JM, Ernstoff MS, Davis CA, Reiss M, Ferraresi R, Rudnick SA (1985) Comparison of intramuscular and intravenous recombinant alpha-2 interferon in melanoma and other cancers. Ann Intern Med 103:32–36

38. Merigan TC, Sikora K, Breeden JH, Rosenberg SA (1978) Preliminary observations on the effect of human leukocyte interferon on non-Hodgkin's lymphoma. N Engl J Med 299:1449–1453

39. Louie AC, Gallagher JG, Sikora K, Levy R, Rosenberg SA, Merigan TC (1981) Followup observations on the effect of human leukocyte interferon on non-Hodgkin's lymphoma. Blood 58:712–718

40. Foon KA, Sherwin SA, Abrams PG, et al. (1984) Treatment of advanced non-Hodgkin's lymphoma with recombinant leukocyte A interferon. N Engl J Med 311:1148–1152

41. Bunn PA, Foon KA, Ihde DC, et al. (1984) Recombinant leukocyte A interferon: an active agent in advanced cutaneous T cell lymphoma. Ann Intern Med 109:484–487

42. Foon KA, Bottino GC, Abrams PG, et al. (1985) A phase II of recombinant interferon for patients with advanced chronic lymphocytic leukemia. Am J Med 78:216–220

43. Quesda JR, Reuben J, Manning JR, Hersh EM, Gutterman JU (1984) Alpha interferon

for induction of remission in hairy-cell leukemia. N Engl J Med 310:15–18

44. Ratain MJ, Golomb HM, Vardiman JW, Vokes EE, Jacobs RH, Daly K (1985) Treatment of hairy cell leukemia with recombinant alpha$_2$ interferon. Blood 65:644–648

45. Jacobs AD, Champlin RE, Golde DW (1985) Recombinant α-2-interferon for hairy cell leukemia. Blood 65:1017–1020

46. Foon KA, Maluish AE, Abrams PG, et al. (1986) Recombinant leukocyte A interferon therapy for advanced hairy cell leukemia: therapeutic and immunologic results. Am J Med 80:351–356

47. Talpaz M, McCredie KB, Mavligit GM, Gutterman JU (1983) Leukocyte interferon-induced myeloid cytoreduction in chronic myelogenous leukemia. Blood 72:689–692

Haematology and Blood Transfusion   Vol. 31
Modern Trends in Human Leukemia VII
Edited by Neth, Gallo, Greaves, and Kabisch
© Springer-Verlag Berlin Heidelberg 1987

IL-2 Receptors in Adult T-Cell Leukemia:
A Target for Immunotherapy

T. A. Waldmann, R. W. Kozak, M. Tsudo, T. Oh-ishi, K. F. Bongiovanni, and C. K. Goldman

A. Introduction

The induction of a T-cell immune response to a foreign antigen requires the activation of T-lymphocytes that is initiated by the interaction of the T-cell antigen receptor with antigen presented in the context of products of the major histocompatibility locus and the macrophage-derived interleukin-1. Following this interaction, T cells express the gene encoding the lymphokine interleukin-2 (IL-2) [1, 2]. To exert its biological effect, IL-2 must interact with specific high-affinity membrane receptors. Resting T cells do not express IL-2 receptors, but receptors are rapidly expressed on T cells after activation with an antigen or mitogen [3–5]. Thus, the growth factor IL-2 and its receptor are absent in resting T cells, but after activation the genes for both proteins become expressed.

Progress in the analysis of the structure, function, and expression of the human IL-2 receptor was greatly facilitated by the production of the anti-Tac monoclonal antibody that recognizes the human receptor for IL-2 [6–8] and blocks the binding of IL-2 to this receptor.

Using quantitative receptor binding studies employing radiolabeled anti-Tac and radiolabeled IL-2, it was shown that activated T cells and IL-2 dependent T-cell lines express 5- to 20-fold more binding sites for the Tac antibody than for IL-2 [9, 10]. Employing high concentrations of IL-2, Robb et al. [11] resolved these differences by demonstrating two affinity classes of IL-2 receptors. One had a binding affinity for IL-2 in the range of 10^{-11}–10^{12} M, whereas the remaining receptors bound IL-2 at a much lower affinity, approximately 10^{-8} or 10^{-9} M. The high-affinity receptors appear to mediate the physiologic responses to IL-2, since the magnitude of cell responses is closely correlated with the occupancy of these receptors. As outlined below, the anti-Tac monoclonal antibody has been utilized to: (a) characterize the human receptor for IL-2; (b) molecularly clone cDNAs for the human IL-2 receptor; (c) analyze disorders of IL-2 receptor expression on leukemic cells; and (d) develop protocols for the therapy of patients with IL-2 receptor-expressing adult T-cell leukemia and autoimmune disorders, and for individuals receiving organ allografts.

B. Chemical Characterization of the IL-2 Receptor

Using the anti-Tac monoclonal antibody, the IL-2 binding receptor on phytohemagglutinin (PHA)-activated normal lymphocytes was shown to be a 55-kd glycoprotein [7, 8]. Leonard and coworkers [7, 8] showed that the IL-2 receptor is composed of a 33-kd peptide precursor that is cotranslationally N-glycosylated to 35-kd and 37-kd forms and then θ-glycosylated to the 55-kd mature form. Furthermore, the IL-2 receptor was shown to be sulfated [12] and phosphorylated on a serine residue [13].

There are a series of unresolved questions concerning the IL-2 receptor that are diffi-

Metabolism Branch, National Cancer Institute, National Institutes of Health, Bethesda, Maryland 20892, USA

cult to answer when only the 55-kd Tac peptide is considered. These questions include: (a) what is the structural explanation for the great difference in affinity between high- and low-affinity receptors; (b) how, in light of the short cytoplasmic tail of 13 amino acids (see below), are the receptor signals transduced to the nucleus; and (c) how do certain Tac-negative cells (e.g., natural killer cells) make nonproliferative responses to IL-2? To address these questions, we have investigated the possibility that the IL-2 receptor is a complex receptor with multiple peptides in addition to the one identified by anti-Tac. A leukemic T-cell line was identified that binds IL-2 yet does not bind four different antibodies (including anti-Tac and 7G7) that react with the Tac peptide. This cell line manifests 6800 receptors per cell with an affinity of 14 nM (Tsudo, Kozak, Goldman, and Waldmann, unpublished observations). On the basis of cross-linking studies using [^{125}I]IL-2, this IL-2-binding receptor peptide was shown to be larger than the Tac peptide with an approximate M_r of 75000. When similar cross-linking studies were performed on human T-lymphotrophic virus I (HTLV-I)-induced T-cell lines (e.g., HUT 102) that manifest both high- and low-affinity receptors, IL-2 binding peptides of both 55 kd and 75 kd were demonstrated.

C. Molecular Cloning of cDNAs for the Human 55-kd Tac IL-2 Receptor Peptide

Three groups [14–17] have succeeded in cloning cDNAs for the IL-2 receptor protein. The deduced amino acid sequence of the IL-2 receptor indicates that this peptide is composed of 251 amino acids and a 21-amino acid signal peptide. The receptor contains two potential N-linked glycosylation sites and multiple possible 0-linked carbohydrate sites. Finally, there is a single hydrophobic membrane region of 19 amino acids and a very short (13-amino acid) cytoplasmic domain. Potential phosphate acceptor sites (serine and threonine, but not tyrosine) are present within the intracytoplasmic domain. However, the cytoplasmic domain of the IL-2 receptor peptide identified by anti-Tac appears to be too small for enzymatic

function. Thus, this receptor differs from other known growth factor receptors that have large intracytoplasmic domains with tyrosine kinase activity. Leonard and co-workers [15] have demonstrated that the single gene encoding the IL-2 receptor consists of eight exons on chromosome 10p14. However, mRNAs of two different sizes approximately 1500 and 3500 bases long have been identified. These classes of mRNA differ because of the utilization of two or more polyadenylation signals [14]. Receptor gene transcription is initiated at two principal sites in normal activated T-lymphocytes [15]. Furthermore, sequence analyses of the cloned DNAs also indicate that alternative messenger RNA splicing may delete a 216-base pair segment in the center of the protein coding sequence encoded by the fourth exon [14, 15]. Using expression studies of cDNAs in COS-1 cells, Leonard and coworkers [14] demonstrated that the unspliced but not the spliced form of the mRNA was translated into the cell surface receptor that binds IL-2 and the anti-Tac monoclonal antibody.

D. Distribution of IL-2 Receptors

As discussed above, the majority of resting T cells, B cells, or macrophages in the circulation do not display IL-2 receptors. Specifically, less than 5% of freshly isolated, unstimulated human peripheral blood T-lymphocytes react with the anti-Tac monoclonal antibody. The majority of T-lymphocytes, however, can be induced to express IL-2 receptors by interaction with lectins, monoclonal antibodies to the T-cell antigen receptor complex, or alloantigen stimulation. Furthermore, IL-2 receptors have also been demonstrated on activated B-lymphocytes [18, 19].

Rubin, Nelson, and their coworkers [20] have demonstrated that in addition to cellular IL-2 receptors, activated normal peripheral blood mononuclear cells and certain lines of T- and B-cell origin release a soluble form of the IL-2 receptor into the culture medium. Using an enzyme-linked immunoabsorbent assay, which employs two monoclonal antibodies that recognize distinct epitopes on the human IL-2 receptor, it was shown that normal individuals have measurable amounts of IL-2 receptors in their plasma and that certain lymphoreticular malignancies are associated with elevated plasma levels of this receptor. The release of soluble IL-2 receptors appears to be a consequence of cellular activation of a variety of cell types that may play a role in the regulation of the immune response. Furthermore, the analysis of plasma levels of IL-2 receptors may provide an important new approach to the analysis of lymphocyte activation in vivo.

E. Disorders of IL-2 Expression in Adult T-Cell Leukemia

A distinct form of mature T-cell leukemia was defined by Takasuki and coworkers [21] and termed adult T-cell leukemia (ATL). ATL is a malignant proliferation of mature T cells that have a propensity to infiltrate the skin. Cases of ATL are associated with hypercalcemia and have a very aggressive course in most cases. They are clustered within families and geographically, occurring in the southwest of Japan, the Caribbean basin, and in certain areas of Africa. Human T-cell lymphotrophic virus I has been shown to be a primary etiologic agent in ATL [22]. All the populations of leukemic cells we have examined from patients with HTLV-I-associated ATL expressed the Tac antigen [23]. The expression of IL-2 receptors on ATL cells differs from that of normal T cells. First, unlike normal T cells, ATL cells do not require prior activation to express IL-2 receptors. Furthermore, when a ^{3}H-labeled anti-Tac receptor assay was used, HTLV-I-infected leukemic T-cell lines characteristically expressed five- to tenfold more receptors per cell (270 000–1 000 000) than did maximally PHA-stimulated T-lymphoblasts (30 000–60 000). In addition, whereas normal human T-lymphocytes maintained in culture with IL-2 demonstrate a rapid decline in receptor number, adult ATL lines do not show a similar decline. Leonard et al. [12] and Wano et al. [24] also demonstrated that some but not all HTLV-I-infected cell lines display aberrantly sized IL-2 receptors owing to differences in glycosylation. It is conceivable that the con-

stant presence of high numbers of IL-2 receptors on ATL cells and/or the aberrancy of these receptors may play a role in the pathogenesis of uncontrolled growth of these malignant T cells.

As noted above, T-cell leukemias caused by HTLV-I, as well as all T-cell and B-cell lines infected with HTLV-I, universally express large numbers of IL-2 receptors. An analysis of this virus and its protein products suggests a potential mechanism for this association between HTLV-I and IL-2 receptor expression. In addition to the presence of typical long-terminal repeats (LTRs), gag, pol, and env genes, and retroviral gene sequences common to other groups of retroviruses, HTLV-I and HTLV-II contain an additional genomic region between env and the LTR referred to as pX or more recently as tat. Sodroski and colleagues [25] demonstrated that this pX or tat region encodes a 42-kd protein, now termed the tat protein, that is essential for viral replication. These authors demonstrated that the tat protein acts on a receptor region within the LTRs of HTLV-I and -II, stimulating transcription. Greene and co-workers [26] have demonstrated that this tat protein could also play a central role in directly or indirectly increasing the transcription of host genes such as the IL-2 receptor gene involved in T-cell activation and HTLV-I-mediated T-cell leukemogenesis.

F. The IL-2 Receptor as a Target for Therapy in Patients with ATL and Patients with Autoimmune Disorders, and Individuals Receiving Organ Allografts

The observation that ATL cells constitutively express large numbers of IL-2 receptors identified by the anti-Tac monoclonal antibody, whereas normal resting cells and their precursors do not, provides the scientific basis for therapeutic trials using agents to eliminate the IL-2 receptor-expressing cells. The agents that have been used or are being prepared include: (a) unmodified anti-Tac monoclonal; (b) toxin (e.g., Pseudomonas toxin) conjugates of anti-Tac; and (c) conjugates of alpha-emitting isotopes (e.g., ^{212}Bis) with anti-Tac.

We initiated a clinical trial to evaluate the efficacy of intravenously administering anti-Tac monoclonal antibody in the treatment of patients with ATL [27]. None of the five patients treated suffered any untoward reactions and none produced antibodies to the mouse immunoglobulin or to the idiotype of the anti-Tac monoclonal antibody. Three of the patients with a very rapidly developing form of ATL had a very transient response. Two of the patients had a temporary partial or complete remission following anti-Tac therapy. In one of these patients, therapy was followed by a 5-month remission, as assessed by routine hematologic tests, immunofluorescence analysis of circulating T cells, and molecular genetic analysis of arrangement of the genes encoding the β-chain of the T-cell antigen receptor. After the 5-month remission, the patient's disease relapsed, but a new course of anti-Tac infusions was followed by a virtual disappearance of skin lesions and an over 80% reduction in the number of circulating leukemic cells. Two months later, leukemic cells were again demonstrable in the circulation. At this time, although the leukemic cells remained Tac-positive and bound anti-Tac in vivo, the leukemia was no longer responsive to infusions of anti-Tac and the patient required chemotherapy. This patient may have had the smoldering form of ATL initially when he responded to anti-Tac therapy wherein the leukemic T cells may still require IL-2 for their proliferation. Alternatively, the clinical responses may have been mediated by host cytotoxic cells reacting with the tumor cells bearing the anti-Tac mouse immunoglobulin on their surface by such mechanisms as antibody-dependent cellular cytotoxicity.

These therapeutic studies have been extended in vitro by examining the ability of toxins coupled to anti-Tac to selectively inhibit protein synthesis and viability of Tac-positive ATL lines. The addition of anti-Tac antibody coupled to *Pseudomonas* exotoxin inhibited protein synthesis by Tac-expressing HUT 102-B2 cells, but not that by the Tac-negative acute T-cell line MOLT-4, which does not express the Tac antigen [28].

The action of toxin conjugates of monoclonal antibodies depends on their ability to be internalized by the cell and released into the cytoplasm. Anti-Tac bound to IL-2 receptors on leukemic cells is internalized slowly into coated pits and then endosomic vesicles. Furthermore, the toxin conjugate does not pass easily from the endosome to the cytosol, as is required for its action. To circumvent these limitations, an alternative cytotoxic reagent was developed that could be conjugated to anti-Tac and that was effective when bound to the surface of leukemic cells. It was shown that ^{212}Bi, an alpha-emitting radionuclide conjugated to anti-Tac by use of a bifunctional chelate, was well suited for this role [29]. Activity levels of 0.5 μCi or the equivalent of 12 rad/ml of alpha radiation targeted by ^{212}Bi-anti-Tac eliminated over 98% of the proliferative capacity of the HUT 102-B2 cells, with only a modest effect on IL-2 receptor-negative lines. This specific cytotoxicity was blocked by excess unlabeled anti-Tac, but not by human IgG. Thus, ^{212}Bi-anti-Tac is a potentially effective and specific immunocytotoxic agent for the elimination of IL-2 receptor-positive cells.

In addition to being used in the therapy of patients with ATL, antibodies to the IL-2 receptors are being evaluated as potential therapeutic agents to eliminate activated IL-2 receptor-expressing T cells in other clinical states, including certain autoimmune disorders and in protocols involving organ allografts. The rationale for the use of anti-Tac in patients with aplastic anemia is derived from the work of Zoumbos and coworkers [30], who have demonstrated that select patients with aplastic anemia have increased numbers of circulating Tac-positive cells. In this group of patients, the Tac-positive but not Tac-negative T cells were shown to inhibit hematopoiesis when cocultured with normal bone marrow cells. Furthermore, we have demonstrated that anti-Tac inhibits the generation of activated suppressor T cells (Oh-ishi and Waldmann, unpublished observations). Studies have been initiated to define the value of anti-Tac in the therapy of patients with aplastic anemia. The rationale for the use of an antibody to IL-2 receptors in recipients of renal and cardiac allografts is that anti-Tac inhibits the proliferation of T cells to foreign histocompatibility antigens expressed on the donor organs and prevents the generation of cytotoxic T cells in allogeneic cell cocultures. Furthermore, in studies by Strom and coworkers [31], the survival of renal and cardiac allografts was prolonged in rodent recipients treated with an anti-IL-2 receptor monoclonal antibody. Thus, the development of monoclonal antibodies directed toward the IL-2 receptor expressed on ATL cells, on autoreactive T cells of certain patients with autoimmune disorders, and on host T cells responding to foreign histocompatibility antigens on organ allografts may permit the development of rational new therapeutic approaches in these clinical conditions.

References

1. Morgan DA, Ruscetti FW, Gallo RC (1976) Selective in vitro growth of T lymphocytes from normal human bone marrows. Science 193:1007–1008
2. Smith KA (1980) T-cell growth factor. Immunol Rev 51:337–357
3. Robb RJ, Munck A, Smith KA (1981) T-cell growth factors: quantification, specificity, and biological relevance. J Exp Med 154:1455–1474
4. Greene WC, Leonard WJ, Depper JM (1985) Growth of human T lymphocytes: an analysis of IL-2 and the IL-2 receptor. In: Brown E (ed) Progress in hematology, vol XIV. Grune and Stratton, New York, pp 283–301
5. Waldmann TA (1986) The structure, function, and expression of interleukin-2 receptors on normal and malignant T cells. Science 232:727–732
6. Uchiyama T, Broder S, Waldmann TA (1981) A monoclonal antibody (anti-Tac) reactive with activated and functionally mature human T cells. J Immunol 126:1393–1397
7. Leonard WJ, Depper JM, Uchiyama T, Smith KA, Waldmann TA, Greene WC (1982) A monoclonal antibody that appears to recognize the receptor for human T cell growth factor: partial characterization of the receptor. Nature 300:267–269
8. Leonard WJ, Depper JM, Robb RJ, Waldmann TA, Greene WC (1983) Characterization of the human receptor for T cell growth factor. Proc Natl Acad Sci USA 80:6957–6961
9. Depper JM, Leonard WJ, Krönke M, Waldmann TA, Greene WC (1984) Augmentation of T-cell growth factor expression in HTLV-I-infected human leukemic T cells. J Immunol 133:1691–1695
10. Depper JM, Leonard WJ, Krönke M, Noguchi P, Cunningham R, Waldmann TA, Greene WC (1984) Regulation of interleukin-2 receptor expression: effects of phorbol diester, phospholipase C, and reexposure to lectin and antigen. J Immunol 133:3054–3061
11. Robb RJ, Greene WC, Rusk CM (1984) Low and high affinity cellular receptors for interleukin 2: implications for the level of Tac antigen. J Exp Med 160:1126–1146
12. Leonard WJ, Depper JM, Waldmann TA, Greene WC (1984) A monoclonal antibody to the human receptor for T cell growth factor. In: Greaves M (ed) Receptors and recognition, vol 17. Chapman and Hall, London, pp 45–46
13. Shackelford DA, Trowbridge IS (1984) Induction of expression and phosphorylation of the human interleukin-2 receptor by a phorbol diester. J Biol Chem 259:11706–11712
14. Leonard WJ, Depper JM, Crabtree GR, Rudikoff S, Pumphrey J, Robb RJ, Krönke M, Svetlik PB, Peffer NJ, Waldmann TA, Greene WC (1984) Molecular cloning and expression of cDNAs for the human interleukin-2 receptor. Nature 311:626–631
15. Leonard WJ, Depper JM, Krönke M, Peffer NJ, Svetlik PB, Sullivan M, Greene WC (1985) Structure of the human interleukin-2 gene. Science 230:633–639
16. Cosman D, Cerretti DP, Larsen A, Park L, March C, Dower S, Gillis S, Urdal D (1984) Cloning, sequence and expression of human interleukin-2 receptor. Nature 312:768–771
17. Nikaido T, Shimizu N, Ishida N, Sabe H, Teshigawara K, Maeda M, Uchiyama T, Yodor S, Honjo T (1984) Molecular cloning of cDNA encoding human interleukin-2 receptor. Nature 311:631–635
18. Waldmann TA, Goldman CK, Robb RJ, Depper JM, Leonard WJ, Sharrow SO, Bongiovanni KF, Korsmeyer SJ, Greene WC (1984) Expression of IL-2 receptors on activated human B-cells. J Exp Med 160:1450–1466
19. Tsudo M, Uchiyama T, Uchino H (1984) Expression of Tac antigen on activated normal human B cells. J Exp Med 160:612–617
20. Rubin LA, Kurman CC, Biddison WE, Goldman ND, Nelson DL (1985) A monoclonal antibody 7G7/B6 binds to an epitope on the human interleukin-2 (IL-2) receptor that is distinct from that recognized by IL-2 or anti-Tac. Hybridoma 4:91–102
21. Takasuki K, Uchiyama T, Sagawa K, Yodoi J (1977) Adult T cell leukemia in Japan. In: Seno S, Takaku F, Irino S (eds) Topics in hematology. Excerpta Medica, Amsterdam, p 73–74

22. Poiesz BJ, Ruscetti FW, Gazdar AF, Bunn PA, Minna JD, Gallo RC (1980) Detection and isolation of type-C retrovirus particles from fresh and cultured lymphocytes of a patient with cutaneous T-cell lymphoma. Proc Natl Acad Sci USA 77:7415–7419

23. Waldmann TA, Greene WC, Sarin PS, Saxinger C, Blayney W, Blattner WA, Goldman CK, Bongiovanni K, Sharrow S, Depper JM, Leonard W, Uchiyama T, Gallo RC (1984) Functional and phenotypic comparison of human T cell leukemia/lymphoma virus positive adult T cell leukemia with human T cell leukemia/lymphoma virus negative Sézary leukemia. J Clin Invest 73:1711–1718

24. Wano Y, Uchiyama T, Fukui K, Maeda M, Ucheno H, Yodoi J (1984) Characterization of human interleukin-2 receptor (Tac expression) in normal and leukemic T-cells: coexpression of normal and azerrant receptor in HUT 102 cells. J Immunol 132:3005–3010

25. Sodroski JG, Rosen CA, Haseltine WA (1984) Trans-acting transcriptional activation of the long terminal repeat of human T-lymphotrophic viruses in infected cells. Science 225:381–385

26. Greene WC, Leonard WJ, Wano Y, Sekaly RP, Long EO, Sodroski JG, Rosen LA, Haseltine WA (1976) The transactivator (*tat*) gene of the human T lymphotrophic virus type II (HTLV-II) induces interleukin-2 receptor, interleukin-2 and Ia cellular gene expression. Clin Res 34:669A

27. Waldmann TA, Longo DL, Leonard WJ, Depper JM, Thompson CB, Krönke M, Goldman CK, Sharrow S, Bongiovanni K, Greene WC (1985) Interleukin-2 receptor (Tac antigen) expression in HTLV-I associated adult T-cell leukemia. Cancer Res 45:4559S–4562S

28. FitzGerald D, Waldmann TA, Willingham MC, Pastan I (1984) Pseudomonas exotoxin-anti-Tac: Cell specific immunotoxin, active against cells expressing the T-cell growth factor receptor. J Clin Invest 74:966–971

29. Kozak RW, Atcher RW, Gansow OA, Friedman AM, Waldmann TA (1986) Bismuth-212 labeled anti-Tac monoclonal antibody: alpha-particle emitting radionuclides as novel modalities for radioimmunotherapy. Proc Natl Acad Sci USA 83:474–478

30. Zoumbos NC, Gascon P, Djeu J, Trost SR, Young N (1985) Circulating activated suppressor T lymphocytes in aplastic anemia. N Engl J Med 312:257–265

31. Strom TB, Banet LV, Gauiton GN, Kelley VG, Thier AY, Diamanstein T, Tilney NL, Kirkman RL (1985) Prolongation of cardiac allograft survival in rodent recipients treated with an anti-interleukin-2 receptor monoclonal antibody. Cancer Res 33:561A

Haematology and Blood Transfusion   Vol. 31
Modern Trends in Human Leukemia VII
Edited by Neth, Gallo, Greaves, and Kabisch
© Springer-Verlag Berlin Heidelberg 1987

Application of Interleukin 2 in Neuroblastoma

R. Handgretinger[1], G. Bruchelt[1], M. Schneider[2], D. Niethammer[1], and J. Treuner[1]

A. Introduction

Neuroblastoma is one of the most common solid tumors in childhood, with some unusual neoplastic behavior depending on the age of the affected children. Patients older than 1 year who have metastatic disease have a very poor prognosis. However, in children younger than 1 year who have disseminated disease, regression of neuroblastoma often occurs after only minimal therapy, or even spontaneously. This latter feature and other observations led to longstanding speculations that cytotoxic effector cells of the tumor-bearing host may contribute to this biological behavior of human neuroblastoma [1]. Recently, Main et al. [2] published data concerning the interaction of human neuroblastoma cell lines with effector cells. They demonstrated that the neuroblastoma cell lines CHP 100 and CHP 126 were lysed by natural killer (NK) cells but not by cytotoxic T-lymphocytes [2]. This was interpreted as a consequence of the weak expression of HLA class-I antigens on neuroblastoma cells [3].

In this study we examined whether other neuroblastoma cell lines are susceptible targets for effector cells from healthy individuals and from patients with neuroblastoma. Since Interleukin 2 (IL-2) has considerable stimulating activity on the cytotoxic functions of lymphocytes, we further investigated whether IL-2 can also stimulate the cytotoxic effects of lymphocytes against the neuroblastoma targets. We next addressed the question of whether the concept of the recently described adoptive immunotransfer of lymphokine-activated killer (LAK) cells as an alternative or additional approach to cancer therapy may also be a new therapeutic approach in human neuroblastoma [4]. Since this requires large amounts of cytotoxic lymphocytes, we tried to optimize the conditions for the in vitro generation of activated killer cells using only IL-2.

B. Materials and Methods

I. Isolation and Preincubation of Effector Cells with IL-2

Peripheral mononuclear blood cells (MNBC) from healthy individuals and from children with neuroblastoma before therapy were isolated by Ficoll-Hypaque gradients. Cells were incubated in a 5% CO_2 incubator at 37 °C for 3 days in RPMI 1640 culture medium, supplemented with either 10% heat-inactivated human AB serum or 10% heat-inactivated fetal calf serum (FCS) in the presence or absence of the indicated concentrations of recombinant IL-2 (rIL-2, Biogen).

II. Cultivation of Lymphocytes with rIL-2

For cultivation of lymphocytes, RPMI 1640 culture medium supplemented with 10% AB serum was used. After isolation, lympho-

---

[1] Universitätskinderklinik, Abtlg. Hämatologie und Onkologie, Rümelinstrasse 19–23, 7400 Tübingen, FRG
[2] Medizinische Universitätsklinik, Otfried Müller Strasse 10, 7400 Tübingen, FRG

cytes were seeded at $3–5 \times 10^5$ cells/ml in the presence of 100 U/ml rIL-2. Fresh culture medium and rIL-2 were added every 3–4 days, and cell concentration was readjusted to 3×10^5 cells/ml.

III. Target Cells

Four established neuroblastoma cell lines with different biological features were used: The well differentiated SK-N-SH, which is dopamine-β-hydroxylase positive and has no N-myc amplification, the only weakly differentiated SK-N-LO, the IMR-5, which has N-myc amplification, and the SK-N-MC, with cholinergic features. For measuring NK activity, the NK-sensitive erythroleukemic cell line K 562 was used.

IV. Proliferation of Lymphocytes

Proliferation of MNBC cultured with different concentrations of rIL-2 for 6 days was quantified with the MTT-proliferation assay [5].

V. Determination of Cell Surface Markers

Lymphocytes were stained with the monoclonal antibodies OKT-3(CD3), OKT-4(CD4), OKT-8 (CD8), Leu-11(CD16), and anti-IL-2 receptor mAb Tü 69(CD25) and were analyzed with a FACS analyzer.

VI. Chromium 51-Release Assay of Cytotoxicity

Briefly, 1×10^6 target cells were labeled with 100 µCi ^{51}Cr for 1 hour, washed, and adjusted to 5×10^4 cells/ml. Aliquots of 0.1 ml were added in triplicates to the effector cells and incubated for 4 hours.

C. Results and Discussion

I. Preincubation of Effector Cells with rIL-2 Stimulates the Cytotoxicity Against Neuroblastoma Targets

MNBC from healthy individuals were preincubated with 100 U/ml rIL-2 for 3 days.

Controls consisted of MNBC cultured only in culture medium. Since it is known that FCS may contain some unspecific lymphocyte-stimulating factors, we additionally compared the influence of culturing the MNBC for 3 days in either 10% FCS or 10% AB serum in the absence of rIL-2. There was a significant difference in the spontaneous cytotoxicity of the effector cells against the neuroblastoma targets. MNBC cultured in RPMI 1640–10% FCS consistently became more cytotoxic compared with the effector cells cultured in RPMI 1640–10% AB serum, which showed only modest or no detectable cytotoxicity against the neuroblastoma cells. However, preincubation of the MNBC with 100 U/ml rIL-2 for 3 days resulted in a considerable augmentation of their cytotoxicity against all four neuroblastoma targets. Figure 1 summarizes the results of these experiments. Since preincubation of MNBC in culture medium supplemented with FCS can stimulate the cytotoxicity of lymphocytes through factors present in FCS, and this may therefore mimic an NK sensitivity of target cells, all further experiments were performed in culture medium supplemented with 10% AB serum.

II. Influence of rIL-2 on Effector Cells from Patients with Neuroblastoma

We next investigated whether rIL-2 can also augment the cytotoxicity of lymphocytes isolated from patients with neuroblastoma before therapy. As shown in Table 1, preincubation of MNBC from all patients with rIL-2 for 3 days resulted in a considerable augmentation of the cytotoxicity of the effector cells against the neuroblastoma targets and against the K 562. Unstimulated effector cells showed almost no detectable cytotoxicity against all targets.

III. Proliferation of MNBC in rIL-2

MNBC were incubated with various concentrations of rIL-2 for 6 days. The optimal conditions for inducing proliferation of MNBC were obtained in the presence of 100 U/ml rIL-2 in the culture medium.

117

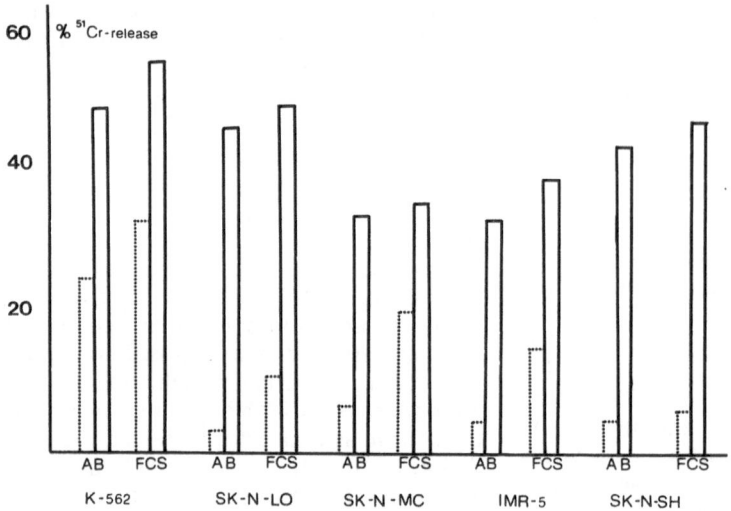

Fig. 1. Susceptibility of different human neuroblastoma cell lines and K 562 as targets for MNBC from healthy individuals preincubated for 3 days with (☐) or without (▒) IL-2. Culture medium was supplemented with either 10% AB serum (*AB*) or 10% fetal calf serum (*FCS*). E:T-ratio = 10:1

Table 1. Percent of specific [51]-Cr-release after 3-day incubation of MNBC with and without IL-2 (E:T = 10:1)

Patient	Target cells							
	SK-N-LO		SK-N-MC		IMR-5		K 562	
	0	100 IL-2	0	100 IL-2	0	100 IL-2	0	100 IL-2
1	0.3% → 54.1%		–		−0.3% → 66.3%		1.4% → 66.6%	
2	–		2.2% → 36.2%		–		3.1% → 30.7%	
3	1.8% → 30.3%		−1.4% → 18.1%		–		5.8% → 36.7%	
4	–		1.1% → 21.9%		–		1.7% → 18.5%	
Healthy person	–		0.9% → 26.1%		–		11.2% → 48.3%	

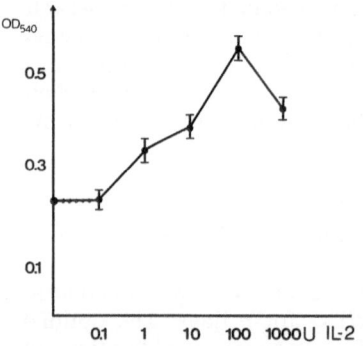

Fig. 2. Proliferation kinetics of MNBC after 6 days' culture with different amounts of IL-2

Higher or lower concentrations of rIL-2 resulted in a lower proliferation rate of lymphocytes, as shown in Fig. 2.

IV. Cultivated Lymphocytes Retain Their Cytotoxic Potential

MNBC from patients with neuroblastoma were cultured in the presence of 100 U/ml rIL-2. Generally, lymphocytes started to proliferate after about 6 days. Starting with 1×10^6 MNBC, about 30×10^6 lymphocytes were obtained after 10–12 days. Cultured lymphocytes were still capable of killing both the neuroblastoma targets and the K 562 cells to the same degree as after 3 days incubation with 100 U/ml rIL-2. After 12–16 days in continuous culture in the presence of 100 U/ml rIL-2, lymphocytes stopped proliferating and started to disintegrate. However, when the rIL-2 concentration was reduced or omitted for a short period at this point, a following restimulation of MNBC with the original rIL-2 concentration resulted in further proliferation. In this way, prolonged survival of cultured lymphocytes for up to 30 days was possible. Surface marker analysis of the cultured lymphocytes revealed only minimal or no expression of T cell markers or NK cell markers. The phenotype of these cells has still to be determined.

In summary, we showed that the four investigated neuroblastoma cell lines are only weakly susceptible targets for spontaneous cell-mediated cytotoxicity by unstimulated MNBC. Preincubation of MNBC with rIL-2 for 3 days, however, resulted in a strong stimulation of their cytotoxicity against the neuroblastoma targets. Furthermore, it is possible to cultivate MNBC for certain periods of time using rIL-2 alone while retaining their cytotoxic potential. It still has to be tested whether MNBC from patients with neuroblastoma activated with IL-2 are also capable of killing autologous neuroblastoma cells. If this is the case, treatment of these patients with IL-2 and the immunotransfer of lymphokine-activated killer cells could be a new therapeutic approach to neuroblastoma, serving as an adjunct to conventional therapy.

References

1. Bill AH, Morgan A (1970) Evidence for immune reaction to neuroblastoma and future possibilities for investigation. J Pediatr Surg 5:111
2. Main EJ, Lampson LA, Hart MK, Kornbluth J, Wilson DB (1985) Human neuroblastoma cell lines are susceptible to lysis by natural killer cells but not by cytotoxic T lymphocytes. J Immunol 135:242
3. Lampson LA, Fisher CA, Whelan JP (1983) Striking paucity of HLA-A,B,C and β_2-microglobulin on human neuroblastoma cell lines. J Immunol 130:2471
4. Rosenberg SA (1985) Lymphokine-activated killer cells: a new approach to immunotherapy of cancer. JNCI 75:595
5. Mosmann T (1983) Rapid colorimetric assay for cellular growth and survival: application to proliferation and cytotoxicity assays. J Immunol Methods 65:55

Haematology and Blood Transfusion   Vol. 31
Modern Trends in Human Leukemia VII
Edited by Neth, Gallo, Greaves, and Kabisch
© Springer-Verlag Berlin Heidelberg 1987

Biologic Agents for the Management of Hematological Disorders: Chronic Myeloid Leukemia

K. B. McCredie[1], M. Talpaz[2], H. Kantarjian[1], M. Rosenblum[2], M. Keating[1], and J. Gutterman[2]

Biological materials, either alone or in combination with cancer chemotherapeutic agents, have been used in treatment for almost 20 years. Initially, agents such as BCG, pseudomonas vaccine, and MER were used in the hopes of enhancing normal immunity and retarding the proliferation of neoplastic cells. In addition, it was felt that these agents might enhance the production of normal hematopoiesis, allowing for early bone marrow recovery and thus enabling increasing doses of chemotherapy to be administered with lower toxicity and a consequent reduction in morbidity and mortality. A number of studies from many institutions using this approach showed a prolongation of complete remission, particularly in leukemia, but there was no clearcut increase in the percentage of patients cured. Additional studies of solid tumors, particularly breast cancer and small-cell carcinoma of the lung, produced similar but less convincing data. No long-term benefit was obtained as related to freedom from disease and eventual survival.

The 1980s have been associated with a rapid increase in the development of naturally occurring compounds that control different aspects of proliferation, differentiation, and immunity (biological response modifiers).

Interferon has long been recognized as the body's front-line defense against viruses. Commercially, it was initially prepared from leukocytes by the Finnish Red Cross for clinical trial. The success of the osteogenic sarcoma program in Sweden led in the early 1980s to a more widespread investigation of human leukocyte interferon. Responses were seen particularly in patients with hairy cell leukemia, renal cell carcinoma, and chronic granulocytic leukemia.

Developed in parallel with the use of the crude interferon preparations, a number of companies, using cloning techniques, have been able to produce purified preparations of alpha, beta, and gamma interferon, and these materials are undergoing extensive clinical trials throughout the world (Table 1).

A number of other materials are now becoming available for clinical testing. Tumor

[1,2] Departments of Hematology and of Clinical Immunology and Biological Therapy, The University of Texas M.D. Anderson Hospital and Tumor Institute, 6723 Bertner Avenue, Houston, Texas 77030, USA

Table 1. Results of clinical investigations of alpha interferon

Sensitive Tumors
Remission rate 75%–90%
Hairy cell leukemia
Cutaneous T-cell lymphoma
Chronic myeloid leukemia
Remission rate 40%–50%
Kaposi's sarcoma
Nodular poorly differentiated lymphoma
Moderately sensitive tumors
Remission rate 20%–30%
Renal cell carcinoma
Multiple myeloma
Relatively resistant tumors
Lung cancer

necrosis factor has advanced to combination clinical trials in a number of centers. Future use of these materials either singly, in combination, or in combination with chemotherapy or other modalities of therapy would add a significant number of new methods for better biological control of tumor proliferation over the next few years. Following is a list of biological agents that are currently used in clinical practice:

Human leukocyte interferon
Alpha recombinant interferon
Gamma recombinant interferon
Tumor necrosis factor
Interleukin 2
Granulocyte-macrophage colony-stimulating factor
Pluripoitin and pluripoitin A
Antidiotypic antibodies

For a number of years we have been investigating the use of the various interferons as a modality of therapy for patients with chronic granulocytic leukemia. The initial studies were done [1] with human leukocyte alpha interferon given intramuscularly to a series of seven patients. Hematological remission obtained in five patients was associated with reduction of their white cell count from an average of 97 to an average of $4.2 \times 10^3/ml^3$. Associated with this fall in peripheral white cell count was normalization of the platelet count and the serum B-12 and LDH levels. Enlarged spleens, seen in half the patients, became smaller again. These patients continued to respond to treatment and showed reduction in the number of cells containing the Philadelphia (Ph) chromosome.

These studies were subsequently extended to use the human recombinant interferon alpha-A in chronic myeloid leukemia (CML) in 17 patients [2]; of these, eight showed hematological remission with cytogenic improvement, five showed hematological remission without cytogenic improvement, and one patient had a partial hematological improvement. Three patients were considered treatment failures, either because of toxic reactions to interferon or because the interferon failed to control the disease [1]. The disappearance of cells containing the translocation and the return of cells of normal karyotype was encouraging. Results of preliminary studies with probes related to the abnormal protein production seen in the Ph-positive leukemias suggest that the abnormal protein and abnormal gene expression disappeared in patients who became Ph negative.

The study has now been extended to 51 patients with previously untreated or minimally treated benign-phase chronic granulocytic leukemia. Eighty percent of the patients demonstrated a response; 71% obtained a complete hematological remission as judged by the criteria previously reported. More than half of the patients showed a reduction in the number of chromosomes. These changes have persisted for periods of 30 or more months, and there appears to be continuing reduction in the Ph-positive metaphases seen over time in these patients. They have been followed up for longer than 2 years, and 28 remain in continued disease-free control on the therapy. The current projected 3-year survival rate is 74% [2].

Risk factors have been defined from our past experience in treating patients with chronic granulocytic leukemia, and these include such adverse blood and bone marrow parameters as anemia with thrombocytosis or thrombopenia, a high proportion of peripheral blasts and promyelocytes or basophils, a high proportion of marrow blasts or basophils, a decrease in bone marrow megakaryocytes, and cytogenetic abnormalities in addition to the Ph chromosome [3]. In a multivariant regression analysis of these features we found that age, blood and marrow basophilia, and additional cytogenetic abnormalities had a strong predictive relationship to survival. Patient groups could be divided into low-, intermediate-, and high-risk groups according to these prognostic factors, their median survivals being 53, 39, and 25 months respectively. As defined by this multivariant prognostic model, patients on alpha interferon did significantly better than those in the control groups.

Ten patients developed blastic transformation without clonal evolution, and of these, six were of lymphoid origin and two had an undifferentiated morphology, which suggests a suppression of the myeloid clone and reversion to the more primitive lymphoid disease. In the blastic phase, this has been easier to treat with intensive chemotherapy.

The use of intensive chemotherapy for the treatment of chronic granulocytic leukemia has been previously reported, and in younger patients it shows a significant advantage over treatment with conventional or single-drug therapy. This type of therapy [3] is now being combined with interferon in an attempt to combine a biological response modifier with intensive chemotherapy and in the hope of substantially prolonging the survival of these patients. In addition to intensive chemotherapy, attempts are being made to render these patients Ph negative for prolonged periods, during which marrows are harvested for use substantially in autologous transplantation, as the disease progresses from the more benign to the accelerated phase.

In an attempt to look at the mechanisms of resistance to interferon, we have correlated interferon receptor binding and induction of 2′,5′-oligoadenylate synthetase. A study of 14 patients treated with partially purified human interferon suggested an association between the absence of clinical response to interferon therapy and a failure of induction of 2′,5′-oligoadenylate synthetase activity. In the sensitive patients, enhancement of enzyme activity was seen during the responsive phases despite reduction of interferon receptor density on the cell surface. The absence of clinical response may in fact be initiated by events subsequent to receptor binding, and thus result in a failure of induction of the enzyme activity which activates interferon and leads to control of proliferative activity [4].

The initiation of new therapies with combinations of interferons and tumor necrosis factor, the use of factors that control proliferation and differentiation of granulocytes and macrophages, and an understanding of the role played by the rearranged chromosome at the ber-abl region and its associated production of an abnormal protein may increase our ability to control CML.

References

1. Talpaz M, McCredie KB, Mavligit GM, Gutterman JU (1983) Leukocyte interferon-induced myeloid cytoreduction in chronic myelogenous leukemia. Blood 62:689–692
2. Talpaz M, Kantarjian HM, McCredie KB, Trujillo JM, Keating MJ, Gutterman JU (1986) Hematologic remission and cytogenetic improvement induced by recombinant human interferon alpha_2 in chronic myelogenous leukemia. N Engl J Med 314:1065–1069
3. Kantarjian HM, Smith TL, McCredie KB, Keating MJ, Walters RS, Talpaz M, Hester JP, Blijham G, Gehan E, Freireich EJ (1985) Chronic myelogenous leukemia: a multivariant analysis of the associations of patient characteristics and therapy with survival. Blood 66:1326–1335
4. Rosenblum MG, Maxwell BL, Talpaz M, Kelleher PJ, McCredie KB, Gutterman JU (1986) In vivo sensitivity and resistance of chronic myelogenous leukemia cells to α-interferon: correlation and receptor binding and induction of 2′,5′-oligoadenylate synthetase. Cancer Res 46:4848–4852

Haematology and Blood Transfusion   Vol. 31
Modern Trends in Human Leukemia VII
Edited by Neth, Gallo, Greaves, and Kabisch
© Springer-Verlag Berlin Heidelberg 1987

Human B-Cell Growth and Differentiation Factors, and Their Effects on Leukemic B-Cells

F. C. Rawle [1,2], R. J. Armitage [1], and P. C. L. Beverley [1]

A. Introduction

A wealth of data on B-cell growth and differentiation factors has been published recently, and so many different factors have been shown to act on B cells [1] that it is difficult to determine which, if any, of these factors are physiologically relevant. Initial models assumed that B-cell activation leads to an ordered expression of receptors for specific growth and then differentiation factors, but these now appear to be incorrect. Firstly, most of the factors with functional effects on B cells are not specific for cells of that lineage. IL2, IL1 and IFNγ have all been shown to have effects on B cells [1, 2]. Secondly, BSF-2 (B-cell differentiation factor BCDFγ), which has recently been cloned [3], has been shown to activate mast cells and basophils, and to cause T-cell proliferation [4], while BCGF II acts as a differentiation factor for eosinophils [5].

The same lymphokine may also have different effects at different stages of B-cell differentiation. BSF-1 acts on resting B cells to induce expression of class II antigens and prime cells for subsequent activation by anti-μ, but also acts on Staphylococcus A Cowan activated B cells to promote switching to production of the IgG1 subclass [3]. Since BSF-1 acts on resting B cells, it also appears that the assumption that antigen-specific activation is required before B cells can respond to non-specific lymphokines derived from T helper cells is not correct.

It is clearly of great importance to define at which stages of maturation and activation B cells express receptors for, and are capable of responding to, the various lymphokines. We have adopted two complementary approaches; first, the use of monoclonal antibodies to define molecules of functional importance on the B-cell surface, and second, the purification of cytokines for use in identifying receptors and in studies of their functional effects.

B. Methods

BCDF activity was measured using the CESS assay [6]. Briefly, 5000 cells per well were cultured in flat-bottomed 96-well microtitre plates for 5 days, and IgG in the supernatant was measured by enzyme-linked immunosorbent assay (ELISA). Peripheral blood lymphocytes from prolymphocytic leukaemia (PLL) patients were cultured at 10^6 per well in 2 ml costar wells, with or without T24 supernatant at 10%. Cells were fixed with 70% ethanol and then subjected to ribonuclease digestion and propidium iodide staining, followed by analysis on the FACS IV (Becton Dickinson). For measurement of IgM secretion, PLL cells were cultured at 10^5 per well in flat-bottomed 96-well microtitre plates; supernatants from triplicate cultures were harvested at day 7, pooled and assayed for IgM by ELISA.

[1] ICRF Human Tumour Immunology Group, Faculty of Clinical Sciences, and [2] Department of Zoology and Comparative Anatomy, University College London, London, UK

Table 1. BCDF activity in supernatants of bladder carcinoma cell lines in the CESS assay

	IgG secreted (ng/ml)	
	Experiment A	Experiment B
Medium control	24	76
MLR[a]	343	988
5637	340	613
T24	426	772
Supernatant concentration	20%	10%

[a] MLR is the supernatant from a 4-day mixed lymphocyte reaction with peripheral blood lymphocytes from three donors, cultured at a total concentration of 2×10^6/ml.

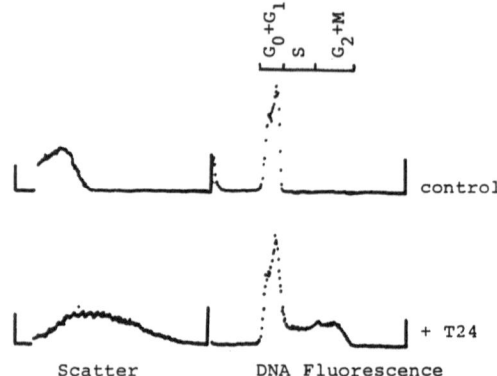

Fig. 1. Cell cycle analysis and cell size (measured by forward-angle light scatter) of PLL cells cultured for 5 days with T24 supernatant (10%) or medium only

C. Results and Discussion

We have found that the human bladder carcinoma cell lines T24 and 5637 secrete BCDF detectable in the CESS assay (Table 1). The factor from T24 is a soluble molecule which elutes from an ACA54 gel filtration column as a single peak with a molecular weight of approximately 25 kD, and has a pI in the range 5.5–6.0 on isoelectric focusing (data not shown). We are in the process of purifying this molecule in order to determine its relation to the T-cell-derived BCDF described by other workers [7].

We have also found that supernatants from these two cell lines cause PLL cells to undergo a significant increase in cell size, as measured by forward-angle light scatter, and to enter cell cycle (Fig. 1). In contrast, chronic lymphocytic leukaemia (CLL) cells do not respond to these supernatants, and preliminary data indicate that normal non-T cells can respond with an increase in size but do not enter cycle. Normal T cells show no response.

PLL cells stimulated with 5637 or T24 supernatant are also induced to secrete IgM (Table 2), and this is accompanied by a decrease in expression of surface IgM detected by staining with monoclonal anti-μ and FACS analysis (data not shown). Thus, the PLL cells appear to differentiate into antibody-producing cells. It is not clear whether this is due to the BCDF or whether proliferation and differentiation are both due to a

Table 2. IgM secretion by PLL cells stimulated with bladder carcinoma supernatants

	IgM secreted (ng/ml)
Control	5
T24 20%	121
T24 2%	97
5637 20%	78
5637 2%	167

single signal, as in the response of murine BCL1 cells to BCGF II [1].

These cell lines had been repeatedly tested for mycoplasma contamination by orcein acetate staining and culture, with negative results. However, recent data suggest that the growth-promoting activity for PLL cells may be associated with a mycoplasma or ureaplasma. It is not yet clear whether production of BCDF is associated with mycoplasm infection.

Regardless of their origin, these factors/activities have clearly defined effects on B cells and are thus likely to be binding to receptors of functional importance. They can therefore be used to investigate the normal function of these receptors and of the signals transmitted through them.

Identification of the receptors should be possible either by receptor-ligand cross-linking or by blocking studies with monoclonal antibodies. We have already used the latter strategy to search for antibodies which interfere with differentiation induced by mixed lymphocyte reaction (MLR) supernatant, and have identified several B-cell surface molecules with functional roles [8, 9].

It is of interest that cells at different stages of differentiation (PLL and CLL cells) differ in responsiveness to bladder carcinoma factors. Clearly, future strategies for treatment of leukaemia, based on manipulation of growth and differentiation, need to define which receptors and factors are important in regulation of each stage of B-cell development. Cytokines and monoclonal antibodies provide powerful tools for approaching these questions.

Acknowledgements. F.C. Rawle is supported by a grant from the Medical Research Council and Celltech Ltd. We thank Professor E. Huehns for use of the FACS and Professor T. Kishimoto for the gift of CESS cells.

References

1. Kishimoto T (1985) Annu Rev Immunol 3:135–159
2. Melchers F, Anderson J (1984) Cell 37:715–720
3. Noma Y, Sideras P, Naito T, Bergstedt-Lindquist S, Azuma C, Severinson E, Tanabe T et al. (1986) Nature 319:640–646
4. Vitetta E (in press) Proceedings of the International Conference on Lymphocyte Activation and Immune Regulation
5. Sanderson CJ, O'Garra A, Warren DJ, Klaus GGB (1986) Proc Natl Acad Sci USA 83:437–440
6. Muraguchi A, Kishimoto T, Miki Y, Kuritani T, Kaieda T, Yoshizaki K, Yamamura Y (1981) J Immunol 127:412–416
7. Hirano T, Taga T, Nakano N, Yasukawa K, Kashiwamura S, Shimizu K, Nakajima K, Pyun H, Kishimoto T (1985) Proc Natl Acad Sci USA 82:5490–5494
8. Golay JT, Rawle FC, Beverley PCL (1985) In: Reinherz EL, Nadler LM (eds) Leucocyte typing II. Springer, Berlin Heidelberg New York Tokyo, pp 463–472
9. Golay JT, Clark EA, Beverley PCL (1985) J Immunol 135:3795–3801

Haematology and Blood Transfusion   Vol. 31
Modern Trends in Human Leukemia VII
Edited by Neth, Gallo, Greaves, and Kabisch
© Springer-Verlag Berlin Heidelberg 1987

Production of Three Monoclonal Antibodies – A01, B05, and C11 – Against B-Cell Leukemia

P. Chen[1], C. Chiu[1], T. Chiou[1], C. Tzeng[1], C. Ho[2], S. Lin[1], R. Hsieh[1], H. Yeh[1], and B. N. Chiang[1]

A. Introduction

The advent of MoAb technology has greatly facilitated the identification of various subsets of lymphoid cells [1, 2]. However, most studies have been concentrated on acute lymphoblastic and myelocytic leukemias [1–4], and relatively few MoAbs that are directed against surface determinants of chronic lymphocytic cells have been reported [5–7]. The reason may be that CLL cell lines are few in number and are not as well characterized as acute lymphocytic or acute myelocytic leukemia cells. In this report we describe the establishment of three hybridomas which secrete MoAbs against an antigen present on malignant B-lymphocytes in the peripheral blood of most CLL and some non-T, non-B ALL patients. These newly established MoAbs have unique patterns of reactivity to normal and leukemic cells distinct from other reported MoAbs and may be useful for the characterization of certain malignant B cells, either for clinical purposes or for the staging of leukemic cells.

B. Methods and Materials

I. Leukemic Cells

All leukemic cell samples were obtained at the onset of disease from patients referred to the Veterans General Hospital (VGH) in

Taipei. Initial diagnosis was based upon the morphology and cytochemistry of cells from bone marrow (BM) aspiration. All samples were first separated on Ficoll-Hypaque gradient and further characterized by differentiation-linked markers. The cells were either used within 24 h after collection or cryopreserved in liquid nitrogen until use. The different types of leukemia/lymphoma cell lines listed in Table 1 were kind gifts of Dr. J. Minowada [8] and were cultured in RPMI 1640 medium supplemented with 10% FBS and antibiotics at 37 °C in 5% CO_2.

II. Normal Cells From Various Sources

Blood and bone marrow cells were donated by healthy volunteers. Thymic biopsies and tonsil cells were obtained from children undergoing cardiovascular surgery and tonsillectomy respectively. In some experiments, leukemic cells were separated into B-lymphocytes by a sequential method of filtration through a nylon-wool column, as described by Aota et al. [9]. Red blood cells, platelets, and granulocytes were obtained from normal blood donors using an IBM 2991 separator. Monocytes were separated by a method previously described [10].

III. Hybridomas

Female balb/c mice 8–10 weeks old were immunized i.p. with 1×10^7 leukemic cells from patients with B-cell CLL, and 3 weeks after the first injection the mice were boosted once

Departments of Medicine[1] and Medical Research[2], Veterans General Hospital and National Yang-Ming Medical College, Taipei, Taiwan, Republic of China

with more of the same cells; fusion was carried out 4 days later using the method of Köhler and Milstein [11]. Mouse spleen cells and NS-1 myeloma cells were induced to fuse in a 50% polyethlene-glycol solution and then cultured in HAT selection medium. After about 4 weeks in culture, supernatants from HAT-resistant cultures were tested for the presence of antibodies reactive to the eliciting CLL cells, leukemic cell lines, and primary leukemic cells by immunofluorescence and immunoperoxidase assays.

IV. Radioimmunoprecipitation

Daudi cells (5×10^7 cells/ml) were surface labeled with 0.5 mCi ^{125}I by the lactoperoxidase technique as described by Lebien et al. [12]. The labeled cells were lysed and added to an equal volume of MoAbs and then incubated overnight at 4 °C. The immune complex formed was adsorbed onto protein A-sepharose CL-4B, and the immunoprecipitated proteins were analyzed by sodium dodecyl sulphate polyacrylamide gel electrophoresis (SDS-PAGE), followed by autoradiography.

C. Results

I. Establishment of MoAbs

Three MoAbs, designated A01, B05, and C11, were obtained from three different clones of cells from a successful fusion experiment. The MoAbs were prepared by immunization against cells from a 39-year-old female patient with B-CLL. The patient was admitted to the VGH in February, 1984, with an initial PB cell count of 12×10^4/ mm^3, 90% of which were sIg$^+$ and Ia$^+$ lymphoid cells. Clones that secreted the MoAbs had been maintained in vitro for over a year with no apparent change in growth characteristics and properties. All MoAbs were of the IgG$_1$ subclass with kappa light chain, as revealed by immunodiffusion.

II. Reactivity to Hematopoietic Cell Lines

Sixteen different established cell lines of various types of leukemia/lymphoma, as listed in Table 1, were examined for their reactivity to MoAbs A01, B05, and C11, and, as shown in the same Table, all three

Table 1. Reactivity of A01, B05, and C11 MoAbs with leukemia/lymphoma cell lines

Cell line	Origin	Compartment at differentiation stage	A01	B05	C11
T cell lines					
Molt-3	ALL	T-blast	–	–	–
CCRF-CEM	ALL	T-blast	–	–	–
B cell lines					
RPMI 6410	ALL	B-blast	–	–	–
BALL	ALL	B-blast	–	–	–
Daudi	BL	B-blast	+	+	+
Nalm-6	ALL	B-blast	–	–	–
Nalmava	ALL	B-blast	–	–	–
SA	ALL	B-blast	–	–	–
Non-T, non cell lines					
NALL	ALL	N-blast	–	–	–
HL-60	APL	Promyelocyte	–	–	–
K562	CML in ABC	Pre-Ery	–	–	–
U-937	Lymphoma	Histiocyte	–	–	–
Kg-1	AML	Myeloblast	–	–	–
CTV-2	AMOL	Monoblast	–	–	–

MoAbs reacted with the B lymphoma cell line Daudi but not with any other cell lines.

III. Reactivity
to Normal Hematopoietic Cells

MoAbs A01, B05, and C11 did not react with peripheral blood lymphocytes (PBL), transformed lymphocytes, granulocytes, monocytes, platelets, RBCs, or thymocytes, and only the C11 MoAb reacted with 3%–9% of tonsil cells. The reactivity of the C11 MoAb to tonsil cells was confirmed by immunoperoxidase staining of frozen sections of the tonsil, which showed that a few cells in the follicular center and the intrafollicular areas were reactive to the C11 MoAb but not to A01 or B05 (data not shown).

IV. Reactivity to Leukemic Cells

Specificity to the A01, B05, and C11 MoAbs was tested against a total of 125 cases of various types of leukemia and lymphoma.

Table 2. Reactivity of A01, B05, and C11 MoAbs to cells from patients with different leukemias and lymphomas

	A01 (%)	B05 (%)	C11 (%)
ALL			
cALL	12/36 (33.3)	9/26 (34.6)	5/27 (18.5)
TALL	0/4	0/5	0/3
NALL	1/10 (10.0)	1/8 (12.5)	1/5 (20.0)
CLL			
B	14/16 (87.5)	14/15 (93.3)	15/18 (83.3)
T	0/1	0/1	0/1
Myeloma	0/1	0/1	0/1
AML	0/24	0/23	1/24 (4.17)
AMOL	0/14	0/13	3/19 (15.8)
CML	0/1	0/1	0/1
CML in ABC	0/3	0/2	0/1
B-Lymphoma	1/8 (12.5)	0/5	0/4

Table 3. Reactivity of A01, B05, and C11 MoAbs to cells from selected cALL patients

Patient no.	MoAbs				
	A01	B05	C11	cALL	Ia
1	90	90	90	90	90
2	99	90	0	95	90
3	99	99	0	90	90
4	80	80	5	72	74
5	99	0	90	99	90
6	90	5	80	90	90
7	90	0	95	95	90
8	70	0	65	75	65
9	90	0	0	85	75
10	98	0	0	98	95
11	0	80	0	85	80
12	0	80	2	90	85
13	0	80	0	85	80
14	0	60	0	75	68

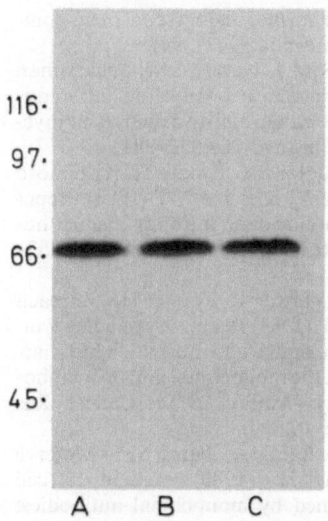

116·
97·
66·
45·

A   B   C

Fig. 1. Autoradiogram of ^{125}I-labeled Daudi cell membrane proteins immunoprecipitated by A01 (*A*), B05 (*B*) and C11 (*C*) monoclonal antibodies. The markers, in descending order, were B-galactosidase (116 K), phosphorylase B (97 K), bovine serum albumin (66 K) and ovalbumin (45 K)

The results (Table 2) showed that most of our B-CLL cells (83%–93%) were reactive to all three MoAbs, and 12% of our B-lymphoma cells were positive for the A01 reactive antigen. Furthermore, 18%–35% of cells from our cALL patients also reacted with one or all of the MoAbs (Table 2). In addition, MoAb C11 reacted with 4% of AML and 16% of AMOL cells (Table 2). Among the positive cALL cases, 14 were selected for more detailed studies. Table 3 shows that cells from only one cALL patient reacted with all three MoAbs, cells from four patients with only one MoAb, and cells from the remaining nine patients with two types of MoAbs. These results suggest that the MoAbs are of different clonal origins and that all three MoAbs are selective for B-lymphocytes.

V. Characterization
of the MoAb Reactive Antigen

In order to determine the molecular weight of the antigen(s) reactive to MoAbs A01, B05, and C11, cell extracts were prepared from surface radiolabeled Daudi cells, mixed with the MoAbs, and sorted out by immunoprecipitation with protein A-Sepharose beads. As shown in Fig. 1, all three MoAbs immunoprecipitated a single protein with an approximate mol.wt. of 66. This suggests that all three MoAbs react with the same surface antigen but presumably with different determinants on Daudi cells.

D. Discussion

This report describes the establishment of three MoAbs, A01, B05, and C11, against cells from a patient with B-CLL. These MoAbs were selected after repeated cloning of hybridomas from different culture wells. All three MoAbs reacted selectively with the B-lymphoma cell line Daudi but not with other tested cell lines (Table 1). This suggests that the MoAbs recognize a unique surface antigen present only on certain B cells. Furthermore, it appears that the antigen reactive to A01, B05, and C11 is not present on normal lymphoid cells, since, with the exception of a few C11-reactive cells in the tonsil, the MoAbs do not react with cells of normal lymphoid tissues (data not shown). Caligaris-Cappio et al. [13] have recently identified an infrequent B-lymphocyte subpopulation in normal tonsil and lymph nodes which carries a 65-K cell-surface determinant. Coincidently, the antigen recognized by C11 as well as by the other two MoAbs has a similar mol.wt. (Fig. 1). Therefore, one might speculate that the few C11-positive cells in the tonsil may be the infrequent B-lymphocytes that are presumably distinct from conventional B-lymphocytes.

When tested against different leukemia and lymphoma cells, the three MoAbs showed distinct patterns of reactivity. The B05 is most selective, in that it recognizes mostly the B-CLL cells and some cALL cells; the A01 reacts with some B-lymphoma cells in addition to B-CLL cells, while the C11 exhibits a more diverse pattern of reactivity, as it can react with both AML (4%) and AMOL (15%) cells other than malignant B cells (Table 2). Furthermore, the three MoAbs react differently to cALL cells from different patients (Table 3). These results strongly suggest that the MoAbs have different clonal origins and identify antigenic determinants present mostly on certain neoplastic B cells or their putative precursors, which may be very heterogeneous in antigenicity. Although, the three MoAbs are obviously distinct from one another, they have many properties in common. Thus, all three react mostly with B-CLL cells and some cALL cells, and they all immunoprecipitate a single surface antigen from Daudi cells with a mol.wt. of about 66 (Fig. 1). Based on these results, it is very likely that A01, B05, and C11 all recognize the same antigen but at different determinant sites.

The MoAbs reported on in the present study are distinct from those described by other investigators. Thus, the B1 [14], B2 [15], T101 [7, 16], Y 29/55 [6, 17] and BA-1 [18] all recognize malignant B cells, but they also react with normal T or B cells from certain tissues. In conclusion, we have been able to establish three MoAbs which react selectively with B-CLL and some cALL cells but not with lymphocytes from normal tissues. These MoAbs may have unique diagnostic value, in that they can distinguish neoplastic from normal B cells, and may be powerful tools in identifying a small number of abnormal B cells in the peripheral blood, either following chemotherapy or at the subleukemic stage of ongoing diseases. Finally, the A01, B05, and C11 MoAbs may also be useful in distinguishing B-cell leukemia from B-cell lymphoma cells since they all react mostly with leukemic cells.

Acknowledgments. This work was supported by grants from the Clinical Research Center, the Institute of Biomedical Sciences, Academia Sinica, and the National Science Council of the Republic of China.

References

1. Greaves MF, Verbi W, Kemshead J, Kennett R (1980) A monoclonal antibody identifying a cell surface antigen shared by common acute lymphoblastic leukemias and B-lineage cells. Blood 56:1141–1148
2. Pirruccello SJ, Lebien TW (1985) Monoclonal antibody BA-1 recognizes a novel human leukocyte cell surface sialoglycoprotein complex. J Immunol 134:3962–3968
3. Griffin JD, Ritz J, Nadler LM, Schlossman SF (1981) Expression of myeloid differentiation antigens on normal and malignant myeloid cells. J Clin Invest 68:932–941
4. Maruyama S, Naito T, Kakita H, Kishimoto S, Yamamura Y, Kishimoto T (1983) Preparation of a monoclonal antibody against human monocyte lineage. J Clin Immunol 3:57–64
5. Hirt A, Baumgartner C, Forster HK, Imbach P, Wagner HP (1983) Reactivity of acute lymphoblastic leukemia and normal bone marrow cells with the monoclonal anti-B-lymphocyte antibody, Anti-Y 29/55. Cancer Res 43:4483–4485
6. Royston I, Majda JA, Baird SM, Meserve BL, Griffiths JL (1980) Human T cell antigens defined by monoclonal antibodies: the 65 000-dalton antigen of T cell (T65) is also found on chronic lymphocytic leukemia cells bearing surface immunoglobulin. J Immunol 125:725–731
7. Stashenko P, Nadler LM, Hardy R, Schlossman SF (1980) Characterization of a human B-lymphocyte-specific antigen. J Immunol 125:1678–1685
8. Minowada J, Sagawa K, Lok MS, Kubonishi I, Nakazawa S, Tatsumi E, Ohnuma T, Goldlum N (1980) A model of lymphoid-myeloid cell differentiation based on the study of marker profiles of 50 human leukemia-lymphoma cell lines. In: Serrou B, Rosenfeld C (eds) International symposium on new trends in human immunology and cancer immunotherapy. Doin, Paris, pp 188–199
9. Aota F, Chang D, Hill NO, Khan A (1983) Monoclonal antibody against myeloid leukemia cell line (KG-1). Cancer Res 43:1093–1096
10. Chen P, Kwan S, Hwang T, Chiang B, Chou C (1983) Insulin receptors on leukemia and lymphoma cells. Blood 62:251–255
11. Kohler G, Milstein C (1975) Continuous cultures of fused cells secreting antibody of predefined specificity. Nature 259:495–497
12. Lebien TW, Boue DR, Bradley JG, Kersey JH (1982) Antibody affinity may influence antigenic modulation of the common acute lymphoblastic leukemia antigen in vitro. J Immunol 129:2287–2292
13. Caligaris-Cappio F, Gobbi M, Bofill M, Janossy G (1982) Infrequent normal B-lymphocytes express features of B-chronic lymphocytic leukemia. J Exp Med 155:623–628
14. Nadler LM, Ritz J, Hardy R, Pesando LM, Schlossman SF (1981) A unique cell surface antigen identifying lymphoid malignancies of B cell origin. J Clin Invest 67:134–140

15. Nadler LM, Stashenko P, Hardy K, van Agthoven A, Terhorst C, Schlossman SF (1981) Characterization of a human B-cell-specific antigen (B2) distinct from B1. J Immunol 126:1941–1948

16. Wormsley SB, Collins ML, Royston I (1981) Comparative density of the human T-cell antigen T65 on normal peripheral blood T cells and chronic lymphocytic leukemia cells. Blood 57:657–662

17. Forster HK, Gudat FG, Girard M-F, Albrecht R, Schmidt J, Ludwig C, Obrecht J-P (1982) Monoclonal antibody against a membrane antigen characterizing leukemic human B-lymphocytes. Cancer Res 42:1927–1934

18. Abramson CS, Kersey JH, Lebien TW (1982) A monoclonal antibody (BA-1) reactive with cells of human B-lymphocyte lineage. J Immunol 126:83–88

131

Haematology and Blood Transfusion Vol. 31
Modern Trends in Human Leukemia VII
Edited by Neth, Gallo, Greaves, and Kabisch
© Springer-Verlag Berlin Heidelberg 1987

Natural Killer Activity in Preleukemic States

P. Obłąkowski [1]

A. Introduction

Natural killer cells (NKC) were first identified by their ability to kill without prior immunization certain tumor target cells grown in vitro [15, 16, 20]. In preliminary observations they were defined only in negative terms: that is, they were not thymus-derived (T) or bone marrow-derived (B)-lymphocytes, nor were they adherent or phagocytes, and they lacked demonstrable surface membrane immunoglobulin [17]. Most human blood NKC bear an $Fc\gamma$ receptor [23]. As with rodents, a number of observations suggested that NKC were not necessarily divorced from the T-cell lineage. For example, they reacted with anti-T serums and anti-T monoclonal antibodies [5, 9, 11]. On the basis of the partial isolation of NKC on Percoll, they were characterized as identical to large granular lymphocytes (LGL) with cytoplasmic azurophilic granules [1, 21]. NKC and their regulation by interferons (IFN) and interleukin-2 (IL-2) are proposed to be one of the important factors in tumor immunosurveillance and tumor resistance [3, 4, 8, 14, 18, 22]. A significant reduction in NKC activity has been demonstrated in patients with various disorders such as the Chédiak-Higashi syndrome which are known for their high incidence of malignant diseases [6, 13]. It was of interest to examine NKC activity in preleukemic states and to determine its influence on the development of the disease.

[1] Department of Internal Medicine, Institute of Hematology, 00-957 Warsaw, Poland

B. Patients and Controls

Natural killer (NK) activity was determined in 20 patients ranging in age from 30 to 79 years (mean 59.9). There were six cases of acquired idiopathic sideroblastic anemia (AISA), nine cases of refractory anemia (RA), four cases of refractory anemia with an excess of blasts (RAEB), and one case of refractory anemia with an excess of blasts in transformation (RAEBt). The patients were

Table 1. Diagnosis in 20 patients examined

	No. of patients	
	Female	Male
Acquired idiopathic sideroblastic anemia (AISA)	5	1
Refractory anemia (RA)	7	2
Refractory anemia with an excess of blasts (RAEB)	3	1
RAEB in transformation	0	1

classified as AISA, RA, RAEB, and RAEBt according to the FAB classification of myelodysplastic (preleukemic) syndromes [2] (Table 1). All patients had less than 10% of blasts in peripheral blood, and none received drugs which might influence NK cell activity. A control group constituted of 56 healthy blood donors.

C. Effector Cells

Effector cells were obtained by sedimentation of heparinized blood on "Lymphoprep". Mononuclear cells were washed and resuspended in MEM supplemented with 10% FCS.

D. Target Cells

Cells of the K562 line derived from a patient with blast crisis in CML were used as targets [7]. K562 cells were cultured in RPMI 1640 medium containing 10% FCS, gentamicin and L-glutamine, under standard conditions.

E. Cytotoxicity Assay

NK activity of mononuclear cells was measured in a 4-h cytotoxicity test with ^{51}Cr-labeled K562 cells as targets [16]. After 4-h incubation of effector cells together with targets in a 20:1 ratio, cells were centrifuged and supernatants were collected for determination of released ^{51}Cr in a gamma scintillation counter.

The percentage of cytolysis was calculated according to the formula:

$$\% \; CTX = \frac{\text{experimental cpm } - \text{ spontaneous cpm}}{\text{maximal cpm } - \text{ spontaneous cpm}} \times 100$$

Maximal cpm was obtained by the incubation of target cells in the presence of 1% Triton X-100; spontaneous cpm was obtained by the incubation of target cells in MEM containing 10% FCS.

The results revealed strong suppression of NK activity in all of the preleukemic patients (11.5% $\pm$ 10.1%) and in each of the diagnosed syndromes, as compared with the control group (30.6% $\pm$ 11.5%; Table 2 and Fig. 1). The difference was statistically significant ($P < 0.01$) in the Wilcoxon–Mann-Whitney test. Similar changes in NK activity in preleukemia have been detected by others [12, 19]. There are reports that suppression of NK activity was not connected with dilution of effector cells by blasts or by a reduced frequency of LGL in mononuclear cells of examined patients. Takagi and co-workers suggested that suppression of NK activity in preleukemic patients was caused by the impaired IFN-linked regulatory system of NKC [19].

In this study, two of the 20 investigated patients developed leukemia 2–3 months after diagnosis. Both cases showed very low NK activity:

1. Patient M.S. (RAEB) %CTX = −4.2%
2. Patient W.M. (RAEBt) %CTX = −1.7%

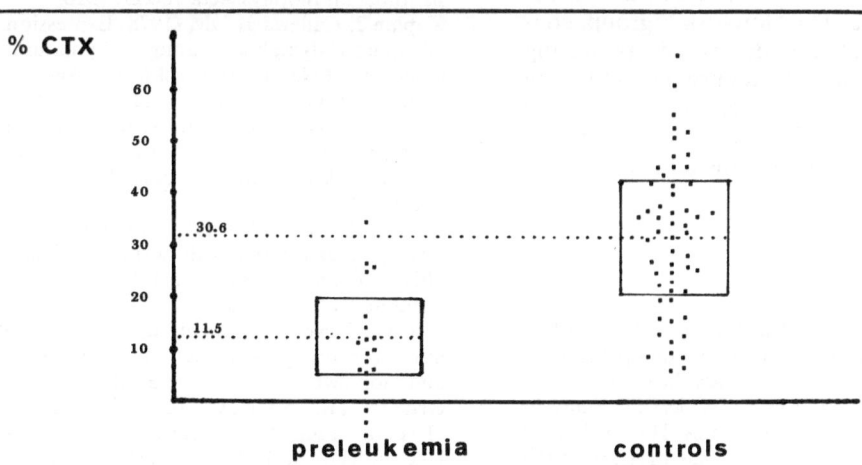

Fig. 1. NK activity in preleukemic patients compared with healthy controls. Mean $\pm$ SD is indicated for each group

Table 2. Percentage of NK activity in 20 patients according to preleukemic syndrome

Patient		AISA	RA	RAEB	RAEB t
Female	Male	Cytotoxicity (%)			
W. L.		8.0			
J. S.		25.9			
S. P.		27.6			
	S. G.	8.6			
K. K.		13.1			
M. W.		10.9			
I. D.			3.9		
	Z. N.		8.7		
K. L.			11.4		
T. S.			11.2		
A. G.			− 8.9		
M. K.			2.4		
J. F.			2.9		
	E. M.		25.7		
M. N.			30.2		
M. S.				− 4.2	
	T. H.			4.9	
H. K.				12.2	
F. D.				25.4	
	W. M.				−1.7
Mean		15.6	9.7	9.5	−1.7

These preliminary observations show that very low NK activity might be connected with a high risk for overt leukemia. Furthermore, the preleukemic patients were divided into two groups on the basis of their risk for leukemic transformation. The "high-risk" group, consisting of patients with RA, RAEB, and RAEBt, showed a mean NK activity of 5.8%. The "low-risk" group, consisting of patients diagnosed as having AISA, which has a better prognosis for long survival, showed a higher mean percentage of NK activity (15.6%), but the difference was not statistically significant (Table 2).

References

1. Babcock GF, Phillips JH (1983) Human NK cells: light- and electron-microscopic characteristics. Surv Immunol Res 2:88–101
2. Benett JR, Catovsky D, Daniel MT, Flandrin G, Galton DAG, Gralnick HR, Sultan C (1982) Proposals for the classification of the myelodysplastic syndromes. Br J Haematol 51:189–199
3. Einhorn S, Blomgren H, Strander H (1978) Interferon and spontaneous cytotoxicity in man. I. Enhancement of the spontaneous cytotoxicity of peripheral lymphocytes by human leukocyte interferon. Int J Cancer 22:405–412
4. Hanna N (1985) The role of natural killer cells in the control of tumor growth and metastasis. Biochim Biophys Acta 780:213–226
5. Kaplan J, Callewaert DM (1978) Expression of human T-lymphocyte antigens by natural killer cells. J Natl Cancer Inst 60:961–964
6. Katz P, Zaytoun AM, Lee JH, Fauci AS (1984) In vivo Epstein-Barr virus – induced augmentation of natural killer cell activity in the Chédiak-Higashi syndrome. J Immunol 132:571–573
7. Lozzio CB, Lozzio BB (1975) Human chronic myelogenous cell line with positive Philadelphia chromosome. Blood 45:321–334
8. Ortaldo JR, Mantovani A, Hobbs D (1983) Effects of several species of human leukocyte interferon on cytotoxic activity of NK cells and monocytes. Int J Cancer 31:285–289
9. Ortaldo JR, Sharrow SD, Timonen T, Herberman RB (1981) Determination of surface antigens on highly purified human NK cells by flow cytometry with monoclonal antibodies. J Immunol 127:2401–2409

10. Perussia B, Trinchieri G, Jackson A, Warner NL, Faust J, Rumpold H, Kraft D, Lanier LL (1984) The Fc receptor for IgG on human natural killer cells: phenotypic, functional, and comparative studies with monoclonal antibodies. J Immunol 133:180–189
11. Potter MR, Moore M (1979) Natural cytotoxic reactivity of human lymphocyte subpopulation. Immunology 37:187–194
12. Porzsolt F, Heimpel H (1982) Impaired T-cell and NK-cell function in patients with preleukaemia. Blut 45:243–248
13. Roder JC, Haliotis T, Klein M (1980) A new immunodeficiency disorder in humans involving NK cells. Nature 284:553–555
14. Roder JC, Pross HF (1982) The biology of the human natural killer cell. J Clin Immunol 2:249–263
15. Rosenberg EB, Herberman RB, Levine PH (1972) Lymphocyte cytotoxicity reactions to leukaemia associated antigens in identical twins. Int J Cancer 9:648–658
16. Rosenberg EB, Mc Coy JL, Green SS (1974) Destruction of human lymphoid tissue-culture cell lines by human peripheral lymphocytes in ^{51}Cr release cytotoxicity assays. J Natl Cancer Inst 52:345–352
17. Santoli O, Trinchieri G, Morelta L (1978) Spontaneus cell-mediated cytotoxicity in humans. Distribution and characterisation of the effector cell. Clin Exp Immunol 33:309–318
18. Shaw ARE, Bleackley RC, Merryweather JP, Barr PJ (1985) Modulation of human natural killer cell activity by recombinant human interleukin 2. Cell Immunol 90:547–554
19. Takagi S, Kitagawa S, Takeda A, Minato N, Takaku F, Miura Y (1984) Natural killer – interferon system in patients with preleukaemic states. Br J Haematol 58:71–81
20. Takasugi M, Mickey MR, Terasaki P (1978) Reactivity of lymphocytes from normal persons on cultured tumor cells. Cancer Res 33:2898–2902
21. Timonen T, Saksela E, Ranki A, Häyry P (1979) Fractionation, morphological and functional characterisation of effector cells responsible for human natural killer activity against cell-line targets. Cell Immunol 48:133–148
22. Trinchieri G, Matsumoto-Kobayashi M, Clark SC, Seehra J, London L, Perussia B (1984) Response of resting human peripheral blood natural killer cells to interleukin 2. J Exp Med 160:1147–1169
23. West WH, Cannon GB, Kay HD (1977) Natural cytotoxic reactivity of effector cells. J Immunol 118:355–361

Haematology and Blood Transfusion Vol. 31
Modern Trends in Human Leukemia VII
Edited by Neth, Gallo, Greaves, and Kabisch
© Springer-Verlag Berlin Heidelberg 1987

Some Karyotypic Aspects of Human Leukemia

H. Van den Berghe and C. Mecucci [1]

A. Introduction

Chromosome abnormalities are found in the vast majority of hematologic malignancies. A great number of these changes are very specific, and some unambiguously identify the nature and type of the malignant disorder in which they are found.

The purposes of this paper are (a) to update the list of characteristic chromosome changes occurring in human hematologic neoplasia; (b) to bring together data presently known about the nature of trisomies found in these disorders; and (c) to review which genes, other than oncogenes, located near the chromosomal breakpoints may play a role in the cellular proliferation and differentiation, as well as in some other phenotypic manifestations.

B. Recently Discovered Characteristic Chromosome Changes in Human Hematologic Malignancies

I. Lymphoproliferative Disorders

Six anomalies are to be added to the existing list of characteristic chromosome changes in lymphoid proliferations (Table 1). A t(1;19) characterizes some cases of pre-B-ALL [1]. All other specific changes were found in T-cell leukemias and lymphomas. The 9p anomaly is found predominantly in child-

Table 1. Recently discovered chromosome changes

Lymphoproliferation

pre-B ALL	t(1;19)(q23;p13)
T-ALL	t(11;14)(p13;q11)
T-cell proliferation	9 p-
T-cell proliferation	inv(14)(q11q32)
T-cell proliferation	t(14;...)(q11;...), several translocations possible
T-cell lymphoma	6p-/t(6;...)(p23;...)
Malignant histiocytosis	t(2;5)(p23;q35)

Myeloproliferation

t(1;7)(p11;p11)	MDS, secondary
t(1;15)(q12;p11)	MDS
t(2;11)(p21;q23)	ANLL
Trisomy 4	ANLL
t(1;3)(p36;q21)	ANLL
t(3;5) (q21-q25;q35)	ANLL
t(3;17)(q26;q22)	Myeloproliferative syndromes

hood ALL [2]. Lymphomas with 9p are found in adults [3]. The T-cell lymphomas with involvement of 6p23 [4] might be the counterpart in man of a T-cell lymphoma occurring in mice with activation of the *pim*-oncogene after insertion of Moloney murine leukemia virus [5]. The other three chromosome changes have one breakpoint in common, 14q11, where the alpha chain of the T-cell receptor is located [6]. Finally, a t(2;5) clearly characterizes a subset of malignant histiocytic proliferations [7].

[1] Center for Human Genetics, University of Leuven, Herestraat 49, B-3000 Leuven, Belgium

II. Myeloproliferative Disorders

An even larger series of characteristic chromosome changes have been discovered recently in myeloproliferative disorders (Table 1). The first of these changes, t(1;7), is invariably found in myelodysplastic syndromes (MDS) occurring as secondary disorders (iatrogenic or environmentally induced). The long arm and centromere of chromosome 7 are lost; the remaining short arm is translocated on the remainder of a chromosome 1 which had lost the short arm. Furthermore, two normal no. 1 chromosomes are present. Therefore, the leukemic cells are trisomic for 1q and monosomic for 7q:t(1;7)(p11;p11) [8]. Partial trisomy of chromosome 1 is also seen in another anomaly, but this time the long arm is translocated upon the short arm of chromosome 15. This t(1;15)(q12;p11) is found in MDS [9].

Chromosome 1 is involved in a t(1;3)(p35;q21), but this time in an apparently balanced rearrangement, found in acute myelogenous leukemia (ANLL) [10]. Two other balanced translocations show a rearrangement between chromosome 3 and either chromosome 5 or chromosome 17. The t(3;17) is found in myeloproliferative syndromes (MPS) and the t(3;5) in ANLL [11, 12].

Some ANLL are characterized by a t(2;11), with the breakpoint in chromosome 11 being at q23 as in monoblastic and myelomonocytic leukemia [13] and also in the t(4;11), which is by now a well-known entity frequently occurring as a congenital leukemia. A very remarkable anomaly is trisomy 4 occurring as the sole anomaly [14]. It is associated with a myelomonocytic leukemia and very clearly constitutes a new entity which, remarkably, was not discovered earlier, despite its conspicuous chromosomal change. It is possible that this type of leukemia may only recently have arisen.

C. Nature of Trisomy Occurring as the Sole Anomaly in Hematologic Malignancies

Trisomy 8 is found ubiquitously in myeloid proliferation and more rarely in lymphoid malignancies. It is found as the sole anomaly in 10% of de novo ANLL; it appears in transformation of CML, as well as in a number of other hematologic conditions.

Trisomy 9 is more than occasionally found as an early event in polycythemia vera. Trisomy 12 characterizes chronic lymphocytic leukemia (CLL). Trisomy 4 identifies a subgroup of ANLL. In the light of oncogene activation by chromosomal changes, one does not readily see how chromosomal trisomies could be instrumental in this respect. Taking the example of chromosome 4, there are three genes on this chromosome which could be proliferation related: T-cell growth factor, epidermal growth factor, and the *Kit*-oncogene. Is a 50% increase in gene product sufficient to cause transformation or increased proliferation? Questions were raised, therefore, with regard to the nature of these trisomies. Could they not be in fact a triplication of one parental chromosome with the other parental chromosome missing? In trisomy 4 we used the G8 probe which detects an RFLP sequence linked to the Huntington gene on 4p and found a $2+1$ and not a 3×1 situation. By a similar approach it was shown in CLL with trisomy 12 that there was a similar situation of $2+1$. By morphological analysis of C-polymorphism in chromosome 9, we were able to show that in trisomy 9 also no parental chromosome was missing and that one of the homologs was duplicated. These preliminary data seem to indicate that if these trisomic changes are crucially important in the malignant process, it could be through a 50% increase of their gene products.

D. Chromosome Breakpoints Involving Genes of Specific Cell Differentiation and/or Functions

I. Differentiation Genes

It has been clearly demonstrated that chromosome breakpoints in B- and T-type lymphoproliferative disorders are related to two groups of genes specifically expressed in B- and T-cell differentiation; the immunoglobulin genes and the T-cell receptor genes. Some additional examples indicating a nonrandom involvement of differentiation genes

Table 2. Differentiation genes

Lymphocytic Cells (Burkitt's lymphoma; non-Hodgkin lymphoma-leukemia)

B-type

14q32	Heavy chain immunoglobulin	t(8;14)(q24;q32); t(11;14)(q13;q32); t(14;18)(q32;q21)
2p11	κ-chain immunoglobulin	t(2;8)(p11;q24)
22q11	λ-chain immunoglobulin	t(8;22)(q24;q11)

T-type (T-cell lymphoma-leukemia)

14q11	α chain T-cell receptor	inv(14)(q11q32); t(11;14)(p13;q11)
7q35	β chain T-cell receptor	t(7; 14)
7p15	γ chain T-cell receptor	t(7;14)
11q23	T3 subunit of T3-T cell receptor	(1;6;11)(p33;q16;q23)
11q22	Thy-1 antigen	(1;6;11)(p33;q16;q23)
10q23	TdT	t(10;...)(q23;...)
2p11	T8 antigen	t(2;17)(p11;p11)
12	T4 antigen	

Erythrocytic cells (Erythroleukemia-ANLL, M6-FAB)

11p15	β globin cluster	t(7;11)(q22;p15) t(9;11)(q11;p15)
16pter-p12	α globin cluster	t(16;17)(p13;q21)

in chromosome aberrations accompanying malignant T-cell proliferations are shown in Table 2.

A single patient with a T-cell lymphoma with T8-positive malignant lymphocytes and a t(2;17) translocation involving the region where the T8 antigen is located has been observed [15]. Additional breakpoints in T-cell lymphomas possibly corresponding to T-stage differentiation genes affect 11q23 at the level of or close to the genes for the T3 subunit of the T-cell receptor and the Thy-1 antigen. Moreover, more than one case has been observed with a chromosome rearrangement in 10q23, where the gene for terminal deoxynucleotydil transferase is located.

In addition, a few chromosome translocations involving the genes for α and β globin have been associated with acute leukemias

Table 3. Growth factors/growth factor receptors

Chromosome localization	Gene	Chromosome aberration	Malignant disorder
3q21-q26/3q26-qter	Transferrin/Transferrin receptor	inv(3)(q21q26)-3q-3q+	ANLL with thrombocytosis
10p14-p15	Interleukin 2 receptor	t(8;10)(q12;p14)	Malignant lymphoma
9pter-p13/p24-p13	Interferon α/β	t(9;11)(p21;q22)	ANLL, M5-FAB
4q25-q27/4q26-q28	EGF/Interleukin 2	trisomy 4	ANLL
19p13.3-p13.2	Insulin receptor	t(1;19)(q23;p13)	pre-B ALL
5q33/5q11-q13	GM-CSF/glucocorticoid Receptor	del(5)(q12q33)	MDS-ANLL
17q	Homeobox region	t(15;17)(q22;q21); iso(17q); t(3;17)(q26;q22)	ANLL-M3 FAB Acute myeloproliferative disorders

Table 4. Metal ions regulating genes

Chromosome localization	Gene	Chromosome aberration	Malignant disorder
16q22	Metallothionein genes	inv(16)(p13q22)	ANLL,M4 with eosinophilia
11q(13?)	Ferritin	del(11)(q14)/ del(11)(q14q23)	Acquired idiopathic sideroblastic anemia

characterized by predominant erythrocytic differentiation [16].

II. Growth Factors and Growth Factor Receptors

There are two lines of evidence supporting an involvement of these genes in neoplastic processes (for review see Goustin et al. [17]).

First, c-*sis* and c-*erb*-B correspond to the platelet-derived growth factor and the epidermal growth factor respectively. Furthermore, it is known that tumor cells may "autocontrol" their own proliferation by producing specific growth-controlling polypeptides.

In the t(9;11) translocation associated with M5-FAB leukemias an oncogene, c-ets-1, moves to the short arm of chromosome 9, adjacent to interferon genes [18]. The insulin receptor gene on 19p13.3-p13.2 corresponds to the breakpoint of the t(1;19) translocation described in pre-B ALL [19].

Other well-established chromosome aberrations in malignant hematologic disorders that possibly involve genes controlling cell growth are indicated in Table 3.

III. Metal Ion Regulating Genes

In acute myelomonocytic leukemias (M4-FAB) with a high eosinophilic marrow component the typically associated pericentric inversion of chromosome 16, breakpoints in p13 and q22, involves the metallothionein genes, which, according to some authors, may be split by the chromosome rearrangement.

Another typical association has been found between a subgroup of myelodysplastic syndromes with sideroblastosis and a deletion of chromosome 11, with breakpoints apparently located in q14 and/or q23, close to the active gene for the subunit H of ferritin (Table 4).

These examples illustrate how several genes important for differentiation and cell proliferation are located on a number of chromosomes, in or near breakpoints specifically known to be involved in malignant hemopoietic cells. Some of these genes are very clearly involved in the mechanism(s) that govern the proliferation and phenotype of the malignant cell. Further work along these lines will undoubtedly lead to more insight into how these genes contribute to the malignant process or to its phenotypic expression.

References

1. Williams DL, Look AT, Melvin SL, Roberson PK, Dahl G, Flake T, Stass S (1984) Cell 36:101
2. Kowalczyk J, Sandberg AA (1983) Cancer Genet Cytogenet 9:383
3. Chilcote RR, Brown E, Rowley JD (1985) N Engl J Med 313:286
4. Mecucci C, Michaux JL, Tricot G, Louwagie A, Van den Berghe H (1985) Leuk Res 9:1139
5. Cuypers HT, Selten G, Quint W, Zijlstra M, Robanus-Maandag E, Boelens W, Van Wezenbeek P, Melief C, Berns A (1984) Cell 37:141
6. Human Gene Mapping 8 (1985) Cytogenet Cell Genet 40:1–4
7. Morgan R, Hecht BK, Sandberg AA, Hecht F, Smith SD (1986) New Engl J Med 314:1322

8. Scheres JMJC, Hustinx TWS, Hodrinet RSG, Geraedts JPM, Hagemeijer A, Van der Blij-Philipsen M (1984) Cancer Genet Cytogenet 12:283

9. Mecucci C, Tricot G, Boogaerts M, Van den Berghe H (1986) Br J Haematol 62:439

10. Bloomfield CD, Garson OM, Volin L, Knuutila S, de la Chapelle A (1985) Blood 66:1409

11. Mecucci C, Michaux JL, Broeckaert-Van orshoven A, Symann M, Boogaerts M, Külling G, Van den Berghe H (1984) Cancer Genet Cytogenet 12:111

12. Rowley JD, Potter D (1976) Blood 47:705

13. de la Chapelle A, Knuutila S, Elonen E (1986) Scand J Haematol 60 (suppl) 1:230

14. Mecucci C, Van Orshoven A, Tricot G, Michaux JL, Delannoy A, Van den Berghe H (1986) Blood 67:1328

15. Mecucci C, Van den Berghe H (1985) New Engl J Med 313:185

16. Kirsch IR, Brown JA, Lawrence J, Korsmeyer SJ, Morton CC (1985) Cancer Genet Cytogenet 18:159

17. Goustin AS, Leof EB, Shipley GD, Moses HL (1986) Cancer Res 46:1015

18. Diaz MO, Le Beau MM, Pitha P, Rowley JD (1986) Science 231:265

19. Yang-Feng TL, Francke U, Ullrich A (1985) Science 228:728

Haematology and Blood Transfusion   Vol. 31
Modern Trends in Human Leukemia VII
Edited by Neth, Gallo, Greaves, and Kabisch
© Springer-Verlag Berlin Heidelberg 1987

Nonisotopic In Situ Hybridization for Mapping Oncogenic Sequences

P. F. Ambros [1], C. R. Bartram [2], O. A. Haas [1], H. I. Karlic [3], and H. Gadner [1]

A. Introduction

In situ hybridization techniques are currently the most direct way of determining the localization and quantification of repetitive sequences or unique genes, e.g. oncogenes, in tissues or on chromosomes. This method involves the annealing of labeled polynucleotide sequences to chromosomal or cellular preparations whose DNA or RNA has been denatured (or otherwise exposed) to enable hybridization with the labeled probe. Along with autoradiographic techniques [5, 6], the use of nonisotopic in situ hybridization methods has brought a better resolution of the signal and a considerable shortening of the procedure.

The rapid biotin/streptavidin method [8] combined with a specific microscopic set up [7] is a powerful tool for locating unique sequences on metaphase chromosomes [1, 2]. Using biotinylated DNA probes and a streptavidin-peroxidase detection system we are now able to trace cellular oncogenes on human chromosomes by in situ hybridization with DNA probes less than 2 kb in size. Sequential staining of the preparations with chromomycin A_3 and DA/DAPI [10] allows unequivocal chromosome identification and an exact assignment of the in situ hybridization signals in the target chromosomes.

In the present study we applied this high-resolution in situ hybridization technique to chromosomes of the human leukemia cell line K562. This cell line, originating from a patient with CML in blast crisis, has turned out to be an ideal model for molecular biological studies: A marker chromosome contains nearly identical amplified c-abl/5'bcr and lambda light-chain constant-region immunoglobulin genes (C_L) [3]. The aim of our study was to analyze the exact positions of the c-abl and 5'bcr sequences in the genome.

B. Material and Methods

Two pUC plasmids (kindly provided by G. Grosveld) were used, one containing a 1.8-kb EcoRI c-abl, and the other one a 2.0-kb Bgl II/HindIII 5'bcr insert. Labeling of the DNA probes was done with biotinylated dUTP (ENZO Biochem., Inc., New York) with an Amersham Nick-Translation Kit.

K562 cells grown according to standard techniques (RPMI 1640 supplemented with 10% FCS) were used for chromosome preparations. The in situ hybridization protocol was performed as described previously in detail [1, 2]. Briefly, after RNase treatment and dehydration of the slides, the hybridization solution was applied. Slides were covered with ethanol-cleaned glass coverslips and sealed with rubber cement. Denaturation was done at 75°–78 °C for 10 min in a humid chamber and followed by overnight incubation at 37 °C in the same chamber. After extensive washing in several steps with 2 × SSC (2xSSC/50% formamide), PBS, and PBS with 0.1% triton, signal detection of the la-

[1] St. Anna Kinderspital, Kinderspitalg. 6, A-1090 Vienna, Austria
[2] Universitätskinderklinik Ulm, Prittwitzstr. 43, D-7900 Ulm, Federal Republic of Germany
[2] Ludwig-Boltzmann Inst. f. Leukämieforschung Hanusch-Krankenhaus Vienna

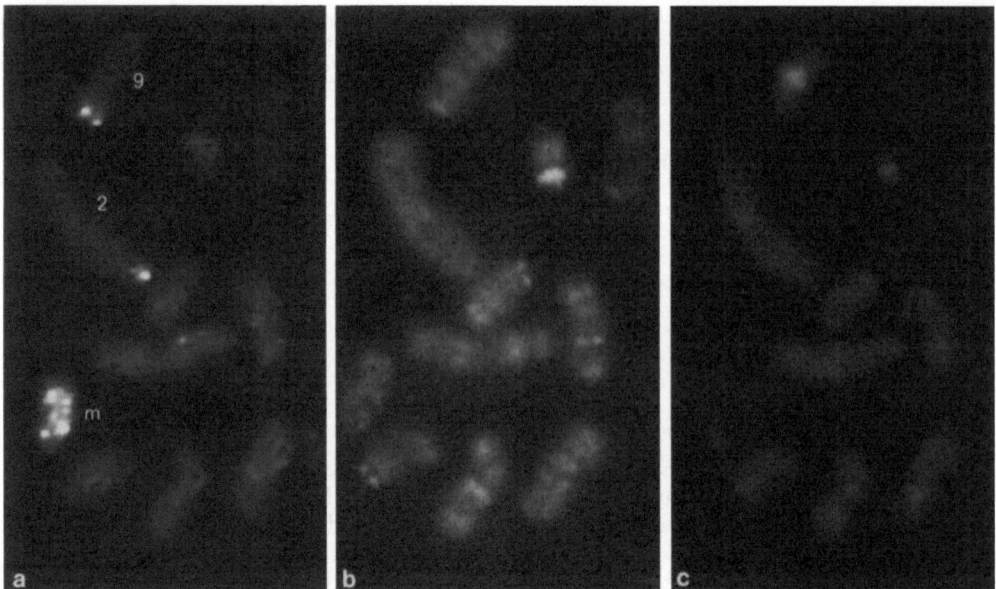

Fig. 1. a Partial chromosome spread from a K562 cell after hybridization with a biotinylated c-abl probe and detection of the signals with peroxidase-labeled streptavidin, which were visualized with a reflection-contrast microscope on chromosome 9 (9q34) chromosome 2 (2q37) and on a marker chromosome. **b** R-banding of the same cell with chromomycin A$_3$. **c** Distamycin A/DAPI banding

beled DNA probes was performed as described in the DETEK I-hrp signal-generating systems instruction manual (ENZO Biochem., Inc., New York). The diaminobenzidine development was carried out for 5 min at room temperature.

After analysis of the slides with reflection-contrast microscopy [7] chromomycin-distamycin-DAPI staining was performed with a slight modification according to Schweizer [10].

C. Results and Discussion

Nonisotopic detection systems such as the rapid biotin/streptavidin system offer marked advantages over autoradiographic methods currently in use: In view of the considerably shortened procedure, in situ hybridization is no longer restricted to research laboratories and has proven to be a reliable tool for diagnostic and routine work. An increased resolving potential, highlighting sin-

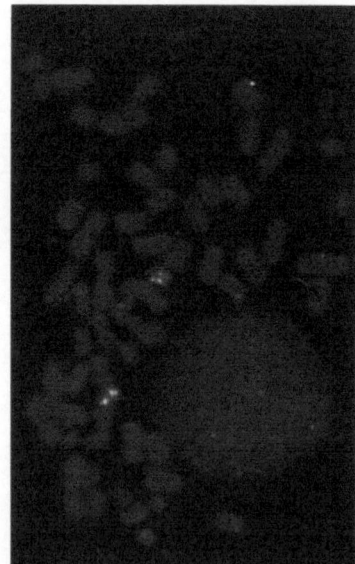

Fig. 2. Chromosome spread from a K562 cell after hybridization with a biotinylated 5'*bcr* probe and peroxidase-streptavidin detection

142

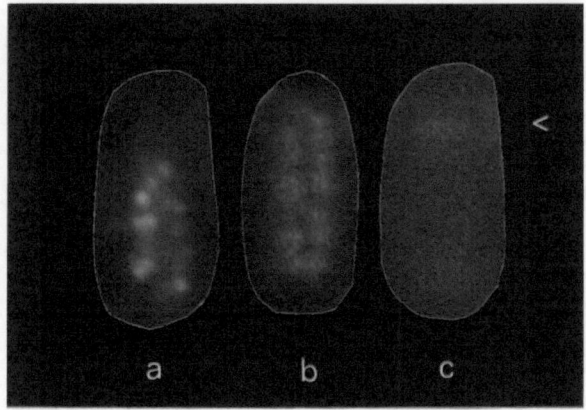

Fig. 3 a–c. Marker chromosome probed with a biotinylated *c-abl* probe **a**, and sequentially stained with chromomycin A₃ **b** and DA/DAPI **c**, indicating the centromere position (*arrow*). The bright spots in **a** represent the saltatory amplified *c-abl* sequences on this chromosome

gle sequences down to less than 2 kb, gives more detailed information about chromosome organization and gene localization.

Using the biotin-HRP-streptavidin/reflection-contrast microscopy technique and sequential staining of the chromosomes with chromomycin/distamycin/DAPI after the signal detection, we demonstrated that both the *c-abl* oncogene (1.8kb *Eco*RI fragment) and the 5'*bcr* (2.0kb *Bgl*II/*Hin*dIII fragment) are located on the same acrocentric marker chromosome (presumably derived from a Ph¹ chromosome) in the human K562 cell line (see Figs. 1–3), amplified four to seven times.

Besides the germline position of the *c-abl* oncogene on chromosome 9 (9q34), this DNA probe hybridized to a specific site on chromosome 2 (2q37), indicating a further translocation in the genome (Fig. 1). In addition to the rearranged position of this gene, the site of 5'*bcr* on 22q was also clearly visible by this technique (data not shown in detail).

In accordance with molecular biological [3] and in situ hybridization data obtained previously with radioactively labeled *c-abl* and c-lambda probes [11], we clearly identified an amplification of the *c-abl* oncogene and 5'*bcr* gene on the Ph¹-like marker chromosome. The most striking information gained from this study is a result of the increased resolution obtained by this specific technique: the amplified *c-abl* sequences also include the second molecular hallmark of CML, the *bcr* sequences [a region on chromosome 22 (22q) within which the majority of Ph¹ breakpoints are clustered], in a saltatory pattern, interspersed with other DNA segments (Fig. 3). A further translocation of the *c-abl* oncogene could be seen in a terminal position of the long arm of chromosome 2 in this specific cell line.

This method has considerable advantages over time-consuming autoradiographic in situ hybridization techniques and expensive molecular biological assays, and recent data show that the methods presented in this study will be useful for future routine diagnosis of unusual translocations in CML or other leukemias and tumors.

Acknowledgement. The authors thank Dr. G. Grosveld for *c-abl* and 5'*bcr* probes. This work was supported by a grant from the *Bundesministerium für Wissenschaft und Forschung,* Vienna, Austria (P.F.A.).

References

1. Ambros PF, Matzke MA, Matzke AJM (1986) Chromosoma 94:11–18
2. Ambros PF, Karlic H (1987) Hum Genet (in press)
3. Collins SJ, Groudine MT (1983) Proc Natl Acad Sci USA 80:4813–4817
4. de Klein A, Geurts van Kessel A, Grosveld G, Bartram CR, Hagemeijer A, Bootsma D, Spurr NK, Heisterkamp N, Groffen J, Stephenson JR (1982) Nature 300:765
5. Gall J, Pardue ML (1969) Proc Natl Acad Sci USA 63:378–383

6. John H, Birnstiel ML, Jones KW (1969) Nature 223:582–587
7. Landegent JE, Jansen in de Wal N, van Ommen GJ-B, Baas F, de Vijlder JJM, van Duijn P, van der Ploeg M (1985) Nature 317:175–177
8. Langer-Safer PR, Levine M, Ward DC (1982) Proc Natl Acad Sci USA 79:4381–4385
9. Leibowitz D, Cubbon R, Bank A (1985) Blood 65:526–529
10. Schweizer D (1981) Hum Genet 57:1–14
11. Selden JR, Emanuel BS, Wang E, Canizzarro L, Palumbo A, Erickson J, Nowell PC, Rovera G, Croce CM (1983) Proc Natl Acad Sci USA 80:7289–7292
12. Shtivelman E, Lifshitz B, Gale RP, Canaani E (1985) Nature 315:550–554

Haematology and Blood Transfusion   Vol. 31
Modern Trends in Human Leukemia VII
Edited by Neth, Gallo, Greaves, and Kabisch
© Springer-Verlag Berlin Heidelberg 1987

Persistence of CML Despite Deletion of Rearranged *bcr/c-abl* Sequences

C. R. Bartram [1], J. W. G. Janssen [1], and R. Becher [2]

A. Introduction

Chronic myelocytic leukemia (CML) is clinically divided into a chronic phase lasting for about 4 years, followed by an acute phase (blast crisis) of a few months' duration [5]. The cytogenetic hallmark of 95% of CML cases is the Philadelphia (Ph) chromosome, resulting from a reciprocal translocation between chromosomes 9 and 22 [21, 22] that places the *c-abl* oncogene into the breakpoint cluster region (*bcr*) on chromosome 22 [7, 11]; this area is part of a gene of yet unknown function [17, 24]. An involvement of *c-abl* and *bcr* sequences in the development of Ph-positive CML has been deduced from (a) the consistent rearrangement of both genes in all cytogenetic subtypes of this leukemia [1, 7, 14, 15], (b) the concurrent detection of a novel 8.5-kb hybrid *bcr/abl* RNA transcript [6, 10, 15], and (c) the expression of an altered *c-abl* protein that differs from its normal counterpart in having a higher associated tyrosine kinase activity [18, 19].

B. Material and Methods

I. Patient

A 49-year-old man developed blast crisis 45 months after diagnosis of Ph-positive CML. Blast cells were of the T-cell phenotype and genotype (Tβ gene rearrangement) and

showed a second Ph chromosome as an additional chromosomal aberration. Both Ph chromosomes in blast crisis were similar in size to the single pH chromosome in the chronic state. Combination chemotherapy achieved clinical remission; the patient has been in the chronic state for 14 months.

II. DNA Analysis

Bone marrow DNA (15 µg) was digested with appropriate enzymes, electrophoresed, blotted, and hybridized to 2-kb 5'*bcr*, 1.2-kb 3'*bcr*, and 1-kb 5'8E *bcr* cDNA probes as described elsewhere [2, 12, 25].

III. RNA Analysis

RNA was isolated from bone marrow cells as described by de Klein et al. [8]; 10 µg of poly-(A)-RNA was electrophoresed in the presence of formaldehyde, blotted, and hybridized to 0.6-kb *c-abl* and 2-kb 5'*bcr* probes as previously described [3].

IV. In Situ Hybridization

Chromosomes obtained from bone marrow were prepared according to standard techniques and treated for in situ hybridization as described [1]. The tritiated probe was a 1:1 mixture of human 1.1-kb 3' and 0.6-kb 5'*c-abl* plasmids [1]. After exposure for 12 days, slides were developed and stained with quinacrine mustard.

[1] Department of Pediatrics II, University of Ulm, D-7900 Ulm, FRG
[2] Department of Internal Medicine, University of Essen, D-4300 Essen, FRG

C. Results

A recombination within the *bcr* gene of this patient was established by Southern blot analysis of acute phase cells to a 3'*bcr* probe (Fig. 1, lane b). However, in contrast to all Ph-positive CML patients investigated to date, 5'*bcr* sequences detected only a 5-kb germline fragment for this man (Fig. 1, lane a). Hybridization of different digests of blast-cell DNAs to a cDNA probe covering most 5'*bcr* sequences known thus far [12]

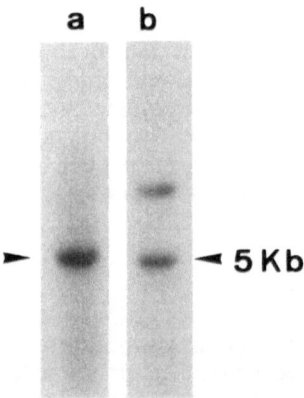

Fig. 1. Southern blot analysis of 15 µg DNA obtained from blast crisis. Bgl II digests were hybridized to a 5'*bcr* probe (*lane a*) and to a 3'*bcr* probe (*lane b*) that detect 5-kb germline bands. Note the rearranged 3'*bcr* fragment in lane b

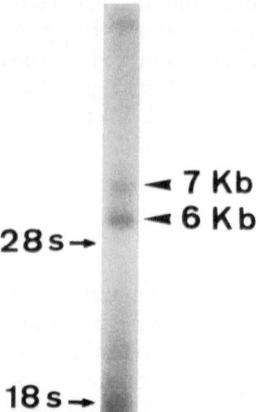

Fig. 2. Northern blot analysis of 10 µg poly-(A)-RNA obtained from blast crisis cells and hybridized to *c-abl* sequences

Table 1. Results of in situ hybridization to *c-abl* probes

Chro-mosome	Chronic phase		Blast crisis	
	Ob-served[a]	Grains Ex-pected[b]	Ob-served	Grains Ex-pected
1	7	9.0	24	18.1
2	12	8.8	14	17.7
3	4	7.3	12	14.6
4	9	7.0	7	14.0
5	6	6.7	11	13.4
6	2	6.3	6	12.6
7	5	5.8	10	11.6
8	2	5.3	8	6.5
9	13———2.5		34——— 5.0	
9q+	5	3.0	7	5.7
10	2	4.9	8	9.7
11	3	5.0	6	10.0
12	0	4.9	11	9.8
13	6	3.9	4	7.8
14	1	3.7	5	7.5
15	2	3.5	2	7.1
16	3	3.2	9	6.5
17	5	3.1	8	6.2
18	0	2.9	5	5.9
19	1	2.3	5	4.5
20	0	2.5	0	5.0
21	0	1.7	1	3.4
22	3	0.9	0	1.8
Ph	9———0.5		4[c]——— 2.2[c]	
X	4	2.8	7	5.6
Y	0	1.0	3	1.9

[a] Grains were counted on complete, well-spread metaphases.
[b] Number of grains expected according to DNA content [26].
[c] On two Ph chromosomes.

likewise failed to detect rearranged fragments (not shown). These results suggested a deletion of rearranged 5'*bcr* sequences on the Ph's in blast crisis. Since cell samples from the chronic state of this patient were not available for Southern blot analysis, we performed in situ hybridization studies of the *c-abl* oncogene to metaphases obtained from both phases to investigate a possible concurrent deletion of *abl* sequences.

Distribution of silver grains was uniform and random on 21 chromosomal spreads obtained from the chronic state, except for specific signals ($P < 0.01$) on chromosomes 9 and 22q− (Table 1). This result demonstrated the expected translocation of *c-abl* sequences to the Ph chromosome. However, 49 metaphases from blast-crisis cells demonstrated a significant ($P<0.01$) grain accumulation only on chromosome 9 (Table 1), and thus established a deletion of *c-abl* sequences from the blast-phase Ph chromosomes.

Northern blot analyses were in agreement with these data. Hybridization to *c-abl* and *bcr* sequences exhibited normal 6-kb and 7-kb *c-abl* (Fig. 2), as well as 4.5-kb and 7-kb *bcr* transcripts (not shown) respectively. Neither probe detected the hybrid 8.5-kb *bcr/abl* RNA species usually observed in Ph-positive CML.

D. Discussion

Various data suggest a multistep pathogenesis of CML, with the development of the cytogenetically visible Ph chromosome as well as the molecularly detectable *bcr/c-abl* rearrangement being a second event in this process [9, 13, 16, 20]. Transition from the chronic to the acute phase of Ph-positive CML would represent a third step, characterized by marked differences in the biology of leukemic cells and additional chromosomal aberrations [23]. The detection of identically rearranged *bcr* fragments as well as of comparable levels of the 8.5-kb *abl/bcr* transcript in blast cells and chronic-state cells of the same patient suggest that genes other than *c-abl* and *bcr* induce this terminal shift of biological properties within leukemic cells [4, 10].

However, the data presented here may indicate a possible modulating effect on the clinical course of this leukemic phase. In this respect it seems to be noteworthy that the patient has survived the acute phase for more than 14 months already in remarkably good condition. A deletion of the rearranged *abl/bcr* sequences, i.e., the withdrawal of the second step on the way to CML blast crisis, may result in the manifestation of a leukemic state different from the more aggressive blast crisis usually observed in CML.

On the other hand, the results of the present study suggest that once a leukemic cell has entered blast crisis, rearranged *abl/bcr* sequences are no longer essential for the maintenance of a leukemic state. In this respect it would be of interest to investigate in vitro the effect of antisense RNA or monoclonal antibodies directed against altered *bcr/abl* sequences in chronic-phase cells of Ph-positive CML patients. While the reported case appears to be a unique in vivo model, it can address only the respective roles of these genes in blast crisis.

Acknowledgements. We thank Drs. A. de Klein and G. Grosveld for probes and helpful discussions, Dr. Brittinger for providing cell samples and clinical information on the patient, and Angela Erkert for help with the preparation of the manuscript. This study was supported by the *Deutsche Forschungsgemeinschaft* and the *Ministerium für Wissenschaft und Kunst, Baden-Württemberg.*

References

1. Bartram CR, Klein A de, Hagemeijer A, Agthoven T van, Geurts van Kessel A, Bootsma D, Grosveld G, Fergusson-Smith MA, Davies T, Stone M, Heisterkamp N, Stephenson JR, Groffen J (1983) Nature 306:277
2. Bartram CR, Kleihauer E, Klein A de, Grosveld G, Teyssier JR, Heisterkamp N, Groffen J (1985) EMBO J 4:683
3. Bartram CR (1985) J Exp Med 162:2175
4. Bartram CR, Klein A de, Hagemeijer A, Carbonell F, Kleihauer E, Grosveld G (1986) Leuk Res 10:221
5. Champlin RE, Golde DW (1985) Blood 65:1039
6. Collins SJ, Kubonishi J, Myoshi J, Groudine MT (1984) Science 225:72
7. Klein A de, Geurts van Kessel A, Grosveld G, Bartram CR, Hagemeijer A, Bootsma D, Spurr NK, Heisterkamp N, Groffen J, Stephenson JR (1982) Nature 300:765
8. Klein A de, Hagemeijer A, Bartram CR, Houwen R, Hoefsloot L, Carbonell F, Chan L, Barnett M, Greaves M, Kleihauer E, Heisterkamp N, Groffen J, Grosveld G (1986) Blood 68:1369
9. Fialkow PH, Martin PJ, Najfeld V, Penfold GK, Jacobson RJ, Hansen JA (1981) Blood 58:158
10. Gale RP, Canaani E (1984) Proc Natl Acad Sci USA 81:5648
11. Groffen J, Stephenson JR, Heisterkamp N, Klein A de, Bartram CR, Grosveld G (1984) Cell 36:93
12. Grosveld G, Verwoerd T, Agthoven T van, Klein A de, Ramachandran KL, Heisterkamp

N, Stam K, Groffen J (1986) Mol Cell Biol 6:607

13. Hagemeijer A, Smit EME, Löwenberg B, Abels J (1979) Blood 53:1

14. Hagemeijer A, Bartram CR, Smit EME, Agthoven AJ van, Bootsma D (1984) Cancer Genet Cytogenet 13:1

15. Hagemeijer A, Klein A de, Gödde-Salz E, Turc-Carel C, Smit EME, Agthoven T van, Grosveld G (1985) Cancer Genet Cytogenet 18:95

16. Hayata J, Sakuri M, Kakati S, Sandberg AA (1975) Cancer 36:1177

17. Heisterkamp N, Stam K, Groffen J, Klein A de, Grosveld G (1985) Nature 315:758

18. Konopka JB, Watanabe SM, Singer JW, Collins SJ, Witte ON (1985) Proc Natl Acad Sci USA 82:1810

19. Konopka JB, Witte ON (1985) Mol Cell Biol 5:3116

20. Lisker R, Caras L, Mutdrinick O, Perez-Chavez F, Labardini J (1980) Blood 56:812

21. Nowell PC, Hungerford DA (1960) Science 132:1497

22. Rowley JD (1973) Nature 243:290

23. Sandberg AA (1980) Cancer Genet Cytogenet 1:217

24. Shtivelman E, Lifshitz B, Gale RP, Canaani E (1985) Nature 315:550

25. Stam K, Heisterkamp N, Grosveld G, Klein A de, Verma RS, Coleman M, Dosik H, Groffen J (1985) N Engl J Med 313:1429

26. Mendelsohn ML, Mayall BH, Bogart E, Moore DH, Perry BH (1973) Science 179:1126

Haematology and Blood Transfusion   Vol. 31
Modern Trends in Human Leukemia VII
Edited by Neth, Gallo, Greaves, and Kabisch
© Springer-Verlag Berlin Heidelberg 1987

Similar Molecular Alterations Occur in Related Leukemias With and Without the Philadelphia Chromosome

L. M. Wiedemann, K. Karhi, and L. C. Chan

A. Introduction

The reciprocal translocation between the long arms of chromosomes 9 and 22, t(9:22), results in the Philadelphia (Ph1) chromosome, the karyotypic hallmark of chronic myeloid leukaemia (CML) [1]. The molecular consequences of this translocation have been well characterized, although their contribution to the disease process is less clear. The translocation creates a hybrid transcription unit consisting of the 5' end of the so-called breakpoint cluster region (*bcr*) gene on ch22q11 and the *c-abl* proto-oncogene on ch9q34 [2]. This new gene is capable of being expressed as a chimeric 8.7 kb mRNA [3] which, when translated, produces a fusion protein (p210) with an enhanced phosphorylating activity [4] compared, in vitro, to the normal *c-abl* protein (p145).

This translocation event can be seen at the DNA level in the *bcr* gene, since it usually occurs within an 5.8 kb region of DNA and can be detected with a specific probe for this region (bcr probe) [2]. Involvement of *c-abl* is more difficult to demonstrate since the break on ch9q34 can occur anywhere within 50 kb or more [5] upstream of the proto-oncogene. We therefore chose to look at the size of the *abl* protein-tyrosine kinase as well as the level of its activity, as an assay for *c-abl* involvement. Using these criteria we analysed two other types of leukaemias (a) Ph1-positive acute lymphoblastic leu-

kaemia, (Ph1$^+$ ALL) and (b) Ph1-negative (Ph1$^-$) CML.

The Ph1 chromosome is present in about 10% of adult ALL and is associated with a poor prognosis. It is not clear, however, whether Ph1$^+$ ALL represents blast crisis of previously undiagnosed Ph1$^+$ CML, whether it is a clinically distinct group, or (what is more likely) a mixture of the two [6].

The Ph1$^-$ CML group, represents 5% of patients diagnosed as CML whose cells do not contain the Ph1 chromosome. However, the need for more accurate assessment of these cases has been demonstrated by Pugh et al. [7], who examined 25 cases originally diagnosed as Ph1$^-$ CML and reclassified all but one as myelodysplastic syndromes including various refractory anaemias, chronic myelomonocytic leukaemia (CMML) and polycythaemia rubra vera.

B. Results

DNA was isolated and purified from peripheral blood and/or bone marrow leukocytes of samples from patients diagnosed on the basis of clinical and haematological criteria by Prof. D. Galton (Royal Postgraduate Medical School, Hammersmith, London) as Ph1$^+$ CML (1 case), bona fide Ph1$^-$ CML (2 cases), atypical Ph1$^-$ CML (aCML) (2 cases) and Ph1$^-$ CMML (1 case). The DNA was digested with the restriction endonuclease *Bgl*II, fractionated by electrophoresis through a 0.7% agarose gel, and blotted onto nitrocellulose according to the method of Southern [8]. Relevant restriction frag-

Leukaemia Research Fund Centre, Institute of Cancer Research, Fulham Road, London SW3 6JB

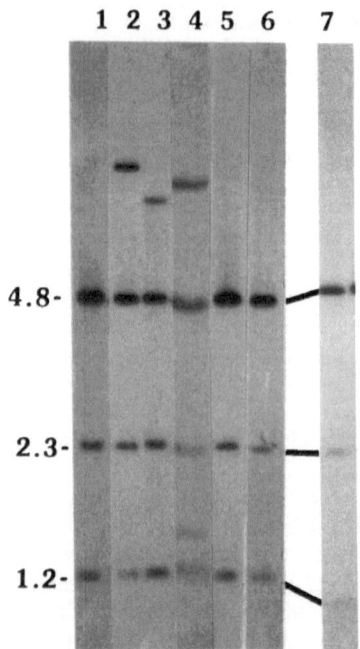

1 2 3 4 5 6   7

4.8-

2.3-

1.2-

Fig. 1. DNA analysis of the breakpoint cluster region (*bcr*) on chromosome 22. The restriction map of the region of chromosome 22 is illustrated in the *lower portion* as well as the probe used for hybridization analysis for rearrangement (kindly supplied by Dr. J. Groffen of Oncogene Sciences, USA). The *dashed region* of the probe was deleted due to the presence of repetitive sequences. The normal size of the *Bgl*II fragments detected by this probe are delineated. The known positions of the bcr exons are also shown. Bg, *Bgl*II; Ba, *Bam*HI; E, *Eco*RI; and H, *Hind*III. *Bgl*II digested DNA from cells with the normal *bcr* configuration, Bri-7, *lane 1;* Ph1$^+$, CML, *lane 2;* Ph1$^-$ CML-1, *lane 3;* Ph1$^-$ CML-2, *lane 4;* Ph1$^-$ aCML-1, *lane 5;* Ph1$^-$ CMML, *lane 6,* and Ph1$^-$ aCML-2, *lane 7,* were hybridized to the bcr probe and autoradiographed. The normal bcr bands are labelled in kb.

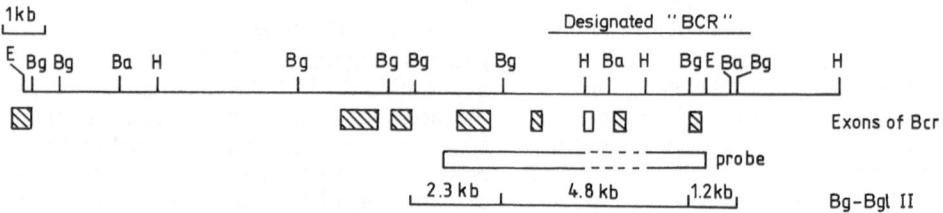

ments were identified by hybridization with the bcr probe (kindly supplied by Dr. J. Groffen, Oncogene Science, USA) and visualized using Kodak XAR-5 film (Fig. 1).

In germline DNA from cells without a Ph1 chromosome, the bcr probe reveals three bands reflecting the normal restriction fragment sizes of the nonrearranged chromosome 22 region (Fig. 1, lane 1). When a translocation occurs in Ph1$^+$ CML, one or two new bands are detected by the probe, (i.e., Fig. 1, lane 2) depending on the position of the break and the retention of the 3' as well as 5' portion of the translocation products (deletion of the 3' region of bcr appears not to be uncommon [6]).

When the DNA from the six patients was analysed, new bands were detected in the Ph1$^+$ CML (Fig. 1, lane 2) as well as two

bona fide Ph1$^-$ CML (Fig. 1, lanes 3 and 4), suggesting that the DNA is rearranged in the bcr locus in the DNA from these leukaemias. DNA samples from the two aCML and the CMML did not give rise to additional bands (Fig. 1, lanes 5–7). This information shows an interesting correlation with the diagnosis based solely on clinical and haematological features and confirms the conclusion reached in a recent report [9] although our data on aCML is in conflict with a study by Ganesan et al. [10]. DNA from the cells from the bona fide Ph1$^-$ CML patients, although karyotypically apparently normal, appear to have a "masked" Ph1 chromosome as analysed by bcr rearrangement and will be refered to as bcr-positive.

To exclude the possibility of polymorphism associated with *Bgl*II in a published

150

report of Ph1⁻ CML [11], several enzymes were used to confirm the rearrangement of bcr in the DNA from bona fide CML patients and the lack of rearrangement in the bcr⁻ group.

Detection of the Abl-Kinase Activity

Mononuclear cells from selected samples were isolated on Ficoll-Hypaque (acute or blast crisis cases) or Percoll density gradients (chronic cases) and analysed by a modification of the in vitro autophosphorylation assay of the abl protein tyrosine kinase [2]. Briefly, 4–10 million cells were lysed in the presence of protease inhibitors and an antiserum raised against a synthetic peptide which was derived from the abl protein tyrosine kinase sequence (a kind gift of Syd Raytner, NIMR, London), was added in the presence or absence of the peptide antigen.

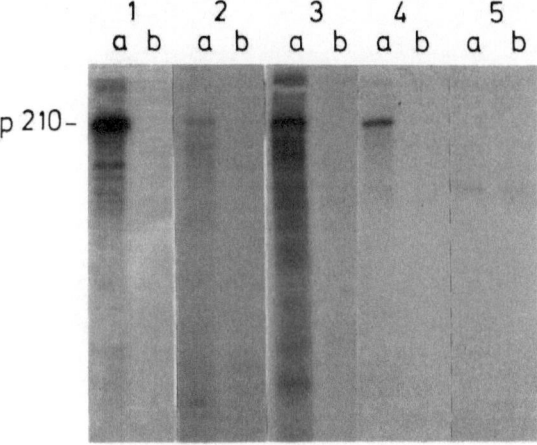

Fig. 2. Analysis of samples for bcr-abl protein tyrosine kinase. Blast cells were purified on density step gradients, *abl*-related proteins were isolated from the lysed cells in the presence (*lanes b*) or absence (*lanes a*) of the synthetic peptide used to generate the antiserum. Proteins were allowed to autophosphorylate in the presence of γ-^{32}P-ATP and were analysed by PAGE. The autoradiographic results shown were from Nalm-1 cells, *lanes 1;* Ph1⁺ CML-myeloid blast crisis, *lanes 2;* Ph1⁻ CML-2, *lanes 3;* Ph1⁺ ALL, *lanes 4,* and Ph1⁻ ALL, *lanes 5.* The position of the p210 protein tyrosine kinase as determined from markers, is indicated.

The lysate was clarified after 15 min and added to Sepharose 4B-CL-protein-A beads. The beads were collected and washed and the bound material was allowed to autophosphorylate in the presence of γ-^{32}P-ATP. The products were analysed by SDS-polyacrylamide gel electrophoresis.

Lysates from a cell line Nalm-1 which bears the Ph1 chromosome and in which bcr is rearranged, were used as positive controls. The addition of the peptide 4 completely eliminated the precipitation and subsequent autophosphorylation of the p210 in Nalm-1 demonstrating specificity of the anti-abl antiserum for this protein (Fig. 2, lane 1 b). The p210 activity was observed in all samples that had been shown to rearrange in the *bcr* locus. These included a Ph1⁺ CML in myeloid blast crisis (Fig. 2, lane 2) the Ph1⁻ CML-2 (Fig. 2, lane 3) and a Ph1⁺ ALL (Fig. 2, lane 4) that had previously been shown to rearrange in the *bcr* locus, (see [6], patient L8), while we were unable to detect any *abl*-related products in Ph1⁻, bcr⁻ samples of aCML (data not shown) or in a Ph1⁻, bcr⁻ All (Fig. 2, lane 5).

C. Conclusion

We have shown the importance of the protein kinase assay as a complementary study to bcr analysis in leukaemias that are related to Ph1⁺ CML. We find that: (a) Ph1⁻ bona fide CML and Ph1⁺ CML appear to be the same disease as measured at the DNA level by bcr rearrangement and at the protein level as measured by the p210 abl protein tyrosine kinase assay (b) Ph1⁺ ALLs which rearrange in bcr also express the p210 kinase activity. Since the protein kinase assay is quick (< 36 h) and requires only 5 million enriched blast cells, it could be used as an alternative to DNA analysis for identification of bcr-positive samples in clinical specimens.

Acknowledgements. We thank the following people who have helped in this study: Dr. D. Bain (St. Mary's Hospital, London), Dr. D. Bevan (St. George's Hospital, London), Dr. A. Lister (St. Bartholomew's Hospital, London), Dr. A. Parker (Royal Infirmary, Edinburgh), Prof. A. Jacobs (University of Wales, Cardiff), and Dr. R. Powles (Royal Marsden Hospital, Sutton) for providing clinical samples. Prof. D. Galton (Royal Postgraduate Medical School, London) for reviewing the haematological slides; Dr. J. Groffen (Oncogene Sciences, USA) for bcr probe; Drs. G. Foulkes, S. Raytner (NIMR, London) and O. Witte (UCLA, USA) for anti-abl antibodies and Ms. G. Parkins for typing of the manuscript. We also thank Prof. M. F. Greaves for helpful discussion and the Leukaemia Research Fund of Great Britain for funding of this project.

References

1. Nowell PC, Hungerford DA (1960) Science 132:1947
2. Groffen J, Stephenson JR, Heisterkamp N, Klein A de, Bartram CR, Grosveld G (1984) Cell 36:93
3. Stam K, Heisterkamp N, Grosveld G, Klein A de, Verma RS, Coleman M, Dosik H, Groffen J (1985) New Engl J Med 313:1429
4. Konopka JB, Watanabe SM, Singer JW, Collins SJ, Witte ON (1985) Proc Natl Acad Sci (USA) 82:1810
5. Grosveld G, Verwoerd T, Agthoven T van, Klein A de, Ramachandran KI, Heisterkamp N, Stam R, Groffen J (1986) Mol Cell Biol 6:607
6. Klein A de, Hagemeijer A, Bartram CR, Houwen R, Hoefsloot L, Carbonell F, Chan L, Barnett M, Greaves MF, Kleihauer E, Heisterkamp N, Groffen J, Grosveld G. Blood (1986)6:1369
7. Pugh WC, Pearson M, Vardiman JW, Rowley JD (1985) Br J Haematol 60:457
8. Southern EM (1975) J Mol Biol 98:503
9. Morris CM, Reeve AE, Fitzgerald PH, Hollings PE, Beard MEJ, Heaton DC (1986) Nature (London) 320:281
10. Ganesan TS, Rassol F, Guo A-P, Young BD, Galton DAG, Goldman JM (In this volume)
11. Bartram CR, Carbonell F (1986) Cancer Genet Cytogenet 21:183
12. Konopka JB, Witte ON (1985) Mol Cell Biol 5:3116

Haematology and Blood Transfusion   Vol. 31
Modern Trends in Human Leukemia VII
Edited by Neth, Gallo, Greaves, and Kabisch
© Springer-Verlag Berlin Heidelberg 1987

Rearrangement of the *bcr* Gene in Philadelphia-Chromosome-Negative Chronic Myeloid Leukemia

T. S. Ganesan[2], F. Rassool[1], A.-P. Guo[1], B. D. Young[2], D. A. G. Galton[1], and J. M. Goldman[1]

A. Introduction

The majority of patients with chronic myeloid leukaemia (CML) have a characteristic deletion of a portion of the long arm of one chromosome 22, the Philadelphia (Ph^1) chromosome, in their myeloid cells. The missing material is reciprocally translocated to chromosome 9 such that the usual karyotype is described as $t(9;22)(q34;q11)$. In Ph^1-positive CML, the oncogene (c-*abl*) normally present on chromosome 9 is translocated to chromosome 22 [1, 2] where it comes into juxtaposition with a region named the "breakpoint cluster region" (*bcr*) [3]. A chimeric *abl*-related mRNA has been identified in cells from patients with CML [4] and is associated with the presence of a fusion protein that has tyrosine kinase activity [5]. Thus, patients with Ph^1-positive CML show evidence of rearrangement of DNA within the *bcr* region.

About 10% of patients regarded on clinical and haematological grounds as having CML lack the Ph^1 chromosome. Some of these have a leukaemia that is totally indistinguishable from Ph^1-positive disease in all other respects, while in other cases clinical and haematological features suggest that the disease is different. We report the results of studying the clinical, haematological, cytogenetic and molecular biological features in seven patients with Ph^1-negative CML. Two

further patients who were classified as having chronic myelomonocytic leukaemia (CMML) are also included.

B. Materials and Methods

I. Patients

We selected for study nine patients who had attended the Hammersmith Hospital within the previous 2 years with a diagnosis of Ph^1-negative CML. Their clinical and haematological features at diagnosis are shown in Table 1.

II. Cytogenetic Analysis

Cytogenetic studies were carried out on fresh bone marrow cells or on fresh or cryopreserved buffy-coat cells collected from the patients at the time of diagnosis. Mononuclear cells were prepared from the blood samples by centrifugation on a Lymphoprep (Nyegaard, Oslo, Norway) density gradient. Cells from marrow or blood were then incubated at 37 °C at a final concentration of 1×10^6/ml in RPMI 1640 medium supplemented with 20% foetal calf serum, L-glutamine and antibiotics for a period of 24–72 h. Colcemid was then added, and the cells were harvested 1 h later. Chromosomes were prepared according to standard methods and analysed after Giemsa banding [6]. In a number of the cultures, mitoses were synchronized by addition of fluorodeoxyuridine (FDU) in accordance with the method of Webber and Garson [7]. For this purpose,

---

[1] The MRC Leukaemia Unit, Hammersmith Hospital and Royal Postgraduate Medical School, London, UK
[2] The ICRF Medical Oncology Unit, St. Bartholomew's Hospital, London, UK

Table 1. Clinical and haematological details of nine patients with Ph¹-negative CML

Patient	Age/sex	Spleen cm	Peripheral blood at diagnosis			Differential (% of 300 cells)									NAP	Treatment and response
			Hb g/dl	WBC ×10.9/1	Platelets ×10.9/1	Bl	Pm	My +Met	Neut	Eos	Baso	Mono	Lymph	NRBCs		
1.	M/24	25+	8.3	174	941	6	6	21	41	6	14	0	4	0	0	HU; PR
2.	M/58	0	11.2	170	53	1	3	28	61	0	0.5	0.5	6	0	0–12	HU; PR
3.	M/31	0	12.1	46	375	0	0	10	56	17	2	1	14	0	NA	BU, Hu; CR. BMT
4.[a]	F/33	0	10.5	77	492	0	0	17	68	4	2	3	6	0	0	BU, HU; CR. BMT
5.[a]	M/62	3	10.6	105	87	0	4	31	58	0	0	1	2	2	NA	SRT; CR
6.	F/43	12	10.3	506	319	2	4	28	59	2	3	1	1	0.3	0	BU; CR
7.	F/54	3	7.0	163	545	2	4	22	58	2	9	1	1	0.3	0	BU, HU; CR
8.[b]	M/63	0	9.4	15	116	9	–	22	28	6	1	12	27	0	94	NYT
9.[b]	M/61	15	14.2	42	74	0	0	6	73	4	1	13	4	4	NA	NYT

HU, hydroxyurea; BU, busulphan; SRT, splenic irradiation; NYT, not yet treated; CR, complete haematological response; PR, partial haematological response; BMT, Bone marrow transplantation; NA, not available; NAP, neutrophil alkaline phosphatase (normal range 30–100 units).
[a] Blood film morphology not typical of Ph¹-positive CML.
[b] Morphological diagnosis: CMML.

154

cultures were incubated for an initial period of either 24 or 48 h, after which FDU was added at a concentration of 0.1 μM. Incubation was continued for a further 18 h, after which thymidine was added to release cells from the FDU-induced block of division. Incubation was continued for a further 6 h, after which colcemid was added and the cells were harvested 30 min later. Chromosomes were prepared as described above.

III. Southern Analysis

Leukaemic cells were isolated from the peripheral blood or marrow samples, and high molecular weight DNA was prepared by standard procedures. All the samples of DNA were digested with restriction enzymes (*Bam*HI, *Bg*III, *Eco*RI, and *Hin*dIII), separated on a 0.8% agarose gel by electrophoresis and transferred to Hybond-N (Amersham) by the Southern technique [8]. The filters were prehybridized and then hybridized [9] at 43 °C with radiolabelled (^{32}P) probe. They were washed twice for 60 min in 0.1 × SSC/0.1% sodium dodecyl sulphate at 43 °C and autoradiographed for 3–5 days at −70 °C.

The 0.6-kb intron fragment (*bcr*-G) was subcloned from a commercially available *bcr* probe (Oncogene Sciences, Mineola, New York) and labelled by the oligonucleotide

priming method to a specific activity of 1–3 × 10^9 cpm/μg [10].

C. Results

I. Haematology

The haematological findings for the nine patients are shown in Table 1. Their leucocyte counts ranged from 46 to 506 × 10^9/l at diagnosis. Minor dysplastic changes were present in the granulocyte series in three cases (patients 2, 5, and 7). The neutrophil alkaline phosphatase score was low in the five patients studied at diagnosis. Two of the patients were thrombocytopenic. In each case the bone marrow in aspirate smears, trephine sections or in both was hypercellular and showed gross granulocytic hyperplasia with maturation and no excess of blast cells. The morphology in five cases (1, 2, 3, 6, and 7) was indistinguishable from that characteristic of *Ph*^{1}-positive chronic granulocytic leukaemia (CGL) [11]; in two cases (4 and 5) it was atypical, and in two others (8 and 9) was characteristic of CMML. In five cases, treatment usually effective in *Ph*^{1}-positive CGL was effective in restoring the patient's blood counts to normal, but in two cases only partial responses were observed. All seven patients were alive at the time of writing. Two patients (3 and 4) had been treated

Table 2. Cytogenetic findings in the nine patients

Patient	Source of cells	Number of metaphases	Karyotype
1.	PB	38	46, *XY* (*n* = 38)
		2	46, *XY, del*(22) (*pter—q*11:)
2.	BM	30	46, *XY del* (16) (*pter→q*22:)
3.	BM[a]	30	46, *XY*
4.	PB	20	46, *XX*
5.	BM[a]	20	46, *XY*
6.	PB	25	46, *XX*
7.	BM	30	46, *XX, t*(4;9;22) (9*pter→*9*q*34::22*q*11→*qter*; 22*pter→*22*q*11::4*p*11→4*pter*)
8.	BM	20	46,*XY*
9.	BM	20	46,*XY*

[a] Except in two cases, blood (PB) or bone marrow (BM) for these studies was collected before any treatment was administered. Marrow cells from patients 3 and 5 were studied after the patients had been treated with chemotherapy and splenic irradiation, respectively.

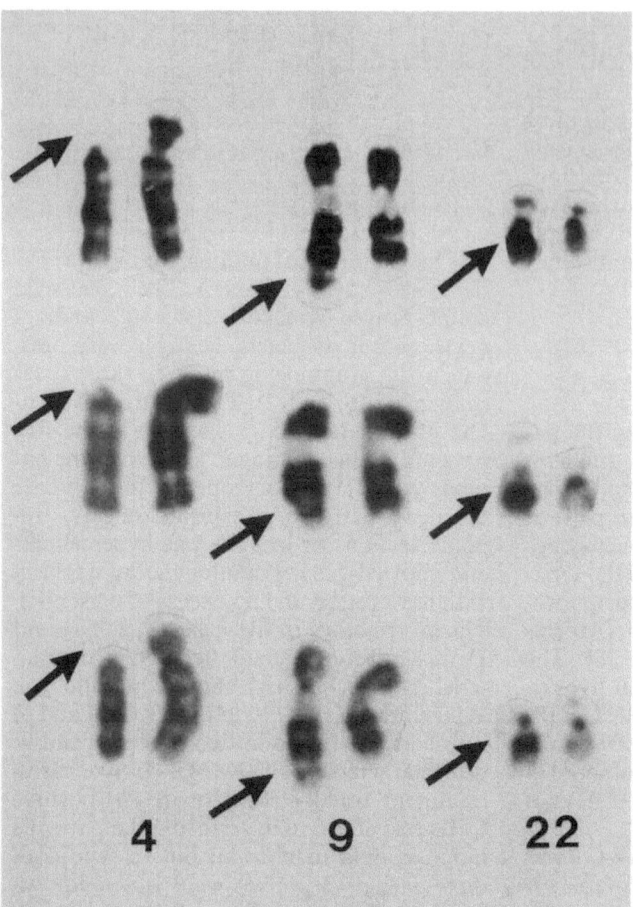

Fig. 1. Partial karyotype of three G-banded metaphases from myeloid cells of patient 1, showing $t(4;9;22)(p11;q34;q11)$. Chromosomal material has been reciprocally translocated between chromosomes 9 and 22, resulting in $9q+$. Moreover, material from the short arm of chromosome 4 has been translocated to the long arm of chromosome 22. These changes are indicated by *arrows*

by allogeneic bone marrow transplantation and were well 6 and 12 months after transplant, respectively.

II. Cytogenetics

The results of cytogenetic studies are summarized in Table 2. Patient 7 had a complex translocation and her karyotype may be regarded as showing a "masked" Ph^1 chromosome (Fig. 1). Patient 2 had a deletion involving chromosome 16, but the karyotype was otherwise normal. A third patient (1) had a minority population of myeloid metaphases that showed $22q-$ (but no $9q+$), but the majority of metaphases were normal.

Table 3. Schematic representation of *bcr* gene rearrangements in the nine patients

Pa-tient	Rearrangement detected with restriction			
	*Bam*HI	*Bg*III	*Eco*RI	*Hind*III
1.	+	+	+	−
2.	−	−	−	+
3.	−	+	−	−
4.	+	−	+	+
5.	−	−	+	−
6.	−	+	+	−
7.	+	+	+	−
8.	−	−	−	−
9.	−	−	−	−

156

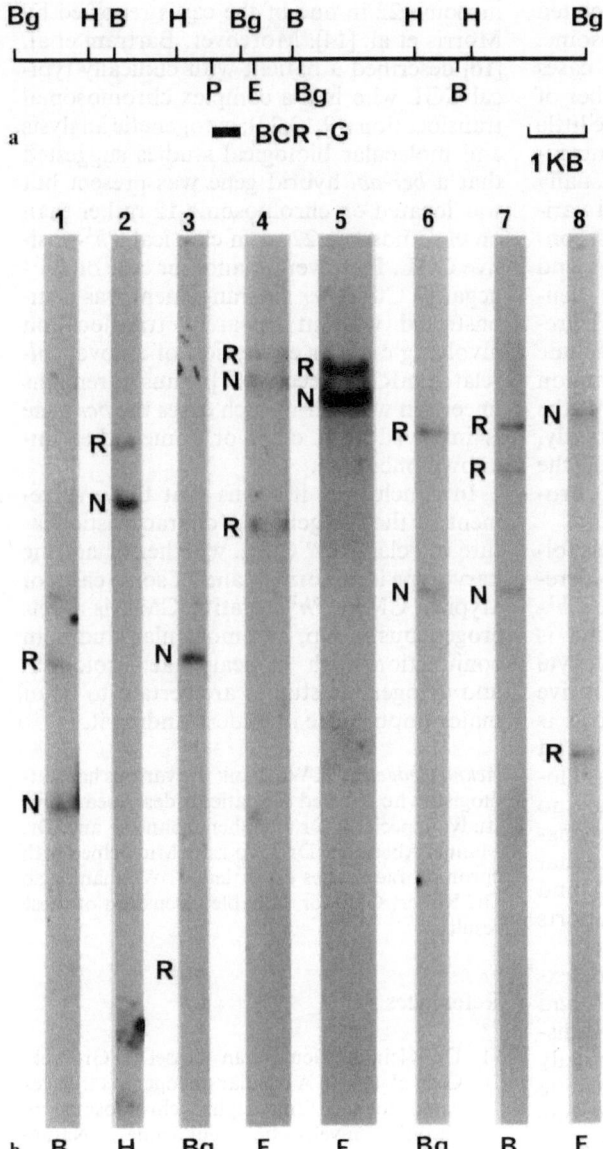

Bg   H B   H   Bg B   H   H   Bg

                    P E Bg   B
a   ■■ BCR-G |___|
                                                 1 KB

       1   2   3   4   5   6   7   8

b   B   H   Bg   E   E   Bg   B   E

Fig. 2. a Schematic representation of the *bcr* region (3), showing the position of the probe (*bcr*-G) used. For the sake of clarity, not all PstI sites are indicated. *E, EcoRI; B, BamHI; Bg, BgIII; H, HindIII; P, PstI.* **b** Composite of Southern blots from the seven patients, showing patterns of rearrangement for each patient. *Lanes 1–7* show blots from each patient using DNA digested with one of the restriction endonucleases that displayed a rearrangement. The numbers correspond to the numbers given to each patient in Table 1. *Lane 8* shows DNA from a patient with *Ph¹*-positive CML, digested with EcoRI and hybridized with the *bcr*-G probe. The enzyme used in each case is indicated below the corresponding lane. *N,* normal band; *R,* rearranged band(s)

The other six patients had entirely normal karyotypes.

III. Southern Analysis

Southern blots prepared from leukaemic cells and probed with the *bcr*-G probe (Fig. 2 A) showed abnormal restriction bands in seven of the nine cases (Table 3). A representative Southern blot for each patient exhibiting rearrangement with one of the restriction enzymes is shown in Fig. 2 B. Patients 8 and 9 did not show any rearrangements of the *bcr* region with multiple enzymes and different probes of that region (data not shown).

D. Discussion

The common form of CML is CGL (90% of cases): it has a highly characteristic clinical and haematological profile and is associated with the presence of the Ph^1 chromosome. The remaining 10% of Ph^1-negative cases are heterogeneous and include a number of possibly unrelated conditions that have little in common, except high leucocyte counts involving the granulocytic lineage and usually enlargement of the spleen. The named variants include juvenile CML, which is confined to children under 4 years of age, and CMML and chronic neutrophilic leukaemia, confined to elderly patients. The remaining cases, found at all ages, include firstly, examples identical with the common Ph^1-positive CGL in all respects except the lack of the Ph^1 chromosome, and secondly, others with atypical features which lead the haematologist to predict that the Ph^1 chromosome will not be found.

The atypical features referred to are as follows: (a) the spleen is often smaller at corresponding leucocyte counts than in the Ph^1-positive disease; (b) thrombocytopenia is common at presentation; (c) the myelocyte "peak" characteristic of the Ph^1-positive disease is often absent; (d) monocytosis is common; (e) basophilia is exceptional; and (f) dysplastic morphology in the granulocytic series is common. Because there are no generally accepted guidelines for the recognition of these latter cases, it is possible that some at least have been called CMML and myelodysplastic syndrome in other reports on Ph^1-negative CML [12, 13, 15].

Two of our patients (4 and 5) are examples of atypical CML, two (8 and 9) had CMML and five (1, 2, 3, 6, and 7) were indistinguishable clinically and haematologically from Ph^1-positive CGL. None of the nine patients had the classical $t(9;22)$, though one (7) had a "masked" Ph^1 chromosome; three had various chromosome abnormalities and six had normal karyotypes. This work suggests that among cases of Ph^1-negative CML, patients whose disease is clinically and haematologically indistinguishable from classical Ph^1-positive CGL are likely to show evidence of bcr rearrangement; the only two "atypical" cases studied also showed rearrangement, but the two cases of CMML did not. We do not know whether c-abl is the oncogene involved in the seven patients with rearranged bcr. abl-related genetic material was demonstrated on chromosome 22 in one of the cases reported by Morris et al. [14]. Moreover, Bartram et al. [16] described a patient with clinically typical CGL who had a complex chromosomal translocation $t(9;12;22)$; cytogenetic analysis and molecular biological studies suggested that a bcr-abl hybrid gene was present but was located on chromosome 12 rather than on chromosome 22 as in classical Ph^1-positive CGL. However, in another case of Ph^1-negative CGL, bcr rearrangement was demonstrated without apparent translocation involving c-abl or expression of a novel abl-related mRNA species [17]. Thus, it remains uncertain whether in such cases the bcr gene is involved with c-abl or some other unknown oncogene.

In conclusion, it seems that the involvement of the bcr gene is a characteristic feature of "classical" CGL, whether or not the karyotype is abnormal, and of some cases of atypical CML. Ph^1-negative CML is a heterogeneous group, and molecular studies in conjunction with clinical, haematological and cytogenetic studies are certain to be of major importance in understanding it.

Acknowledgements. We thank the various haematologists who referred the patients described in this study, especially Dr. Stephen Johnson and Dr. Manuel Abecassis. Dr. Gao Ling Min helped with chromosome studies on patient 7. We thank also Dr. Robert Gale for valuable discussion of these results.

References

1. De Klein A, Geurts van Kessel A, Grosveld G, et al. (1982) A cellular oncogene is translocated to the Philadelphia chromosome in chronic myelocytic leukaemia. Nature 300:765–767
2. Bartram CR, Klein A de, Hagemeijer A, et al. (1983) Translocation of c-abl oncogene correlates with the presence of a Philadelphia chromosome in chronic myelocytic leukaemia. Nature 306:277–280
3. Groffen J, Stephenson JR, Heisterkamp N, Klein A de, Bartram CR, Grosveld G (1984) Philadelphia chromosomal breakpoints are clustered within a limited region – bcr – on chromosome 22. Cell 36:93–99
4. Shtivelman E, Lipshitz B, Gale RP, Canaani E (1985) Fused transcript of abl and bcr genes in chronic myelogenous leukaemia. Nature 315:550–554

5. Konopka JB, Watanabe SM, Singer JW, Collins SJ, Witte ON (1985) Cell lines and clinical isolates derived from Ph[1]-positive chronic myelogenous leukaemia patients express c-abl proteins with a common structural alteration. Proc Natl Acad Sci USA 85:1810–1818

6. Seabright M (1983) A rapid banding technique for human chromosomes. Lancet 2:971–972

7. Webber LM, Garson OM (1983) Fluorodeoxyuridine synchronization of bone marrow cultures. Cancer Genet Cytogenet 8:123–132

8. Southern EM (1975) Detection of specific sequences among DNA fragments separated by gel electrophoresis. J Mol Biol 98:503–517

9. Anderson MLM, Szajnert MF, Kaplan JC, McColl L, Young BD (1984) The isolation of a human Ig V_λ gene from a recombinant library of chromosome 22 and estimation of its copy number. Nucleic Acids Res 12:6647–6661

10. Feinberg AP, Vogelstein B (1983) A technique for radiolabeling DNA restriction endonuclease fragments to high specific activity. Anal Biochem 132:6–13

11. Galton DAG (1984) Chronic leukaemia. In: Hardisty RM, Weatherall DG (eds) Blood and its disorders. Blackwell, Oxford, pp 877–917

12. Pugh WC, Pearson M, Vardiman JW, Rowley JD (1985) Philadelphia chromosome-negative chronic myelogenous leukaemia: a morphological reassessment. Br J Haematol 60:457–468

13. Travis LB, Pierre RV, DeWald GW (1986) Ph[1]-negative chronic granulocytic leukaemia: a nonentity. Am J Clin Pathol 85:186–193

14. Morris CM, Reeve AE, Fitzgerald PH, Hollings PE, Beard MEJ, Heaton DC (1986) Genomic diversity correlates with clinical variation in Ph[1]-negative chronic myeloid leukaemia. Nature 320:281–283

15. Bartram CR, Carbonell F (1986) bcr Rearrangement in Ph-negative CML (letter). Cancer Genet Cytogenet 21:183–184

16. Bartram CR, Kleihauer D, Klein A de, Grosveld G, Teyssier JR, Heisterkamp N, Groffen J (1985) c-abl and bcr are rearranged in a Ph[1]-negative CML patient. EMBO J 4:683–686

17. Bartram CR (1985) bcr Rearrangement without juxtaposition of c-abl in chronic myelocytic leukaemia. J Exp Med 162:2175–2179

Haematology and Blood Transfusion   Vol. 31
Modern Trends in Human Leukemia VII
Edited by Neth, Gallo, Greaves, and Kabisch
© Springer-Verlag Berlin Heidelberg 1987

Rearrangement of *bcr* and *c-abl* Sequences in Ph-positive Acute Leukemias and Ph-negative CML – an Update

C. R. Bartram [1]

A. Introduction

The molecular hallmark of the Philadelphia (Ph) translocation in CML is a rearrangement between the *c-abl* oncogene and a gene provisionally called *bcr* [7, 11, 13, 19]. As a consequence of this genomic recombination on the Ph chromosome, CML cells transcribe a chimeric 8.5-kb RNA species, consisting of both 5'*bcr* and *c-abl* sequences [6, 10, 20], that is translated into a p 210 *abl* protein [15, 16]. As yet the normal cellular functions of *c-abl* and *bcr* have not been characterized. However, *c-abl* belongs to a family of genes coding for proteins with associated tyrosine kinase activity; it is tempting to speculate that the *bcr* moiety of the hybrid *bcr/abl* molecule has altered the structure of the *abl* protein and thus changed its tyrosine kinase activity. Recently, we extended the analyses of *c-abl* and *bcr* sequences to Ph-negative CML and Ph-positive acute leukemias. The results are summarized below.

B. Ph-negative CML

About 5% of all CML patients exhibit no Ph chromosome in leukemic cells. While Ph-negative CML is associated with a generally less favorable course, it is widely accepted that this entity constitutes a heterogeneous group of prognostically distinct disorders [21]. In our studies we included only cases

that met stringent criteria of CML [5]. As listed in Table 1, these patients usually lack *c-abl* and *bcr* rearrangements in Southern blot and in situ hybridization studies. However, in seven cases an involvement of both genes was established. Among these seven patients, two exhibited an involvement of chromosome region 9q34 on the cytogenetic level, i.e., t(8;9) and t(9;12) and this may represent masked complex Ph translocations.

Table 1. Ph-negative CML ($n = 31$ [a])

I	No *bcr* rearrangement, no *c-abl* translocation	23
II	*bcr/c-abl* rearrangement	7
III	*bcr* rearrangement, no *c-abl* translocation	1

[a] Data of some patients have been published elsewhere [1–5, 7, 11, 13].

The other cases showed no chromosomal abnormality, even when high-resolution banding techniques were used. Yet Southern blots revealed a *bcr* rearrangement, and in situ hybridization studies demonstrated a *c-abl* translocation toward chromosome 22. In one patient, Northern blot analysis exhibited the 8.5-kb *abl/bcr* transcript. Similar results have recently been reported by Morris et al. [17]. Leukemic cells of only one Ph-negative CML patient showed a *bcr* rearrangement without juxtaposition of *c-abl* sequences [3]. In leukemic cells of this patient Northern blots revealed a novel 7.3-kb *bcr* transcript.

Department of Pediatrics II, University of Ulm, D-7900 Ulm, FRG

C. Ph-positive ALL and AML

Initially considered specific for CML, the Ph chromosome has been described in other hematopoietic neoplasias; in adult ALL the Ph translocation is the most frequent detectable chromosomal aberration, with an incidence of about 20% (van den Berghe, this volume). The question of whether Ph-positive acute leukemias represent distinct clinical entities or comprise CML patients initially diagnosed in the acute phase is still a matter of controversy [14]. Since Ph chromosomes in CML and acute leukemias are indistinguishable cytogenetically, we applied molecular approaches to further elucidate this problem.

Ten Ph-positive ALL patients exhibited a *bcr/c-abl* rearrangement comparable to Ph-positive CML (Table 2); moreover, Northern blots showed the 8.5-kb *abl/bcr* transcript in two of these ten cases that could be investigated. It may be sensible to assume that those patients are suffering from CML blast crisis. Three other Ph-positive ALLs likewise revealed a *bcr* rearrangement, but 3'*bcr* sequences, usually transferred to chromosome 9q+, have been deleted. The biological meaning of this observation remains obscure, but similar deletions have never been detected in Ph-positive CML.

Despite the presence of a Ph chromosome, a third group of ALL patients showed no *bcr* rearrangement (Table 2). Similar results have recently been reported by other investigators [9, 18]. In situ hybridization studies exhibited a *c-abl* translocation in three of our patients. The possibility remains that at least in some of the patients *c-abl* translocated to 5' sequences of the *bcr* gene mapping outside the CML-specific cluster region. Since the entire *bcr* gene has recently been cloned (Mes-Masson et al., this volume), this problem can now be investigated directly. However, the observation that Northern blots of one of our ALL patients and of an ALL cell line [8, 9] detect normal-size *bcr* and *abl* transcripts argues against this interpretation.

Thus far we have analyzed four Ph-positive AML patients (Table 2). As in Ph-positive ALL, two cases exhibited *abl/bcr* rearrangements and thus may be regarded as in CML blast crisis. In situ hybridization studies of one variant Ph-positive AML patient lacking a *bcr* recombination showed *c-abl* sequences exclusively on chromosome 9 [12]. This case may be an example of yet another leukemic subgroup comprising cytogenetically defined "Ph-like" leukemias that exhibit no alteration of either *c-abl* or *bcr* sequences.

D. Discussion

These data, although still preliminary, emphasize the possible value of *c-abl* and *bcr* sequences in the subclassification of heterogeneous leukemic entities as Ph-negative CML or Ph-positive acute leukemias. However, these differences on the molecular level cannot readily be correlated with specific clinical, morphological, or immunological features. Thus, in contrast to a recent report based on five cases [17], we detected no significant distinctions in the clinical course of our 31 Ph-negative CML patients. The same holds true for Ph-positive ALL. While nine cases of childhood Ph-positive ALL investigated by us and others [8, 9, 18] exhibited no *bcr* rearrangement, the demonstration of a similar genomic configuration in four adult

Table 2. Ph-positive ALL and AML

Molecular hallmark	Ph-pos ALL ($n=23$[a])	Ph-pos AML ($n=4$[a])
I *c-abl/bcr* rearrangement as in Ph-positive CML	10	2
II Rearrangement of 5'*bcr* and *c-abl*, deletion of 3'*bcr*	3	–
III No *bcr* rearrangement	10	2

[a] Data of some patients have been published elsewhere [8, 12].

cases [8] at least rules out a restriction of this molecular pattern to pediatric patients. Nevertheless, investigation of more cases with longer follow-up may finally unravel the possible clinical importance of molecular differences among these heterogeneous leukemic entities and supplement our rather incomplete understanding of what overall biological consequences are triggered by such genomic rearrangements as those discussed above.

Acknowledgements. I thank Drs. A. de Klein and G. Grosveld for close cooperation and helpful discussions, as well as Drs. R. Becher, F. Carbonell, O. A. Haas, and H. Heimpl for cytogenetic analyses and cell samples. This study was supported by the *Deutsche Forschungsgemeinschaft* and the *Ministerium für Wissenschaft und Kunst, Baden-Württemberg.*

References

1. Bartram CR, Klein A de, Hagemeijer A, Agthoven T von, Geurts van Kessel A, Bootsma D, Grosveld G, Fergusson-Smith MA, Davies T, Stone M, Heisterkamp N, Stephenson JE, Groffen J (1983) Nature 306:277
2. Bartram CR, Kleihauer E, Klein A de, Grosveld G, Teyssier JR, Heisterkamp N, Groffen J (1985) EMBO J 4:683
3. Bartram CR (1985) J Exp Med 162:2175
4. Bartram CR, Klein A de, Hagemeijer A, Carbonell F, Kleihauer E, Grosveld G (1986) Leuk Res 10:221
5. Bartram CR, Carbonell F (1986) Cancer Genet Cytogenet 21:183
6. Collins SJ, Kubonishi J, Myoshi J, Groudine MT (1984) Science 225:72
7. Klein A de, Geurts van Kessel A, Grosveld G, Bartram CR, Hagemeijer A, Bootsma D, Spurr NK, Heisterkamp N, Groffen J, Stephenson JR (1982) Nature 300:765
8. Klein A de, Hagemeijer A, Bartram CR, Houwen R, Hoefsloot L, Carbonell F, Chan L, Barnett M, Greaves M, Kleihauer E, Heisterkamp N, Groffen J, Grosveld G (1986) Blood 68:1369
9. Eriksson J, Griffin CA, Ar-Rushdi A, Valtieri M, Hoxie J, Finau J, Emanuel BS, Rovern G, Nowell PC, Croce CM (1986) Proc Natl Acad Sci USA 83:1807
10. Gale RP, Canaani E (1984) Proc Natl Acad Sci USA 81:5648
11. Groffen J, Stephenson JR, Heisterkamp N, Klein A de, Bartram CR, Grosveld G (1984) Cell 36:93
12. Haas OA, Bartram CR, Panzer S, Bettelheim P (1987) Cancer Genet Cytogenet (in press)
13. Heisterkamp N, Stam K, Groffen J, Klein A de, Grosveld G (1985) Nature 315:758
14. Jacobs AD, Gale RP (1984) N Engl J Med 311:1219
15. Konopka JB, Watanabe SM, Singer JW, Collings SJ, Witte ON (1985) Proc Natl Acad Sci USA 82:1810
16. Konopka JB, Witte ON (1985) Mol Cell Biol 5:3116
17. Morris CM, Reeve AE, Fitzgerald PH, Hollings PE, Beard MEJ, Heaton DC (1986) Nature 320:281
18. Rodenhuis S, Smets LA, Slater RM, Behrendt H, Veerman AJP (1985) N Engl J Med 313:51
19. Shtivelman E, Lifshitz B, Gale RP, Canaani E (1985) Nature 315:550
20. Stam K, Heisterkamp N, Grosveld G, Klein A de, Verma RS, Coleman M, Dosik H, Groffen J (1985) N Engl J Med 313:1429
21. Pugh WC, Pearson M, Vardiman JW, Rowley JD (1985) Br J Haematol 60:457

Haematology and Blood Transfusion   Vol. 31
Modern Trends in Human Leukemia VII
Edited by Neth, Gallo, Greaves, and Kabisch
© Springer-Verlag Berlin Heidelberg 1987

Molecular Cloning and Serological Characterization of an Altered *c-abl* Gene Product Produced in *Ph*¹ CML Patients

A.-M. Mes-Masson, J. McLaughlin, and O. Witte

Summary

The reciprocal translocation between human chromosomes 9 and 22, termed the Philadelphia chromosome (Ph^1), is observed in more than 90% of patients with chronic myelogenous leukemia. This translocation fuses sequences from a variable distance 5' to the c-*abl* locus on chromosome 9 to sequences in a breakpoint cluster region (*bcr*) on chromosome 22. The appearance of the Ph^1 chromosome is correlated with the production of a novel 8.7-kb RNA transcript containing both *bcr* and c-*abl* sequences as well as with a 210-kd phosphoprotein ($p210^{c-abl}$) representing non-*abl* polypeptide sequences fused to c-*abl*-derived sequences. Antibodies prepared to a number of different c-*abl* domains and to *bcr* determinants were employed to characterize the normal and altered c-*abl* gene products. By combining a variety of cDNA cloning techniques, we have isolated *bcr/abl* clones representing 8.7 kb of contiguous mRNA sequence.

A. Introduction

The c-*abl* gene is the normal cellular homolog of v-*abl* (p160), the transforming gene of Abelson murine leukemia virus (A-MuLV) (Witte et al. 1979; Goff et al. 1980). A-MuLV is a replication-defective, rapidly transforming retrovirus which can transform early B lymphoid and other hematopoietic cell types both in vitro and in vivo

Molecular Biology Institute, University of California, Los Angeles, CA 90024, USA

(Rosenberg et al. 1975; Rosenberg and Baltimore 1976; Whitlock and Witte 1986). The v-*abl* protein is a chimeric protein in which the amino terminal sequences of the protein are derived from the group antigen gene (*gag*) of the Moloney murine leukemia virus, while the remaining carboxy terminal sequences of the protein are derived from a large protein of the murine c-*abl* gene (Witte et al. 1979; Reddy et al. 1983; Wang et al. 1984). Several lines of evidence have shown that the tyrosine-specific kinase activity of the v-*abl* protein, encoded by c-*abl*-derived sequences, mediates the ability of A-MuLV to cause neoplastic transformation (Witte et al. 1980; Rosenberg et al. 1980; Prywes et al. 1983).

Recently, c-*abl* cDNA cloned from both human and mouse cell lines (Shtivelman et al. 1985; Ben-Neriah et al. 1986a) has been used to map the c-*abl* locus. The mature c-*abl* mRNA represents the assembly of 11 different exons whose sequences are brought together by virtue of an RNA splicing mechanism (Fig. 1). Exons 1, 2, and part of exon 3 represent 5' c-*abl* sequences not found in v-*abl*. In addition, four different exon 1 species, which are individually spliced to the remaining exons, have been found in murine cells (exon 1/types 1–4) (Ben-Neriah et al. 1986a). Exon 1/type 1 and exon 1/type 4 are the most common forms of exon 1 found in mature murine c-*abl* mRNA. To date, exon 1/type 1 has been identified in human cells and shares extensive sequence homology with the murine form of exon 1/type 1.

Chronic myelogenous leukemia (CML) is a disease of the pluripotent stem cell which progresses through a series of stages

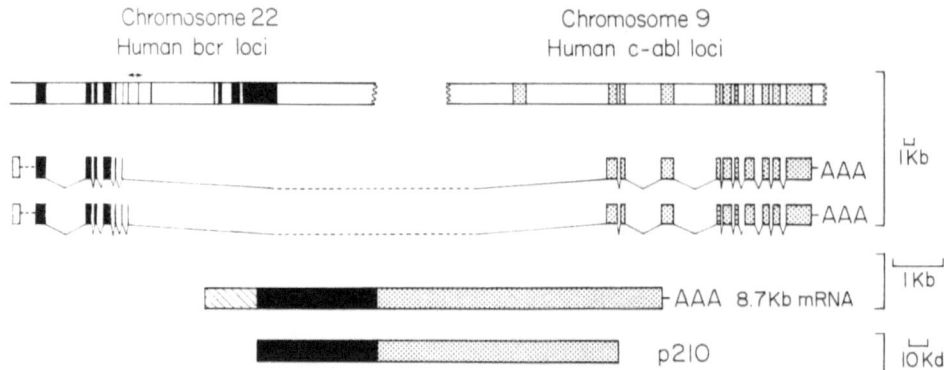

Fig. 1. Model for generating the CML-specific 8.7-kb mRNA and P210$^{c\text{-}abl}$. The *bcr* locus on chromosome 22 (Heisterkamp et al. 1985) and the c-*abl* locus on chromosome 9 (Shtivelman et al. 1985) are partners in the Ph^1 translocation whose breakpoints occur within a 5.8-kb region on chromosome 22 within the *bcr* gene (↔) and at a more variable distance 5′ to the c-*abl* gene (Groffen et al. 1984; Heisterkamp et al. 1983). The variable breakpoint and intron sequences are removed by splicing to generate the 8.7-kb mRNA. As indicated in the figure, microheterogeneity in the splicing pattern of the 8.7-kb mRNA has been observed (Shtivelman et al. 1985). cDNA cloning results demonstrated the presence of approximately 1 kb of novel sequence at the 5′ end of the 8.7-kb mRNA (*hatched box*) which does not form part of the normal *bcr* gene transcript (Mes-Masson et al. 1986). The 8.7-kb mRNA gives rise to an altered form of c-*abl*, P210$^{c\text{-}abl}$, which has a structurally altered amino terminus (Konopka et al. 1984a)

(chronic, accelerated, and blast crisis) where cells become less regulated in their growth and differentiation properties (for review see Koeffler and Golde 1981). Translocation of the c-*abl* gene from chromosome 9 to 22 (t9:22), resulting in the Philadelphia chromosome (Ph^1), occurs in over 90% of CML patients (Rowley 1973). The translocation breakpoint generally occurs within a limited region in a gene on chromosome 22 (termed the *bcr* gene) and at a variable distance 5′ to the c-*abl* gene on chromosome 9 (Heisterkamp et al. 1983; Groffen et al. 1984). Analysis of RNA expression in Ph^1-positive CML cell lines has detected a unique 8.7-kb c-*abl* mRNA (Cananni et al. 1984; Collins et al. 1984). cDNA cloning of a portion of this 8.7-kb mRNA suggests that transcription begins on chromosome 22 and continues through the junction with chromosome 9 to some point downstream of the c-*abl* gene (Shtivelman et al. 1985; Grosveld et al. 1986). RNA splicing joins exons from the *bcr* gene on chromosome 22 to the first common exon of c-*abl* (exon 2) in such a way as to preserve the reading frame of the c-*abl* gene (Fig. 1). A structurally altered c-*abl* protein (P210$^{c\text{-}abl}$), with an in vitro kinase

activity similar to that of the v-*abl* protein, has been detected in a number of Ph^1-positive CML cell lines and direct clinical specimens (Konopka et al. 1984a; Konopka and Witte 1985). These results have strongly implicated c-*abl* in the pathogenesis of CML.

B. P145 and P210 Protein Structure

Large regions of the v-*abl* protein, expressed as fusion proteins in bacteria, were used as immunogens to prepare antisera specific for different regions of the v-*abl* protein (Konopka et al. 1984b). Since v-*abl*-specific antisera displayed cross-reactivity to c-*abl* and P210$^{c\text{-}abl}$, these immunological reagents were used to characterize both forms of the *abl* protein (Konopka et al. 1984a; Konopka and Witte 1985). The P210$^{c\text{-}abl}$ form has acquired new amino acids at its N-terminus, while C-terminal sequences remain indistinguishable from c-*abl*, a configuration reminiscent of the relationship between v-*abl* and c-*abl*. A similar, if not identical, protein is seen in a number of CML lines and patient samples, despite the wide range of different t9:22 breakpoints. In vivo tyrosine phosphorylation has been observed for P210$^{c\text{-}abl}$ but not P145, although both display in vitro tyrosine activity. Although either protein can act as its own substrate in the in vitro tyrosine kinase assay, c-*abl* appears to be phosphorylated at one or two major sites, whereas P210 is phosphorylated at two to three major sites and a number of minor sites. The direct relationship between the 8.7-kb mRNA and P210 has recently been demonstrated using antiserum prepared against *bcr* determinants (Ben-Neriah et al. 1986 b). This antiserum was able to immunoprecipitate P210 and a 190-kd protein which is a candidate for the normal *bcr* protein.

C. Hybrid 8.7-kb mRNA Structure

The CML-specific 8.7-kb mRNA has been shown, by partial cDNA cloning, to be a hybrid transcript of *bcr* and c-*abl* sequences (Shtivelman et al. 1985; Grosveld et al. 1986). While a portion of the hybrid gene had been cloned, we were interested in isolating a clone which represented the entire mRNA, with special attention to clones reaching the 5′ end. To enhance recovery of *abl*-related mRNA, poly (A) selected RNA from K562 cells, a CML-derived cell line, was initially size selected over a sucrose gradient generating a ten fold enrichment of the CML-specific mRNA. Since the hybrid 8.7-kb mRNA represents a long transcript, a cDNA cloning protocol which optimized the recovery of large cDNA clones was established. Although this protocol is described in more detail elsewhere (A.-M. Mes-Masson, J. McLaughlin and O. N. Witte, in preparation), a few features stand out as being important in the recovery of large cDNA clones. These include optimizing conditions for first-strand cDNA synthesis, priming first-strand synthesis with both oligo d(T) and an internal oligonucleotide from the conserved tyrosine kinase domain of c-*abl*, and, after second-strand synthesis and the addition of EcoRI linkers, size-selecting the resulting cDNA library over a sucrose gradient before ligation to lambda arms. When this cDNA library was initially screened with a v-*abl* homologous probe, over 1000 phage plaques scored positive. In

order to concentrate our efforts on clones which would provide information on upstream sequences of the hybrid mRNA, a subset (300) of the phage DNA was tested for its ability to hybridize to a number of probes, including exon 1, exon 2, and exon 3 of c-*abl*, as well as to oligonucleotides complementary to known *bcr* mRNA sequences. In this manner, clones which putatively represent the entire CML-specific 8.7-kb mRNA were isolated.

In order to establish the identity of the isolated cDNA clones, we sequenced regions corresponding to those reported to be found in *bcr*- and c-*abl*-specific sequences. Partial sequence analysis confirmed the identity of these clones. In addition, we determined the sequence at the 5′ end of various cDNA clones, which will be reported elsewhere (Mes-Masson et al. 1986). The cDNA clones were analyzed by using various portions of the cDNA clones as probes in a Northern analysis of RNA from two different CML-derived cell lines, K562 and EM2, as well as from HL60, a promyelocytic leukemia cell line. Sequences derived from the c-*abl* gene (approximately 5.7 kb at the 3′ end of the 8.7 mRNA) hybridized with the CML-specific 8.7-kb mRNA in K562 and EM2 cells, in addition to the normal 7-kb and 6-kb c-*abl* mRNA in all cell lines. Sequences from the 5′ end of the mRNA up to, but not including, the first kb of sequence were also able to hybridize with the 8.7-kb mRNA in K562 and EM2 cells, as well as to normal 4.5- and 6.7-kb *bcr* mRNA in all cell lines. A different pattern of hybridization was observed when the first Kilobases of 5′ cDNA sequences were used to probe the Northern blot. In this instance, while hybridization still occurred with the ⸮ 7-kb mRNA in K562 and EM2 cells, the seque⸮⸮ failed to hybridize with either of the norm⸮⸮ *bcr* mRNAs. However, this sequence does appear to hybridize strongly to an RNA species of approximately 4 kb in length in all three cell lines tested. The identity of this 4-kb RNA is presently being investigated. These results suggest the presence of non-*bcr* sequences at the 5′ end of the 8.7-kb mRNA (Fig. 1).

We are presently attempting to express the P210$^{c\text{-}abl}$ protein produced by the 8.7-kb mRNA in normal cell lines in order to assess the role of P210^{c-abl} in oncogenic transformation. We hope that eventually the overexpression of the P210^{c-abl} protein in either eukaryotic or prokaryotic vectors will allow us to study the function of this protein in greater detail.

Acknowledgements. This work was supported by research grants from the USPHS-NCI. O.W. is a faculty scholar of the American Cancer Society. A.-M.M.-M. is a research fellow of the National Cancer Institute of Canada.

References

1. Ben-Neriah Y, Bernards A, Paskind M, Daley GQ, Baltimore D (1986a) Cell 44:577–586
2. Ben-Neriah Y, Daley GQ, Mes-Masson A-M, Witte ON, Baltimore D (1986b) Science (to be published)
3. Cananni E, Gale RP, Steinder-Saltz D, Berrebi A, Aghai E, Januszewicz E (1984) Lancet I:593–595
4. Collins S, Kubonishi I, Myoshi I, Groudine MT (1984) Science 225:72–74
5. Goff SP, Gilboa E, Witte ON, Baltimore D (1980) Cell 22:777–785
6. Groffen J, Stephenson JR, Heisterkamp N, Klein A de, Bartram A, Bartram CR, Grosveld G (1984) Cell 36:93–99
7. Grosveld G, Verwoerd T, Agthoven T van, Klein A de, Ramachandran KL, Heisterkamp N, Stam K, Groffen J (1986) Mol Cell Biol 6:607–616
8. Heisterkamp N, Stephenson JR, Groffen J, Hansen PF, Klein A de, Bartram CR, Grosveld G (1983) Nature 306:239–242
9. Heisterkamp N, Stam K, Groffen J, Klein A de, Grosveld G (1985) Nature 315:758–761
10. Koeffler MD, Golde DW (1981) N Engl J Med 304:1201–1209, 1269–1274
11. Konopka JB, Witte ON (1985) Mol Cell Biol 5:3116–3123
12. Konopka JB, Watanabe SM, Witte ON (1984a) Cell 37:1035–1042
13. Konopka JB, Davis RL, Watanabe SM, Ponticelli AS, Schiff-Maker L, Rosenberg N, Witte ON (1984b) J Virol 51:223–232
14. Prywes R, Foulkes JG, Rosenberg N, Baltimore D (1983) Cell 34:569–579
15. Reddy EP, Smith MJ, Srinivasan A (1983) Proc Natl Acad Sci USA 80:3623–3627
16. Rosenberg N, Baltimore D (1976) J Exp Med 147:1126–1141
17. Rosenberg N, Baltimore D, Scher CD (1975) Proc Natl Acad Sci USA 75:3974–3978
18. Rosenberg N, Clark DR, Witte ON (1980) J Virol 36:766–774
19. Rowley JD (1973) Nature 243:290–291
20. Shtivelman E, Lifshitz B, Gale RP, Canaani E (1985) Nature 315:550–554
21. Wang JYJ, Ledley F, Goff S, Lee R, Groner Y, Baltimore D (1984) Cell 36:349–356
22. Whitlock CA, Witte ON (1986) Adv Immunol (to be published)
23. Witte ON, Rosenberg N, Baltimore D (1979) Nature 281:396–398
24. Witte ON, Dasgupta A, Baltimore D (1980) Nature 283:826–831

Haematology and Blood Transfusion Vol. 31
Modern Trends in Human Leukemia VII
Edited by Neth, Gallo, Greaves, and Kabisch
© Springer-Verlag Berlin Heidelberg 1987

Human Follicular Lymphomas:
Identification of a Second t(14;18) Breakpoint Cluster Region

N. Galili, M. L. Cleary, and J. Sklar

A. Introduction

Most follicular lymphomas, which comprise nearly two-thirds of the non-Hodgkin's lymphomas occurring in U.S. adults, have been shown by cytogenetic analyses to contain a t(14;18) translocation [1, 2]. This breakpoint on chromosome 14 has been localized to band 14q32, the site of the immunoglobulin heavy chain genes. It was thus possible to use human *Ig* gene fragments to clone out a breakpoint DNA fragment (pFL-1) from tissue biopsy specimens of these lymphomas and from cell lines containing this translocation. When used as a hybridization probe, rearranged pFL-1 containing DNA was detected in approximately 60% of follicular lymphomas. Thus, a significant percentage of follicular lymphomas failed to show a breakpoint on chromosome 18 within 15–20 kb on either side of the breakpoint region. We describe here the cloning of a chromosome 18 DNA fragment (pFL-2) that detects t(14;18) rearranged DNA in most of these negative follicular lymphomas.

B. Materials and Methods

I. Tumor Tissues and Cell Lines

Lymphoma tissues serving as a source of DNA for cloning were obtained from a single patient with follicular lymphoma. The

Laboratory of Experimental Oncology, Department of Pathology Stanford University, Stanford, California 94305, USA

hybrid cell lines UV20 HL21-7 (containing human chromosomes 4, 8, 18, and 21) and UV20 HL 21-27 (human chromosomes 4, 8, and 21) have been described previously [3]. The cell line SU-DUL-5 was provided by Jean Jang and Dr. H. Kaplan (Stanford University).

II. Genomic Southern Blot Analyses

DNA was extracted from lymph node biopsy specimens and cultured cell lines and subjected to Southern blot analysis using procedures previously described [4].

III. Construction and Screening of Genomic DNA Libraries

To isolate rearranged IgH genes, follicular lymphoma DNA was digested to completion with the appropriate restriction enzyme, and size-fractionated in 0.8% ⌐⸗arose gel. Regions of the gels that contained DNA fragments of 3–6 kb for *Hind* III (producu.⸗ Ig allele) and from 20–23 kb for *Eco*RI (translocated allele) were excised. DNA was electroeluted from the gel slices, purified, and ligated into appropriate phage vectors as described previously [4]. The recombinant DNAs were packaged in vitro and ~10^6 recombinant phages were plated and screened using a radiolabeled J_H hybridization probe according to methods previously described [4]. Hybridizing plaques were purified by three successive platings.

IV. Nucleotide Sequencing

Nucleotide sequences were obtained using the dideoxy chain termination method [5], using DNA fragments subcloned into M13 phages [6].

C. Results and Discussion

All t(14;18) breakpoints that have been analyzed [4, 7–9] occur in chromosome 14 DNA adjacent to or within the heavy chain J region segment. Thus, using the probe specific for the human J_H region, the breakpoint of a follicular lymphoma lacking the previously described breakpoint cluster region pFL-1 chromosome 18 rearrangement was molecularly cloned from genomic DNA.

The cloned DNAs are shown in Fig. 1. As expected, each was homologous in part to the human J_H region. The homology is terminated 5' of the joining segment J4 for both alleles. In addition, C_μ has been deleted from one allele and replaced by C_γ sequences. Since the malignant cells of the lymphoma expressed μ-containing Ig, the C_γ allele must represent the nonproductive (i.e., translocated) Ig gene. This apparent class switch is, in our experience [2], a frequent but unexplained finding in follicular lymphomas.

In order to see whether this nonproductive allele DNA fragment contained a t(14;18) breakpoint, a 5' subclone (fragment B in Fig. 1) was used as a hybridization probe on genomic Southern blots of DNA from a series of hamster/human hybrid cell lines (Fig. 2 B). The 3' half of this 5 kb DNA probe contained sequences derived from the J_H region, while the 5' end contained sequences of unknown origin. Two *Eco*RI fragments were detected in human germline DNA (lane 1). The 19 kb band corresponds to the expected *Eco*RI germline J_H region. The 4 kb *Eco*RI band resulted from hybridization with the 5' end of this probe. No cross-hybridization was seen with the parent hamster cell line UV20 (lane 2). The human/hybrid cell line UV20HL21-7 DNA in lane 3 lacks the human chromosome 14, but has chromosome 18 [3]. This lane correspondingly lacks the 19 kb band but contains the 4 kb band. The hybrid UV20HL21-27 in lane 4 has lost chromosome 18 and thus no hybridizing sequences can be detected. These results indicated, therefore, that the 5' half of this probe contains DNA from chromosome 18. The nonproductive IgH allele thus contained a t(14;18) breakpoint.

Restriction enzyme mapping of the cloned breakpoint DNA fragment indicated that the site of t(14;18) fusion had occurred near the joining segment J4. Nucleotide sequencing was thus carried out on fragments subcloned into M13 phages. As seen in Fig. 3, the breakpoint DNA sequence diverged from germline J_H immediately 5' of J4. The sequence also showed that the D-J joint in

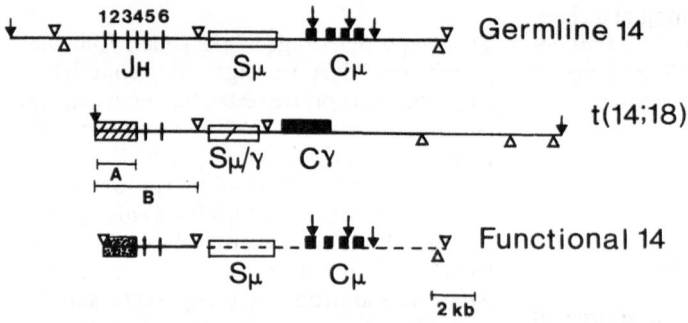

Fig. 1. Graphic depiction of the cloned DNA fragments representing the two rearranged heavy chain alleles shown along with the germline configuration for comparison. The cloned DNAs are oriented 5' to 3'. *Solid boxes* represent C_H-containing regions, the *open boxes* denote switch region sequences, and the *stippled box* represents V_H-containing sequences of the productive *Ig* gene. The *cross-hatched box* represents DNA sequences derived from chromosome 18. **A** indicates the chromosome 18-specific probe pFL-2; **B** indicates the breakpoint DNA fragment used as a probe on the human/hamster cell lines. Restriction sites as follows: *Eco*RI (↓), BamHI (△), *Hind*III (▽)

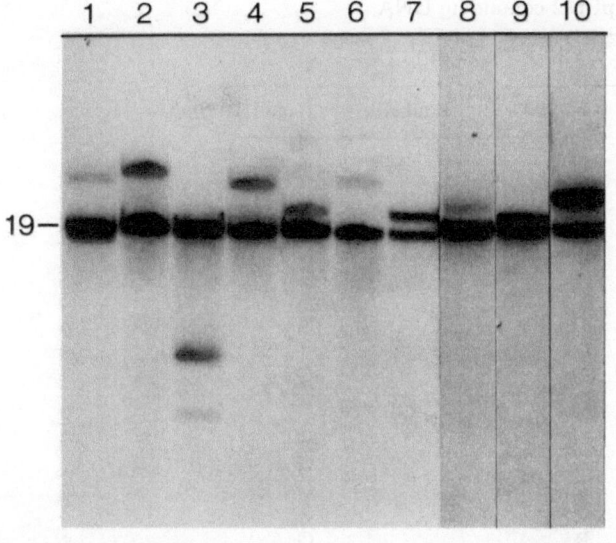

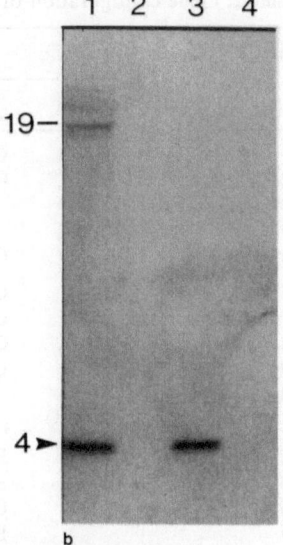

Fig. 2. a Southern blot analyses of genomic DNAs containing pFL-2 (fragment A) as shown in Fig. 1. Germline *Bam*HI and *Hind*III containing pFL-2 bands are ~17 kb each. *Lane 8,* lymphoid cell line SU-DUL-5; all *other lanes,* follicular lymphomas.

b Southern blot analyses of hamster/human hybrid cell line DNAs digested with *Eco*RI and probed with a t(14;18) DNA probe. *Lane 1,* germline human DNA; *lane 2,* UV20; *lane 3,* UV20HL21-7; *lane 4,* UV20HL21-27

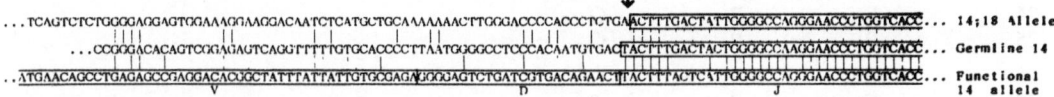

Fig. 3. Nucleotide sequences of the t(14;18) breakpoint DNA and the productive V-D-J joint isolated from a follicular lymphoma. Orientation is 5' to 3'. *Arrow* indicates presumed point of translocation

the functional allele has occurred at J4 in a position nearly identical to the breakpoint on the translocated allele. We have reported similar patterns of nearly identical t(14;18) breakpoint and D-J joint in the productive allele for two other lymphomas using the pFL-1 probe [4]. These structural similarities implicate D-J recombination enzymes as mediators of t(14;18) translocations.

Follicular lymphomas negative for rearranged pFL-1 containing DNA fragments were screened by genomic Southern analyses using the subcloned pFL-2 fragment (fragment A in Fig. 1) as the probe. Ten of these lymphoma DNAs are shown in Fig. 2A. A significant fraction of follicular lymphomas

contained a chromosome 18 DNA rearrangement detectable with pFL-2, thereby defining a second breakpoint cluster region for this translocation. Table 1 summarizes our results with 30 follicular lymphoma DNA biopsy specimens and cell lines examined with pFL-1 and/or pFL-2. More than 90% of these randomly selected samples contained a chromosome 18 DNA rearrangement falling within one or the other cluster region. This correlates well with the reported [2] frequency of cytologic t(14;18) translocations.

In order to determine a possible linkage relationship of pFL-1 and pFL-2 on chromosome 18, the pFL-2 fragment was used as

Table 1. Gene configuration of pFL-1 or pFL-2 containing DNA

Patient	pFL-1			pFL-2	
	Bam HI	Hind III	Eco RI	Bam HI	Hind III
1	G	G	G	R	R
2	G	G	G	R	
3			G	R	
4			G	R	
5		G	G	R	R
6		G	G	R	R
7		G	G	R	G
8		G	G	G	
9		G	G	G	G
10			R		
11		G	G		R
12		R	R		G
13		R	R		G
14		G	G		R
15		R	R		G
16		G	R		G
17		R	G		G
18		R	R		G
19		G			R
20			R		
21	R	R	G		
22	R	R	G		
23	R	G	G		
24	R	R	G		
25	R	R	G		
26	R	R	G		
27	G	R	G		
28	R		G	G	G
Cell line					
SU-DHL-4	R	R		G	G
SU-DUL-5	G	G		R	R

R, rearrangement of pFL-1 or pFL-2 containing DNA, respectively; G, germline configuration.

a probe against recombinant phages whose inserts contained ~40 kb of germline chromosome 18 DNA flanking pFL-1 [4]. No hybridization was detected (not shown), indicating that the cluster region defined by pFL-2 is not within 20 kb on either side of pFL-1.

The finding of two major cluster regions for the t(14;18) translocation suggests two different outcomes of such crossovers. Breakpoints in either region may, in some as yet unknown way, affect the transcription of the same gene product despite the distance (>20 kb) between them. Alternatively, each cluster region may affect different transcriptional units. The use of the two DNA probes pFL-1 and pFL-2 will enable further study of the biological or clinical significance of these two classes of t(14;18) translocations and may be useful for the diagnosis of this type of lymphoma.

References

1. Fukuhara S, Rowley JD, Variakojis D, Golomb HM (1979) Chromosome abnormalities in poorly differentiated lymphocytic lymphoma. Cancer Res 39:3119

2. Yunis JJ, Oken N, Kaplan ME, Ensrud KM, Howe RR, Theoligides A (1982) Distinctive chromosomal abnormalities in histologic subtypes of non-Hodgkin's lymphoma. N Engl J Med 307:1231
3. Thompson LH, Mooney CL, Burkhart-Schultz K, Carrano AV, Siciliano MJ (1985) Correction of a nucleotide-excision-repair mutation by human chromosome 19 in hamster-human hybrid cells. Somatic Cell Mol Genet 11:87
4. Cleary ML, Sklar J (1985) Nucleotide sequence of a t(14;18) chromosomal breakpoint in follicular lymphoma and demonstration of a breakpoint-cluster region near a transcriptionally active locus on chromosome 18. Proc Natl Acad Sci USA 82:7439
5. Sanger F, Nicklen S, Coulson AR (1977) DNA sequencing with chain-terminating inhibitors. Proc Natl Acad Sci USA 74:5463
6. Norrander J, Kempe T, Messing J (1983) Construction of improved M13 vectors using oligo-deoxy-nucleotide-directed mutagenesis. Gene 26:101
7. Bakhshi A, Jensen JP, Goldman P, Wright JJ, McBride DW, Epstein AL, Korsmeyer SJ (1985) Cloning the chromosomal breakpoint of t(14;18) human lymphomas: clustering around J_H on chromosome 14 and near a transcriptional unit on 18. Cell 41:899
8. Tsujimoto Y, Finger LR, Yunis JJ, Nowell P, Croce CM (1984) Cloning of the chromosome breakpoint of neoplastic B cells with the t(14;18) chromosome translocation. Science 226:1097
9. Tsujimoto Y, Gorham J, Cossman J, Jaffe E, Croce CM (1985) The t(14;18) chromosome translocations involved in B-cell neoplasms result from mistakes in VDJ joining. Science 229:1390

Haematology and Blood Transfusion   Vol. 31
Modern Trends in Human Leukemia VII
Edited by Neth, Gallo, Greaves, and Kabisch
© Springer-Verlag Berlin Heidelberg 1987

Amino Acid Substitution at Position 13 of the N-*ras* Gene in a Non-Hodgkin's Lymphoma Patient

A. Wodnar-Filipowicz [1,2], H.-P. Senn [1], J. Jiricny [1], E. Signer [2], and Ch. Moroni [1]

A. Introduction

In many human tumors, cellular proto-on-cogenes are structurally modified by gene translocation, gene amplification, or point mutations. Modification by the latter is observed in members of the *ras* gene family. Single-base substitutions occurring at defined positions and resulting in a change in the corresponding amino acid significantly alter the biological properties of *ras*-encoded p21 protein [1]. The relevance of "activated" p21 in the neoplastic development of the cell is not yet understood, but it is thought that such mutations contribute to the develop-ment of malignancy. *Ras* genes activated by point mutations have been demonstrated in 10%–20% of certain human tumors, e.g., acute leukemias [2, 3]. Here one observes mainly mutations in the N-*ras* gene at positions 12 and 61 [1, 4]. More recently, an altered codon 13 of N-*ras* leading to Gly → Val or Asp substitution was reported in acute myeloid leukemia (AML) cases [5]. A novel point mutation at codon 13 of N-*ras*, leading to Gly → Cys change, which was detected in a T-cell malignancy is described in this paper.

[1] Friedrich Miescher Institute, PO Box 2543, 4002 Basel, Switzerland
[2] Children's Hospital, University of Basel, 4058 Basel, Switzerland

B. Results and Discussion

The NIH/3T3 transfection assay combined with a direct in vivo selection of transfected

Table 1. Tumorigenicity of DNA-transfected NIH/3T3 cells in nude mice

DNA used for transfection	Experiment	Number of tumors/inoculation sites	Latency period (days)
Calf thymus/pSV$_2$neo	A	0/6	–
	B	1/8	·?
Patient DNA/pSV$_2$neo	A	7/12	39–53
	B	12/18	21–35
Calf thymus/pEJ$^{(H-ras)}$/pSV$_2$neo	A	4/4	14
	B	2/2	10

Results from two independent experiments (A and B) are presented. 37.5 μg of cellular DNA and 0.375 μg of plasmids were precipitated with calcium phosphate into 100-mm plates seeded 1 day previously with 5×10^5 NIH/3T3 cells. After 6 h, the precipitate was washed off and cells incubated in Dulbecco's modified Eagle's medium + 10% calf serum for 20 h. Cells were then trypsinized and each plate seeded into 3, containing selective medium with 1 mg of G418. After 12 days, colonies were pooled and 2.5×10^6 cells were injected subcutaneously into each of 2 sites in nude mice.

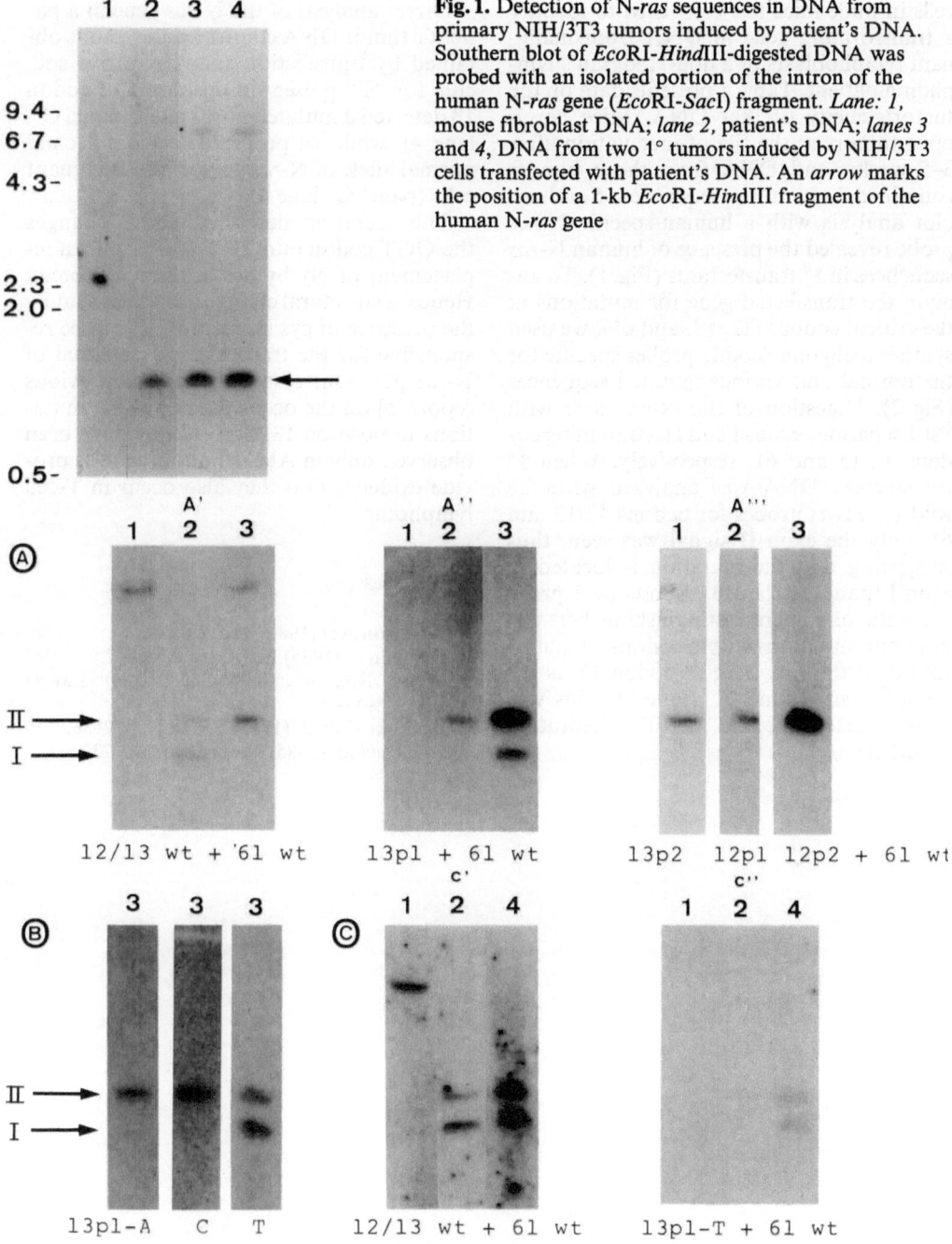

Fig. 1. Detection of N-*ras* sequences in DNA from primary NIH/3T3 tumors induced by patient's DNA. Southern blot of *Eco*RI-*Hind*III-digested DNA was probed with an isolated portion of the intron of the human N-*ras* gene (*Eco*RI-*Sac*I) fragment. *Lane: 1,* mouse fibroblast DNA; *lane 2,* patient's DNA; *lanes 3* and *4,* DNA from two 1° tumors induced by NIH/3T3 cells transfected with patient's DNA. An *arrow* marks the position of a 1-kb *Eco*RI-*Hind*III fragment of the human N-*ras* gene

Fig. 2. Hybridization of synthetic oligonucleotide probes to genomic DNA from NIH/3T3 primary tumor induced by patient's DNA (*panels A and B*) and to DNA isolated from patient's malignant lymphoblasts (*panel C*). *Pst*I-digested DNA was hybridized directly in agarose gel to the synthetic oligomer probes. *Lane 1,* mouse fibroblast DNA, *lane 2,* human fibroblast DNA; *lane 3,* DNA from the primary NIH/3T3 tumor; *lane 4,* DNA from patient's malignant lymphoblasts. Probes: wt 12/13 and 61 – nonmutated exons I and II; 12 and 13, p1 and p2 – mutated exon I at codons 12 or 13, base 1 or 2. *Arrows* mark positions of human *Pst*I N-*ras* gene fragments (exons I and II)

cells in nude mice has been used to identify a transforming gene in DNA from malignant lymphoblasts of a non-Hodgkin's lymphoma patient. Table 1 presents data on the tumorigenicity of that DNA. Mice developed tumors at the site of inoculation after 3–5 weeks, and DNA from those tumors contained human *alu* sequences. Southern blot analysis with a human-specific N-*ras* probe revealed the presence of human N-*ras* sequences in 1° transfectants (Fig. 1). To analyze the transfected gene for mutations at the critical codons (12, 13, and 61), we used synthetic oligonucleotide probes specific for the normal and various mutated sequences (Fig. 2). Digestion of the N-*ras* gene with Pst I separates exons I and II, containing codons 12/13 and 61, respectively. When 1° transfectant DNA was analyzed with the wild-type (wt) probes for codons 12/13 and 61, only the exon II signal was seen, thus suggesting that the mutation is located in exon I (panel A', lane 3). Subsequent probing with oligomers distinguishing between different mutations within codons 12 and 13 identified the first base of codon 13 as the mutation site (panel A", lane 3). This was further determined as G→T substitution (panel B).

Direct analysis of the N-*ras* gene in a patient's tumor DNA confirmed the results obtained by transfection assay. A probe specific for "T" present in position 1 of codon 13 detected a mutated N-*ras* allele (panel C", lane 4), while wt probes detected a second normal allele of N-*ras* gene of the malignant cells (panel C', lane 4).

The mutation described above changes the GGT codon into TGT and results in replacement of gly by cys in the *ras* protein. Hence, a structural change brought about by the presence of cys in position 13 can be responsible for the transforming potential of N-*ras* p21. Our results extend the previous report [5] on the occurrence of N-*ras* mutations in position 13. So far, they have been observed only in AML, but our results provide evidence that they also occur in T-cell lymphoma.

References

1. Levinson AD (1986) TIG 2:81–85
2. Balmain A (1985) Br J Cancer 51:1–7
3. Weiss RA, Marshall ChJ (1984) Lancet 17:1138–1142
4. Gambke C et al. (1985) PNAS 82:879–882
5. Bos JL et al. (1985) Nature 315:726–730

Haematology and Blood Transfusion Vol. 31
Modern Trends in Human Leukemia VII
Edited by Neth, Gallo, Greaves, and Kabisch
© Springer-Verlag Berlin Heidelberg 1987

Loss of Hematopoietic Progenitor Cells CFU-GEMM, BFU-E, CFU-Mk, and CFU-GM in the Acquired Immunodeficiency Syndrome (AIDS)? *

A. Ganser [1], C. Carlo Stella [3], B. Völkers [1], K. H. Brodt [2], E. B. Helm [2], and D. Hoelzer [1]

A. Introduction

Hematological abnormalities have been found in the majority of patients with AIDS, in addition to immunological derangements [1]. Furthermore, treatment of opportunistic infections with folic acid antagonists and of neoplasms with cytostatic drugs is frequently complicated by profound thrombocytopenia, neutropenia, and anemia, thus resulting in the withdrawal of the drugs.

In the present study we therefore analyzed the hematopoietic progenitor cell compartments, using an in vitro culture system that allows colony formation by the pluripotent progenitor cells CFU-GEMM and by the unipotent erythroid progenitors BFU-E, the megakaryocytic progenitors CFU-Mk, and the granulocytic-monocytic progenitors CFU-GM [2].

B. Materials and Methods

Bone marrow cells from patients with AIDS and from normal controls were obtained from the posterior iliac crest after informed consent. Light-density cells (< 1.077 g/ml) or cells that had been depleted of T cells by a rosetting technique with AET-treated sheep red blood cells [3] were cultured at 10^5 cells/ml in Iscove's modified Dulbecco's me-

dium supplemented with 30% fresh frozen human plasma, 5%–10% PHA-leukocyte – conditioned medium, 50 μM 2-mercaptoethanol, and 1 U/ml erythropoietin (Connaught, Step III). After 14 days at 37 °C and 5% CO_2 in air, colonies were counted using an inverted microscope [4].

C. Results and Discussion

A total of nine patients with AIDS ($n = 7$) or advanced lymphadenopathy syndrome ($n = 2$) were analyzed. All of the patients with AIDS had Kaposi's sarcoma. T4-lymphocytes in the blood were reduced to 149/mm^3 (range 11–681; normal 1100–1300) and T8-lymphocytes increased to 533/mm^3 (range 107–1308; normal 350–450). At the time of bone marrow aspiration, anemia was observed in six of the patients, thrombocytopenia in two, and neutropenia in one.

In all patients, the in vitro colony formation was reduced for all four types of progenitor cells (Table 1). To find out whether the reduction in colony formation was due to an actual deficiency of progenitor cells or due to their impaired in vitro proliferation resulting from altered "accessory" T-cell subsets [5], T-cells were depleted from the bone marrow cells prior to culture. In contrast to normal controls, T-cell depletion from AIDS-derived bone marrow cells was followed by a significant increase in colony formation of all four types of progenitors; however, normal values were obtained only in three out of nine patients. Colony formation significantly increased from 1.0 ± 0.3 to 3.4 ± 1.3 (mean $\pm$ standard error of mean)

---

* Supported by a grant from the Bundesgesundheitsamt.
Departments of Hematology [1] and Infectious Disease [2], University of Frankfurt, FRG
[3] Department of Internal Medicine, University of Pavia, Italy

Table 1. Growth of hematopoietic progenitors in AIDS (colonies per 10^5 cells $\pm$ SEM)

	CFU-GEMM	CFU-Mk	BFU-E	CFU-GM
AIDS ($n=9$)	1.0 ± 0.3	1.4 ± 0.7	5.3 ± 2.5	18 ± 5
Normal ($n=24$)	15 ± 4	15 ± 2	117 ± 42	84 ± 16
P value	<0.01	<0.05	<0.001	<0.001

per 10^5 cells for CFU-GEMM; from 5.3 ± 2.5 to 19.9 ± 8.7 for BFU-E; from 1.4 ± 0.7 to 5.6 ± 2.2 for CFU-Mk; and from 17.9 ± 5.2 to 42.8 ± 13.2 for CFU-GM.

Readdition of the previously isolated T cells to the autologous T-cell-depleted marrow cells at a 1:1 ratio again resulted in a significant decrease in colony formation which was not observed in the normal controls. Since the percentage of inhibition was inversely correlated to the T4:T8 ratio, the reduced in vitro growth of the hematopoietic progenitor cells can partially be explained by growth inhibition due to the T4:T8 imbalance.

To exclude impairment of in vitro colony growth of AIDS-derived progenitor cells by soluble factors, cocultures of AIDS-derived bone marrow cells with irradiated or nonirradiated normal bone marrow cells were carried out. However, no change in the in vitro growth of normal or AIDS-derived progenitor cells was observed in either case. While inhibition by soluble factors, e.g., interferons, is unlikely, inhibition by cell-cell interaction could still account for the effects observed, because these interactions might depend on autologous coculture conditions [6].

However the inability in the majority of our cases to completely restore colony formation by T-cell depletion might indicate that in more advanced infections with HTLV-III/LAV the number of pluripotent and unipotent hematopoietic progenitor cells is reduced owing to a still unknown mechanism which might include infection of stem cells by HTLV-III/LAV, leading to failure of the hematopoietic system in situations of stress.

References

1. Fauci AS, Masur G, Gelman EP, Markham PD, Hahn BH, Clifford Lane H (1985) Ann Intern Med 102:800–813
2. Messner HA, Jamal N, Izaguirre C (1982) J Cell Physiol [Suppl] 1:45–51
3. Minden MD, Buick RN, Mc Culloch EA (1979) Blood 54:186–195
4. Ganser A, Hoelzer D (1984) Exp Hematol 12:712–716
5. Zoumbos HC, Gascon P, Dieu JY, Trost SR, Young N (1985) N Engl J Med 312:257–265
6. Li S, Champlin R, Fitchen JH, Gale RP (1984) J Clin Invest 75:234–241

Haematology and Blood Transfusion   Vol. 31
Modern Trends in Human Leukemia VII
Edited by Neth, Gallo, Greaves, and Kabisch
© Springer-Verlag Berlin Heidelberg 1987

Sensitivity of Stromal Elements from Human Bone Marrow Cells to Cytosine Arabinoside In Vitro

E. Elstner, H. Goldschmidt, M. Wächter, and R. Ihle

A. Introduction

Cytosine arabinoside (Ara-C) is one of the most effective agents in the treatment of acute myelogenous leukemia (AML). Recently, low-dose Ara-C therapy has been the subject of topical interest in view of its differentiation-inducing effect on leukemic blast cells. Many patients, however, develop severe aplasia with low-dose Ara-C therapy [1, 6, 10, 11]. The aim of our study was to obtain some information about causes of this aplasia, i.e., to determine whether the lesion is primarily in the hemopoietic stem cells or whether there is any additional damage done to stromal elements.

Bone marrow cells (BMC) were exposed to concentrations of Ara-C in cultures, reflecting the plasma Ara-C concentrations in low-dose-treated patients (10^{-6}–10^{-8} M) [9].

University Hospital (Charité), Department of Internal Medicine, Division of Hematology, Berlin, GDR

B. Material and Methods

Human BMC were obtained from normal volunteers. Iliac bone marrow aspirates were used, diluted with the same volume of McCoy's 5A medium containing preservative-free heparin. Cultures of granulocyte-macrophage colony-forming cells (GM-CFC) were performed with mononuclear BMC from eight normal volunteers in double-layer agar cultures [7]. To study hemopoietic stroma (stroma cell layer), we used the Dexter culture [2] modified for human BMC [3, 4]. Briefly, after spontaneous sedimentation of erythrocytes without washing, the diluted BMC were added to the culture medium (McCoy's 5A supplemented with 10% fetal calf serum SIFIN, GDR, and 10% horse serum, Flow) in order to obtain a cell concentration of 5×10^5 cells per milliliter suspension. The cells were cultivated in Petri dishes at 37 °C in 7.5% CO_2 for 14 days without feeding.

All dilutions of Ara-C were freshly made from a stock solution of Alexan (Mack) and were added to the agar or Dexter cultures on

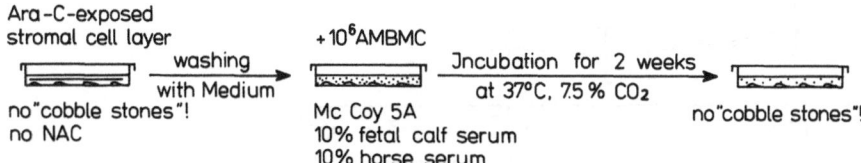

Fig. 1. The influence of Ara-C exposure on the ability of stromal elements to induce active hemopoiesis. Schematic presentation of a cultivation from autologous mononuclear bone marrow cells (AMBMC) over a marrow stromal layer formed during exposure to Ara-C at concentrations of 10^{-6} M, 10^{-5} M

day 0. The influence of Ara-C on the ability of stromal elements to induce active hemopoiesis was studied in suspension cultures. Fresh autologous mononuclear BMC from five normal volunteers were given over a stromal layer formed during exposure to Ara-C at concentrations of $10^{-6}-10^{-5}\,M$ (Fig. 1).

C. Results

Figure 2 shows that GM-CFC were damaged at a concentration of $10^{-8}\,M$ Ara-C and completely disappeared at a concentration of $10^{-5}\,M$ Ara-C. In the modified 2-week-old Dexter culture, we found a decreased ability of Ara-C-exposed BMC to

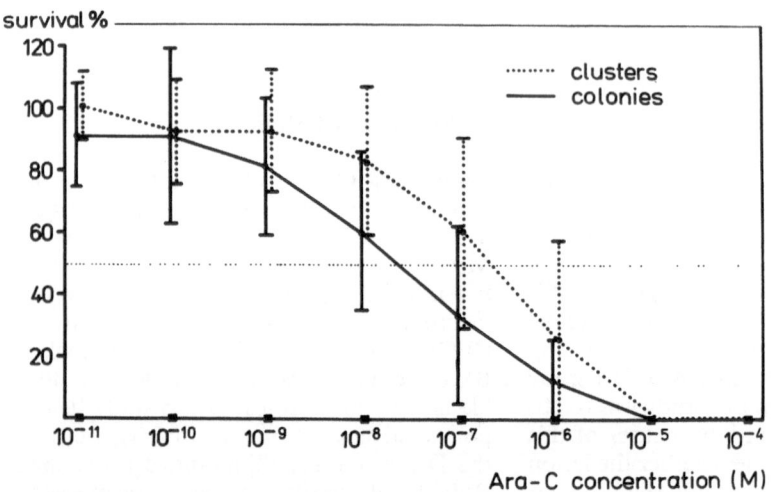

Fig. 2. Sensitivity of GM-CFC from human bone marrow to long-term exposure (7 days) at different concentrations of Ara-C

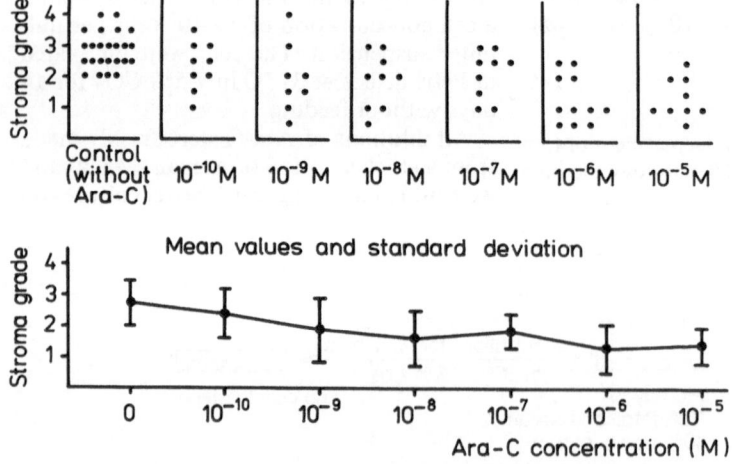

Fig. 3. Sensitivity of stromal layer (Stroma grade) from human bone marrow cells to long-term exposure (14 days) at different concentrations of Ara-C. SG: stromal grade. Each Petri dish was assigned a score from 1 to 4, corresponding to a stromal layer covering from 25% to 100% of the area of the culture dish

Table 1. Effects of different Ara-C concentrations on growth characteristics of bone marrow cells in the modified 2-week-old Dexter culture

Ara-C concentration (M)	NAC	F	CS
0	24/24[a]	24/24	24/24
10^{-10}	8/9	9/9	9/9
10^{-9}	4/8	8/8	6/8
10^{-8}	3/9	9/9	2/9
10^{-6}	1/11	11/11	0/11
10^{-5}	0/9	9/9	0/9

NAC, nonadherent cells (trypan-blue – negative); F, fibroblasts; CS, cobblestones.
[a] Number of growth characteristics present/number of investigations.

establish an adherent stromal layer (Fig. 3). The formation of active hemopoietic areas ("cobblestones") was rapidly affected at a concentration of 10^{-8} M, and no cobblestones were detectable at concentrations from 10^{-6} M Ara-C and upward. Fibroblasts, however, could still be observed at a concentration of 10^{-5} M Ara-C (Table 1). After 2 weeks of 10^{-5}–10^{-6} M Ara-C treatment, adherent stromal cells were unable to support cobblestone formation from fresh autologous mononuclear BMC added after removal of the drug (Fig. 1).

D. Discussion

During the last 5 years, low-dose Ara-C therapy of patients with AML and preleukemic syndromes has been assessed optimistically and with increasing interest among clinicians, because Ara-C in low dosage might exert a differentiation-inducing effect on leukemic blast cells, in addition to its cytotoxic action. Many patients, however, develop severe aplasia with this therapy. Although the dose of Ara-C in low-dose therapy is about ten times lower than conventional intravenous dosages, it is, however, administered for a much longer period. Furthermore, the effect of Ara-C on GM-CFC in vitro is more dependent on time than on dosage [8]. We showed that long-term exposure (7 days) to Ara-C concentrations of 10^{-8}–10^{-6} M produces toxic effects on GM-CFC. The latter completely disappear at an Ara-C concentration of 10^{-5} M.

There is some evidence that normal hemopoiesis is dependent on intact stromal cells, and vice versa. Thus, busulfan-related aplasia is connected with damage to the stroma cells [5]. It has also been demonstrated that the ability of BMC from patients with aplastic anemia to form a stromal layer in Dexter culture is defective [3].

The results presented here indicate that Ara-C concentrations reflecting the plasma Ara-C concentrations in low-dose-treated patients produce toxic effects on the ability of BMC to form a stromal layer. Moreover, the marrow stromal cell layer formed by BMC continuously exposed to Ara-C at concentrations of 10^{-5} or 10^{-6} M lost the ability to support normal hemopoiesis. Whether our results can be extrapolated to the in vivo situation has still to be proved, because the stromal progenitors with usually low proliferation in vivo proliferate during Ara-C exposure in our system.

References

1. Degos L, Castaigne S, Tilly H, Sigaux F, Daniel MT (1985) Treatment of leukemia with low-dose Ara-C. A study of 160 cases. Semin Oncol [Suppl 3] 12(2):196–199
2. Dexter TM, Allen TD, Lajtha LG (1977) Conditions controlling the proliferation of haemopoietic stem cells in vitro. J Cell Physiol 91:335–344
3. Elstner E, Schulze E, Ihle R, Stobbe H, Grunze S (1985) Stromal progenitor cells in bone marrow of patients with aplastic anemia. In: Neth R, Gallo R, Greaves MF,

Janka G (eds) Haematology and blood transfusion. Springer, Berlin Heidelberg New York Tokyo, pp 168–171 (Modern trends in human leukemia 6)

4. Gartner S, Kaplan HS (1980) Long-term culture of human bone marrow cells. Proc Natl Acad Sci USA 77:4756–4759

5. Hays E, Hale L, Villarreal B, Fitchen JM (1982) "Stromal" and hemopoietic stem cell abnormalities in long-term cultures of marrow from busulfan-treated mice. Exp Hematol 10:383–392

6. Jehn U, Bock R de, Haanen C (1984) Clinical trial of low-dose Ara-C in the treatment of acute leukemia and myelodysplasia. Blut 48:255–261

7. Pike BL, Robinson WA (1970) Human bone marrow colony growth in agar-gel. J Cell Physiol 76:77–84

8. Raijmakers R, Witte T de, Linssen P, Wessels J, Haanen C (1986) The relation of exposure time and drug concentration in their effect on cloning efficiency after incubation of human bone marrow with cytosine arabinoside. Br J Haematol 62:447–453

9. Spriggs D, Griffin J, Wisch J, Kufe D (1985) Clinical pharmacology of low-dose cytosine arabinoside. Blood 65:1087–1089

10. Tilly H, Castaigne S, Bordessoule D, Sigaux F, Faniel M, Monconduit M, Degos L (1985) Low-dose cytosine arabinoside treatment for acute nonlymphocytic leukemia in elderly patients. Cancer 55:1633–1636

11. Tricot G, Bock R de, Dekker AW, Boogaerts MA, Pettermans M, Punt K, Verwilghen RL (1984) Low-dose cytosine arabinoside (Ara-C) in myelodysplastic syndromes. Br J Haematol 58:231–240

Haematology and Blood Transfusion Vol. 31
Modern Trends in Human Leukemia VII
Edited by Neth, Gallo, Greaves, and Kabisch
© Springer-Verlag Berlin Heidelberg 1987

The Secretion of Plasminogen Activators by Human Bone Marrow Progenitor Cells

E. L. Wilson [1] and G. E. Francis [2]

A. Introduction

Leukaemic cells from patients with acute myeloid leukaemia (AML) and chronic myeloid leukaemia (CML) secrete plasminogen activators either of the urokinase (u-PA) or of the tissue plasminogen activator (t-PA) type. The enzyme has prognostic significance in that those individuals with AML whose cells secreted only t-PA failed to respond to combination chemotherapy, whereas those whose cells released u-PA alone or a combination of u-PA and t-PA could be induced to remission (Wilson et al. 1983).

Poor responses to chemotherapy are also seen when leukaemic cells display features of the early progenitor phenotype (Francis et al. 1979, 1981 a, b). It seemed likely, therefore, that secretion of the two species of plasminogen activator by haemopoietic cells might be differentiation-linked and that the association between u-PA secretion and favourable therapeutic outcome would reflect the tendency of early cells to release t-PA, whereas later cells would release u-PA.

B. Materials and Methods

Bone marrow cells were separated on the basis of differences in buoyant density in continuous Ficoll-Isopaque gradients (Loos

[1] Department of Clinical Science and Immunology, University of Cape Town Medical School, Observatory, Cape Town, South Africa
[2] Department of Haematology, Royal Free Hospital, Pond Street, Hampstead, London, England

and Roos 1974). Granulocyte-macrophage colony-forming cells (CFU-GM) were cultured using the method of Pike and Robinson (1970). The culture method for CFU-GM was that of Fauser and Messner (1978). Plasminogen activator and caseinolytic plaque assays have previously been described in detail (Wilson et al. 1980, 1983; Wilson and Francis 1987).

C. Results

Marrow samples from 11 normal subjects were fractionated by equilibrium density centrifugation, and cells from each fraction were examined to determine the type and rate of plasminogen activator that they produced. Representative results from two experiments are presented in Fig. 1 in two ways. In the first (Fig. 1 a, b), the rate of enzyme synthesis by all the cells in each gradient fraction is plotted as a function of gradient density. In the second (Fig. 1 c, d), the rate of synthesis has ᵇᵉᵉn corrected for the number of cells in each fraction and is expressed in terms of milliunits of enzyme/10^7 cells for 24 h. It is evident from both graphic presentations that the low-density cells (approximately $1.045–1.065^{-3}$ g cm^{-3}) synthesized exclusively t-PA. More mature, higher density cells (approximately $1.07–1.085$ g cm^{-3}) released a mixture of t-PA and u-PA. It can also be noted from the profiles plotted in Fig. 1a and b that the cells which produced t-PA comprised two populations. When they were corrected for cell number, only one peak of t-PA production (density

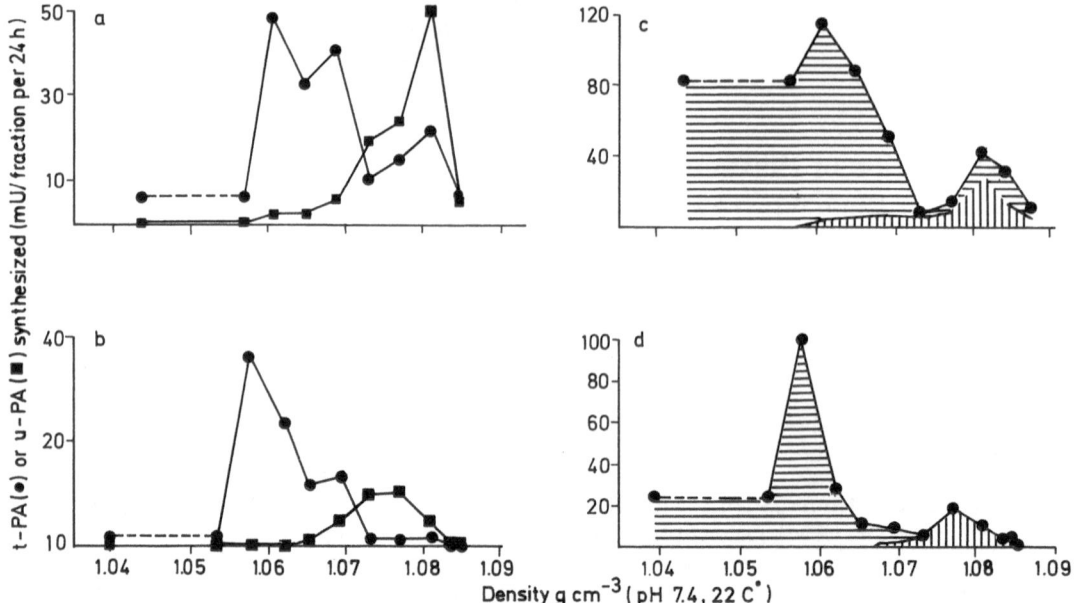

Fig. 1. a and **b** Equilibrium density distribution profiles of two normal marrow specimens, showing t-PA (●) and u-PA (■) expressed as units of enzyme per fraction per density increment. Cells producing t-PA have a relatively lower density than those producing u-PA. In both cases, the t-PA peaks were biphasic. **c** and **d** Density distribution profiles of the same marrow specimens, showing the relationship between total units of plasminogen activator/10^7 cells produced in 24 h and buoyant density. *Vertical hatching* indicates u-PA and *horizontal hatching* indicates t-PA (*dashed lines* represent adjacent fractions which have been pooled)

approximately 1.060 g cm^{-3}) was observed, thus indicating that although these cells can be divided into two populations on the basis of their density, they constituted a single population on the basis of the rate of enzyme production per cell.

The bimodal distribution in the t-PA-producing cell populations was observed in 7 out of 11 cases. The mean densities for the two t-PA-containing peaks were 1.063 and 1.072 g cm^{-3}, respectively.

The u-PA, in contrast, was produced by cells which fractionated in either a single peak or one which had a low broad profile. The mean density of the u-PA-producing cells was 1.076 g cm^{-3}. In vitro agar bone marrow cultures of the cells in the different gradient fractions revealed that the first and second t-PA-producing cell populations most closely resembled CFU-GM and cluster-forming cells, respectively. The modal density for myeloblasts was found to

be between the two t-PA-producing cell peaks. Promyelocytes and myelocytes had modal densities of 1.069 and 1.072 g cm^{-3}, respectively. These populations appeared to correspond to the second peak of t-PA, which had a density of 1.072 g cm^{-3}. The u-PA-producing cells with a density of 1.076 g cm^{-3} corresponded to the neutrophil-granulocyte population.

In order to assess more directly the cellular species secreting each enzyme type, the low-density bone marrow cells (less than 1.063 g cm^{-3}) were cultured in semi-solid agar for varying periods of time. Developing clones were examined for the species of enzyme produced. Developing clones on day 3 produced t-PA exclusively. Clones examined on days 6–9 secreted both enzyme species; by day 11, large neutrophil and/or macrophage colonies were present and all the secreted enzyme was u-PA. Macrophages were also found to produce u-PA.

D. Discussion

These results showed that the secretion of t-PA and u-PA by haemopoietic cells was a differentiation-linked property, with t-PA being produced by primitive progenitors and u-PA being secreted by more differentiated cells (Wilson and Francis 1987).

It has been shown that a variety of human cells release plasminogen activators of either the t-PA or the u-PA type (Tucker et al. 1978; Vetterlein et al. 1979; Wilson et al. 1980). Apart from the involvement of t-PA in the fibrinolytic system (Collen et al. 1983), the physiological role of these two enzymes is obscure. The enzymes are produced by a wide variety of cells, including macrophages (Vassali et al. 1977) and neutrophil polymorphonuclear leucocytes (Granelli-Piperno et al. 1977; Wilson et al. 1983), where they may be involved in a number of processes, including proteolysis of inflammatory exudates, generation of chemotactic peptides and processes that require regulated local proteolysis (Reich 1978).

Tissue plasminogen activator was secreted by two populations of bone marrow cells, one with a mean density of $1.063\ \mathrm{g\,cm^{-3}}$ and the other with one of $1.072\ \mathrm{g\,cm^{-3}}$. The first population corresponds to the modal density for CFU-GM. We cannot exclude the possibility that other progenitor types also produce t-PA. Analysis of the density distribution of the fractionated cells suggested that myelocytes and possibly promyelocytes were responsible for the second t-PA peak. Urokinase was secreted by cells with a density of between 1.067 and $1.082\ \mathrm{g\,cm^{-3}}$. Promyelocytes, myelocytes and neutrophil granulocytes are present in these fractions. It thus appears either that the promyelocytes and myelocytes produce both types of enzyme or that the switch from t-PA to u-PA production occurs over a range of maturation stages.

The functional properties of AML clonogenic cells have been shown to relate to response to chemotherapy (Moore et al. 1974; Francis et al. 1981 b; McCulloch et al. 1982). The results indicating that early normal progenitor cells secrete t-PA (Wilson and Francis 1987), together with the previous observation (Wilson et al. 1983) that patients whose AML cells secreted t-PA alone failed to respond to chemotherapy, suggest that these patients have an accumulation of a primitive t-PA progenitor secreting cell population.

While it appears that neutrophils and macrophages require u-PA for their role in inflammation, the reason why primitive haemopoietic cells produce t-PA is less readily apparent. The production of proteases by progenitor cells may be necessary to provide a local proteolytic mechanism for generating biologically active peptides. In addition, stem cells are endowed with the capacity for migration and implantation in specific haemopoietic sites, and this process could also require proteolytic enzyme secretion.

References

1. Collen D, Stassen JM, Verstraete M (1983) Thrombolysis with human extrinsic (tissue-type) plasminogen activator in rabbits with experimental jugular vein thrombosis. J Clin Invest 71:368–376
2. Fauser AA, Messner HA (1978) Granuloerthyopoeitic colonies in human bone marrow, peripheral blood and cord blood. Blood 52:1243–1248
3. Francis GE, Berney JJ, Chipping M, Hoffbrand AV (1979) Stimulation of human haemopoeitic cells by colony stimulating factors; sensitivity of leukemic cells. Br J Haematol 41:545–566
4. Francis GE, Boll SJL, Berney JJ (1981 a) Clone size potential and sensitivity to colony stimulating activity: differentiation linked properties of granulocyte – macrophage progenitor cells. Stem Cells 1:124–139
5. Francis GE, Tuma GA, Berney JJ, Hoffbrand AV (1981 b) Sensitivity of acute myeloid leukemia cells to colony stimulating activity: relation to response to chemotherapy. Br J Haematol 49:1259–1267
6. Granelli-Piperno A, Vassali J-D, Reich E (1977) Secretion of plasminogen activator by human polymorphonuclear leucocytes. J Exp Med 146:1693–1706
7. Loos JA, Roos D (1974) Ficoll-isopaque gradients for the determination of density distribution of human blood lymphocytes and other reticulo-endothelial cells. Exp Cell Res 86:331–341
8. McCulloch EA, Curtis JE, Messner HA, Senn JS, Germanson TP (1982) The contribution of blast cell properties to outcome variation in AML. Blood 59:601–608

9. Moore MAS, Spitzer G, Williams M, Metcalf D, Buckley J (1974) Agar culture studies in 127 cases of untreated leukemia: the prognostic value of reclassification of leukemia according to in vitro growth characteristics. Blood 44:1–8

10. Pike BL, Robinson WA (1970) Human bone marrow colony growths in agar gel. J Cell Physiol 76:77–84

11. Reich E (1978) Activation of plasminogen: a general mechanism for producing localized extracellular proteolysis. In: Berlin RD, Herman H, Lepow IH, Tanzer JM (eds) Molecular basis of biological degradative processes. Academic, New York, pp 155–169

12. Tucker WS, Kirsch WM, Martinez-Hernandez A, Fink LM (1978) In vitro plasminogen activator activity in human brain tumours. Cancer Res 38:297–302

13. Vassali J-D, Hamilton J, Reich E (1977) Macrophage plasminogen activator; induction by concanavalin A and phorbol myristate acetate. Cell 11:695–705

14. Vetterlein D, Young PL, Bell TE, Roblin R (1979) Immunological characterization of multiple molecular weight forms of human cell plasminogen activators. J Biol Chem 254:575–578

15. Wilson EL, Kirsch WM, Martinez-Hernandez A, Fink LM (1978) In vitro plasminogen activator activity in human brain tumours. Cancer Res 38:297–302

16. Wilson EL, Becker MLB, Hoal EG, Dowdle EB (1980) Molecular species of plasminogen activators secreted by normal and neoplastic human cells. Cancer Res 40:933–938

17. Wilson EL, Jacobs P, Dowdle EB (1983) The secretion of plasminogen activators by human myeloid leukemic cells in vitro. Blood 61:568–574

18. Wilson EL, Francis GE (1987) Differentiation linked secretion of urokinase and tissue plasminogen activator by normal human haemopoetic cells. J Exp Med 165:1609–1629

Haematology and Blood Transfusion   Vol. 31
Modern Trends in Human Leukemia VII
Edited by Neth, Gallo, Greaves, and Kabisch
© Springer-Verlag Berlin Heidelberg 1987

Leukemic Colony-Forming Cells in Acute Myeloblastic Leukemia: Maturation Hierarchy and Growth Conditions *

F. Herrmann [1], W. Oster [1], A. Lindemann [1], A. Ganser [1], B. Dörken [2], W. Knapp [3], J. D. Griffin [4], and R. Mertelsmann [4]

A. Introduction

Despite their primitive morphological appearance, the majority of leukemic blasts in acute myeloblastic leukemia (AML) are endstage, nonproliferating cells. Only a small subset of AML blasts are capable of a sufficient number of divisions to form colonies in semisolid medium [1, 2]. It has been suggested that these leukemic colony-forming cells (L-CFC) may act in vivo as progenitor cells to maintain the rest of the leukemic cell population [3, 4]. L-CFC share several properties with normal myeloid progenitor cells, including self-renewal potential and high thymidine suicide index [2, 3]. As in the case of normal myeloid progenitor cells (NMPC), colony growth of L-CFC from most patients requires exogenous colony-stimulating factors (CSF) which are routinely supplied by the addition of media conditioned by activated T cells, placental tissue, or media derived from various tumor cell lines, including GCT [5], MO [6], or 5637 [7]. As NMPC proliferate in the presence of CSF, differentiate, and acquire new differentiation-associated surface antigens during this process, so L-CFC have the capacity to undergo at least limited, although abnor-

mal, differentiation to nonproliferative cells [3, 8].

It has previously been shown that in some AML samples the majority of leukemic blasts expressed differentiation-associated antigens not present on L-CFC from the same donors [8–10], thus suggesting immaturity of L-CFC. In this study, we tested the presence of L-CFC in 62 patients with AML, using a standard agar colony assay system [11] and GCT-conditioned medium as source of CSF. Under these conditions, 21 leukemic samples did not grow in vitro, 22 formed clusters of fewer than 20 cells per aggregate, and 19 formed blast-like colonies with a buoyant density greater than 20 cells per aggregate. These 19 leukemic samples provided the basis for further studies with the goal of (a) comparing L-CFC with the majority of the leukemic cells in each sample; (b) comparing L-CFC with normal bone marrow colony-forming cells; (c) replacing GCT medium, which is known to contain a multiplicity of hematopoietic growth factor, by recombinant granulocyte-macrophage colony-stimulating factor (GM-CSF) [12] and HPLC-purified G-CSF [7] in order to identify specific L-CFC growth factors; and (d) exploring the possibility of autocrine secretion of CSF by the leukemic blast cells of some AML samples.

B. Material and Methods

I. Leukemic Cells

Peripheral blood or bone marrow aspirates were obtained at diagnosis. Leukemic cells,

* Supported in part by a grant (He 1380-2/1) from the Deutsche Forschungsgemeinschaft.
[1] Departments of Hematology, Johannes Gutenberg University, Mainz, FRG, Johann Wolfgang Goethe University, Frankfurt, FRG
[2] Ruprecht-Karls University, Heidelberg, FRG
[3] Immunological Institute, University of Vienna, Austria
[4] Dana Farber Cancer Institute, Division of Tumor Immunology, Boston, Massachusetts, USA

recovered by Ficoll-Diatrizoate density gradient centrifugation, were further enriched by rosetting with AET-treated sheep red blood cells to remove T cells, and by plastic adherence at 37 °C to remove monocytes. All samples tested contained more than 90% blasts. The diagnosis of AML was established by morphology, cytochemical staining, and surface antigen analysis, using a panel of monoclonal antibodies (mcAbs).

II. Colony Assay

Colonies derived from normal marrow colony-forming unit granulocyte-macrophage (CFU-GM) and L-CFC were assayed in a double-layer agar system in quadruplicate by a modification of the method of Pike and Robinson as described [13]. In this system, either highly purified NMPC (2×10^3/ well) or leukemic blasts (5×10^4/well) were incorporated in the agar overlayer. CFU-GM were enumerated on days 7 and 14, L-CFC on day 10.

III. Growth Factors

GCT-conditioned medium (GCT-CM) was obtained from Gibco (Grand Island, New York). Recombinant GM-CSF was obtained from Behring (Marburg, FRG) and HPLC-purified G-CSF was a gift from Dr. K. Welte (Sloan-Kettering Cancer Center, New York, NY). In selected experiments, media conditioned by short-time (3 days)-cultured AML blasts (AML-CM) was used. Growth factors were incorporated in the agar underlayer (GCT-CM: 10% v/v; recombinant GM-CSF: 1 µg/ml; HPLC-purified G-CSF: 500 U/ml; AML-CM: 1–10% v/v).

IV. Complement Lysis

To determine the surface antigen phenotype of the CFU-GM and L-CFC, aliquots of 10^6 cells were incubated with lytic antimyeloid mcAb (1 : 250 dilutions of ascites) for 30 min at 4 °C. After two wash steps, cells were suspended in baby rabbit complement (Pel-

Freez, Rogers, AR) at a dilution of 1 : 5 for 90 min at 37 °C. After two further wash steps, cells were resuspended in Iscove's modified Dulbecco's medium containing 20% fetal calf serum. Negative controls included treatment with complement alone and treatment with a lytic but nonbinding IgG monoclonal antibody (MZ4; F. Herrmann, unpublished results) and complement. Monoclonal anti-beta-2 microglobulin antibody HD46 (B. Dörken and F. Herrmann, unpublished results) was used as a positive control.

VII. Immunofluorescence Staining

Antibody reactivity with the whole leukemic cell population was determined by indirect immunofluorescence staining using a flow cytometer (Coulter Epics C) as described [13]. Negative and positive controls included the same mcAb as described above.

VIII. Monoclonal Antibodies

Besides MZ4 and HD46, a panel of five lytic antimyeloid mcAbs was used, including anti-MY9, -MZ17, -VIM2, -VIM D5, and -MY3. The reactivity of anti-MY9, -VIM2, VIM D5, and -MY3 has been described before [14]. MZ17, produced in the own laboratory, is an IgM murine mcAb which is reactive with 95% of AML samples and all permanent myeloid leukemia lines tested, including Kg1, Kg1a, HL60, HL60BII, and U937. MZ17 reacts with granulocytes, monocytes, and 3% of ALL samples but does not react with resting T cells or B cells. Preliminary biochemical data suggest that MZ17 binds to a carbohydrate moiety.

IX. Northern Blot Hybridization

In selected experiments, Northern blot hybridization of leukemic cell mRNA with complementary oligonucleotide probes corresponding to GM-CSF and G-CSF (kindly provided by Dr. D. Blohm, BASF, Ludwigshafen, FRG) was performed using standard procedures [15]. In additional experiments,

Table 1. Surface antigen phenotypes of the total AML population and of L-CFC

Patient no.	HD46 Total	HD46 L-CFC[a]	MY9 Total	MY9 L-CFC	MZ17 Total	MZ17 L-CFC	VIM2 Total	VIM2 L-CFC	VIMD5 Total	VIMD5 L-CFC	MY3 Total	MY3 L-CFC	MZ4 Total	MZ4 L-CFC
1	++	+++[b]	++	+++	+++	+++	++	++	−	−	−	−	−	−
2	+++	++++	+	+++	++	+++	+++	+++	−	−	−	−	−	−
3	++++	++++	+++	++++	+	+	++	+	−	−	+	−	−	−
4	++++	++++	+++	++++	+	+	+	++	++	−	−	−	−	−
5	++++	++++	++	++	+	+	++	+	++	−	+	−	−	−
6	+++	++++	+	+++	++	+++	++	+++	+	−	−	−	−	−
7	+++	++++	++	+++	++	+++	++	+++	−	−	−	−	−	−
8	++++	++++	++	+++	++	+++	+++	+++	−	−	−	−	−	−
9	++++	++++	++	+++	+	+	++	+++	++	−	−	−	−	−
10	++++	++++	+	+++	++	+++	+++	+++	+++	−	+	−	−	−
11	++++	++++	++	+++	++	+++	++	+++	++	−	+	−	−	−
12	++++	++++	+	+++	++	+++	+	+++	−	−	−	−	−	−
13	++++	++++	++	+++	++	+++	+++	+++	−	−	+	−	−	−
14	++++	++++	+	++	++	++	+++	+++	−	−	−	−	−	−
15	++++	++++	++	++	+++	+++	++++	++++	−	−	+	−	−	−
16	+++	++++	++	+++	+++	+++	+++	+++	+	++	++	+	−	−
17	+++	++++	++	+++	+++	+++	++	+++	−	++	−	−	−	−
18	+++	++++	+++	+++	+++	+++	++	+++	−	+++	+	+	−	+
19	+++	++++	+++	+++	+++	+++	+	+	−	−	+	−	−	−

ᵃ L-CFC were plated at 5 × 10⁴/well. Results are expressed as the mean of quadruplicate cultures. Total number of L-CFC per 5 × 10⁴ cells counted at day 10 ranged from 132±17 to 148±46.

ᵇ +, 25%–50% antigen-positive cells; ++, 50%–75% antigen-positive cells; +++, >75% antigen-positive cells.

hybridized blots were washed with boiling $0.1 \times SSC/0.1\%$ sodium dodecyl sulfate and rehybridized with a probe for the constant region of the alpha chain of the T-cell antigen receptor (kindly provided by Dr. H. D. Royer, DFCI, Boston, Massachusetts).

C. Results and Discussion

Clonogenicity of leukemic cells from 62 patients with AML was investigated in an agar culture system. In 19 of the AML samples tested, L-CFC giving rise to clonal growth into blast-like colonies was detectable. Expression of myeloid surface antigens on these L-CFC was monitored by complement lysis experiments using antimyeloid mcAb described above, and L-CFC phenotypes were compared with phenotypes of surface antigens obtained from normal bone marrow (day 7 and day 14 CFU-GM), which were assayed in an identical agar system. To investigate the relationship between L-CFC and the total leukemic cell population, immunofluorescence studies of all the leukemic populations were performed. As shown in Table 1, L-CFC formed a distinct subset of cells in AML that could be separated from the majority of the AML blasts in the same patient by immunological analysis of the surface antigen phenotype. Furthermore, surface antigen phenotypes of L-CFC showed a considerable heterogeneity among different patients. L-CFC from 3 out of 19 cases studied expressed only HD46, MY9 and MZ17; a second group of 13 cases expressed HD46, MY9, MZ17 and VIM2; in a third group of 2 cases, L-CFC were lysed with HD46, MY9, MZ17, VIM2, VIM D5, and complement, and in one case MY3 was additionally expressed.

Comparison of the phenotypes of NMPC (days 7 and 14 CFU-GM; Table 2) with L-CFC revealed that these antigens are acquired in both the normal and the malignant ontogeny in an analogous maturation-associated sequence, thus suggesting that AML can arise at multiple stages corresponding to the normal differentiation pathway. In vitro testing of L-CFC biology may be of value for the clinical evaluation of patients with AML. The identification of L-

Table 2. Surface antigen phenotypes of NMPC

Donor no.	Percent antigen-positive cells													
	Day 7–CFU-GM[a]							Day 14–CFU-GM						
	HD46	MY9	MZ17	VIM2	VIMD5	MY3	MZ4	HD46	MY9	MZ17	VIM2	VIMD5	MY3	MZ4
1	+++[b]	+++	++	–	–	–	–	+++	++	++	–	–	–	–
2	+++	+++	++	+	+	–	–	++++	+++	+++	–	–	–	–
3	+++	+++	++	–	–	–	–	+++	++	++	–	–	–	–
4	+++	+++	+++	–	–	–	–	++++	+++	+++	–	–	–	–
5	+++	+++	++	–	+	–	+	+++	++	+++	–	–	–	–
6	+++	+++	++	+	+	–	+	+++	++	+++	–	–	–	–

[a] Purified NMPC were plated at 20×10^3/well. Results are expressed as the mean of quadruplicate cultures. Total number of colonies derived from day 7 CFU-GM ranged from 89 ± 4 to 181 ± 8. Number of day 14 CFM-GM ranged from 179 ± 7 to 281 ± 22.
[b] For explanation of symbols, see first footnote to Table 1.

188

Table 3. Presence of biologically CSF with GM-CSF properties in a medium conditioned by fresh AML cells with autonomous L-CFC growth

Source of CSF	Concentration of CSF	CFU-GM (day 14)/2×10^3 purified NMPC[a]		
		CAE+ colonies	ANAE+ colonies	LFB+ colonies
AML-CM 5	1% v/v	99	82	15
	5% v/v	100	81	15
	10% v/v	105	76	17
GCT-CM	10% v/v	101	88	17
Recombinant GM-CSF	1 µg/ml	86	75	14
HPLC-purified G-CSF	500 U/ml	150	48	1

[a] CFU-GM were enumerated at day 14. Values are expressed as colonies of quadruplicate cultures. Colonies were stained in situ for chloroacetate esterase (*CAE*; granulocytes), alpha-naphthyl acetate esterase (*ANAE*; monocytes), and Luxol fast blue (*LFB*; eosinophils).

CFC has the potential to predict effective drug combinations in cases of resistance and could also play a role in the preclinical setting of new therapies. This may be important in the evaluation of monoclonal antibodies as therapeutic in vivo agents or for in vitro purging of leukemic clonogenic cells from autologous bone marrow transplants. As in the case of normal CFU-GM, L-CFC colony growth requires the addition of exogenous growth factors, in most cases provided by CSF-containing media, although

some L-CFC may be independent of exogenous CSF, probably owing to production of CSF by leukemic cells in an autocrine pathway.

We tested the L-CFC growth of 16 out of 19 AML samples in response to various sources of CSF, including GCT-CM, recombinant GM-CSF, and HPLC-purified G-CSF. In all cases, L-CFC growth occurred in the presence of GCT-CM. In each of those cases which required exogenous growth factors for L-CFC growth, recombinant GM-

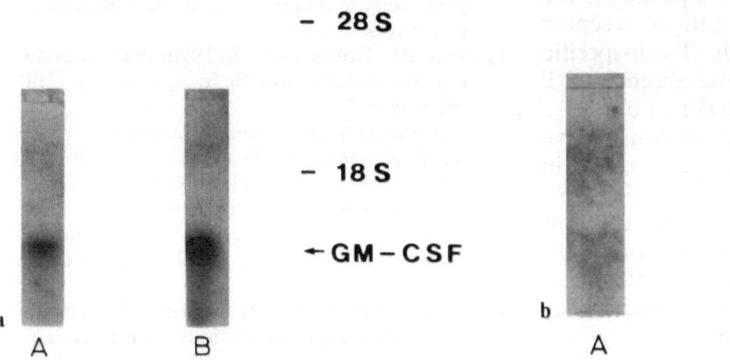
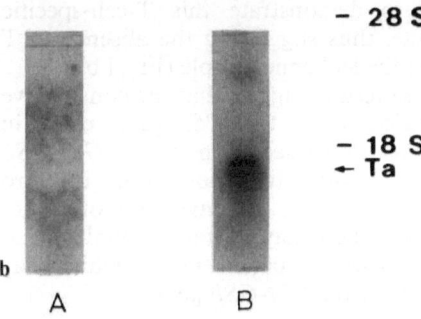

Fig. 1. a GM-CSF message of 1.0-Kb length in Northern blot analysis. Total cellular RNA (10 µg) was glyoxilated and then fractionated in a 0.8% agarose gel. RNA was transferred to a nylon membrane and hybridized to a complementary oligonucleotide (GM-CSF probe) labeled with X^{32} ATP, using T4 oligonucleotide kinase, or to a complementary Tα-DNA labeled with p^{32} dCTP, using the random primer method. *Lane A:* AML with autonomous L-CFC growth; *lane B:* phorbol myristate acetate stimulated T-lymphocytes. **b** The same blot as shown in Fig. 1a was washed and rehybridized with a probe for the α-chain constant region of the T-cell antigen receptor, thus demonstrating the absence of this T-cell-specific message in the AML case (*lane A*) and presenting the 1.7 Kb mRNA in phorbol myristate acetate T-lymphocytes (*lane B*)

189

CSF but not HPLC-purified G-CSF could fully replace GCT-CM, thus suggesting that GM-CSF provides a major growth support for L-CFC in vitro (data not shown). However, in two cases, L-CFC growth occurred autonomously (patient no. 5: M2-type AML according to FAB classification; patient no. 17: M5-type AML).

It was found that medium conditioned by leukemic cells from patient no. 5 (AML-CM 5) supported normal bone marrow granulocyte, monocyte, and eosinophil colony growth (Table 3), whereas AML-CM derived from patient no. 17 (AML-CM 17) did not (data not shown). Since induction of eosinophil colony growth by AML-CM 5 suggested similarity between AML-CM 5 and GM-CSF (G-CSF and M-CSF do not induce eosinophil colony growth), we performed Northern blot hybridization of leukemic cell mRNA from this patient, using a complementary oligonucleotide for the *GM-CSF* and *G-CSF* gene respectively as probes. As shown in Fig. 1 a, Northern blot hybridization experiments with leukemic cells of patient no. 2 revealed, using the GM-CSF probe, a 1-Kb message which was indistinguishable in size from the GM-CSF message detected in phorbol myristate acetate stimulated T cells. No GM-CSF mRNA was detected in patient no. 17. G-CSF mRNA was absent in both cases (data not shown). Rehybridization of the blots with a probe for the alpha chain of the T-cell antigen receptor failed to demonstrate this T-cell-specific message, thus suggesting the absence of T cells in the leukemic sample (Fig. 1 b).

These results suggest that the constitutive expression of the *GM-CSF* gene results in the constitutive secretion of the *GM-CSF* protein, leading to autonomous in vitro growth of L-CFC in some cases of AML. However, there may exist additional mechanisms, as seen in patient no. 17, which may not involve the *GM-CSF* gene.

References

1. Moore MAS, Williams N, Metcalf D (1977) In vitro colony formation by normal and leukemic human hematopoietic cells: characterization of the colony forming cells. JNCI 50:603

2. Buick RN, Till JE, McCulloch EA (1977) Colony assay for proliferative blast cells circulating in myeloblastic leukemia. Lancet 1:862

3. Minden MD, Till JE, McCulloch EA (1978) Proliferative state of blast cell progenitors in acute myeloblastic leukemia. Blood 52:592

4. Wouters R, Löwenberg B (1984) On the maturation order of AML cells: A distinction on the basis of self-renewal properties and immunologic phenotypes. Blood 63:684

5. Brennan JK, di Persio JF, Abboud CN, Lichtman MA (1979) The exceptional responsiveness of certain human myeloid leukemia cells to colony stimulating activity. Blood 54:1230

6. Golde DW, Quan SG, Cline MJ (1978) Human T lymphocyte cell line producing colony-stimulating activity. Blood 52:1068

7. Welte K, Platzer E, Lu L, Gabrilove JL, Levi E, Mertelsmann R, Moore MAS (1985) Purification and biochemical identification of human pluripotent hematopoietic colony stimulating factor. Proc Natl Acad Sci USA 82:1526

8. Griffin JD, Larcom P, Schlossman SD (1983) Use of surface markers to identify a subset of acute myelomonocytic leukemia cells with progenitor cell properties. Blood 62:1300

9. Lange B, Ferrero D, Pessano S, Columbo A, Faus J, Meo P, Rovera G (1984) Surface phenotype of clonogenic cells in acute myeloid leukemia defined by monoclonal antibodies. Blood 64:693

10. Sabbath KD, Ball ED, Larcom P, Davis RB, Griffin JD (1985) Heterogeneity of clonogenic cells in acute myeloblastic leukemia. J Clin Invest 75:746

11. Pike BL, Robinson WA (1970) Human bone marrow colony growth in agar gel. J Cell Physiol 76:77

12. Cantrell MA, Anderson D, Ceretti DP, Price V, McKereghan K, Tushinski R, Mochizuki DY, Larsen A, Grabstein K, Gillis S, Cosman D (1985) Cloning, sequence, and expression of a human granulocyte/macrophage colony-stimulating factor. Proc Natl Acad Sci USA 82:6250

13. Herrmann F, Cannistra SA, Griffin JD (1986) T cell monocyte interactions in the production of humoral factors regulating human granulopoiesis in vitro. J Immunol 136:2856

14. Reinherz EL, Haynes BM, Nadler LM, Bernstein ID (eds) (1985) Human myeloid and hematopoietic cells. Springer, Berlin Heidelberg New York (Leukocyte typing 2)

15. Maniatis T, Fritsch EF, Sambrook J (1982) Molecular cloning, a laboratory manual. Cold Spring Harbor Laboratory publication, Cold Spring Harbor

Haematology and Blood Transfusion   Vol. 31
Modern Trends in Human Leukemia VII
Edited by Neth, Gallo, Greaves, and Kabisch
© Springer-Verlag Berlin Heidelberg 1987

Hexosaminidase I Indicates Maturation Disarrangement in Acute Leukemias *

J. R. Novotny[1], S. Brendler[2], H. J. Kytzia[2], K. Sandhoff[2], and G. Gaedicke[1]

A. Introduction

For a number of lysosomal hydrolases, abnormally expressed forms have been found to occur in childhood and adult leukemia. Most of these abnormalities are confined to the physicochemical properties of the enzymes, e.g., abnormal electrophoretic mobility, change of isoelectric point, and alteration of isoenzyme pattern. All this has been described for the hexosaminidase system in human leukemia cells. The most-investigated phenomenon is the occurrence of hexosaminidase I [1–3, 5, 6, 19]. Other abnormalities, such as the anodic shift of the Hex A isoenzyme [2, 6] or a relative decrease of the Hex B form [1], are found in various leukemia subtypes.

In our study, we found that the Hex I isoenzyme is present in excess in cells from typical cALL, pre B-ALL, AUL, and AML. This has also been described in T-ALL, pre T-ALL, T-CLL, and multiple myeloma cells. However, this isoenzyme has so far not been found to be raised in CML and B-CLL. An anodic shift of Hex A and a decrease in Hex B activity appeared independently in a few cases from among all investigated leukemia forms.

In normal leukocytes, hexosaminidases occur in two isoenzymatic variants: Hex A

and Hex B. Hex A is a heteropolymer enzyme composed of one alpha subunit and one beta subunit, whereas Hex B is a homopolymer enzyme consisting of two beta subunits [16, 17].

Since there are only few data available about the nature of the hexosaminidase I or the "shifted" hexosaminidase A in human leukemia cells, we have investigated their subunit composition and enzymatic properties.

B. Methods

All methods used are described elsewhere [4, 7, 8, 10–15].

C. Results

I. Biochemical and physicochemical properties of hexosaminidase I demonstrate that Hex I belongs to the hexosaminidase system and behaves like Hex B whereas the "shifted" hexosaminidase A resembles Hex A. cALL cells and REH-6 cells contain an excess of hexosaminidase I isoenzyme, as compared to normal lymphocytes.

II. Immunochemical analysis of preparations from such cells shows that Hex I is a homopolymer of beta subunits. Since the molecular weight is about 100 000 daltons, it must be made up of two beta subunits. The "shifted" Hex A is a heteropolymer of one alpha and one beta subunit.

III. The processing of the enzyme subunits in REH-6 cells shows striking differ-

* Supported by the Deutsche Forschungsgemeinschaft (Grants SFB 112, Project B10 and Project Ga 167/4-1).
[1] Abteilung Pädiatrie II, Universitäts-Kinderklinik, Prittwitzstraße 43, 7900 Ulm/Donau, FRG
[2] Institut für Organische Chemie und Biochemie der Universität, Gerhard-Domagk-Straße 1, 5300 Bonn, FRG

Table 1. Comparison of hexosaminidase I and "shifted A" hexosaminidase from leukemia cells with the hexosaminidase isoenzymes A and B

Property	Hexosaminidase A	Hexosaminidase B	Hexosaminidase I	"Shifted" hexosaminidase A
Isoelectric point	5.0	7.3	about 6.5	about 4.6
Stability at 50 °C	−	+	+	−
Precipitation with antibodies to hexosaminidase B	+	+	+	+
Precipitation with specific antibodies to hexosaminidase A	+	−	−	+
Molecular weight	About 100 000	About 100 000	About 100 000	Not determined
Proposed composition	Alpha/beta	Beta/beta	Beta/beta	Alpha/beta
Hydrolysis of:				
MUF-/pNP-Glc-NAc	+	+	+	+
MUF-/pNP-Gal-NAc	+	+	+	+
MUF-/pNP-Glc-NAc-6-S	+	−	−	+
Ganglioside GM_2*	+	−	−	+

* In presence of the physiological activator

Table 2. Molecular weights of precursor proteins, intermediate forms, and "mature" polypeptides of beta hexosaminidase from human cells (modified from 9, 18)

Enzyme	Cell system	Enzyme precursor	Intermediate form	"Mature" enzyme subunit
Beta hexosaminidase Alpha subunit	Fibroblasts Macrophages Monocytes Lymphocytes Granulocytes Smooth-muscle cells Endothelial cells	67		54
Beta hexosaminidase Beta subunit	Fibroblasts Macrophages Monocytes Lymphocytes Granulocytes Smooth-muscle cells Endothelial cells	63	52	29
	Leukemia cells (REH-6 cell line)	66	51.5	Not formed

In leukemia cells (REH-6 cell line), hexosaminidase alpha precursors and mature alpha subunits are formed only in traces.

ences in quantitative and qualitative synthesis, in comparison to normal fibroblasts. Thus, an abnormal precursor of the hexosaminidase beta chain (about 1000 daltons larger than the regular beta precursor) and an abnormal beta subunit (slightly smaller than the regular one) are formed, while no normal alpha or beta precursors or alpha subunits occur in REH-6 cells. Mature beta chains do not appear in these cells.

D. Discussion

Although a raised Hex I level has been found in most cases of cALL, pre B-ALL, AML, and roughly half of the cases of AUL, it has also been demonstrated in cases of other leukemia subtypes (e.g., T-ALL, T-CLL, and multiple myeloma). The above-mentioned abnormalities, such as the shifted Hex A or the decreased Hex B, seem not to be strictly confined to certain leukemia subtypes. It is therefore suggested that the abnormalities described might be more general, as they affect a number of lysosomal enzymes in various leukemia subtypes.

Hexosaminidase I is an isoenzyme which shows a different physicochemical behavior, as compared to isoenzymes A and B. Our results from heat inactivation of isoenzyme I activity, as well as the lack of any specific activity against sulfated synthetic substrates or ganglioside GM_2, clearly demonstrate that hexosaminidase I must be largely composed of beta subunits. This is further strongly supported by our immunodiffusion assays using antisera against pure hexosaminidase B and specific antibodies against hexosaminidase A. Thus, we conclude from our data that hexosaminidase I from cALL cells is a homopolymer polypeptide like hexosaminidase B and is composed of hexosaminidase beta units only. In contrast, shifted hexosaminidase A is a heteropolymer enzyme like the normal Hex A and consists of one alpha and one beta unit.

Data from determination of apparent molecular weight by gel filtration do not reveal major differences. On the basis of these findings, we favor the hypothesis that the difference may be due to an abnormal post-translational processing of the beta subunits of isoenzyme I, as compared to that of the regular isoenzyme B. This view is supported by labeling experiments in which we were able to show an abnormal beta precursor and beta subunit of Hex I, as well as a lack of mature beta chains in cALL cells. These differences could be due to an altered composition of the carbohydrate chains of the molecules. Corresponding mechanisms may lead to the anodic shift of hexosaminidase A. In summary, we conclude that the findings described may indicate maturation disarrangement in acute leukemias.

References

1. Besley GTN, Moss SE, Bain AD, Dewar AE (1983) Correlation of lysosomal enzyme abnormalities in various forms of adult leukaemia. J Clin Pathol 36:1000–1004
2. Broadhead DM, Besley GTN, Moss SE, Bain DA, Eden OB, Sainsbury CPQ (1981) Recognition of abnormal lysosomal enzyme patterns in childhood leukemia by isoelectric focusing, with special reference to some properties of abnormally expressed components. Leuk Res 5:29–40
3. Dewji N, Rapson N, Greaves M, Ellis R (1981) Isoenzyme profiles of lysosomal hydrolases in leukaemic cells. Leuk Res 5:19–27
4. Drexler HG, Gaedicke G, Novotny JR, Minowada J (1986) Occurrence of particular isoenzymes in fresh and cultured leukemia – Lymphoma cells. II. Hexosaminidase I isoenzyme. Cancer 58:245–251
5. Dunn NL, Maurer HM (1982) Enzyme alterations in leukemic cells. Am J Hematol 13:343–351
6. Ellis RB, Rapson NT, Patrick DA, Greaves MF, Path MRC (1978) Expression of hexosaminidase isoenzymes in childhood leukemia. N Engl J Med 298:476–480
7. Gaedicke G, Novotny JR, Raghavachar A, Drexler HG (1985) Hexosaminidase isoenzyme: an early marker of hematopoietic malignancy. In: Neth R, Gallo R, Greaves MF, Janka G (eds) Haematology and blood transfusion. Springer, Berlin Heidelberg New York Tokyo, pp 187–190 (Modern trends in human leukemia 6)
8. Geiger B, Calef E, Arnon R (1978) Biochemical and immunochemical characterization of hexosaminidase P. Biochemistry 17:1713–1717
9. Hasilik A, von Figura K (1984) Processing of lysosomal enzymes in fibroblasts. In: Dingle JT, Dean RT, Sly WS (eds) Lysosomes in biology and pathology. Elsevier, Amsterdam, pp 3–16
10. Kresse H, Fuchs W, Glössl J, ʌˉltfrerich D, Gilberg W (1981) Liberation of N-aˌˌylglucosamine-6-sulfate by human beta-N-acetylhexosaminidase A. J Biol Chem 256:12926–12932
11. Kytzia HJ, Hinrichs U, Sandhoff K (1984) Diagnosis of infantile and juvenile forms of G gangliosidosis variant 0. Residual activities toward natural and different synthetic substrates. Hum Genet 67:414–418
12. Novotny JR, Drexler HG, Raghvachar A, Gaedicke G (in preparation) Hexosaminidase isoenzyme profiles in various leukemia subtypes

13. Novotny JR, Kytzia HJ, Brendler S, Conzelmann E, Gaedicke G (in preparation) Biochemical properties of hexosaminidase I from common ALL cells
14. Novotny JR, Brendler S, Gaedicke G, Schedel R, Sandhoff K (in preparation) Defective processing of beta-hexosaminidase subunits in common ALL-leukemia cells
15. Proia RL, d'Azzo A, Neufeld EF (1984) Association of alpha- and beta-subunits during the biosynthesis of beta-hexosaminidase in cultered human fibroblasts. J Biol Chem 259:3350–3354
16. Sandhoff K, Christomanou H (1979) Biochemistry and genetics of gangliosidoses. Hum Genet 50:107–143
17. Sandhoff K, Conzelmann E (1984) The biochemical basis of gangliosidosis. Neuropediatrics 15:85–92
18. Skudlarek MD, Novak EK, Swank RT (1984) Processing of lysosomal enzymes in macrophages and kidney. In: Dingle JT, Dean RT, Sly WS (eds) Lysosomes in biology and pathology. Elsevier, Amsterdam, pp 17–43
19. Tanaka T, Kobayshi M, Saito O, Kamada N, Kuramoto A, Usui T (1983) Hexosaminidase isoenzyme profiles in leukemic cells. Clin Chim Acta 128:19–28

Haematology and Blood Transfusion Vol. 31
Modern Trends in Human Leukemia VII
Edited by Neth, Gallo, Greaves, and Kabisch
© Springer-Verlag Berlin Heidelberg 1987

Membrane-Microfilament Interactions in the Cells of B-Chronic Lymphocytic Leukemia

F. Caligaris-Cappio, L. Bergui, G. Corbascio, L. Tesio, F. Malavasi, P.C. Marchisio, and F. Gavosto

In the present study we have investigated the association between cell surface molecules and the cytoskeleton in malignant B-chronic lymphocytic leukaemia (B-CLL) cells. The rationale was the observation that close interactions between surface receptors and cytoskeletal proteins are involved in the regulation of several major lymphocyte functions, including activation and recirculation [1]. B-CLL cells were selected for this study for three reasons. First, B-CLL monoclonal B cells have a well-characterized phenotype [2]: they express on the membrane the monoclonal-antibody (MoAb)-defined cluster differentiation (CD) 19, 20, 21, 24 and 5 structures. Second, they have abnormalities that suggest defects of cytoskeleton function, such as the inability to cap surface immunoglobulins (sIg) and other ligand receptors [3]. Finally, these cells have a peculiar organization of F-actin that is predominantly associated with dot-shaped close-contact adhesion sites which have recently been characterized and described as podosomes [4, 5]. On those bases, our experimental approach was devoted to answering the following questions: (a) Can the different CDs present on the B-CLL cell surface be capped? (b) If such a phenomenon occurs, does it modify the cytoskeleton organization? (c) Can the perturbation of membrane-cytoskeleton interactions lead to any functional change in B-CLL cells?

Monoclonal B cells from 12 patients with typical B-CLL were studied utilizing RFT1, B4 (Coulter), RFB7, RFB6 and BA1 (Menarini) to characterize CD5, 19, 20, 21 and 24, respectively. The analysis of cytoskeleton structures was performed as detailed in [5]; F-actin-containing microfilamentous structures were identified by means of rhodamine-isothiocyanate-labelled phalloidin (R-PHD). Short-term cultures were set up at 37 °C in air containing 5% CO_2 with RPMI medium and 10% fetal calf serum. The results indicate that CD5 can be capped on the surface of B-CLL cells by treating the cells with anti-CD5. The capping phenomenon becomes evident after 2 h of incubation, is maximal after 24 h and is more prominent when CD5 is cross-linked with an anti-mouse Ig Ab. In contrast, the CD5 molecules on the surface of normal and B-CLL T-lymphocytes cannot be capped. CD21 (C3d receptor) is the only other CD which can be capped on the surface of B-CLL cells. CD5 and CD21 co-cap on the surface of B-CLL cells and co-modulate. Finally, the incubation of B-CLL cells with anti-CD5 and/or anti-CD21 either abolishes or largely inhibits the organization of intracellular F-actin into podosomes.

The above data indicate that the lateral movements of CD5 and CD21 on the surface of B-CLL cells interfere with the organization of F-actin in the cytoplasm, and point to the existence of a strict spatial relationship on the membrane between CD5 and CD21. The possible functional significance of CD21 has been investigated in four cases. The in vitro stimulation of B-CLL cells with anti-CD21 does not modify their morphol-

Dipartimento di Scienze Biomediche e Oncologia Umana, Sezione Clinica e Istologia, Istituto de Genetica Medica, Università di Torino, Italy

195

ogy and phenotype. The picture changes drastically when anti-CD21 Sepharose-linked MoAb is used. After 72 h of stimulation, B-CLL cells transform into large blast-like elements with nucleoli, become CD5⁻, $CD10^+$ and lose sIg. These activated cells are not proliferating, as they are unable to incorporate bromodeoxyuridine ($BUDR^-$). However, a very active wave of proliferation can be obtained by culturing B-CLL cells preactivated with Sepharose-linked anti-CD21 in the presence of 10% B-Cell Growth Factor (BCGF; CPI). The vast majority of cells enter the S phase of the cell cycle ($BUDR^+$) and reach a peak ($>20\%$) after 72 h of culture. The same BCGF-induced proliferative activity can be observed in B-CLL cells preactivated with Sepharose-linked CB04 MoAb which detects the receptor for the C3b fraction of complement [6]. These data indicate that B-CLL cells may be a valuable model for investigating the interactions between surface receptors, i.e. complement receptors, and cytoskeleton. Their abnormalities may help in understanding the differentiation and proliferative properties of malignant B-lymphocytes.

Acknowledgements. This work was supported by PF Oncologia, CNR, Rome, and partly by AIRC, Milan. L.B. is the recipient of a fellowship of the Comitato G. Ghirotti. We thank Professor G. Janossy, London, for providing RFT1, RFB6 and RFB7 monoclonal antibodies, and Professor Th. Wieland, Heidelberg, for providing R-PHD.

References

1. Braun J, Unanue ER (1983) The lymphocyte cytoskeleton and its control on surface receptor function. Semin Haematol 20:322–333
2. Caligaris-Cappio F, Janossy G (1985) Surface markers in chronic lymphoid leukemias of B cell type. Semin Haematol 22:1–11
3. Cohen HJ (1975) Human lymphocyte surface immunoglobulin capping. Normal characteristics and anomalous behaviour of chronic lymphocytic leukaemia antigens. J Clin Invest 55:84–93
4. Caligaris-Cappio F, Bergui L, Tesio L, Corbascio G, Tousco F, Marchisio PC (1986) Cytoskeleton organization is aberrantly rearranged in the cells of B chronic lymphocytic leukemia and hairy cell leukemia. Blood 67:233–239
5. Tarone G, Cirillo D, Giancotti FG, Comoglio PM, Marchisio PC (1985) Rous sarcoma virus transformed fibroblasts adhere primarily at discrete protrusions of the ventral membrane called podosomes. Exp Cell Res 159:141–157
6. Malavasi F, Funaro A, Bellone G, Caligaris-Cappio F, Berti E, Tetta C, Dellabona P, De-Maria S, Campogrande M, Cappa APM (1985) Functional and molecular characterization by the CB04 monoclonal antibody of a cell surface structure exerting C3-complement receptor activity. J Clin Immunol 5:412–420

Cell Biology

Haematology and Blood Transfusion Vol. 31
Modern Trends in Human Leukemia VII
Edited by Neth, Gallo, Greaves, and Kabisch
© Springer-Verlag Berlin Heidelberg 1987

ts-Oncogene-Transformed Erythroleukemic Cells: A Novel Test System for Purifying and Characterizing Avian Erythroid Growth Factors

E. Kowenz [1,2], A. Leutz [1,2], G. Döderlein [1], T. Graf [1], and H. Beug [1]

A. Introduction

An emerging, important characteristic of many leukemic cell types is their altered dependence on and/or response to hematopoietic growth factors [6, 17]. In mammals, many of these growth-regulatory proteins have been purified and the respective genes molecularly cloned [16, 26], but the mechanism by which they regulate growth and differentiation of normal hematopoietic precursors is still poorly understood. This is due partly to the fact that such hematopoietic precursors do not self-renew in vitro and constitute only a minor fraction of bone marrow cells, precluding their purification in large numbers [25]. One particularly successful approach to circumventing this problem was the use of avian retroviral oncogenes that transform hematopoietic precursors [10].

For instance, avian retroviruses containing tyrosine kinase oncogenes such as v-*erbB*, v-*sea*, or v-*src,* as well as the v-Ha-*ras* oncogene, readily transform avian erythroid progenitor cells [late BFU-E (burst-forming unit erythroid) to early CFU-E (colony-forming unit erythroid)] from chick bone marrow [8, 11]. By transformation, these precursors are induced to self-renew and thus to grow into mass cultures of immature, precursor-like cells. The transformed cells, however, retain the ability to undergo terminal differentiation at low frequency [3, 7, 12]. At the same time, they become independent of an activity present in anemic chicken serum that induces CFU-E-like colonies in chicken bone marrow and probably represents avian erythropoietin (EPO) [1, 21].

Recently, our laboratory described the use of erythroblasts transformed with temperature-sensitive mutants of v-*erbB* (*ts* AEV) and v-*sea* (*ts* S13) containing retroviruses as novel systems for studying differentiation of normal and leukemic erythroid cells. Upon a shift to the nonpermissive temperature, *ts*-AEV and *ts*-S13 erythroblasts are induced to differentiate synchronously into erythrocytes. At the same time, the cells regain their dependence on a factor(s) from anemic chicken serum [1–3] (H. Beug et al., unpublished work).

Since little information was available on the nature of this avian erythropoietin-like factor(s) and its possible relationship to mammalian erythropoietin [5, 20], we were interested in using *ts*-oncogene-transformed erythroblasts to attempt its purification and characterization. Here we describe two simple assay systems for avian erythroid growth factors and their use in partially purifying and characterizing chicken erythropoietin, which is shown to be a glycoprotein of 38 kd, resembling mammalian EPO in many respects.

B. Materials and Methods

I. Viruses and Cells

A temperature-sensitive mutant of the S13 strain of avian erythroblastosis virus [2], re-

[1] European Molecular Biology Laboratory, Postfach 10.2209, 6900 Heidelberg, FRG
[2] Present address: University of New York at Stonybrook, Dept. of Microbiology, Life Sciences Bldg., Stonybrook, NY 11790

ferred to as *ts*1-S13, was obtained from Peter Vogt (Los Angeles) and biologically cloned by preparing nonproducer erythroblasts [2]. Its properties will be described elsewhere (Knight et al., manuscript in preparation). *ts*1-S13 erythroblast clones were generated as described below and grown in CFU-E medium [19] in the absence of anemic serum.

II. Selection of *ts-S13* Test Cell Clones

Colonies of *ts*1-S13-transformed erythroblasts were induced from infected SPAFAS chick bone marrow cells as described earlier [2]. A large number of colonies were picked into CFU-E medium and clones were propagated for 3 days in 96-well plates (Falcon). Equal aliquots of each clone were then distributed to two 96-well plates; one was kept at 37 °C in CFU-E medium, whereas the other was kept at 42 °C after addition of differentiation medium plus anemic serum (see below). Three days later, a small aliquot of each clone was stained for hemoglobin with acid benzidine [9]. Clones exhibiting >95% benzidine-positive cells were centrifuged onto slides, stained with neutral benzidine and histological dyes, and evaluated for the presence of terminally differentiated cells, as described earlier [1]. Finally, those clones that contained more than 95% erythrocytes plus late reticulocytes [1] were tested for their response in both EPO assays (see below) and for their in vitro lifespan by repeated passage (1 in 3) in CFU-E medium. One clone (clone 30), which showed a particularly prominent response to anemic serum in both assays and exhibited a lifespan of >45 generations in vitro, was frozen in many aliquots in liquid nitrogen and used for the experiments described in this paper.

III. Production of Anemic Serum

Chickens (5–12 months, SPAFAS) were made severely anemic by bleeding them by heart puncture on 3 consecutive days (15–30 ml/day/kg). They were then bled on day 4 to generate anemic serum. Since EPO titers generated by this method proved to be highly variable, we changed to phenylhy-drazine injection. Four grams of phenylhy-drazine (p.A., Merck, Darmstadt) were dissolved in 400 ml of aq bidest, the pH was adjusted to 7.0 with $2N$ NaOH, and the solution was immediately frozen and kept at -40 °C. Thawed solutions were used for injection within 15 min. Chickens were injected i.m. with 2 ml solution/kg on day 1, with 1 ml/kg on day 2, with 0.3–0.5 ml/kg on day 3, and were bled on day 4. Sera were allowed to clot for only 1–2 h and the clots were then spun at 40 000 g (15 000 rpm, SS34 for 30 min) to obtain the anemic serum.

IV. Assays for Erythropoietin Activity from Anemic Serum

In both assays, anemic serum or test samples (for instance column fractions) appropriately diluted with modified Iscove's DMEM (see below) were applied to the wells of 96-well multidishes (Falcon) in duplicate or triplicate, not exceeding a volume of 10 µl. Then 90 µl of differentiation medium were added [consisting of 16.4 ml of Iscove's modification of Dulbecco's modified Eagles (Iscove's DMEM, Gibco, minus mercaptoethanol and selenite; salt concentrations changed according to the recipe for DMEM); 4.28 ml sterile distilled water; 32 µl 10^{-1} M mercaptoethanol; 150 µl iron-saturated ovotransferrin (15 mg/ml; Conalbumin, Sigma); 690 µl detoxified BSA (20% w/v solution; Behring-Werke, Marburg/Lahn [2]); 920 µl NaHCO$_3$, 5.6%; 3 ml fetal calf serum (pretested batch); and 12 µl porcine insulin (Actrapid, Bayer-Leverkusen, 1.7 mg/ml), if not stated otherwise]. Then the test cells (:-S13 c130) were separated from spontaneousiy differentiated cells by centrifugation through Percoll (density 1.072) and 30 000–50 000 cells were seeded per well, suspended in 5–10 µl differentiation medium.

For the DNA synthesis assay, ^{3}H-thymidine (0.2–0.4 µCi in 5 µl DMEM per well) was added after 40–48 h of incubation at 42 °C and 5% CO$_2$. The labeled cells were then harvested onto fiberglass filters using a Skatron cell harvester, the filters were dried, and the cells were counted in a beta-counter (Fig. 2).

For the photometric hemoglobin assay (measuring accumulated hemoglobin in viable cells) cells were incubated for 50–72 h at 42 °C and 5% CO_2. They were then transferred to 96-well, V-bottomed microtiter plates and washed twice with Hanks' balanced salt solution containing 0.1% detoxified BSA. Cells were lysed in 20 µl H_2O for 20 min, and 200 µl of developing reagent was added (0.5 mg/ml 0-phenylenediamine in 0.1 M citrate/phosphate buffer, pH 5.0, containing 5 µl/ml 30% H_2O_2 added just prior to use). The color was allowed to develop for 15–30 min in the dark at room temperature, and the solutions were transferred to a flat-bottomed 96-well microtiter plate containing 30 µl of 4 M sulphuric acid per well to stop the reaction and enhance the color. Absorbances were read at 492 in a Kontron SLT210 ELISA photometer, using 630 mm as the reference wavelength (Fig. 1).

V. Partial Purification of Chicken Erythropoietin

We centrifuged 200 ml of pooled anemic chicken sera for 90 min at 150 000 g (Ti45 rotor Beckman, 40 000 rpm). The clear supernatant was then applied to a Sephadex G25 column (Sephadex G25 fine; 5 cm in diameter, 50 cm long, equilibrated with 50 mM $(NH_4)_2CO_3$ buffer, pH 8.0). Protein-containing fractions eluting before or at the exclusion volume were then directly applied to a DEAE ion-exchange column (DEAE Sephacel; 6 cm in diameter, 25 cm long, equilibrated with 50 mM $(NH_4)_2CO_3$ buffer, pH 8.0). After washing with 500 ml of starting buffer the column was eluted with a linear gradient of 50–400 mM $(NH_4)_2CO_3$; pH 8.0; gradient volume 2 l. Active fractions eluting at 150–200 mM $(NH_4)_2CO_3$ were combined and lyophilized.

For size-exclusion chromatography, the lyophilized fractions from DEAE ion-exchange chromatography were dissolved in 10 ml of 50 mM $(NH_4)_2CO_3$ buffer, pH 8, and applied to a size-exclusion column (Biogel P60, BioRad; 200–400 mesh, 5 cm in diameter, 90 cm long, 20 ml/h). The activity eluted behind the main protein peak (at a mol. wt.) range of 50 000–30 000). Active fractions were pooled and lyophilized.

For affinity chromatography, the lyophilized material was dissolved in 50 ml phosphate-buffered saline plus 0.1 mM $MnCl_2$ and 0.1 mM $CaCl_2$, pH 7.4, and applied to two connected columns containing immobilized lentil-lectin (Affi-Gel P10, 8 mg lentil-lectin/ml gel, column volume 50 ml) and immobilized wheat-germ agglutinin (WGA, Pharmacia, Sepharose 4B, 10 mg lectin/ml gel, column volume 20 ml). After application of the sample and washing with 1 l of the above buffer, the two columns were separated. The lentil-lectin column was eluted with 100 mM methyl-alpha-D-mannopyranoside, the WGA column with 200 mM N-acetyl glucosamine in the same buffer. No biological activity was found in the flowthrough of both columns or in the lentil-lectin eluate. The WGA eluate containing all the biological activity was concentrated by ultrafiltration (Amicon, PM10), dialyzed against 50 mM $(NH_4)_2CO_3$, and lyophilized. It was then dissolved in PBS and chromatographed on a small Sephadex G25 column (10 ml) in PBS to remove traces of N-acetyl glucosamine, which were toxic in the bioassays.

VI. Characterization of Chicken Erythropoietin by High-pressure Liquid Chromatography (HPLC)

1. Reversed-phase HPLC

An aliquot of partially purified chicken EPO (250 µl from a total of 5 ml) was adjusted to 100 mM Tris-HCl, pH 6.8, and applied to a C-3 column (Ultrapore, RPSC, Altex, 0.5 ml/min). The column was washed consecutively with HPLC-water and 0.1% trifluoroacetic acid (TFA) in water (buffer A) and eluted with an acetonitrile gradient as follows: 10 min 0%–45% buffer B (75% acetonitrile in 0.1% TFA), 60 min 45%–70% buffer B. Fractions (2 ml) were collected during the second phase of the gradient elution, lyophilized, and dissolved in DMEM for testing of their activity.

2. Size-exclusion HPLC

Another aliquot of partially purified EPO was adjusted to 100 mM sodium phosphate buffer, pH 6.8, and applied to two coupled size-exclusion columns (Pre-column, LKB TSK 4000, 0.7 cm in diameter, 10 cm long, plus two separation columns, LKB, TSK 3000, 0.7 cm in diameter, 60 cm long). Columns were eluted at 0.5 ml/min and fractions (1 ml, 2 min/fraction) were collected 40 min after injection. Fractions were diluted appropriately with DMEM before testing in both available EPO assays.

C. Results and Discussion

I. Assay Systems for Avian Erythroid Growth Factors Using *ts*-Oncogene-transformed Leukemic Erythroblasts

Previous work had shown that erythroblasts transformed by temperature-sensitive mu-

tants of v-*erbB* or v-*sea* required factors in anemic chicken serum for terminal differentiation in vitro after a shift to the nonpermissive temperature. Pilot experiments designed to test the usefulness of these cells in possible assay systems for erythroid growth factors quickly demonstrated that *ts-sea* erythroblasts were much more suitable for such assays than *ts-erbB* cells (probably because of the presence of v-*erbA* in the latter) [13]. In addition, it soon became evident that suitable test-cell clones had to be selected, exhibiting the potential for complete in vitro differentiation as well as an extended in vitro lifespan [1] (see Materials and Methods).

Investigation of the differentiation behavior of such a selected *ts*-S13 erythroblast clone (clone 30) after shift to 42 °C with and

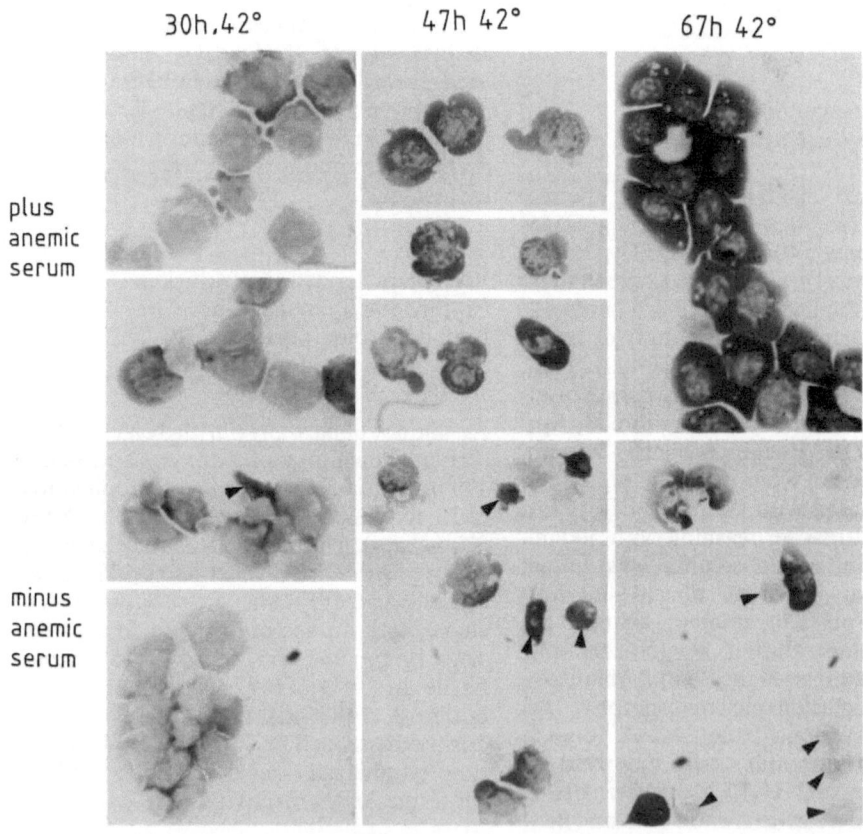

Fig. 1. Differentiation of *ts*-S13 erythroblasts in the presence and absence of anemic serum. *ts*-S13 erythroblasts (clone 3O) were incubated at 42° in differentiation medium plus or minus anemic serum. At the times indicated, aliquots were cy- tocentrifuged onto slides, stained with neutral benzidine plus histological dyes, and photographed under blue light (480 μm) to reveal histochemical hemoglobin staining [1]. *Arrowheads* indicate lysed and moribund cells

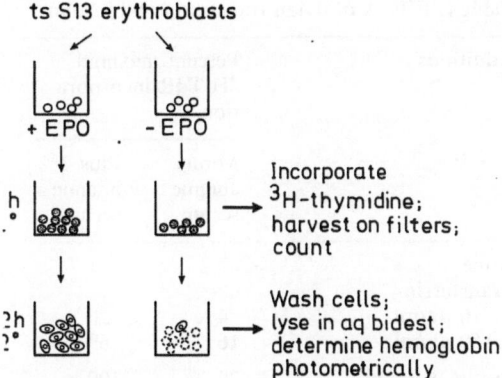

ts S13 erythroblasts

+ EPO   - EPO

h

?h
?

→ Incorporate
³H-thymidine;
harvest on filters;
count

→ Wash cells;
lyse in aq bidest;
determine hemoglobin
photometrically

Fig. 2. Essential features of two assay systems for chicken erythroid growth factors employing *ts*-S13 erythroblasts. Erythroblasts (*open circles*) are seeded into 96-well tissue culture plates with (*+EPO*) or without (*−EPO*) anemic serum or samples to be assayed. After 48 h at 42 °C the cells start to differentiate (*dotted circles*) but still proliferate in the presence, but not in the absence of EPO, allowing assessment of EPO activity by measurement of ³H TdR incorporation (DNA-synthesis assay). After 72 h at 42 °C, cells have differentiated into late reticulocytes in the presence of EPO, whereas they have mostly disintegrated (*broken circles*) in the absence of EPO and therefore released their hemoglobin into the supernatant. At this point, photometric determination of hemoglobin accumulated in viable cells therefore constitutes a second, independent measurement of EPO activity (photometric assay)

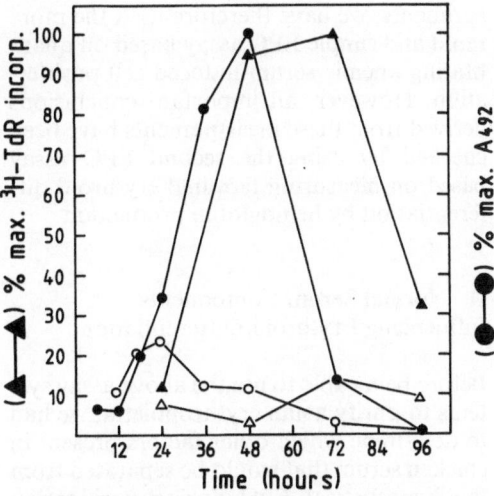

Fig. 3. Time course of proliferation and hemoglobin accumulation during differentiation of *ts*-S13 erythroblasts at 42 °C. *ts*-S13 cells were incubated in the presence (*closed symbols*) or the absence (*open symbols*) of anemic serum and assayed for ³H TdR incorporation (●—●) or hemoglobin accumulation (▲—▲) at the times indicated, using the two assay systems described in legend to Fig. 2. Data were normalized with respect to the maximum values obtained in the two assays after 48 and 72 h respectively

without anemic serum revealed that the cells continued to proliferate in the presence of anemic serum for at least 2 days, whereas they rapidly withdrew from the cell cycle in the absence of anemic serum, being essentially at rest after 36–48 h. Furthermore, in the presence of anemic serum, very few cells died during differentiation, whereas anemic serum-deprived cells mostly disintegrated within 24–48 h after shift, then being at the early-to-late reticulocyte stage (Fig. 1). However, for those cells which survived in the absence of anemic serum differentiation into erythrocytes was only slightly slower than for control cells in the presence of anemic serum (Fig. 1) [24].

These observations enabled us to devise two assay systems for avian erythroid growth factors, the principles of which are schematically depicted in Fig. 2. The first as-

say exploited the fact that anemic serum stimulates cell proliferation of *ts*-S13 cells for 48–55 h, whereas cells kept without anemic serum ceased to proliferate after 24–30 h (Fig. 3). The second assay was based on the observation that anemic serum-treated *ts*-S13 erythroblasts reached a maximum of hemoglobin accumulated in viable cells at a time when most of the cells that were shifted to 42 °C in the absence of anemic serum had lysed and therefore released their accumulated hemoglobin into the medium (Figs. 2 and 3; see Materials and Methods).

The availability of these two different assay systems for erythroid growth factor(s) facilitated the study of whether the initial proliferation and the terminal differentiation of *ts*-S13 erythroblasts are regulated by one or more than one active molecule in anemic serum. To simplify matters, we have assumed in the following that the putative avian erythropoietin, like mammalian hematopoietic growth factors, stimulates both proliferation and differentiation. In most experiments, we have therefore used the more rapid and simple EPO assay based on quantitating anemic serum-induced cell proliferation. However, all important conclusions derived from these measurements have been checked by using the second EPO assay based on measuring terminal erythroid differentiation by hemoglobin production.

II. Normal Serum Components Influencing Erythroid Differentiation

Before being able to use the above assay systems to purify avian erythropoietin, we had to determine which other factors present in chicken serum that would be separated from the hypothetical EPO during purification would affect proliferation/differentiation of *ts-sea* erythroblasts. An obvious candidate was avian transferrin, since erythroid differentiation requires massive iron uptake mediated through iron-saturated transferrin [24]. Furthermore, we had observed that insulin seemed to stimulate proliferation/differentiation of both normal and *ts*-oncogene-transformed erythroid cells (J. Schmidt, personal communication; H. Beug et al., unpublished). We therefore titrated the effects of these two proteins, either alone or in combination with each other and with anemic serum, using a medium devoid of other chicken proteins and containing as essential components detoxified bovine serum albumin, mercaptoethanol, and a preselected batch of fetal calf serum that did not stimulate erythroid differentiation on its own (see Material and Methods). The essential features of these results are summarized in Table 1. As expected, high concentrations of *avian,* iron-saturated transferrin were absolutely essential for both proliferation and differentiation of *ts-sea* erythroblasts. On its own, however, transferrin exhibited only weak, if not absent growth factor-like activity. Similarly, insulin had only a weak growth-promoting ability in the absence of anemic serum, but it significantly enhanced erythroid cell proliferation in the presence of anemic serum (Table 1). More careful inspection of this phenomenon revealed that insulin enhanced early proliferation of *ts-sea* erythroblasts shifted to 42 °C and prolonged their lifespan in the absence of anemic

Table 1. Effects of avian transferrin and insulin

Additions	Percent maximal ^{3}H TdR incorporation	
	Minus anemic serum	Plus 2% anemic serum
None	< 0.2	1
Transferrin		
10 µg/ml	4	20
150 µg/ml	16	69
Insulin 1 µg/ml plus transferrin 150 µg/ml	29	100
Insulin plus transferrin plus normal chicken serum (10%)	25	94

* Many batches of normal chicken serum were toxic at this concentration.

serum, leading to disintegration of the cells at the late rather than the early reticulocyte stage and to formation of some malformed erythrocyte-like cells (data not shown).

To test whether we had in fact optimized our test conditions sufficiently to rule out effects of normal chicken serum proteins, we titrated a high-titer batch of anemic chicken serum (Table 1) or purified chicken erythropoietin (data not shown) in the presence or the absence of 10% normal chicken serum. From more than 20 batches tested, no serum could be found that further stimulated *ts-sea* erythroblast proliferation/differentiation in the presence or absence of anemic serum, many batches being in fact inhibitory (Table 1).

III. Partial Purification of an Erythropoietin-like Activity from Anemic Serum

Adult chickens were made anemic by repeated heart puncture (or, more recently, by injection of phenylhydrazine; see Materials and Methods), and the anemic sera obtained were tested individually for activity. High-titer anemic sera were then pooled, ultracentrifuged to remove aggregated protein, and

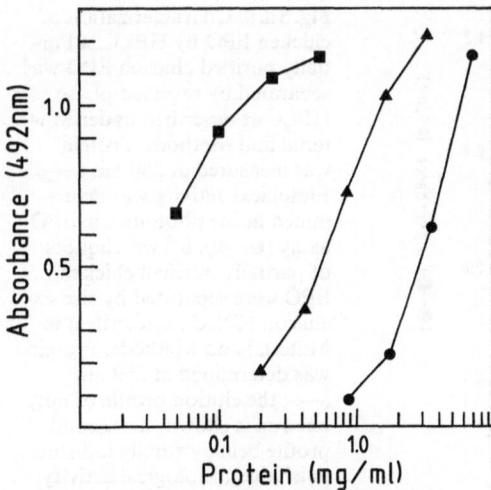

Fig. 4. Partial purification of chicken erythropoietin. Unfractionated anemic serum (●) and pooled, active fractions after DEAE ion-exchange and size-exclusion chromatography (▲) and after combined lentil – lectin–WGA affinity chromatography (■) were assayed for their biological activity by titration in the photometric EPO assay and plotted against protein concentration

consecutively subjected to DEAE ion-exchange chromatography, size-exclusion chromatography, and affinity chromatography on plant lectins (see Materials and Methods). The main difficulty in these experiments was substantial loss of EPO activity during the first steps of the purification procedure. This was probably due to proteases liberated by platelets during serum clotting (data not shown) and could be partially overcome by addition of protease inhibitors, rapid performance of the purification steps, and use of lyophilizable buffers for concentration of column fractions.

Figure 4 shows the result of a typical purification procedure. Starting with about 200 ml of anemic serum, the erythropoietin-like activity could be purified about 80-fold, recovering 25% of the original activity. The most effective purification step was the combination of lentil-lectin and wheat – germ – agglutinin affinity chromatography (see Materials and Methods). Most serum glycoproteins, but not EPO, bound to the first column, containing immobilized lentil lectin, whereas the EPO activity was effectively

bound to the second column, containing immobilized WGA, from which it could be eluted with *N*-acetyl glucosamine.

IV. EPO Activity in Anemic Serum Probably Due to a Single Glycoprotein of About 38 kd

The partial purification of chicken erythropoietin described above yielded enough activity to further characterize this avian erythroid growth factor by HPLC. Figure 5a demonstrates that the activity eluted as a single sharp peak after separation of the partially purified EPO preparation of a reversed-phase HPLC column (see Materials and Methods). Figure 5a also shows that reversed-phase HPLC resulted in a further 20-fold purification of chicken EPO without further significant losses of biological activity.

In a different approach, two aliquots of partially purified EPO were separated by size-exclusion HPLC in two separate experiments. Fractions from the first size-exclusion run were assayed by the photometric EPO assay, whereas those from the second run were assayed by the DNA-synthesis assay. Figure 5b shows that the EPO activity again eluted as a single sharp peak at about 38 kd, regardless of whether *ts*-S13 erythroblast proliferation or differentiation was used to determine EPO activity. Furthermore, size-exclusion HPLC also resulted in a 20-fold further purification of chicken EPO.

Titration of the HPLC-purified EPO preparation on *ts-sea* erythroblasts together with unfractionated anemic serum demonstrated that the activity in the purified material was indistinguishable from the activity in anemic serum in both assay systems (Fig. 6a). Furthermore, the purified EPO allowed formation of healthy, mature erythrocytes to an even larger extent than anemic serum did (Fig. 6b), indicating that a single, acidic glycoprotein of approximately 38 kd is responsible for the erythropoietin-like activity in anemic chicken serum. Finally, the purified EPO preparation stimulated the formation of normal erythroid colonies (CFU-E) from chick bone marrow at dilutions similar to those active on *ts*-S13 erythroblasts (data not shown), further con-

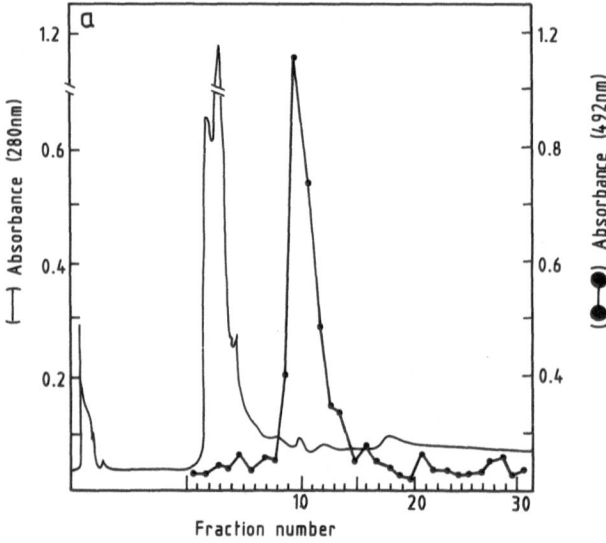

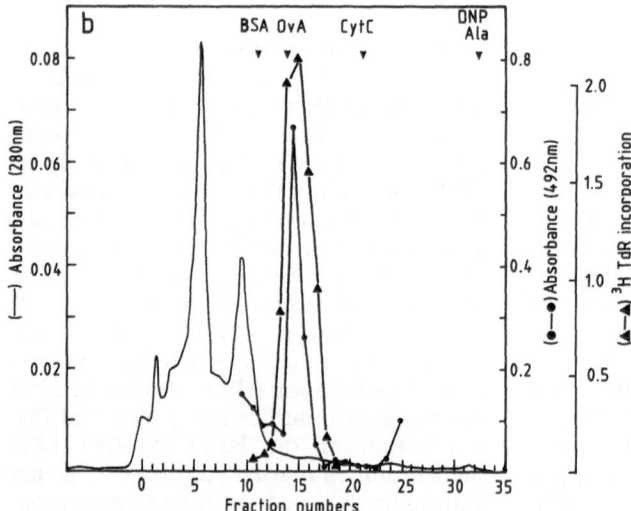

Fig. 5 a, b. Characterization of chicken EPO by HPLC. **a** Partially purified chicken EPO was separated by reversed-phase HPLC as described under Material and Methods. Protein was measured at 280 nm (——). Biological activity was determined in the photometric EPO assay (●—●). **b** Two aliquots of partially purified chicken EPO were separated by size-exclusion HPLC as described in Material and Methods. Protein was determined at 280 nm (——; the elution profile of only one run is shown, the second profile being virtually indistinguishable). Biological activity was determined photometrically (●—●) or by measuring DNA synthesis (▲—▲). The positions at which molecular weight standards (*BSA*, bovine serum albumin; *OvA*, ovalbumin; *CytC*, cytochrome C; *DNP Ala*, dinitrophenylalanine) eluted are indicated by *arrowheads*

firming that the growth factor required by temperature-induced *ts-sea* erythroblasts indeed represents chicken EPO.

V. Chicken EPO Is Species Specific and Acts Like a Typical Hematopoietic Growth Factor

Comparison of purified chicken EPO with mammalian EPO reveals several striking similarities: Like human EPO, the chicken factor represents an acidic glycoprotein of 34–39 kd that binds to wheat-germ lectins, but not to concanavalin A or lentil lectin [22, 23]. It was therefore interesting that, despite this similarity, the chicken EPO was unable to induce CFU-E colony formation in mouse bone marrow cultures under conditions where human EPO was fully active. Conversely, human and mouse EPO were completely inactive in chicken CFU-E assays, even at high concentrations (>10 U) (data not shown), indicating major differences in the receptor binding domain(s) of both molecules.

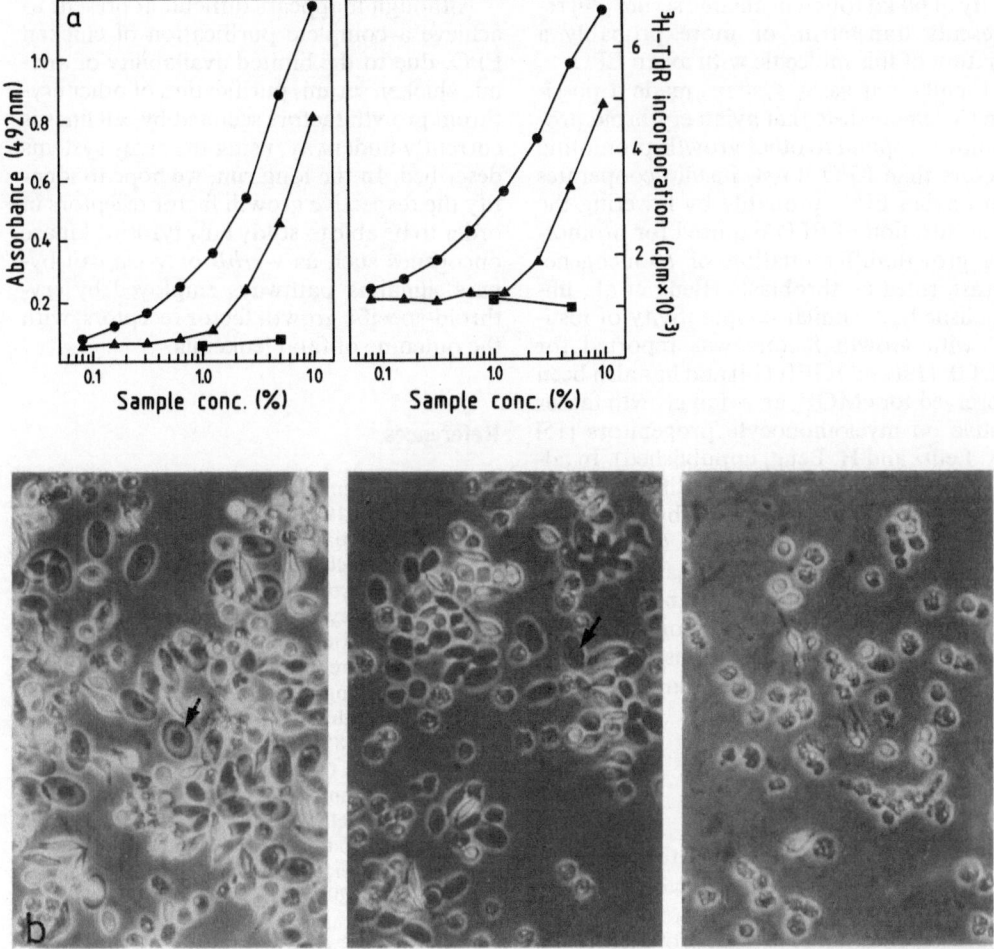

Fig. 6 a, b. Comparison of the biological activities of anemic serum and purified chicken erythropoietin. **a** Unfractionated anemic serum (▲—▲), purified EPO (after reversed-phase HPLC; ●——●), and normal chicken serum (■--■) were titrated for biological activity by measuring hemoglobin accumulation (photometric assay, *left panel*) or ³H-TdR incorporation (DNA-synthesis assay, *right panel*). **b** Phase-contrast micrographs of *ts*-S13 erythroblasts kept for 3 days at 42 °C in the presence (highest concentrations shown in **a**) of purified EPO (*left panel*), anemic serum (*middle panel*), or normal chicken serum (*right panel*) are shown. Note well-differentiated erythrocytes formed in purified EPO and anemic serum (*arrows*)

Our studies using homogeneous, synchronously differentiating erythroid cells as targets for chicken EPO demonstrate, however, that chicken EPO acts like a typical hematopoietic growth factor, in that it is required for both survival and proliferation of hormone-dependent progenitor cells preprogrammed to undergo erythroid differentiation. In addition, the studies presented here help to resolve some ambiguities in the literature concerning avian EPO. Our finding that differentiating avian erythroid cells absolutely require high concentrations of *avian* Fe-transferrin explains why this molecule was claimed to represent an avian erythroid growth factor in a nonoptimized test system [5]. For the same reason, the possibility cannot be excluded that an EPO-like activity of 60 kd found in anemic serum [20] represents transferrin, or more probably a mixture of this molecule with avian EPO.

Finally, our assay systems made it possible to demonstrate that avian erythroid progenitors respond to other growth-promoting factors than EPO. First, insulin cooperates with avian EPO, probably by lowering the concentration of EPO required for promoting growth/differentiation of *ts*-oncogene-transformed erythroblasts (Beug et al., unpublished). A similar cooperativity of insulin with growth factors was reported for PDGF [18] and IGFII [14] and has also been observed for cMGF, an avian growth factor active on myelomonocyte progenitors [15] (A. Leutz and H. Beug, unpublished). In addition, we have recently identified an erythroid growth factor secreted by avian leukemic pre-B, pre-T cells (REV$_T$-lymphoblasts; [1] that stimulates early proliferation of *ts-sea* erythroblasts and promotes terminal erythroid differentiation only in the presence of low concentrations of chicken EPO (A. Leutz and H. Beug, unpublished).

D. Conclusions

In this paper we have shown that *ts*-oncogene-transformed erythroleukemic cells can be successfully used to assay, purify, and characterize avian erythroid growth factors. Although these erythroid leukemic cells appear to be completely growth-factor independent at the permissive temperature, when the oncogene is fully active, they become dependent for survival, growth, and differentiation on specific erythroid growth factors as soon as the oncogene product is temperature inactivated. Our studies also clearly show that chicken EPO does not induce or modulate the erythroid differentiation program, but rather controls the cell's ability to undergo a series of preprogrammed differentiation events. Since no growth factor detectable in the two assay systems described or in CFU-E assays is secreted by the leukemic cells [2, 3], the oncogene seems to induce factor independence by an intrinsic mechanism, for instance by producing a constitutive signal normally generated by the EPO receptor after ligand binding [4].

Although it appears difficult at present to achieve a complete purification of chicken EPO, due to the limited availability of anemic chicken serum, purification of other erythroid growth factors secreted by cell lines is currently underway, using the assay systems described. In the long run, we hope to identify the respective growth factor receptors in order to be able to study how tyrosine kinase oncogenes such as v-*erbB* or v-*sea* can bypass signaling pathways employed by erythroid-specific growth factor receptors, with the outcome of fatal leukemia.

References

1. Beug H, Palmieri S, Freudenstein C, Zentgraf H, Graf T (1982) Hormone-dependent terminal differentiation in vitro of chicken erythroleukemia cells transformed by *ts* mutants of avian erythroblastosis virus. Cell 28:907–919
2. Beug H, Hayman MJ, Graf T, Benedict SH, Wallbank AM, Vogt PK (1985) S13, a rapidly oncogenic replication-defective avian retrovirus. Virology 145:141–153
3. Beug H, Kahn P, Doederlein G, Hayman MJ, Graf T (1985) Characterization of hematopoietic cells transformed in vitro by AEV-H, an erbB-containing avian erythroblastosis virus. In: Neth R, Gallo R, Greaves M, Janka K (eds) Modern trends in human leukemia, VI. Springer, Berlin Heidelberg New York Tokyo, pp 290–297
4. Beug H, Kahn P, Vennstroem B, Hayman MJ, Graf T (1985) How do retroviral oncogenes induce transformation in avian erythroid cells? Proc R Soc London [Biol] 226:121–126
5. Coll J, Ingram VM (1981) Identification of ovotransferrin as a heme-, colony- and burst-stimulating factor in chick erythroid cell cultures. Exp Cell Res 131:173–184
6. Cook WD, Metcalf D, Nicola N, Burgess A, Walker F (1985) Malignant transformation of a growth factor-dependent myeloid cell line by Abelson virus without evidence of an autocrine mechanism. Cell 41:677–683
7. Frykberg L, Palmieri S, Beug H, Graf T, Hayman MJ, Vennstroem B (1983) Transforming capacities of avian erythroblastosis virus mutants deleted in the *erb*A or *erb*B oncogenes. Cell 32:227–238
8. Gazzolo L, Moscovici C, Moscovici MG, Samarut J (1979) Response of hemopoietic cells to avian acute leukemia viruses: effects on the differentiation of the target cells. Cell 16:627–638

9. Graf T, Ade N, Beug H (1978) Temperature-sensitive mutant of avian erythroblastosis virus suggests a block of differentiation as mechanism of leukaemogenesis. Nature 257:496–501

10. Graf T, Beug H (1978) Avian leukemia viruses: interaction with their target cells in vivo and in vitro. BBA Revs Cancer 516:269–299

11. Graf T, von Kirchbach A, Beug H (1981) Characterization of the hematopoietic target cells of AEV, MC29 and AMV avian leukemia viruses. Exp Cell Res 131:331–343

12. Kahn P, Adkins B, Beug H, Graf T (1984) Src- and fps-containing avian sarcoma viruses transform chicken erythroid cells. Proc Natl Acad Sci USA 81:7122–7126

13. Kahn P, Frykberg L, Brady C, Stanley IJ, Beug H, Vennstroem B, Graf T (1986) V-erbA cooperates with sarcoma oncogenes in leukemic cell transformation. Cell 45:349–356

14. King GL, Kahn CR (1981) Non-parallel evolution of metabolic and growth-promoting function of insulin. Nature 292:644–646

15. Leutz A, Beug H, Graf T (1984) Purification and characterization of cMGF, a novel chicken myelomonocytic growth factor. EMBO J 3:3191–3197

16. Nicola NA, Metcalf D (1984) Binding of the differentiation-inducer, granulocyte-colony-stimulating factor to responsive but not unresponsive leukemia cell lines. Proc Natl Acad Sci USA 81:3765–3769

17. Pierce JH, DiGiore PP, Aaronson SA, Potter M, Pumphrey J, Scott A, Ihle JN (1985) Neoplastic transformation of mast cells by Abelson-MuLV: abrogation of IL-3 dependence by a nonautocrine mechanism. Cell 41:685–693

18. Petrides PE, Bohler P (1980) The mitogenic activity of insulin: an intrinsic property of the molecule. Biochem Biophys Res Commun 95:1138–1141

19. Radke K, Beug H, Kornfeld S, Graf T (1982) Transformation of both erythroid and myeloid cells by E26, an avian leukemia virus that contains the myb gene. Cell 31:643–653

20. Samarut J (1978) Isolation of an erythropoietic stimulating factor from the serum of anemic chicks. Exp Cell Res 115:123–126

21. Samarut J, Gazzolo L (1982) Target cells infected by avian erythroblastosis virus differentiate and become transformed. Cell 28:921–929

22. Spivak JL, Small D, Shaper JH, Hollenberg MD (1978) Use of immobilized lectin and other ligands for the partial purification of erythropoietin. Blood 52:1178–1186

23. Spivak JL, Small D, Hollenberg MD (1977) Erythropoietin: isolation by affinity chromatography with lectin-agarose derivates. Proc Natl Acad Sci USA 74:4633–4635

24. Schmidt JA, Marshall J, Hayman MJ, Ponka P, Beug H (1986) Control of erythroid differentiation: possible role of the transferrin cycle. Cell 46:41–51

25. van Zant G, Goldwasser E (1984) Erythropoietin and its target cells. In: Guroff G (ed) Growth and maturation factors, vol 2. Wiley, New York

26. Walker F, Burgess AW (1985) Specific binding of radioiodinated granulocyte-macrophage colony stimulating factor to hematopoietic cells. EMBO J 4:933–939

Haematology and Blood Transfusion   Vol. 31
Modern Trends in Human Leukemia VII
Edited by Neth, Gallo, Greaves, and Kabisch
© Springer-Verlag Berlin Heidelberg 1987

Biological Activities of Recombinant Human Granulocyte Colony Stimulating Factor (rhG-CSF) and Tumor Necrosis Factor: In Vivo and In Vitro Analysis *

M. A. S. Moore [1], K. Welte [2], J. Gabrilove [1], and L. M. Souza [3]

A. Introduction

Within the family of hematopoietic growth factors, murine G-CSF was first recognised as acting predominantly upon mature neutrophils and neutrophil progenitors, stimulating murine neutrophil colonies characterized by small size, maturity, and relative infrequency [1, 2]. G-CSF is synthesized in many murine tissues and organs, possibly by common populations of macrophages or endothelial cells [3], and the factor has been purified from the lung tissue of endotoxin-treated mice as a 24 000–25 000 M_r glycoprotein [4]. In contrast to GM-CSF and interleukin-3 (IL-3), G-CSF exerts a potent differentiation-inducing action on myeloid leukemic cells such as the WEHI-3 myelomonocytic leukemic cell line [4–6] and the M1 myeloblastic leukemic line [7]. Characterization of human CSF in human placental [8] and bladder carcinoma cell line [9] conditioned medium by hydrophobic chromatography or by ion-exchange chromatography and reversed phase-high performance liquid chromatography (RP-HPLC) [10, 11] revealed two species. The least hydrophobic activity, called CSF-alpha [8, 9] or pluripoietin alpha [11], is structurally and functionally homologous to murine GM-CSF (al-

though not species cross-reactive), and the hydrophobic species called CSF-beta [8, 9] or pluripoietin [2, 10] is the human analogue of murine G-CSF since these two CSFs exhibit similar activities on murine and human cells [2, 8, 10] and are fully cross-reactive with each other's specific cellular receptors [8]. This latter CSF species was purified to homogeneity from the conditioned medium of the human bladder carcinoma cell line 5637 and was shown to be O-glycosylated and to have a molecular weight of 19 600 [10]. The gene encoding this pluripotent human G-CSF was subsequently cloned and expressed in *E. coli* [12]. The *E. coli* rhG-CSF was comprised of 174 amino acids with a deduced molecular weight of 18 700 and it had no significant homology with any other previously sequenced growth factors. Recently, the cDNA sequence coding for murine G-CSF has been isolated from a cDNA library prepared with mRNA derived from murine fibrosarcoma NFSA cells, which produce G-CSF constitutively [13]. The nucleotide sequence and the deduced amino acid sequence of murine G-CSF cDNA were 69% and 73% homologous, respectively, to the corresponding sequences of human G-CSF cDNA.

Native and recombinant G-CSF had comparable biological activity, stimulating neutrophil granulocyte colonies of mouse and man with a specific activity of 1×10^8 units/mg of pure protein [12]. Our earlier observations with purified G-CSF, showing that at high concentrations the factor stimulated BFU-E and CFU-GEMM in methylcellulose cultures of adherent and T-cell-depleted human marrow [10], were confirmed using

* Supported by grants CA 20194, CA 32516 and KO8-CA 00966 (JG) from the National Cancer Institute, ACS CH-3I from the American Cancer Society, and the Gar Reichman Foundation
[1] Laboratory of Developmental Hematopoiesis
[2] Laboratory of Molecular Hematology, Memorial Sloan-Kettering Cancer Center, New York, USA
[3] Amgen, Thousand Oaks, USA

rhG-CSF [12]. More recent studies in our laboratory [14], using highly enriched hematopoietic progenitor cells, failed to demonstrate a direct effect of human G-CSF on BFU-E and CFU-GEMM, suggesting that the earlier observations may have been the consequence of an indirect mechanism involving non-T accessory cells. In this context, sequential observations in mouse bone marrow culture indicate that murine G-CSF can initiate proliferation in many progenitor cell populations, including multipotential and erythroid progenitors, but fails to sustain proliferation in these lineages beyond 2–4 days [15]. The action of G-CSF on mature hematopoietic cells appears to be confined to an action on neutrophils involving increased expression of chemotactic receptors, enhanced phagocytic ability, cellular metabolism associated with the respiratory burst, antibody-dependent cell killing, and the expression of function-associated cell surface antigens [2, 16]. The action of G-CSF on leukemic cells is receptor mediated, and competitive binding studies with ^{125}I-labeled hG-CSF [12] or murine G-CSF [9] revealed receptors on fresh human leukemic marrow cells classified as M2, M3, and M4 and on murine WEHI-3 and human HL-60 and U937 leukemic cell lines. Furthermore, these leukemic cell lines and receptor-positive human leukemic cells were induced by recombinant G-CSF to undergo terminal differentiation to macrophages and granulocytes [12].

The ability of endotoxin to elicit production of G-CSF can account for most reports of the leukemia-differentiating action of postendotoxin serum in mouse and man [6, 17]. However, the elevation of bioactive G-CSF in postendotoxin serum is partially masked at high serum concentrations by an inhibitory activity which is particularly evident in postendotoxin sera of mice primed with bacille Calmette-Guérin (BCG) or *C. parvum* [6, 17]. This hematopoietic or colony inhibitory activity was shown to be directed at both normal CFU-GM and myeloid leukemic cells, and biochemical characterization showed that it copurified with an activity with both in vitro L-cell cytotoxicity and in vivo tumor necrosis action [6, 17]. Subsequent studies distinguished between the antiproliferative effects of tumor necrosis

factor (TNF) on CFU-GM and myeloid leukemic cells and the proliferation- and differentiation-inducing action of the G-CSF co-induced with similar kinetics in the serum of *C. parvum*-endotoxin-treated mice [17]. With the availability of recombinant human TNF alpha [18], it was possible to demonstrate that human CFU-GM, BFU-E,and CFU-GEMM were inhibited by relatively low concentrations of TNF (<100 units/ml) and that the inhibition was potentiated by the addition of gamma interferon [19]. We have explored the antagonism between CSF species and TNF alpha in both short-term clonogenic assays and long-term bone marrow cultures and have obtained evidence that TNF may play a physiological role in antagonising G-CSF action in generation of neutrophil granulocytes.

B. Methods

I. CFU-GM Colony Assay

For human assay, 2.5×10^4–1×10^5 low-density, nonadherent, and T-cell-depleted normal marrow or unseparated cells from long-term bone marrow culture (LTBMC) were cultured in 0.3% agar in 1 ml supplemented McCoy's medium in the presence of 200–1000 units rhG-CSF or rhGM-CSF. In some studies, 5% 5637 cell line CM, or G- or GM-CSF purified from this source were used as sources of stimuli. Colonies were scored at days 7 and 14. For murine assay, 2.5×10^4 marrow cells or 1×10^5 spleen cells were cultured in Iscove's Modified Dulbecco's medium containing 15% fetal calf serum (FCS) and 0.3% agarose. Cultures were stimulated with interleukin-3 (IL-3) purified from WEHI-3 CM, CSF-1 purified from L-cell CM, GM-CSF purified from mouse lung CM, and rhG-CSF at 200–1000 units/ml. Cultures were scored at 5–7 days and in some studies, colony morphology was determined on fixed, stained agar plate preparations.

II. WEHI-3 Leukemic Colony Differentiation Assay

The differentiation-inducible D+ subline of the WEHI-3B murine myelomonocytic leukemic cell line was used to monitor the differentiation-inducing action of G-CSF [6, 10]. 3×10^2 WEHI-3 cells were incubated in 0.3% agar in supplemented McCoy's medium containing 12.5% FCS with 0.2 ml/ well in 24-well tissue culture trays (Costar, Cambridge, MA) and in replicates at 37 °C in 5% CO_2 in air. Cultures were scored on day 7 for induction of dispersed, differentiated colonies or tight, blast-cell colonies. Total cloning efficiency was close to 30% at 7 days of culture and was not changed significantly in the presence of G-CSF.

III. Long-term Human Bone Marrow Cultures

Obtained by aspiration from the posterior iliac crest of healthy volunteers who had given informed consent, 10^7 normal human bone marrow nucleated cells were inoculated into 25 cm tissue culture flasks in 10 ml McCoy's medium containing 15% FCS, 15% horse serum, and 10^{-6} M hydrocortisone ("Gartner's medium"). After being gassed with 5% CO_2 in air, the cultures were incubated at 37 °C for 3 days, all suspension cells removed and Ficoll-Hypaque (Pharmacia) separated, and were returned to the culture flasks, together with fresh medium and the appropriate concentration of rhTNF-alpha (a generous gift from Cetus, Inc.) or rhG-CSF (provided by Amgen). Long-term cultures were subject to demidepopulation of suspension cells and medium at weekly intervals and assayed for total cells, differential count, and CFU-GM at days 7 and 14 in agar assays stimulated with G- or GM-CSF.

IV. In Vivo Studies of rhG-CSF

C3H/HeJ mice, 8-12 weeks old, purchased from Jackson Laboratories and maintained in our Institute in laminar air-flow rooms were injected intraperitoneally twice daily with 1.5 µg rhG-CSF in 0.2 ml hydroxethyl-piperazine ethanesulphonic acid (HEPES) buffered balanced salt solution (BSS) containing 1.5 µg purified bovine serum albumin (BSA). Control inocula consisted of buffer containing 3 µg BSA and 1.5 ng E.

coli endotoxin (Difco). The endotoxin contamination of the rhG-CSF was <0.5 µg/ mg of protein. Mice were bled retro-orbitally for total white blood cell count (WBC) and hematocrit, and a smear was obtained for a blood differential. After 1 or 2 weeks of G-CSF treatment, groups of three mice were killed and cell suspensions prepared from femurs, spleen, and thymus. In addition, peritoneal lavage with 10 ml ice-cold BSS containing 10 units/ml heparin was used to obtain unstimulated peritoneal exudate suspensions. Liver hematopoietic cell populations were obtained by collagenase treatment of a minced liver preparation, with subsequent passage through a wire mesh sieve and percoll separation to remove debris and hepatocytes. Cytocentrifuge preparations of lymphohematopoietic tissues were made for morphological assessment, and cell suspensions were assayed for CFU-GM, BFU-E and CFU-GM in standard clonogenic assays. In addition, hematopoietic (CFU-S) determinations were made by injecting 10^5 cells intravenously into groups of 5 C3H/HeJ mice lethally irradiated with 950 rad gamma irradiation. Mice were killed after 12 days and colonies enumerated on Bouin's-fixed spleens.

C. Results

I. Interaction Between G-CSF, GM-CSF and TNF Alpha on Human Myeloid Colony Formation

As previously reported [11], colonies stimulated by GM-CSF were maximal at day 14 of culture, when approximately one third of colonies contained eosinophils and the remainder were neutrophil or mixed neutrophil-macrophage, and at day 7 most clones were of subcolony size (<40 cells). In contrast, with rhG-CSF, neutrophil clones of colony size were present at day 7 and their numbers remained approximately constant to day 14, when the majority were neutrophil and a minority (<20%) were neutrophil-macrophage mixed. Synergism between G-CSF and GM-CSF was noted in the context of increased colony size and number. Dose-response analysis revealed that a more

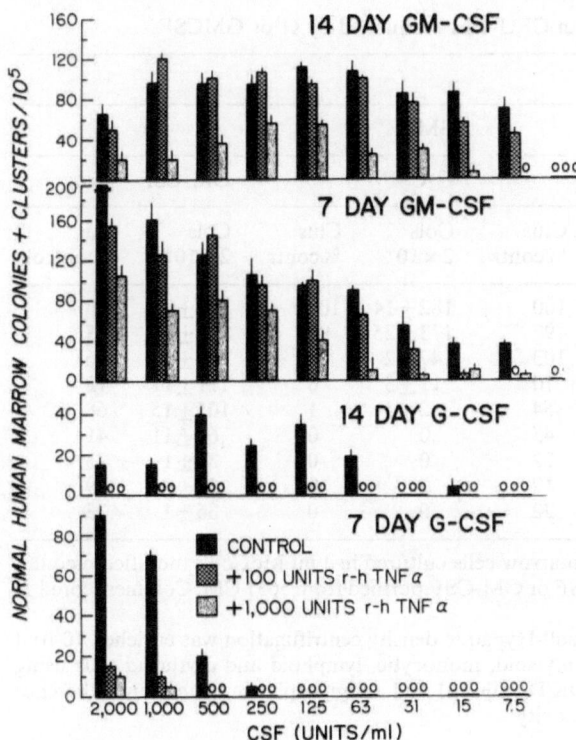

NORMAL HUMAN MARROW COLONIES + CLUSTERS / 10^5

14 DAY GM-CSF

7 DAY GM-CSF

14 DAY G-CSF

7 DAY G-CSF

■ CONTROL
▦ +100 UNITS r-h TNF α
▨ +1,000 UNITS r-h TNF α

CSF (UNITS/ml)
2,000 1,000 500 250 125 63 31 15 7.5

Fig. 1. Colony and cluster formation in agar cultures of 1×10^5 normal human bone marrow cells stimulated by 1000 units rhG-CSF or GM-CSF per milliliter and inhibited by 100 or 1000 units rhTNF alpha per milliliter. Triplicate cultures were scored at days 7 or 14

shallow titration of response was evident when day 14 was the endpoint, and at both days 7 and 14 the G-CSF dose-response curve was steeper than that of GM-CSF when either colonies or colonies plus clusters were used as the endpoint (Fig. 1).

The inhibitory influence of rhTNF alpha on the CFU-GM assay has been reported elsewhere [19], but we have observed additional variables that determine the degree of inhibition, specifically the quantity and species of CSF used to stimulate the assay and the influence of accessory cell populations. With unseparated normal human marrow, colony formation was not significantly inhibited by 100 units/ml TNF when cultures were stimulated with 30–2000 units GM-CSF, and with 1000 units TNF 20%–80% inhibition was seen; in both instances, comparable inhibition was seen at days 7 and 14 of culture (Fig. 1). With G-CSF as a source of stimulus, >80% inhibition of colony and cluster formation was seen at day 7 with 100 units TNF even in the presence of high concentrations of stimulus, and at day 14 total inhibition of colony formation was ob-

served. Particularly evident in the case of G-CSF at concentrations of <500 units and to a lesser extent with GM-CSF at <30 units, the degree of TNF inhibition was amplified at these lower, nonplateau levels of stimulation. Removal of mature granulocytes and monocyte-macrophage populations by adherence and density separation did not significantly alter the TNF dose-response curve since 50% day-14 colony inhibition was seen with 50 units rhTNF in cultures stimulated with 1000 units G-CSF and 400 units TNF was required to give comparable inhibition in cultures stimulated with 1000 units GM-CSF (Table 1). Additionally, while all colony formation was inhibited in G-CSF-stimulated cultures with 500 units TNF, a substantial number of colonies (22%) were found to be resistant to TNF even at concentrations of 10000 units in GM-CSF-stimulated cultures. Further depletion of accessory cells and enrichment for progenitor cell populations using immunoadherence "panning" and complement-mediated cytotoxicity increased the sensitivity of G-CSF-stimulated CFU-GM to TNF inhibition but did

213

Table 1. Inhibitory activity of TNF on human CFU-GM stimulated by G or GMCSF

rh-TNFα (units)	Accessory cell depleted							
	NALD BM[a]				BM[b]			
	G-CSF		GM-CSF		G-CSF		GM-CSF	
	Cols 1×10^5	Clus %contr	Cols 1×10^5	Clus %contr	Cols 2×10^4	Clus %contr	Cols 2×10^4	Clus %control
0	22±1	100	37±2	100	182±14	100	154±29	100
1	24±3	109	36±2	97	173±25	95	128±28	83
10	18±1	82	38±2	103	47±2	26	117±6	76
50	10±1	45	26±3	70	11±3	6	111±11	72
100	4±1	18	20±1	54	2±1	1	105±15	68
500	0	0	16±2	43	0	0	63±11	41
1000	0	0	12±2	32	0	0	36±1	23
5000	0	0	7±1	19	0	0	30±4	19
10000	0	0	8±1	22	0	0	36±1	23

[a] Nonadherent light density normal human marrow cells cultured in 1 ml McCoy's modified medium and 0.3% agar in the presence of 1000 U G-CSF or GM-CSF purified from 5637 CM. Colonies scored at day 14.
[b] Low density bone marrow separated by Ficoll-Hypaque density centrifugation was enriched 10-fold for progenitor cells by depletion of mature myeloid, monocytic, lymphoid and erythroid cells using mAbs Mol, MY8, MY3, N901, B4, OKT4, OKT8, OKT11 and antiglycophorin by immunoadherence "panning" and complement-mediated cytotoxicity.

not alter the sensitivity of the GM-CSF-stimulated colonies (Table 1). Fifty percent inhibition of G-CSF-stimulated colonies in such accessory cell-depleted marrow was now evident with 5 units TNF, a 2-log lower concentration than required to produce comparable inhibition in GM-CSF-stimulated cultures.

II. Action of G-CSF and TNF in Human Long-term Bone Marrow Culture

The inoculation of 10^7 normal human marrow cells in 10 ml of Gartner's medium, with weekly demidepopulation and no additional recharging, resulted in the establishment of a confluent, adherent layer of marrow stromal cells with extensive adipocyte development and sustained hematopoiesis. After an initial falloff from the maximum cellularity in the 1st week, total cells were produced at a level of 7.4×10^5 per flask for the first 2 months with polymorphonuclear neutro-

phils (PMN) comprising 12%–52% of total cells (mean of 35%, Fig. 2). CFU-GM responsive to GM-CSF fell from a maximum of 29000 per flask at 1 week to 1600 after 2 months, and G-CSF-responsive CFU-GM were 28800 at 1 week and 2200 at 2 months. Neutrophil and CFU-GM production persisted for 14 weeks. The weekly addition of rhG-CSF (10000 units/ml) resulted in a marked, sustained elevation of neutrophil production. Between 2 and 8 weeks of culture, cell production averaged 4.0×10^6 neutrophils per flask, a level of neutrophil production ten times higher than in control cultures, sustained for 2 months. CFU-GM production in the early stages of culture in the presence of G-CSF exceeded control values by approximately a factor of 2 regardless of whether the colonies were stimulated by G- or GM-CSF, and no evidence was found for depletion or premature exhaustion of G-CSF-stimulated long-term marrow cultures, since despite the chronic elevation of mature neutrophil production, total CFU-GM produced by 2 months were

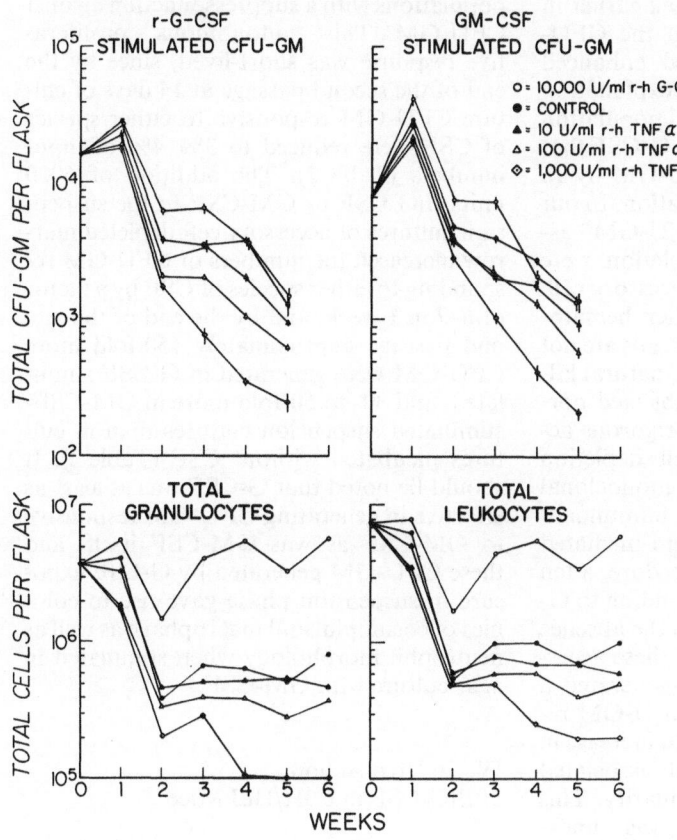

Fig. 2. Long-term cultures of 1×10^7 normal human bone marrow cells were established in 10 ml of Gartner's medium and subject to weekly demidepopulation and weekly addition of rhG-CSF (10 000 units/ml), rhTNF alpha (10–1000 units/ml), or control media to groups of three flasks. Colony assays were established at weekly intervals and CFU-GM responsive to 1000 units rG-CSF or GM-CSF per milliliter were quantitated. Numbers expressed as total per culture flask. Note the log scale

comparable in control and G-CSF-stimulated culture.

In contrast to the proliferative stimulus provided by G-CSF, TNF inhibited neutrophil production and CFU-GM production. At concentrations of 1000 units/ml TNF alpha, cell production was 50% of control in the first 3 weeks, 25% by 4 weeks and only 7% of control with no neutrophil production by 9 weeks; no CFU-GM were produced after 5–6 weeks. At 100 units/ml TNF no difference from control cultures was evident till 8–9 weeks, but by 9 weeks cellularity was 7.5% of control and PMN production was 2% of control with no CFU-GM produced. The lowest concentration of TNF tested (10 units/ml) produced an average 50% reduction in PMN production, otherwise no difference in either CFU-GM production or culture longevity was found. These observations were reproduced in four

subsequent experiments and in one study (data not shown), attempts to reverse the TNF-mediated suppression of myelopoiesis by coaddition of G-CSF were unsuccessful.

III. Ability of G- and GM-CSF to Generate CFU-GM in Suspension Cultures of Accessory Cell-Depleted Human Marrow

The preceding studies on G-CSF action in long-term marrow culture indicated that in the first few weeks of culture the total number of CFU-GM responsive to either G-CSF or GM-CSF was increased substantially over control values. This observation, together with earlier studies indicating that G-CSF could generate CFU-GM in simple 1-week suspension cultures of human mar-

215

row in a "pre-CFU-GM assay" [2], suggested that G-CSF acted on a cell earlier in the developmental lineage than the CFU-GM or alternatively promoted enhanced CFU-GM self-renewal. A third explanation could be that some accessory cell population produced a factor in response to G-CSF that caused recruitment of new CFU-GM by an action on a precursor cell population. In our earlier studies using the "pre-CFU-GM" assay, adherence and T-cell depletion were used to remove some types of accessory cell; however, it is known that other hematopoietic growth factor-producing cells are not removed by this procedure, e.g., natural killer (NK) cells. We therefore subjected normal human marrow to a more rigorous accessory and differentiating cell depletion procedure using a spectrum of monoclonal antibodies in conjunction with immunoadherence panning and complement-mediated cytotoxicity [14]. With this procedure, a ten fold increase in CFU-GM responding to G-CSF or GM-CSF was found. In the absence of exogenous CSF, 2.5×10^5 of these accessory cell-depleted populations generated a doubling in total numbers of CFU-GM responsive to G-CSF and a fivefold increase in GM-CSF-responsive CFU-GM associated with a fourfold increase in cellularity. This factor-independent response was unexpected and was not observed with unseparated marrow. It is possible that the accessory

cell depletion procedure also removes cell populations with a suppressor action against CFU-GM. This "autonomous" proliferative response was short-lived, since by the end of the second passage at 14 days of culture CFU-GM responsive to either species of CSF were reduced to 3%–4% of input numbers (Table 2). The addition of 5000 units rhG-CSF or GM-CSF to the suspension cultures of accessory cell-depleted marrow increased the numbers of CFU-GM responding to either species of CSF by a factor of 6–7 in 1 week, and by the end of the second passage approximately 150-fold more CFU-GM were generated in G-CSF-stimulated, and 30- to 50-fold more in GM-CSF-stimulated suspension cultures than in cultures incubated without CSF (Table 2). It should be noted that G-CSF was at least as effective in generating CFU-GM responsive to GM-CSF as was GM-CSF itself, and these CFU-GM generated by G-CSF exposure in suspension phase gave rise to colonies of eosinophil and macrophage as well as neutrophil morphology when stimulated in agar culture with GM-CSF.

IV. In Vivo Action of rhG-CSF in C3H/HeJ Mice

In order to substantiate the role of G-CSF as a true physiological regulator of granulopoi-

Table 2. Suspension culture of accessory cell depleted normal human bone marrow

7-Day passages of 2.5×10^5 CELLS/ml	Stimulus 5000/ml	Total CELLS $\times 10^5$	Total CFU-GM (G-CSF stimulated)	Total CFU-GM (GM-CSF stimulated)
Input	0	2.50	9950 ± 560	6500 ± 1300
1st Passage	0	9.45	22500 ± 1900	34400 ± 2000
1st Passage	G-CSF	35.50	56500 ± 2400	9000 ± 2200
1st Passage	GM-CSF	12.80	55600 ± 2300	56600 ± 1900
2nd Passage	0	2.10	345 ± 15	250 ± 40
2nd Passage	G-CSF	5.60	54520 ± 1700	34000 ± 1500
2nd Passage	GM-CSF	2.70	10250 ± 930	12000 ± 1000

Cells separated by panning procedure as in Table 1 and incubated in suspension cultures at 2.5×10^5 cells per ml in Iscoves modified Dulbecco's medium with 20% fetal calf serum. At 7-day intervals cells were recovered, washed, and assayed for CFU-GM (day 14) in agar cultures stimulated by 1000 U of rh-G-CSF or natural GM-CSF purified from 5637 CM. Passage was undertaken with 2.5×10^5 cells at day 7 and day 14.
Suspension cultures were incubated with control medium or 5000 U/ml of rh G-CSF or GM-CSF with fresh stimulus added at each passage.

esis, we investigated the action of rhG-CSF in normal endotoxin-hyporesponsive C3H/HeJ mice. The almost complete biological and receptor cross-reactivity of normal and leukemic hematopoietic cells to murine and human G-CSF [9] indicated that the human recombinant molecule should have biological activity in vivo in the murine system. Indirect evidence for this has been obtained in clinical situations where tumor-associated neutrophil leucocytosis could be transferred to nude mice bearing G-CSF-producing human tumor implants [20–23]. Injection of rhG-CSF intravenously into mice, with monitoring of serum levels by a human marrow or WEHI-3 leukemic colony assay, revealed a biphasic decay curve with a rapid initial decline and a subsequent slower rate of decay with a half-life of >2.5 h. Intraperitoneal injections of 1.5 µg of rhG-CSF twice daily produced serum levels of 50 000–75 000 units/ml serum after 1 h and plateau levels were maintained for 6–8 h. Within 48 h of initiation of daily G-CSF therapy, blood neutrophil numbers doubled and then rose progressively to 26 000/mm³ by day 5 and fluctuated between 11 000 and 54 000/mm³ thereafter. The average increase in blood neutrophils was ninefold over control injected mice and the number of blood monocytes, while variable, increased on average threefold from days 5 to 14. The absolute number of eosinophils remained unchanged and a persisting mild lymphocytosis was induced with a twofold increase from 4 to 14 days of treatment.

The influence of G-CSF therapy on hematopoietic tissue was particularly evident in the spleen, whose cellularity increased three- to fourfold by day 7 of G-CSF treatment with a conversion from a lymphoid tissue to a myeloid organ with >50% neutrophilic granulocytes at all stages of differentiation, extensive erythropoiesis and marked megakaryocyte development (Fig. 3). Marrow cellularity was not changed following G-CSF treatment but the marrow population became almost exclusively granulopoietic with loss of marrow lymphopoiesis and marked suppression of marrow erythropoietic activity. Total neutrophil granulopoietic mass in treated animals increased 4.5-fold by day 7 and the decrease in marrow erythropoiesis was more than compensated for by an increase in splenic erythropoiesis, with total erythroid mass more than doubling in treated mice. Megakaryocyte numbers fell progressively in the marrow of treated mice, but the marked increase in splenic megakaryocytes resulted in a threefold increase in total body megakaryocytes. The increase in immature erythroid and megakaryocytic cells was not associated with changes in hematocrit or platelet levels. The total splenic lymphocyte population remained unchanged and there was no evi-

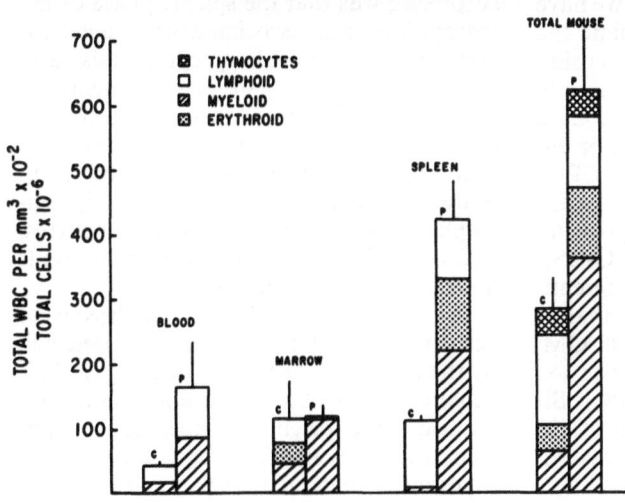

7 DAYS x 2 DAILY i.p. TREATMENT OF C3H/HeJ MICE WITH 1.5 µg r-h-PLURIPOTENT G-CSF

THYMOCYTES
LYMPHOID
MYELOID
ERYTHROID

TOTAL WBC PER mm³ x 10⁻²
TOTAL CELLS x 10⁻⁶

Fig. 3. Hematological parameters in C3H/HeJ mice treated for 7 days with 1.5 µg rhG-CSF administered intraperitoneally twice per day. Three mice were assayed in the treated (*p*) and control (*c*) groups. Total marrow calculated by multiplying total femoral cellularity by 20. Total WBC based on calculated blood volume of 2 ml. Morphology based on Wright-Giemsa-stained cytocentrifuge preparations

dence of stress-induced involution of thymic lymphopoiesis.

Analysis of the various progenitor populations responsive in colony assay to IL-3, CSF-1, GM-CSF, and G-CSF revealed little change in the marrow compartment in G-CSF-treated mice, but a dramatic increase in the splenic CFU-GM population (50- to 150-fold) resulted in an overall increase of IL-3-responsive CFU-GM (fourfold) and of CSF-1-, GM-CSF-, and G-CSF-responsive CFU-GM (threefold). Pluripotential stem cells detected in the day-12 CFU-S assay showed that this compartment remained unchanged in the marrow, but the marked increase in splenic CFU-S resulted in a 2.5-fold total body increase in these stem cells.

D. Discussion

In vitro studies using accessory cell-depleted marrow indicate that the direct action of hG-CSF is restricted primarily to proliferation and differentiation in the neutrophil granulocyte lineage [14] and the factor does not support directly differentiation into the erythroid, megakaryocytic or eosinophil lineage. Evidence for a possible direct action on early stem-cell proliferation and subsequent generation of BFU-E, CFU-GEMM, and megakaryocyte (CFU-M) is equivocal [15] and awaits a demonstration of G-CSF receptors on enriched populations of these cells or a proliferative response involving pure populations of such cells. Here we have documented that G-CSF can stimulate the generation of new CFU-GM in suspension culture of accessory cell-depleted human marrow, suggesting a recruitment action on some pre-CFU-GM population and/or enhanced self-renewal of preexisting CFU-GM, capable of responding to both G-CSF and GM-CSF. This observation provides evidence for a stimulatory action of G-CSF on a progenitor population with a differentiation potential more extensive than that of neutrophil lineage-restricted CFU-GM, since the CFU-GM generated in suspension cultures with G-CSF responded to GM-CSF in colony assay by a normal pattern of differentiation into eosinophils and macrophages as well as neutrophils.

In vivo administration of G-CSF by the intraperitoneal route led to sustained serum levels of bioactive G-CSF comparable to those found 3–6 h post injection of endotoxin in endotoxin-responsive strains of mice [6]. The use of highly purified recombinant G-CSF, the absence of significant contamination of our G-CSF with endotoxin, and the use of C3H/HeJ mice allow us to conclude that the in vivo responses seen were due to the action of G-CSF, rather than any contaminant acting directly or synergistically on neutrophil production. The predominant response involved elevation of peripheral blood neutrophils by a factor of 6–9 in C3H/HeJ mice, which was somewhat lower than we have observed in other strains, since up to a 20-fold increase in blood neutrophils can be obtained in Balb/c mice. Studies in hamsters also indicated a specific action on the neutrophil lineage with a three- to sixfold increase in peripheral blood neutrophils [24], and in monkeys receiving 10 µg rhG-CSF per kilogram per day, neutrophil counts rose fivefold, and up to 12-fold with 100 µg/kg per day [25]. In mice, demand for increased hematopoiesis following such insults as endotoxin treatment, irradiation, or cytotoxic drug treatment is met by a marked expansion of splenic hematopoiesis with little absolute change in marrow cellularity. Thus, it was not surprising that the major expansion of neutrophil production elicited by chronic G-CSF treatment was met by a rapid onset of extensive splenic myelopoiesis. What was surprising was that the splenic phase of hematopoiesis was associated with increased erythropoiesis, megakaryocytopoiesis, and elevated numbers of pluripotential stem cells and progenitors of all hematopoietic lineages. Indeed, the splenic increase led to an absolute total body expansion of production of these cell populations, although only neutrophils and to a lesser extent monocytes, and not red cells, platelets, and eosinophils increased in the circulation.

It is possible that G-CSF acts directly to activate pluripotential stem cells, detected by the day-12 CFU-S assay, leading to their enhanced proliferation, mobilization, migration to the spleen, and subsequent expansion. In this scenario, progenitors for lineages other than neutrophil could be generated in increased numbers as a result of stochastic mechanisms believed to operate at the level of pluripotential stem-cell self-renewal and differentiation. Alternatively, indirect mechanisms may operate, whereby G-CSF-induced differentiation depletes a population of neutrophil progenitors, which in turn triggers activation of the pluripotential stem-cell pool and expansion of the marrow microenvironment. A third possibility is that G-CSF acts in vivo upon an accessory-cell population to induce release of other hematopoietic growth factors known to influence multiple hematopoietic lineages. This third possibility was suggested by the original observations that G-CSF stimulated BFU-E and CFU-GEMM in marrow cultures depleted of T cells but not otherwise depleted of accessory cells. Indirect induction of a growth factor acting on pluripotential stem cells has been invoked as a mechanism to explain the marked stimulation of splenic hematopoiesis following administration of endotoxin [26]. Staber et al. [26] reported a mouse serum factor induced following endotoxin treatment, that, when injected into normal mice, elicited splenomegaly and a marked rise in splenic CFU-GM by 5 days, with concordant elevation of erythroid and megakaryocytic progenitors. The serum factor was thought not to be GM-CSF or residual endotoxin, although its peak appearance in the serum between 30 min and 3 h after endotoxin injection would coincide with the kinetics of endotoxin-induced G-CSF. This serum factor stimulating murine splenic hematopoiesis could be G-CSF itself or a molecule induced by G-CSF and mediating the more general effects on stem-cell proliferation and mobilization seen in the in vivo studies.

The stimulation of increased granulopoiesis persists as long as G-CSF is administered in vivo, although the duration of studies to date has been limited to 4–5 weeks. In long-term marrow culture much longer periods, up to 4 months with sustained high levels of G-CSF, have been obtained with persisting elevation of neutrophil production relative to control cultures, and no evidence was obtained for premature exhaustion of stem cells or accelerated depletion of cultures.

The ability of low concentrations of TNF alpha to counteract the proliferative action of G-CSF in vitro in clonal assay and long-term bone marrow cultures suggests a physiological role for TNF as a natural inhibitor of neutrophil granulopoiesis. The coordinate inducibility of G-CSF and TNF alpha following endotoxin activation of macrophages may provide a mechanism self-limiting the chronic generation of neutrophils from marrow progenitors following bacterial infection. Alternatively, the relative resistance to TNF inhibition of myeloid progenitors stimulated by GM-CSF may provide an alternate pathway for the generation of neutrophils in the face of elevated TNF levels. The interrelationship of TNF and CSF in the production and function of neutrophils is further emphasized by the observation that TNF can enhance both the phagocytic ability and the antibody-dependent cytotoxicity of neutrophils, increase their superoxide anion production, and stimulate their adherence to endothelial cells [27]. In addition, TNF has been shown to stimulate growth factor production by endothelial cells, due in part to activation of transcription of the GM-CSF gene [28]. The interplay of direct marrow-suppressive action of TNF and its role in mature neutrophil activation and induction of CSF production by accessory cells such as endothelium must be considered when extrapolating to an in vivo action of TNF in granulopoiesis.

References

1. Metcalf D, Nicola NA (1983) Proliferative effects of purified granulocyte colony-stimulating factor (G-CSF) on normal hemopoietic cells. J Cell Physiol 116:198
2. Platzer E, Welte K, Gabrilove J, Lu L, Harris P, Mertelsmann R, Moore MAS (1985) Biological activities of a human pluripotent hemopoietic colony-stimulating factor on normal and leukemic cells. J Exp Med 162:1788
3. Metcalf D (1986) Review: the molecular biology and function of the granulocyte-macrophage colony-stimulating factors. Blood 67:257
4. Nicola NA, Metcalf D, Matsumoto M, Johnson GR (1983) Purification of a factor inducing differentiation in murine myelomonocytic leukemia cells: identification as granulocyte colony-stimulating factor (G-CSF). J Biol Chem 258:9017

5. Burgess AW, Metcalf D (1980) Characterization of a serum factor stimulating the differentiation of myelomonocytic leukemic cells. Int J Cancer 26:647

6. Moore MAS (1982) G-CSF: its relationship to leukemia differentiation-inducing activity and other hemopoietic regulators. J Cell Physiol [Suppl] 1:53

7. Tsuda H, Neckers LM, Pluznik EH (1986) Colony-stimulating factor-induced differentiation of murine M1 myeloid leukemia cells is permissive in early G_1 phase. Proc Natl Acad Sci USA 83:4317

8. Nicola NA, Metcalf D, Johnson GR, Burgess AW (1979) Separation of functionally distinct human granulocyte-macrophage colony-stimulating factors. Blood 54:614

9. Nicola NA, Begley CG, Metcalf D (1985) Identification of the human analogue of a regulator that induces differentiation in murine leukaemic cells. Nature 314:625

10. Welte K, Platzer L, Lu L, Gabrilove JL, Levi E, Mertelsmann R, Moore MAS (1985) Purification and biochemical characterization of human pluripotent hematopoietic colony-stimulating factor. Proc Natl Acad Sci USA 82:1526

11. Gabrilove JL, Welte K, Harris P, Platzer E, Lu L, Levi E, Mertelsmann R, Moore MAS (1986) Pluripoietin alpha: a second human hematopoietic colony-stimulating factor produced by the human bladder carcinoma cell line 5637. Proc Natl Acad Sci USA 83:2478

12. Souza LM, Boone TC, Gabrilove J, Lai PH, Zsebo KM, Murdock DC, Chazin VR, Bruszewski J, Lu H, Chen KK, Barendt J, Platzer E, Moore MAS, Mertelsmann R, Welte K (1986) Recombinant human granulocyte colony-stimulating factor: effects on normal and leukemic myeloid cells. Science 232:61

13. Tsuchiya M, Asano S, Kaziro Y, Nagata S (1986) Isolation and characterization of the cDNA for murine granulocyte colony-stimulating factor. Proc Natl Acad Sci USA 83:7633

14. Ottmann OG, Welte K, Souza LM, Moore MAS (in press) Proliferative effects of a recombinant human granulocyte-colony stimulating factor (rG-CSF) on highly enriched hematopoietic progenitor cells. This volume

15. Metcalf D, Nicola NA (1983) Proliferative effects of purified granulocyte colony-stimulating factor (G-CSF) on normal mouse hemopoietic cells. J Cell Physiol 116:198

16. Vadas MA, Lopez AF (1985) Regulation of granulocyte function by colony-stimulating factors and monoclonal antibodies. Lymphokines 12:179

17. Shah RG, Green S, Moore MAS (1978) Colony-stimulating and inhibiting activities in mouse serum after *C. parvum*-endotoxin treatment. J Reticuloendothel Soc 23:29

18. Aggarwal BB, Kohr WJ, Hass PE, Moffat B, Spencer SA, Henzel WJ, Bringman TS, Nedwin GE, Goeddel DV, Harkins RN (1985) Human tumor necrosis factor: production, purification and characterization. J Biol Chem 260:2345

19. Broxmeyer HE, Williams DE, Lu L, Cooper S, Anderson SL, Beyer GS, Hoffman R, Rubin BY (1986) The suppressive influence of human tumor necrosis factors on bone marrow hematopoietic progenitor cells from normal donors and patients with leukemia: synergism of tumor necrosis factor and interferon-gamma. J Immunol 136:4487

20. Asano S, Urabe A, Okabe T, Sato N, Kondo Y, Ueyama Y, Chiba S, Ohsawa S, Kosaka K (1977) Demonstration of granulopoietic factor(s) in the plasma of nude mice transplanted with human lung cancer and in tumor tissue. Blood 49:845

21. Sato N (1979) Granulocytosis and colony-stimulating activity (CSA) by a human squamous cell carcinoma. Cancer 43:605

22. Mizoguchi H, Suda T, Miura Y, Kubota K, Takaku F (1982) Hemopoietic stem cells in nude mice transplanted with colony-stimulating-factor-producing tumors. Exp Hemat 10:874

23. Motoyoshi K, Suda T, Takaku F, Miura Y (1983) Regulatory mechanism of granulopoiesis in the bone marrow of CSF-producing tumor-bearing nude mice. Blood 62:980

24. Zsebo KM, Cohen AM, Murdock DC, Boone TC, Inoue H, Chazin VR, Hines D, Souza LM (1987) Recombinant human granulocyte colony-stimulating factor: molecular and biological characterization. Immunobiology (in press)

25. Welte K, Bonilla MA, Gillio AP, Boone TC, Potter GK, Gabrilove JL, Moore MAS, O'Reilly RJ, Souza LM (1987) Recombinant human G-CSF: effects on hematopoiesis in normal and cyclophosphamide-treated primates. J Exp Med (in press)

26. Staber FG, Burgess AW, Nicola NA, Metcalf D (1984) Biological and biochemical properties of a serum factor that stimulates splenic hemopoiesis in mice. Exp Hematol 12:107

27. Shalaby MR, Pennica D, Palladino MA Jr (1986) An overview of the history and biological properties of tumor necrosis factor. Springer Semin Immunopathol 9:33

28. Broudy VC, Kaushansky K, Segal GM, Harlan JM, Adamson JW (1986) Tumor necrosis factor type alpha stimulates human endothelial cells to produce granulocyte/macrophage colony-stimulating factor. Proc Natl Acad Sci USA 83:7467

Haematology and Blood Transfusion   Vol. 31
Modern Trends in Human Leukemia VII
Edited by Neth, Gallo, Greaves, and Kabisch
© Springer-Verlag Berlin Heidelberg 1987

Molecular Properties and Biological Activity of Human Macrophage Growth Factor, CSF-1

P. Ralph[1]

A. Introduction

CSF-1 belongs to a family of colony-stimu-lating factors (CSF) that regulate the pro-duction of the blood cells (Metcalf 1986). CSF-1 is a specific growth and differenti-ation factor for bone marrow progenitor cells of the mononuclear phagocyte lineage and also promotes the proliferation of ma-ture macrophages via specific receptors on the responding cells (Das et al. 1981; Das and Stanley 1982). CSF-1 also has a variety of stimulatory effects on the function of macrophages and monocytes. This paper summarizes the cloning of the cDNA and the genomic structure of human CSF-1, and describes properties of the macrophage growth factor that may make it a useful drug in several clinical settings.

B. Results

I. Genomic and cDNA Structure

Genomic clones for human CSF-1 were identified using DNA probes based on N-terminal sequence data of the human uri-nary protein. The human pancreatic carci-noma line MIA PaCa-2 was used as a source of CSF-1 protein and mRNA during induc-tion with phorbol myristate in serum-free medium (Ralph et al. 1986a). A cDNA li-brary was constructed from size-fraction-

ated mRNA which was positive for a nucleo-tide probe and for directing the production of bone marrow growth activity in oocytes. Using a genomic probe, a cDNA clone was obtained that codes for bioactive CSF-1 upon transfection of the primate COS cell line (Kawasaki et al. 1985). CSF-1 appears to be encoded by a single-copy gene, which is about 18 kb in length and contains nine exons (Kawasaki et al. 1985; Ralph et al. 1986 b), as shown in Table 1. The signal pep-tide is encoded by segments of exons 1 and 2. The mature polypeptide is encoded by exons 2–8.

The cDNA specifies a 32 amino-acid leader peptide followed by a 224 residue polypeptide. There are two potential N-linked glycosylation sites. At residue 59 of the mature protein, the cDNA codes for tyrosine, whereas the genomic codon is as-partic acid. This could be due to a natural polymorphism or to a reverse transcriptase error when making the cDNA library. The

[1] Department of Cell Biology, Cetus Corpor-ation, 1400 Fifty-Third Street, Emeryville, CA 94608, USA

Table 1. Exon-intron structure of the human CSF-1 gene

Exon	Size (bp)	Intron	Size (kb)
1	217	I	3.0
2	123	II	1.4
3	63	III	1.7
4	171	IV	4.5
5	148	V	2.0
6	131	VI	0.7
7	53	VII	0.3
8	56	VIII	0.7
9	670		

cDNA predicts an unusual structure for a secreted protein, namely a very hydrophobic region of 23 amino acids (residues 166 to 188 of the mature protein) followed by Arg-Trp-Arg-Arg-Arg. This is typical of membrane proteins which have a transmembrane hydrophobic domain followed by three positively charged residues acting as an anchor on the cytoplasmic side (Sabatini et al. 1982). Exon 6 ends exactly after the Arg triplet, further suggesting that the gene is designed to code for a membrane protein.

II. Protein Structure and Amino Acid Homology with Murine CSF-1

Three CSF-1 molecules have been purified to homogeneity and partially sequenced: from murine L929 cells (Kawasaki et al. 1985; Ben-Avram et al. 1985; Ben-Avram 1985), human urine (Kawasaki et al. 1985), and the MIA PaCa cell line (Csejtey and Boosman 1986; Boosman et al. 1986). The sequence data to date show that the human molecules are identical to each other and to the protein predicted from the cDNA and genome (Table 2). The human and murine molecules show 74% amino acid identity over the 65 residues of the regions which have been sequenced, and are thus highly homologous.

Native human and murine CSF-1s are heavily glycosylated dimer proteins of 45 000 to 70 000 daltons. The unglycosylated subunits of murine and human urinary CSF-1 are reported to have a size of 14.5 daltons (Das and Stanley 1982), whereas the human cDNA predicts a polypeptide of 26 daltons. Thus, the larger translated product may have another function as a membrane-bound molecule, with intracellular protein processing or perhaps a differently spliced mRNA used to produce the secreted CSF-1. There is evidence for a cell-surface bound form of CSF-1 (Stanley et al. 1976).

III. Human CSF-1 as a Growth Factor for Human Bone Marrow Progenitors

The activity of purified human CSF-1 has been controversial. Das et al. (1981) reported that urinary CSF-1 supported the growth in agar of diffuse colonies of macrophages which were difficult to detect unless

Table 2. Homology between human and murine CSF-1 proteins

Source	Position				
	1	11	21		
Human urine	E E V S E Y * S				
Human MIA PaCa	E E V S E Y * S H M	I G S G H	L Q S L Q	R L I D S	Q M E T S
Human cDNA	E E V S E Y C S H M	I G S G H	L Q S L Q	R L I D S	Q M E T S
Murine L cell	× ×	×	× ×	×	
	31	41			
MIA PaCa	* Q I T F E F V D Q	E Q L			
cDNA	C Q I T F E F V D Q	E Q L			
L cell	× × * *				
	65	71	81	88	
MIA PaCa	(M)(R)F(R)D N	T P N A (I)	A(I)(V)(Q)L	Q E(L)S(L)(R)**	
cDNA	M R F R D N	T P N A I	A I V Q L	Q E L S L R L K	
L cell	( )(×) ×	× × × ×	× × ×	× × ×	

Murine protein to human cDNA homology: 48/65 = 74% identity. Human MIA PaCa and murine L-cell CSF-1 proteins were purified to homogeneity and partially sequenced (Boosman et al. 1986). Amino acid residues are shown from the N-terminus to position 88 in single letter code. *Blanks* indicate identity to the translation of the cDNA. Residues not determined (*) and residues different from the cDNA (×) are also shown. Residues from position 44 to 64 in the native protein not been determined. *Empty parentheses* indicate a tentative identification agreeing with the cDNA. *Parentheses containing* × indicate a tentative identification different from the cDNA.

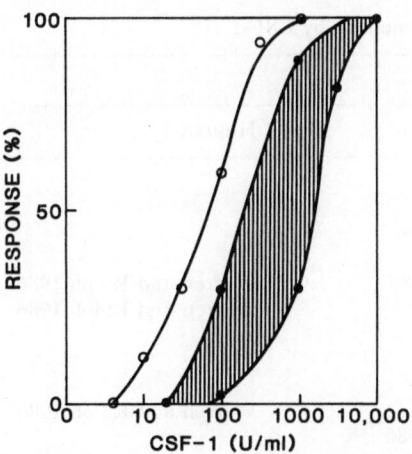

Fig. 1. Dose titration of human CSF-1 in colony formation by human and murine bone marrow cells. Bone marrow cells were cultured in agar with varying concentrations of purified human MIA PaCa CSF-1 (s.a. varying from 2×10^5 to 2×10^7 U/mg) and colonies scored at day 14 for human (range shown by *closed circles*) and day 7 for murine bone marrow cells (*open circles*) as described by Ralph et al. (1986a). Maximum colony numbers were 30–70 per 10^5 for human and 150–300 per 10^5 for mouse bone marrow cells. The variation in the human data depended on the donor response. The range of human data was seen with both partially purified CSF-1 and highly purified (about 40% pure protein, less than 0.1 ng LPS per 20 000 U). Approximately 90% of the human and mouse colonies were macrophage type

persisting cells in the adherent fraction of the bone marrow population were first removed. Waheed and Shadduck (1982) found no colony-stimulating activity of human urinary CSF-1 like factor on human marrow cells, whereas Wu et al. (1981) showed that a similar factor from MIA PaCa cells stimulated human colony formation at 5% of that seen with murine cells at day 7 of culture, and at 34% by day 13 of culture. Motoyoshi et al. (1982) described a urinary protein similar to CSF-1 which stimulated granulocyte colony formation by human marrow cells through the induction of a myeloid CSF in monocytes/macrophages.

We find that purified MIA PaCa CSF-1 does induce bone marrow colonies of intensely staining macrophages (Ralph et al. 1986a). Colonies of 50 or more cells can be

scored at day 14, but not day 7 of culture; they are disperse with no central concentration of cells, so that 10^5 or fewer cells should be plated. Colony formation is similar with total marrow mononuclear cells or the nonadherent fraction, and half-maximum colony formation for human progenitors occuring at 10 to 100 times the concentration required for murine cells (Fig. 1). Several of these conditions may explain why no human activity was detected in the previous studies.

IV. Effects of CSF-1 on Mature Monocytes and Macrophages

CSF-1 has direct stimulating effects on the mature monocyte and macrophage, in addition to being a growth and differentiation factor for bone marrow precursors (Table 3). It stimulates the production of prostaglandins and interferon (IFN), the intracellular killing of Candida, the production of plasminogen activator, interleukin-1, oxygen metabolites, ferritin, and a G-CSF (reviewed in Ralph et al. 1986a). Table 4 shows that CSF-1 had no immediate effect on macrophage tumoricidal activity. However, pretreatment of murine macrophages for one day with murine CSF-1 stimulated the spontaneous killing and greatly augmented the lymphokine-induced killing of TU5 sarcoma targets. The timing of the two signals was important. Pretreating macrophages with lymphokine (LK) and adding CSF-1 at the time of the cytotoxic assay did not show augmented killing (Ralph and Nakoinz 1986).

One or two days of pretreatment of macrophages with CSF-1 were optimal for the stimulation of spontaneous and LK-induced killing. Pretreatment of macrophages with 300 U/ml CSF-1 or more augmented tumor lysis induced with LK or LK plus CSF-1 in the killing assay, whereas 1200 U/ml CSF-1 was required for a large increase in spontaneous killing. The stimulatory activity in L-cell conditioned medium copurified with CSF-1 on a monoclonal immunoabsorbent column. The activity was not due to lipopolysaccharide (LPS) because the preparations had low LPS content, were active on LPS-hyporesponder C3H/HeJ macro-

Table 3. Stimulation of mature macrophage and monocyte functions by CSF-1

Function	References	
	Mouse	Human
Plasminogen activator production	Lin and Gordon 1979	
PGE production	Ralph 1984	
Ferritin production	Broxmeyer et al. 1985 a	
IL-1 production	Moore et al. 1980	
Myeloid CSF production	Metcalf and Nicola 1985	Warren and Ralph 1986
IFN production	Ralph 1984	Warren and Ralph 1986
Oxygen metabolites	Wing et al. 1985	
Intracellular killing of Candida	Ralph 1984	
Tumor cytostatic activity	Wing et al. 1982	
Tumor cytotoxin		Warren and Ralph 1986
Tumor cytotoxic activity	Ralph and Nakoinz 1986	
Resist viral infection	Warren and Lee 1986	

Table 4. Tumoricidal activity of 1-day cultured but not freshly harvested macrophages is enhanced by CSF-1

Treatment		Day of assay	Cytotoxicity (%)	Effect of CSF-1
Day 0				
0		0	8	
CSF-1		0	8	No effect
LK		0	34	
LK + CSF-1		0	35	No effect
Day 0–1	*Day 1*			
0	0	1	10	
CSF-1	0	1	16	Moderate stimulation
0	LK	1	19	
CSF-1	LK	1	58	Strong stimulation
CSF-1	CSF-1	1	22	Moderate stimulation
CSF-1	LK + CSF-1	1	66	Moderate stimulation by additional CSF-1

Adherent peritoneal exudate cells from proteose peptone-injected C3H/HeN mice were tested without preincubation or after 1-day preincubation with medium or CSF-1 (300 U/ml in conditioned medium of L929 cells) for killing ^{3}H-thymidine labeled TU5 sarcoma cells at 40:1 in a 48-h assay (Ralph et al. 1982). At the time of tumor lysis assay, replicate wells received 10% v/v lymphᴏᴋine (LK, 2-day concanavalin A-spleen supernate). Background radiolabel release of 7% from tumor ceɪɪ alone was subtracted

phages, and were not inhibited by LPS-neutralizing polymyxin B (Ralph and Nakoinz 1986). In fact, incubation of macrophages with LPS decreased their cytotoxic activity. We have also observed protection of macrophages by CSF-1 from lytic infection by vesicular stomatitis virus (Warren and Lee 1986).

The effects of CSF-1 on human mononuclear phagocytes are just being discovered (Warren and Ralph 1986). Table 5 shows that CSF-1 treatment of human monocytes stimulates their production of IFN in response to poly I · C and the production of tumor necrosis factor and a myeloid CSF in response to LPS and PMA.

Table 5. Stimulation of human monocyte secretion of TNF, IFN, and myeloid CSF by CSF-1

Monocytes	TNF		IFN		Myeloid CSF
	LPS	LPS+PMA	pIC 10	pIC 50	LPS
Donor 1	6	12	< 6	12	0
+CSF-1	108	486	38	100	700
Donor 2	< 6	6	< 6	38	40
+CSF-1	< 6	162	400	1600	200
Donor 3	6	162	< 31	25	103
+CSF-1	18	486	38	100	377

Adherent peripheral blood mononuclear cells were incubated 3 days in DME medium containing fetal calf serum in the presence or absence of 1000 U/ml human CSF-1. CSF-1 was purified from the MIA PaCa cell line (Ralph et al. 1986a) to a specific activity of approximately 2.5×10^7 U/mg, >40% pure, <0.2 ng lipopolysaccharide (LPS)/1000 U. The cells were washed and 2.5×10^5 cells in 0.5 ml were recultured for 2 days with 1 µg/ml LPS (*Salmonella typhimurium*, Sigma), LPS+20 ng/ml phorbol myristic acetate (PMA, Sigma), or 10 or 50 µg/ml polyinosinic polycytidylic acid (pIC, Sigma). Supernatants were assayed for tumor necrosis factor (TNF), interferon (IFN), and a myeloid growth factor (myeloid CSF) as described (Warren and Ralph 1986), expressed in U/ml. The activity of CSF-1 was not blocked by LPS-neutralizing polymyxin B, and 0.1–1 ng/ml LPS (the maximum possible contamination in the CSF-1) did not stimulate monocyte production of the three factors

V. Pharmacologic Effects of CSF-1

A factor possibly identical to CSF-1 has been isolated from human urine. It induced in human monocytes the production of a G-CSF that promotes the growth of neutrophil colonies from human bone marrow precursors (Motoyoshi et al. 1982). Treatment of normal human donors with the urinary material revealed an increased production of G-CSF by peripheral blood monocytes and increased numbers of blood neutrophils and

Table 6. Expected pharmacologic uses of CSF-1

o Restore monocyte numbers (and indirectly neutrophils and other blood cells) reduced:
   – By myelosuppressive chemotherapy and gamma-irradiation for cancer and bone marrow transplantation
   – In naturally occurring anemias
o Improve resistance to infection in patients at risk:
   – Cancer, bone marrow transplantation
   – Immunodeficiencies and leukopenias
   – Elderly
   – During major surgery
o Anticancer therapy via direct stimulation of macrophages

bone marrow myeloid precursors (Ishizaka et al. 1985). Studies with murine CSF-1 also demonstrated in vivo stimulation of monocytes and neutrophils as well as early pleuripotent progenitors (granulocyte/macrophage/erythrocyte/megakaryocyte-colony forming units) in mice (Broxmeyer et al. 1985 b). These clinical and preclinical results showing CSF-1 stimulation of myelopoietic events outside the mononuclear phagocyte lineage are presumably due to an indirect effect of promoting the endogenous production of G-CSF and pleuripoietins in the body. The cloning of the gene for human CSF-1 will make large amounts of this protein available for further studies.

We therefore anticipate (Table 6) that CSF-1 may find clinical utility in restoring white and red blood cell numbers that have been reduced by myelosuppressive chemotherapy or gamma irradiation for cancer treatment or bone marrow transplantation, and in naturally occurring leukopenias. CSF-1 may also have direct activating effects on mononuclear phagocytes that will improve the body's resistance to infectious diseases – viral, bacterial, and fungal – and that will stimulate the macrophages within or near tumors to destroy the neoplastic cells.

Acknowledgements. I thank I. Nakoinz, M.-T. Lee, M. K. Warren, L. McConlogue, E. S. Kawasaki, and A. Boosman for advice and unpublished experimental information; and R. Bengelsdorf for editorial assistance

References

1. Ben-Avram CH (1985) Correction. Proc Natl Acad Sci USA 82:7801
2. Ben-Avram CH, Shively JE, Shadduck RK, Waheed A, Rajavashisth T, Lusis AJ (1985) Amino-terminal amino acid sequence of murine colony-stimulating factor 1. Proc Natl Acad Sci USA 82:4486
3. Boosman A, Strickler JE, Wilson KJ, Stanley ER (1987) Partial amino acid sequences and composition of human and murine CSF-1. Biochem Biophys Res Comm 144:74
4. Broxmeyer HE, Juliano L, Waheed A, Shadduck RK (1985a) Release from mouse macrophages of acidic isoferritins that suppress hematopoietic progenitor cells is induced by purified L cell colony stimulating factor and suppressed by human lactoferritin. J Immunol 136:3224
5. Broxmeyer HE, Williams DE, Cooper S, Shadduck RK, Gillis S, Waheed A, Urdal D (1985b) The effects in vivo of pure murine CSF-1 and recombinant *IL-3*. Blood 66 [Suppl 1]:146a
6. Csejtey J, Boosman A (1986) Purification of human macrophage colony-stimulating factor (CSF-1) from medium conditioned by pancreatic carcinoma cells. Biochem Biophys Res Comm 138:238
7. Das SK, Stanley ER (1982) Structure-function studies of a colony-stimulating factor (CSF-1). J Biol Chem 257:13679
8. Das SK, Stanley ER, Guilbert LJ, Forman LW (1981) Human colony stimulating factor (CSF-1) radioimmunoassay: resolution of three subclasses of human colony-stimulating factors. Blood 58:630
9. Huebner K, Isobe M, Croce CM, Golde DW, Kaufman SE, Gasson JC (1985) The human gene encoding GM-CSF is at 5q21-q32, the chromosome region deleted in the 5q⁻ anomaly. Science 230:1282
10. Ishizaka Y, Moyoyoski K, Saito M, Miura Y, Takaku F (1985) Mode of action of human urinary colony-stimulating factor in granulopoiesis in vivo and in vitro. J Leukocyte Biol 38:168
11. Kawasaki ES, Ladner MB, Wang AM, Van Arsdell J, Warren MK, Coyne MY, Schweickart VL, Lee M-T, Nikoloff DM, Tal R, Weaver JF, Brindley L, Wilson KJ, Boosman A, Innis MA, Stanley ER, Ralph P, White TJ, Mark D (1987) Human macrophage colony stimulating factor (CSF-1): isolation of genomic and complementary DNA clones. UCLA Symp Mol Cell Biol 41:387
12. Kawasaki ES, Ladner MB, Wang AM, Van Arsdell J, Warren MK, Coyne MY, Schweickart VL, Lee M-T, Wilson KJ, Boosman A, Stanley ER, Ralph P, Mark DF (1985) Molecular cloning of a complementary DNA encoding human macrophage-specific colony stimulating factor (CSF-1). Science 230:291
13. Lin HS, Gordon S (1979) Secretion of plasminogen activator by bone marrow-derived mononuclear phagocytes and its enhancement by colony stimulating factor. J Exp Med 150:231
14. Metcalf D (1986) The molecular biology and functions of the granulocyte-macrophage colony-stimulating factors. Blood 61:251
15. Metcalf D, Nicola NA (1985) Synthesis by mouse peritoneal macrophages of G-CSF, the differentiation inducer for myeloid leukemia cells: stimulation by endotoxin, M-CSF and multi-CSF. Leuk Res 9:35
16. Moore RN, Oppenheim JJ, Farrar JJ, Carter CS Jr, Waheed A, Shadduck RK (1980) Production of lymphocyte-activating factors (interleukin 1) by macrophages activated with colony-stimulating factors. J Immunol 125:1302
17. Motoyoshi K, Suda T, Kusumoto K, Takaku F, Miura Y (1982) Granulocyte-macrophage colony-stimulating and binding activities of purified human urinary colony-stimulating factor to murine and human bone marrow cells. Blood 60:1378
18. Ralph P (1984) Activating factors for nonspecific and antibody-dependent cytotoxicity by human and murine mononuclear phagocytes. Lymphokine Res 3:153
19. Ralph P, Nakoinz I (1987) CSF-1 stimulates macrophage tumoricidal activity. Cell Immunol 105:270
20. Ralph P, Warren MK, Lee M-T, Csejtey J, Weaver JF, Broxmeyer HE, Williams DE, Stanley ER, Kawasaki E (1986a) Inducible production of human macrophage growth factor, CSF-1. Blood 68:633
21. Ralph P, Warren MK, Ladner MB, Kawasaki ES, Boosman A, White TJ (1986b) Molecular and biological properties of human macrophage growth factor, CSF-1. Cold Spring Harbor Symp Quant Biol 51:679
22. Ralph P, Williams N, Nakoinz I, Jackson H, Watson JS (1982) Distinct signals for antibody-dependent and nonspecific killing of tumor target mediated by macrophages. J Immunol 129:427

23. Sabatini DD, Kreibich G, Morimoto T, Adesnik M (1982) Mechanism for the incorporation of proteins in membranes and organelles. J Cell Biol 91:1

24. Stanley ER, Cifone M, Heard PM, Defendi V (1976) Factors regulating macrophage production and growth: identity of colony-stimulating factor and macrophage growth factor. J Exp Med 143:35

25. Warren MK, Lee MT (1986) CSF-1 induces resistance to lytic infection by vesicular stomatitis virus in murine macrophages. J Immunol 137:2281

26. Warren MK, Ralph P (1986) Macrophage growth factor CSF-1 stimulates human monocyte production of interferon, tumor necrosis factor, and myeloid CSF. J Immunol 137:2281

27. Wing EJ, Ampel NM, Waheed A, Shadduck RK (1985) Macrophage colony-stimulating factor (M-CSF) enhances the capacity of murine macrophages to secrete oxygen reduction products. J Immunol 135:2052

28. Wing EJ, Waheed A, Shadduck RK, Nagle LS, Stephenson K (1982) Effect of colony-stimulating factor of murine macrophages: induction of anti-tumor activity. J Clin Invest 69:270

Haematology and Blood Transfusion   Vol. 31
Modern Trends in Human Leukemia VII
Edited by Neth, Gallo, Greaves, and Kabisch
© Springer-Verlag Berlin Heidelberg 1987

Regulatory Control of the Epidermal Growth Factor Receptor Tyrosine Kinase

R. J. Davis and M. P. Czech

A. Regulation of the EGF Receptor Tyrosine Protein Kinase Activity by EGF

The epidermal growth factor (EGF) receptor has been shown to posses an intrinsic tyrosine protein kinase activity that is stimulated by the binding of EGF [1]. In addition, two other ligands for the EGF receptor can stimulate the tyrosine protein kinase activity in intact cells: TGF-α (transforming growth factor α) and a soluble biosynthetic precursor of TGF-α [2, 3]. Analysis of the kinetics of autophosphorylation and of the activity of the receptor to phosphorylate exogenous substrates indicates that the autophosphorylation of the receptor causes an increase in its tyrosine protein kinase activity [4]. This increase in the tyrosine protein kinase activity of the receptor caused by phosphorylation represents a mechanism by which amplification of the signaling mechanism of the EGF receptor can occur subsequent to the binding of EGF to the receptor.

B. Phosphorylation of the EGF Receptor by Protein Kinase C

Protein kinase C is regulated by diacylglycerol and the cytosolic concentration of Ca^{++} [5]. It has recently been demonstrated that protein kinase C is a major cellular receptor for tumor-promoting phorbol

diesters (e.g., PMA[1]) which bind to protein kinase C at the diacylglycerol binding site [5]. Treatment of cells with either PMA or diacylglycerol results in activation of the phosphotransferase activity of protein kinase C [5], the association of cytosolic protein kinase C with the inner surface of the plasma membrane [6, 7], and an increase in the phosphorylation state of the EGF receptor on serine and threonine residues [8–13]. The increased phosphorylation of the EGF receptor occurs at a site that is a substrate for protein kinase C (Fig. 1) and at additional sites [9, 10].

C. Substrate Specificity of Protein Kinase C

The protein kinase C phosphorylation site on the EGF receptor has been identified as threonine^{654} [9, 12]. It is located in a highly basic region of the EGF receptor that is close to the cytoplasmic surface of the plasma membrane. Similar locations of protein kinase C phosphorylation in the primary structure of pp60$^{c\text{-}src}$ [14] and in the interleukin 2 (IL-2) receptor [15] have been reported (Fig. 2). The marked similarity between the protein kinase C phosphorylation sites on the EGF receptor, pp60$^{c\text{-}src}$, and the IL-2 receptor suggests that the proximity of a potential phosphorylation site to the plasma membrane surface may be an important factor in determining the substrate specificity of protein kinase C. Recently, we

Department of Biochemistry, University of Massachusetts Medical School, Worcester, MA 01605, USA

---

[1] *PMA*, 4-phorbol 12β-myristate 13α-acetate

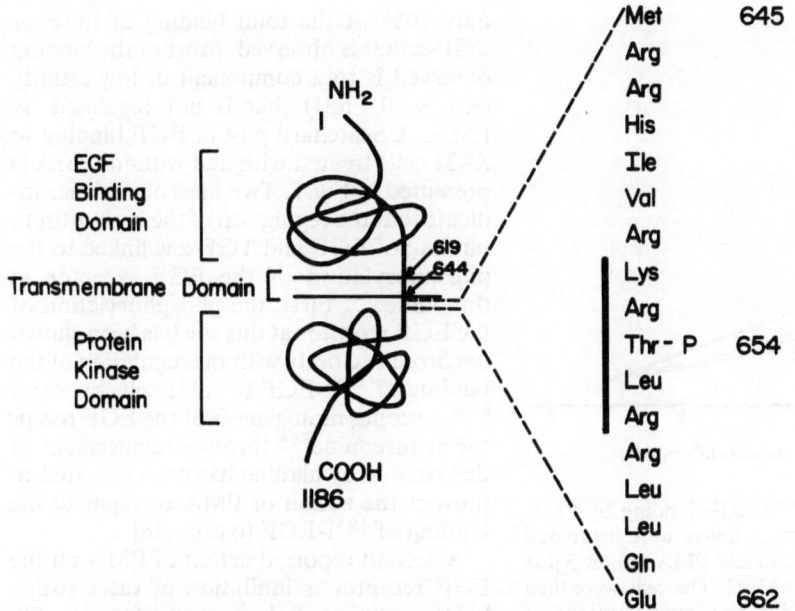

Met	645
Arg	
Arg	
His	
Ile	
Val	
Arg	
Lys	
Arg	
Thr - P	654
Leu	
Arg	
Arg	
Leu	
Leu	
Gln	
Glu	662

Fig. 1. Structure of the protein kinase C phosphorylation site on the EGF receptor (threonine[654]), presented schematically. The deduced structure of the tryptic phosphopeptide containing threonine[654] is indicated by a *bar*. (Reprinted, with permission, from Davis and Czech [9])

identified the protein kinase C phosphorylation site on the transferrin receptor as serine[24] [16]. Inspection of the primary structure of the transferrin receptor indicates that serine[24] is not located close to the

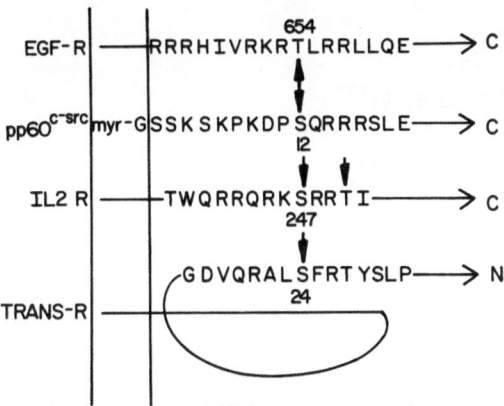

Fig. 2. Substrate specificity of protein kinase C. Protein kinase C phosphorylation sites on the EGF receptor (threonine[654] [9, 12]), pp60[c-src] (serine[12] [14]), IL-2 receptor (serine[247] and threonine[250] [15]), and transferrin receptor (serine[24] [16])

transmembrane domain of the receptor in the primary sequence (Fig. 2). However, it is possible that the tertiary structure of the transferrin receptor is arranged so that serine[24] is located close to the cytoplasmic surface of the plasma membrane. We conclude that the protein kinase C phosphorylation site on many integral membrane proteins may not have a primary structure that is homologous to the protein kinase C phosphorylation site on the EGF receptor (threonine[654]). However, the hypothesis that similarity may exist in the tertiary structure of integral membrane proteins around the protein kinase C phosphorylation site remains to be tested.

D. Regulation of the EGF Receptor by Phorbol Diesters

Addition of the tumor-promoting phorbol diester PMA to A431 cells causes an inhibition of the high-affinity (Kd = 30–50 pM) binding of EGF [8] and TGF-α [2]. This high-affinity component of binding to A431 cells regulated by phorbol diesters represents

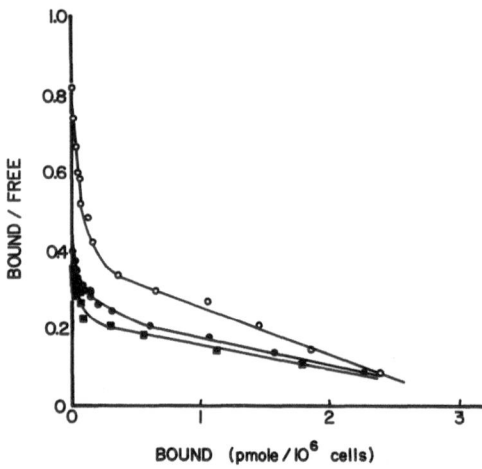

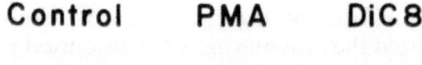

Fig. 3. Inhibition of ^{125}I-EGF binding by PMA and diC$_8$. A431 cell monolayers were incubated with no treatment (○), 10 nM PMA (■), or 3 μM diC$_8$ (●) for 30 min at 37 °C. The cells were then cooled to 0 °C, and different concentrations of ^{125}I-EGF were added for 4 h. The monolayers were then washed with cold medium and solubilized with 0.4 M NaOH, and radioactivity associated with the cells was measured with a gamma counter. Nonspecific binding was measured in the presence of a 500-fold excess of EGF. The data are plotted according to the method of Scatchard. (Reprinted, with permission, from Davis et al. [20])

only 10% of the total binding of EGF or TGF-α that is observed. Most of the binding observed is to a component of low affinity (Kd = 0.3 nM) that is not regulated by PMA. A Scatchard plot of EGF binding to A431 cells treated with and without PMA is presented in Fig. 3. Two lines of evidence indicate that the regulation of the high-affinity binding of EGF and TGF-α is linked to the phosphorylation of the EGF receptor at threonine[654]. First, the phosphorylation of the EGF receptor at this site has been shown to correlate closely with the regulation of the binding of ^{125}I-EGF to A431 cells by PMA [17]. Second, mutagenesis of the EGF receptor at threonine[654] through replacement of this residue by alanine has been reported to prevent the action of PMA to regulate the binding of ^{125}I-EGF to cells [18].

A second reported action of PMA on the EGF receptor is inhibition of the tyrosine kinase activity of the receptor [11, 19, 20]. This is illustrated by the experiment presented in Fig. 4. It has been shown that this decrease in the tyrosine protein kinase activity of the EGF receptor is a result of the phosphorylation of the EGF receptor at threonine[654] by protein kinase C [11].

The molecular basis of the perturbation of the EGF receptor (ligand binding and

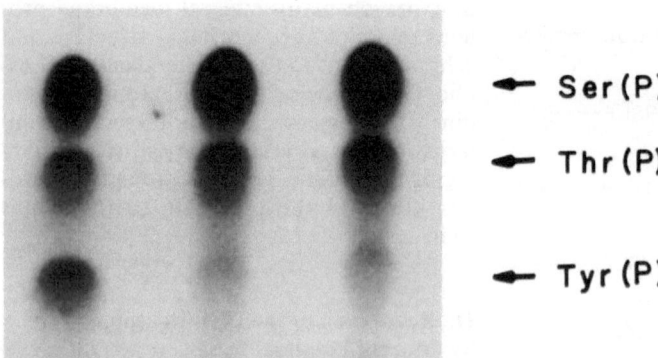

Control   PMA   DiC8

← Ser(P)

← Thr(P)

← Tyr(P)

Fig. 4. Inhibition of tyrosine kinase activity of the EGF receptor by diC$_8$ and PMA. A431 cells labeled with [^{32}P]phosphate were treated with 10 nM PMA or 3 μM diC$_8$ for 30 min. All the cells were then treated with 10 nM EGF for 10 min, and the EGF receptors were isolated by immunoprecipitation and polyacrylamide gel electropho-resis. Phosphoamino acid analysis was performed by partial acid hydrolysis and thin-layer electrophoresis (pH 3.5) of the [^{32}P] phosphoamino acids. Shown is an autoradiograph of the resolved [^{32}P]phosphoamino acids. (Reprinted, with permission, from Davis et al. [20])

tyrosine protein kinase activity) by phosphorylation at threonine[654] by protein kinase C is not understood. However, this phosphorylation site is in an interesting region of the EGF receptor (Fig. 1). The site is nine amino acids from the cytoplasmic side of the predicted transmembrane domain of the EGF receptor, in a region that links the EGF receptor ligand-binding domain to the receptor tyrosine protein kinase domain. If a conformational change occurs subsequent to the binding of EGF to the receptor, the sequence surrounding the transmembrane domain will be of great importance for the transmission of this signal to the tyrosine kinase domain. The very basic sequence around threonine[654] may be involved in the interaction of the receptor with other proteins or phospholipids by an electrostatic mechanism. The introduction of a phosphate group into this sequence could be expected to alter these interactions and may be sufficient to perturb the function of the EGF receptor.

E. Regulation of the EGF Receptor by Diacylglycerol

Diacylglycerol is able to stimulate the activity of protein kinase C [5]. It has been shown that the addition of exogenous diacylglycerol to A431 cells mimics the actions of PMA on the EGF receptor [20–22]. Thus, treatment of A431 cells with diacylglycerol causes an inhibition of the high-affinity binding of ^{125}I-EGF (Fig. 3) and decreases the tyrosine protein kinase activity of the EGF receptor (Fig. 4). These effects of diacylglycerol are associated with the phosphorylation of the EGF receptor at the same sites observed after treatment of the cells with PMA [20]. The structural requirements for diacylglycerols to regulate the EGF receptor have been investigated in detail. It was found that for symmetric sn-1,2-diacylglycerols with saturated acyl chains the optimal responses were observed with sn-1,2-dioctanoylglycerol (diC$_8$), and that the 3′ hydroxyl group was essential for the biological activity of the diacylglycerol [21].

We have recently investigated the hypothesis that the EGF receptor is regulated physiologically by changes in the activity of protein kinase C caused by alterations in the level of endogenous diacylglycerol. In these experiments the regulation of the EGF receptor by platelet-derived growth factor (PDGF) was examined in WI-38 human fetal lung fibroblasts [23, 23]. It has been reported that PDGF rapidly stimulates the hydrolysis of phosphatidyl inositol 4,5 bisphosphate which results in an increase in the level of diacylglycerol [25] and inositol-1,4,5-trisphosphate. The inositol-1,4,5-trisphosphate causes the release of Ca^{++} from intracellular stores and results in an increased cytosolic free Ca^{++} concentration [26, 27]. The dual action of PDGF to increase the level of diacylglycerol and free Ca^{++} would be expected to stimulate the activity of protein kinase C. We confirmed this by demonstrating that PDGF caused the phosphorylation of the EGF receptor at threonine[654] [23]. The functional consequences of this action of PDGF were the inhibition of the tyrosine protein kinase activity of the EGF receptor and the inhibition of the high-affinity binding of ^{125}I-EGF to the fibroblasts [23].

Acknowledgements. We thank Karen Donahue for her assistance in preparing this manuscript. This work was supported by grant AM 30648 from the National Institutes of Health and grant CA 39240 from the National Cancer Institute.

References

1. Ushiro H, Cohen S (1980) J Biol Chem 255:8363–8365
2. Davis RJ, Like B, Massague J (1985) J Cell Biochem 27:23–30
3. Ignotz R, Kelly B, Davis RJ, Massague J (1986) Proc Natl Acad Sci USA 83:6307–6311
4. Bertics PJ, Gill GN (1985) J Biol Chem 260:14642–14647
5. Nishizuka Y (1984) Nature 308:693–698
6. Kraft AS, Anderson WB (1983) Nature 301:621–623
7. McCaffrey PG, Friedman B, Rosner MR (1984) J Biol Chem 259:12502–12507
8. Davis RJ, Czech MP (1984) J Bio Chem 259:8545–8549
9. Davis RJ, Czech MP (1985) Proc Natl Acad Sci USA 82:1974–1978
10. Iwashita S, Fox CF (1985) J Biol Chem 259:2559–2567

11. Cochet C, Gill GN, Meisenhelder J, Cooper JA, Hunter T (1984) J Biol Chem 259:2553–2558

12. Hunter T, Ling N, Cooper JA (1984) Nature 311:480–483

13. Decker S (1984) Mol Cell Biol 4:1718–1723

14. Gould KL, Woodgett JR, Cooper JA, Hunter T (1985) Cell 42:849–857

15. Gallis B, Lewis A, Wignall J, Alpert A, Mochizuki DY, Cosman D, Hopp T, Urdal D (1986) J Biol Chem 261:5075–5080

16. Davis RJ, Johnson GL, Kelleher DJ, Anderson JK, Mole JE, Czech MP (1986) J Biol Chem 261:9034–9041

17. Davis RJ, Czech MP (1986) Biochem J 233:435–441

18. Lin CR, Chen WS, Lazar CS, Carpenter CG, Gill GN, Evans RM, Rosenfeld MG (1986) Cell 44:839–848

19. Friedman BA, Frackelton AR Jr, Ross A, Connors JM, Fujiki H, Sugimura T, Rosner MR (1984) Proc Natl Acad Sci USA 81:3034–3038

20. Davis RJ, Ganong BR, Bell RM, Czech MP (1985) J Biol Chem 260:1562–1566

21. Davis RJ, Ganong BR, Bell RM, Czech MP (1985) J Biol Chem 260:5315–5322

22. McCaffrey PG, Friedman B, Rosner MR (1984) J Biol Chem 259:12502–12507

23. Davis RJ, Czech MP (1985) Proc Natl Acad Sci USA 82:4080–4084

24. Davis RJ, Czech MP (1985) Cancer Cells 3:101–108

25. Habenicht AJR, Glomset JA, King WC, Nist C, Mitchell CD, Ross R (1981) J Biol Chem 256:12329–12335

26. Berridge MJ, Heslop JP, Irvine RF, Brown KD (1984) Biochem J 222:195–201

27. Moolenaar WH, Tertoolen LG, deLaat SW (1984) J Biol Chem 259:8066–8069

Haematology and Blood Transfusion Vol. 31
Modern Trends in Human Leukemia VII
Edited by Neth, Gallo, Greaves, and Kabisch
© Springer-Verlag Berlin Heidelberg 1987

Cellular Specificity and Molecular Characteristics of the Binding of Colony-Stimulating Factors to Normal and Leukemic Cells

N. A. Nicola [1]

A. Introduction

The colony-stimulating factors (CSFs) form a family of hemopoietic growth factors controlling the survival, proliferation and differentiation of hemopoietic progenitor cells as well as the functional activities of the mature cells in the tissues [1]. In the mouse, four distinct CSFs controlling granulocyte and macrophage production have been identified, purified and, in two cases, molecularly cloned – multi-CSF or interleukin-3, GM-CSF, M-CSF or CSF-1, and G-CSF [2, 3]. Human equivalents of GM-CSF (CSFα, NIF-T or pluripoietin α), G-CSF (CSFβ or pluripoietin) and M-CSF have also been

[1] The Walter and Eliza Hall Institute of Medical Research, P.O. Royal Melbourne Hospital 3050, Victoria, Australia

purified and recently cloned [2–6] although no convincing equivalent of murine multi-CSF has yet been identified (Table 1).

A great deal is now known about the biological activities of each of these CSFs in vitro and more recently in vivo [7, 8], and these activities raise some interesting questions. First, some CSFs have broad cellular specificites (multi-CSF and GM-CSF) while other CSFs have very restricted or single-lineage specificities (M-CSF and G-CSF) (Table 1). How is this overlap in cellular specificities mediated and how do the CSFs co-ordinate to control individual cell populations? Second, some of the CSFs show a concentration dependence in the types of colonies stimulated – for example, at low concentrations GM-CSF stimulates the formation of only macrophage colonies, but at higher concentrations it also stimulates granulocyte

Table 1. Murine and human colony-stimulating factors[a]

Murine CSF	Other names	Cell source	Cellular specificity	Human equivalent
Multi-CSF	Interleukin-3, PSF HCGF, MCGF, BPA	T cells WEHI-3B	G, M, Eo, E, Meg, Blast	?
GM-CSF	MGI-1GM, CSF-2	T cells Endothelial cells Macrophages	G, M, Eo	CSF-α, pluri-poietin-α, NIF-T
M-CSF	MGI-1M, CSF-1	Fibroblasts	M > G	M-CSF, CSF-1
G-CSF	MGI-1G, DF	Macrophages	G > M	CSF-β, pluripoietin

G, Granulocyte; *M*, macrophage; *Eo*, eosinophil; *Meg*, megakaryocyte; *Mast*, mast cell; *MGI*, macrophage, granulocyte inducer; *HCGF*, hemopoietic cell growth factor; *MCGF*, mast cell growth factor; *BPA*, burst-promoting activity; *PSF*, P-cell-stimulating factor; *DF*, differentiation factor.
[a] For a list of references see Metcalf [2].

colony formation [9], while the reverse situation holds for G-CSF [10]. What is the cellular and molecular basis for this altered cell specificity with CSF concentration? Third, for normal hemopoietic progenitor cells the action of CSF results in a tight coupling between cell proliferation and cell differentiation, yet in factor-dependent cell lines the actions of multi-CSF and GM-CSF are associated only with cell proliferation [11] and in myeloid leukemias cell proliferation and differentiation are uncoupled or loosely coupled [12]. In some types of murine myeloid leukemias, G-CSF (but not the other CSFs) is able to overcome this uncoupling and induce terminal differentiation [13]. How is the coupling between proliferation and differentiation in normal progenitor cells mediated by CSFs, how does uncoupling occur in cell lines and leukemias, and why does G-CSF have a special role among the CSFs in differentiation induction? It was to try and answer some of these questions that we undertook a systematic study of the cellular specificities of CSF-binding interactions and a molecular analysis of the cross-interactions of CSFs at the receptor level.

B. Molecular Characteristics of CSF Receptors and Their Binding Interactions

Using radioiodinated derivatives of purified or recombinant murine CSFs the molecular nature of all four CSF receptors has now been determined by chemical cross-linking. The M-CSF receptor is a mol.wt. 165000 [14] single-chain glycoprotein closely related or identical to the *c-fms* proto-oncogene [15], and the G-CSF receptor is a single-chain protein of mol.wt. 150000 [16]. The GM-CSF receptor is a smaller (mol.wt. 55000) protein [17] and, while the multi-CSF receptor is also relatively small, experiments have revealed cross-linking to two non-covalently attached subunits with mol.wt. of 75000 and 60000 [16] (Fig. 1). There is no evidence for different forms of these receptors on different normal cell populations, continuous cell lines or leukemic cells.

Binding studies at 4 °C and 37 °C have revealed that for all four CSFs the apparent

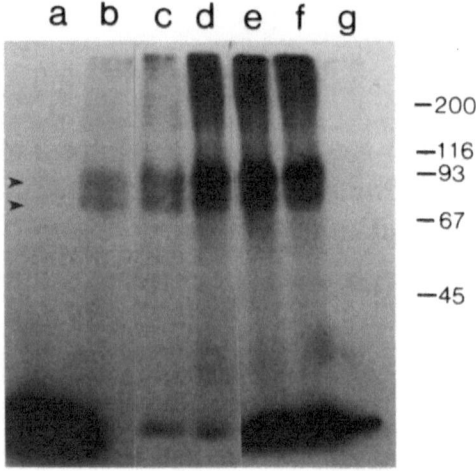

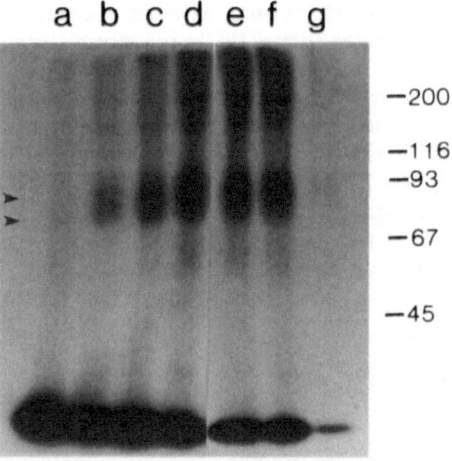

Fig. 1 Chemical cross-linking of ^{125}I multi-CSF to receptors on FDCP-1 cells. After binding of ^{125}I multi-CSF to FDCP-1 cells at 4 °C the cells were washed and incubated with increasing concentrations of the cross-linker disuccinimidyl suberate (DSS) at 4 °C (*a–f*, 0–10 m*M* DSS). Cell pellets were extracted with sodium dodecyl sulfate sample buffer, electrophoresed on 8% polyacrylamide gels in the presence (*upper panel*) or absence (*lower panel*) of dithiothreitol, and exposed for autoradiography. The position of molecular-weight markers (45–200 Kd) is shown on the right. After subtraction of the mol.wt. of cross-linked multi-CSF (15 Kd), the two proteins have mol.wts. of 75000 and 60000. Comparison of upper and lower panels indicates that these two proteins are not disulfide linked

dissociation constant is low (20 pM to 1 nM) and for most CSFs the number of receptors on responsive cells is low (less than a thousand receptors per cell) [17–22]. M-CSF is the exception, with some normal macrophages displaying up to 50000 receptors per cell [23]. On normal cells or cell lines each receptor binding site appears to be unique and specific for its cognate ligand, with no cross-reactivity with other CSFs or several other growth factors tested when binding competition experiments are performed at temperatures of less than 10 °C. Based on the apparent dissociation constants for CSF binding and the known CSF concentrations required for half-maximal biological activity, it might be concluded that biological effects of the CSFs are exerted at low levels of receptor occupancy (i.e. there are spare receptors). This is especially surprising in view of the low levels of CSF receptors on responding cells, but this interpretation is complicated by the kinetic aspects of CSF binding interactions.

The kinetic rates of association of CSFs with their receptors are very fast, reflecting an essentially diffusion-controlled process. For G-CSF at 40 pM and 37 °C the half-time for association with receptors on murine leukemic WEHI-3B D$^+$ cells is about 7 min and the kinetic association constant is 2.6×10^9 M^{-1} min^{-1}. In contrast, the kinetic dissociation rate is very slow ($T\frac{1}{2}$ of 6 h at 0 °C and apparent $T\frac{1}{2}$ of 5 h at 37 °C) even at high dilution of the cells with excess unlabeled G-CSF to prevent re-binding of ^{125}I G-CSF. Calculation of the dissociation constant from the ratio of kinetic dissociation to association constants gives a value of 1 pM for G-CSF binding to WEHI-3B D$^+$ cells at 37 °C, a result much lower than that determined by Scatchard analysis of pseudo-equilibrium binding data (70 pM) but much closer to the concentration required for half-maximal biological effect (differentiation induction) on WEHI-3B D$^+$ cells. This situation parallels that already described for M-CSF binding to macrophages [23, 24].

At 37 °C the apparent kinetic dissociation rate does not reflect only ligand dissociation from its receptor, and Scatchard analysis does not reflect a true equilibrium between ligand and receptor. This is because the

CSFs, like most other growth factors, are internalized along with their receptors after binding at 37 °C and are degraded intracellularly [24]. The binding data at 37 °C thus reflect a steady state (achieved within 1–6 h) where the rate of internalization and degradation of CSF-receptor complexes is balanced by the rate of expression of new receptors at the cell surface. The rates of internalization and degradation of CSF-receptor complexes vary for the different CSFs and for the same CSF in different cell types [24]. For example, M-CSF is rapidly internalized and degraded in macrophages ($T\frac{1}{2}$ of several minutes), while multi-CSF is much more slowly internalized in bone marrow cells ($T\frac{1}{2}$ of 1 h).

The slow dissociation kinetics of CSF-receptor complexes and their relatively rapid internalization at 37 °C mean that measurement of receptor levels on cells obtained from mice or on cell lines that need to be maintained continuously in CSF-containing media need to be interpreted with caution, since they will depend on the past history of the cells.

C. Cellular Specificity of CSF Binding

Several cell lines have been described that display receptors for one or more murine CSF. In principle, these cell lines should provide a homogeneous population of cells with which to study CSF-receptor interactions, but in practice autoradiographic analysis has revealed considerable intraclonal heterogeneity in receptor content not clearly rated to cell cycle or differentiation status.

Of several murine cell lines tested, only two displayed specific binding of ^{125}I G-CSF – the J774 macrophage cell line and WEHI-3B D$^+$ murine myelomonocytic leukemic cells which respond to G-CSF by differentiation induction. These two cell lines displayed very similar receptor numbers and apparent binding affinities for G-CSF [25]. Of special interest was the observation that the derived cell line WEHI-3B D$^-$, which does not respond to G-CSF, had lost nearly all detectable binding sites for G-CSF, providing a ready explanation for its lack of inducibility for differentiation [18]. Cell au-

235

toradiographic analysis of the binding of ^{125}I G-CSF to murine bone marrow cells [19] revealed a cellular pattern of receptor distribution highly consistent with its biological specificity. Binding was restricted to neutrophilic granulocytes and their precursors and to a lesser extent to monocytic cells but was absent from eosinophils, erythroid cells and lymphocytes. Interestingly, receptor numbers were higher on neutrophils than on monocytes, were present on essentially all neutrophils and their precursors, and increased in number with cell differentiation [19]. The ability of G-CSF to stimulate functional activities of neutrophils is consistent with the presence of these receptors on post-mitotic cells [26].

G-CSF, unlike the other three murine CSFs, is fully cross-reactive on human cells, and this allowed a study of the distribution of human G-CSF receptors on human bone marrow cells and human leukemic samples [20]. On human cells binding was again restricted to neutrophilic granulocytes and their precursors and to a lesser extent, monocytic cells, but, in contrast to the situation in the mouse, receptor numbers decreased somewhat with neutrophil differentiation. This cellular specificity was maintained with human leukemias, in that all myeloid leukemias showed specific binding of ^{125}I G-CSF while lymphoid leukemias did not. The receptor content of myeloid leukemic cells was related to the granulocytic or monocytic nature of the leukemias, acute promyelocytic leukemias having the highest receptor content and monocytic leukemias having the lowest. Quantitative binding-competition studies revealed that murine and human G-CSF (CSFβ) competed for the same binding sites on murine or human cells and that their relative binding affinities for all receptors were nearly the same when their respective concentrations were normalized with respect to a common bioassay [19].

M-CSF binds to a variety of monocytic cell lines (including WEHI-3B D$^+$ and J774) and to all normal populations of monocytic cells or macrophages but not to eosinophils, lymphocytes or erythroid cells [27]. There is some controversy about whether M-CSF binds to neutrophils and their precursors [27, 28], but if it does the receptor levels are lower than on monocytic cells. There is some evidence that M-CSF receptors increase with differentiation of monocyte/macrophages [27, 28].

Multi-CSF binds to all factor-dependent continuous hemopoietic cell lines tested (FDCP-1, 32D Cl.3, DA-3. NSF-60) as well as some independent cell lines (P815 mastocytoma and WEHI-3B D$^+$) [21, 22], but the apparent binding affinities and receptor numbers vary widely. Multi-CSF also binds to all neutrophilic and eosinophilic granulocytes and all monocytes and their precursors but not to lymphocytes and erythroid cells [22]. In contrast to the binding patterns seen with G-CSF and M-CSF, there were similar multi-CSF receptor levels on neutrophils, monocytes and eosinophils, and in each case receptor numbers decreased with differentiation. ^{125}I multi-CSF binding to murine bone marrow cells was also characterized by the presence of a very small number (less than 1%) of cells of various morphologies (blasts, promonocytes, metamyelocytes, eosinophils) that displayed very high receptor levels similar to those seen on factor-dependent continuous cell lines [22].

GM-CSF also binds to several cell lines, including some factor-dependent cell lines (FDCP-1), some macrophage cell lines (J774, WR19, RAW 264, R309), and WEHI-3B D$^+$ myelomonocytic leukemic cells [17]. The distribution of receptors for GM-CSF on bone marrow cells is very similar to that of multi-CSF receptors, except that there are fewer GM-CSF receptors on eosinophils than on neutrophils or monocytes and there is no population of bone marrow cells with a very high GM-CSF receptor content (F. Walker, D. Metcalf, N. A. Nicola and A. W. Burgess, unpublished).

It is of special relevance that the majority of non-erythroid bone marrow cells display multiple CSF receptors. All neutrophilic granulocytes and their precursors display simultaneously receptors for multi-CSF, GM-CSF, G-CSF and possibly lower numbers of M-CSF receptors. All monocytic cells display receptors for multi-CSF, GM-CSF, and M-CSF, and a majority display lower numbers of G-CSF receptors. Eosinophils display multi-CSF and GM-CSF receptors but not G-CSF or M-CSF receptors. Lymphocytes and erythroid cells do not display measurable levels of any of these CSF receptors. The display of multiple CSF receptors on granulocytes and macrophages means that they can respond to all of the CSFs directly and the possibility exists for receptor interactions on the same cell.

D. Indirect Receptor Modulations by the CSFs

Despite the fact that the four murine CSF receptors are distinct in both their molecular characteristics and their cellular distribution and that the binding of each CSF to bone marrow cells at 0 °C is not competed for by any of the other CSFs, there is evidence for indirect interactions between CSF receptors. When bone marrow cells were preincubated with one CSF at 37 °C the binding of other CSFs to their own receptors was reduced. This is an example of non-isologous receptor down-modulation, and it has been described for other growth factor receptor systems (for example, platelet-derived growth factor [29] and transforming growth factor β [30] both down-modulate epidermal growth factor receptors on some cell types).

The pattern of CSF-induced receptor down-modulations on bone marrow cells was quite striking, with multi-CSF being able to down-modulate all other CSF receptors, GM-CSF being able to down-modulate M-CSF and G-CSF receptors, and M-CSF being able to down-modulate GM-CSF receptors; G-CSF was able to down-modulate M-CSF receptors only at high concentrations. These down-modulations occurred at 37 °C but not at 0 °C, were generally rapid ($T\frac{1}{2}$ 10–20 min) and were CSF-dose dependent [31] (Fig. 2). The common interpretation of receptor down-modulation is that it serves to limit the response of a cell to that receptor's growth factor. However, we were struck by several correlations between the ability of CSFs to down-modulate receptors and their ability to express certain biological activities that suggested an alternative interpretation.

First, CSFs with the ability to induce multiple types of differentiated cells had the broadest capacity to down-modulate CSF receptors (multi-CSF down-modulated all CSF receptors and GM-CSF down-modu-

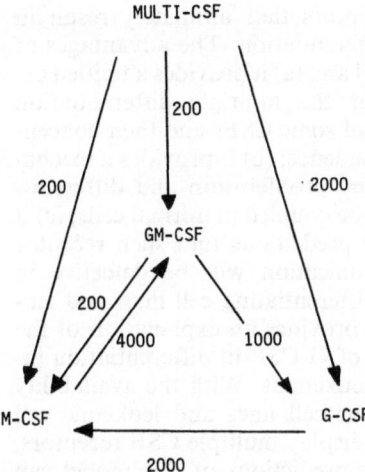

Fig. 2. Pattern and concentration dependence of CSF-induced receptor down-modulators on murine bone marrow cells at 37 °C. The *arrows* indicate the directionality of the ability of a particular CSF to down-modulate another CSF's receptor after pre-incubation of bone marrow cells at 37 °C. The numbers associated with each arrow are the concentrations of the CSFs (in bone marrow colony-stimulating units/ml) that result in 50% of the maximal down-modulation

lated G- and M-CSF receptors, while no CSFs other than multi-CSF down-modulated multi-CSF receptors). Second, the concentration dependence of CSF-induced differentiation matched the concentration dependence of that CSF's ability to down-modulate the appropriate CSF receptors (GM-CSF down-modulated M-CSF receptors at low concentrations and G-CSF receptors at high concentrations, G-CSF down-modulated M-CSF receptors at high concentrations). Third, certain agents that activate neutrophils also down-modulate G-CSF receptors on neutrophils (the chemotactic peptide N-formyl methione leucine phenylalanine and bacterial lipopolysaccharide) [32].

These observations suggested that receptor down-modulation might result in activation of at least some of the biological activities of that receptor just as if it were occupied by the isologous ligand. Such a model proposes that multi-CSF and GM-CSF receptors deliver a mitogenic signal to a cell but, at the same time, indirectly activate lineage-

237

specific receptors that ultimately result in terminal differentiation. The advantages of such a model are: (a) it provides a unified explanation of the multiple differentiation specificities of some CSFs and their concentration dependence; (b) it provides a mechanism whereby proliferation and differentiation might be coupled in normal cells; (c) it makes clear predictions that such receptor cross-communication will be defective in some non-differentiating cell lines and leukemias and provides an explanation of the special role of G-CSF in differentiation induction of leukemias. With the availability of continuous cell lines and leukemic cell lines which display multiple CSF receptors, some of the predictions of this model can now be tested.

Acknowledgements. The original work reported here was supported by N.I.H. Grant CA-22556, the J.D. and L. Harris Trust Fund, the National Health and Medical Research Council of Australia and the Carden Fellowship Fund of the Anti-Cancer Council of Victoria. The technical assistance of Luba Oddo and Linda Peterson is gratefully acknowledged.

References

1. Metcalf D (1984) The hemopoietic colony-stimulating factors. Elsevier, Amsterdam
2. Metcalf D (1986) The molecular biology and functions of the granulocyte-macrophage colony-stimulating factors. Blood 67:257
3. Nicola NA, Vadas M (1984) Hemopoietic colony-stimulating factors. Immunol Today 5:76
4. Nomura M, Imazeki I, Oheda M, Kubota N, Tamura M, Ono M, Ueyama Y, Asano S (1986) Purification and characterization of human granulocyte colony-stimulating factor (G-CSF). EMBO J 5:871
5. Nagata S, Tsuchiya M, Asano S, Kaziro Y, Yamazaki T, Yamamoto O, Hirata Y, Kubota N, Oheda M, Nomura M, Ono M (1986) Molecular cloning and expression of cDNA for human granulocyte colony-stimulating factor. Nature 319:415
6. Souza LM, Boone TC, Gabrilove J, Lai PH, Zsebo KM, Murdock DC, Chasin VR, Bruszewski J, Lu H, Chen KK, Barendt J, Platzer E, Moore MAS, Mertelsman R, Welte K (1986) Recombinant human granulocyte colony-stimulating factor: effects on normal and leukemic myeloid cells. Science 232:61
7. Kindler V, Thorens B, de Kossodo S, Allet B, Eliason JF, Thatcher D, Farber N, Vassali P (1986) Stimulation of hematopoiesis in vivo by recombinant bacterial murine interleukin-3. Proc Natl Acad Sci USA 83:1001
8. Metcalf D, Begley CG, Johnson GR, Nicola NA, Lopez AF, Williamson DJ (1986) Effects of purified bacterially synthesized murine multi-CSF (IL-3) on hemopoiesis in normal adult mice. Blood 68:46
9. Burgess AW, Metcalf D (1977) Colony-stimulating factor and the differentiation of granulocytes and macrophages. In: Baum SJ, Ledney GD (eds) Experimental hematology today. Springer-Verlag, Berlin Heidelberg New York, p 135
10. Metcalf D, Nicola NA (1983) Proliferative effects of purified granulocyte colony-stimulating factor (G-CSF) on normal mouse hemopoietic cells. J Cell Physiol 116:198
11. Dexter TM, Garland J, Scott D, Scolnick E, Metcalf D (1980) Growth of factor-dependent hemopoietic precursor cell lines. J Exp Med 152:1036
12. Sachs L (1975) Control of normal cell differentiation and the phenotypic reversion of malignancy in myeloid leukemia. Nature 274:535
13. Nicola NA, Metcalf D, Matsumoto M, Johnson GR (1983) Purification of a factor inducing differentiation in murine myelomonocytic leukemia cells: identification as granulocyte colony-stimulating factor (G-CSF). J Biol Chem 258:9017
14. Morgan CJ, Stanley ER (1984) Chemical cross-linking of the mononuclear phagocyte-specific growth factor CSF to its receptor at the cell surface. Biochem Biophys Res Commun 119:35
15. Scherr CJ, Rettenmier CN, Sacca R, Roussel MF, Look AT, Stanley ER (1985) The *c-fms* proto-oncogene product is related to the receptor for the mononuclear phagocyte growth factor, CSF-1. Cell 41:665
16. Nicola NA, Peterson L (1986) Identification of distinct receptors for two hemopoietic growth factors (granulocyte-colony stimulating factor and multipotential colony stimulating factor) by chemical cross-linking. J Biol Chem 261:12384
17. Walker F, Burgess AW (1985) Specific binding of radioiodinated granulocyte-macrophage colony-stimulating factor to hemopoietic cells. EMBO J 4:933
18. Nicola NA, Metcalf D (1984) Binding of the differentiation inducer, granulocyte colony-stimulating factor to differentiation responsive but not unresponsive leukemic cell lines. Proc Natl Acad Sci USA 81:3765

19. Nicola NA, Metcalf D (1985) Binding of ^{125}I-labeled granulocyte colony-stimulating factor to normal murine hemopoietic cells. J Cell Physiol 124:313

20. Nicola NA, Begley CG, Metcalf D (1985) Identification of the human analogue of a regulator that induces differentiation in murine leukaemic cells. Nature 314:625

21. Palaszynski EW, Ihle JN (1984) Evidence for specific receptors for interleukin-3 on lymphokine-dependent cell lines established from long-term bone marrow cultures. J Immunol 132:1872

22. Nicola NA, Metcalf D (1986) Binding of iodinated multipotential colony-stimulating factor (interleukin-3) to murine bone marrow cells. J Cell Physiol 128:180

23. Stanley ER, Guilbert LJ (1981) Methods for the purification, assay, characterization and target cell binding of a colony-stimulating factor (CSF-1). J Immunol Methods 42:253

24. Guilbert LJ, Stanley ER (1986) The interaction of ^{125}I colony-stimulating factor-1 with bone marrow-derived macrophages. J Biol Chem 261:4024

25. Nicola NA, Metcalf D (1984) Differentiation induction in leukemic cells by normal growth regulators: molecular and binding properties of purified granulocyte colony-stimulating factor. In: Genes and Cancer. Liss, New York, p 591

26. Lopez A, Nicola NA, Burgess AW, Metcalf D, Battye FL, Sewell WA, Vadas M (1983) Activation of granulocyte cytotoxic function by purified mouse colony-stimulating factors. J Immunol 131:2983

27. Byrne PV, Guilbert LJ, Stanley ER (1981) Distribution of cells bearing receptors for a colony-stimulating factor (CSF-1) in murine tissues. J Cell Biol 91:848

28. Shadduck RK, Pigoli G, Caramatti C, Degliontoni G, Rizzoli V, Porcellini A, Waheed A, Schiffer L (1983) Identification of hemopoietic cells responsive to colony-stimulating factor by autoradiography. Blood 62:1197

29. Bowen-Pope DF, Dicorletto PE, Ross R (1983) Interactions between the receptors for platelet-derived growth factor and epidermal growth factor. J Cell Biol 96:679

30. Assoian RK, Frolik CA, Roberts AB, Miller DM, Sporn MB (1984) Transforming growth factor-β controls receptor levels for epidermal growth factor in NRK fibroblasts. Cell 36:35

31. Walker F, Nicola NA, Metcalf D, Burgess AW (1985) Hierarchical down-modulation of hemopoietic growth factor receptors. Cell 43:269

32. Nicola NA, Vadas MA, Lopez AF (1986) Down-modulation of receptors for granulocyte colony-stimulating factor on human neutrophils by granulocyte-activating agents. J Cell Physiol 128:501

Haematology and Blood Transfusion   Vol. 31
Modern Trends in Human Leukemia VII
Edited by Neth, Gallo, Greaves, and Kabisch
© Springer-Verlag Berlin Heidelberg 1987

Fractionation of CSF Activities
from Human Placental Conditioned Medium

J. Boyd [1] and G. R. Johnson [2]

A. Introduction

Colony stimulating factors (CSFs) are required for the survival, proliferation and differentiation of hemopoietic progenitor cells in vitro and possibly in vivo. Recently, several human CSFs have been purified and molecularly cloned from human tumor cell lines. These include granulocyte colony stimulating factor (G-CSF), from the bladder carcinoma cell line 5637 [1, 2] and the squamous cell carcinoma cell line CHU-2 [3], and granulocyte-macrophage colony stimulating factor (GM-CSF), from the Mo T-lymphoblast cell line [4, 5] and the monocytic cell line U937 (personal communication, Dr. J. DeLamarter). In addition, human erythroid potentiating activity (EPA) has been purified and molecularly cloned from the Mo T-lymphoblast cell line [6, 7]. The relationship between these CSFs and those contained in media conditioned by normal human tissues has not been established. We have therefore fractionated human placental conditioned medium (HPCM) to determine the number of CSFs produced by this tissue able to stimulate human progenitors in vitro. Furthermore, the biological relationship of these factors to the known CSFs has been determined by comparing their ability to stimulate human and murine colony formation with the prolifer-

[1] Department of Clinical Haematology and Oncology, Royal Children's Hospital, Melbourne, Victoria 3050, Australia
[2] The Walter and Eliza Hall Institute for Medical Research, P.O. 3050, Royal Melbourne Hospital, Victoria, Australia

ation of murine factor-dependent cell lines in vitro.

B. Results

Cultures of low-density non-adherent bone marrow (3×10^4 cells/ml) or peripheral blood cells (2×10^5 cells/ml) were established in 35-mm Petri dishes containing Iscove's Modified Dulbecco's Medium, 25% fetal calf serum (FCS) and 0.3% agar and were scored after 14 days' incubation (5% CO_2, 37 °C). Murine (CBA) bone marrow cultures (5×10^4 cells/ml) in 35-mm Petri dishes containing Dulbecco's Modified Eagle's Medium with 20% FCS and 0.3% agar were incubated for 7 days. Cultures were scored under a dissecting microscope and then stained with Luxol-Fast-Blue and hematoxylin. Cellular proliferation of the murine cell lines 32D Cl.3 (IL-3-responsive) and FDC-P1 (IL-3 and GM-CSF-responsive) was assessed in 15-µl suspension cultures containing 200 FDC-P1 or 32D Cl.3 cells. Viable cells were counted after 2 days of incubation.

Initial fractionation of HPCM by phenyl-Sepharose chromatography [8] allowed separation of CSFα from CSFβ. While CSFβ, the human analogue of murine G-CSF [9], only stimulated neutrophil and some neutrophil-macrophage or macrophage colony formation by human progenitor cells in vitro, CSFα stimulated neutrophil, neutrophil-macrophage, macrophage and eosinophil colony formation and, in the presence of erythropoietin (Epo), also stimulated multi-

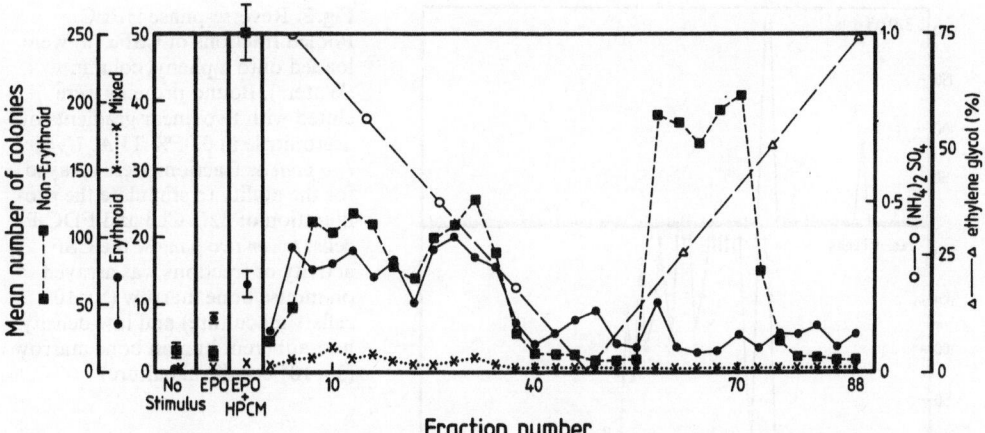

Fig. 1. Phenyl-Sepharose chromatography. Tenfold concentrated HPCM equilibrated in 1 M ammonium sulfate was loaded on a Pharmacia phenyl-Sepharose CL4B column (2.6 × 20 cm). First CSFα was eluted with a linear gradient from 1 M ammonium sulfate to water; this was followed by CSFβ, which eluted during a second linear gradient from water to 75% ethylene glycol. Cultures of low-density non-adherent human peripheral blood cells (2 × 10⁵/ml) were scored after 14 days

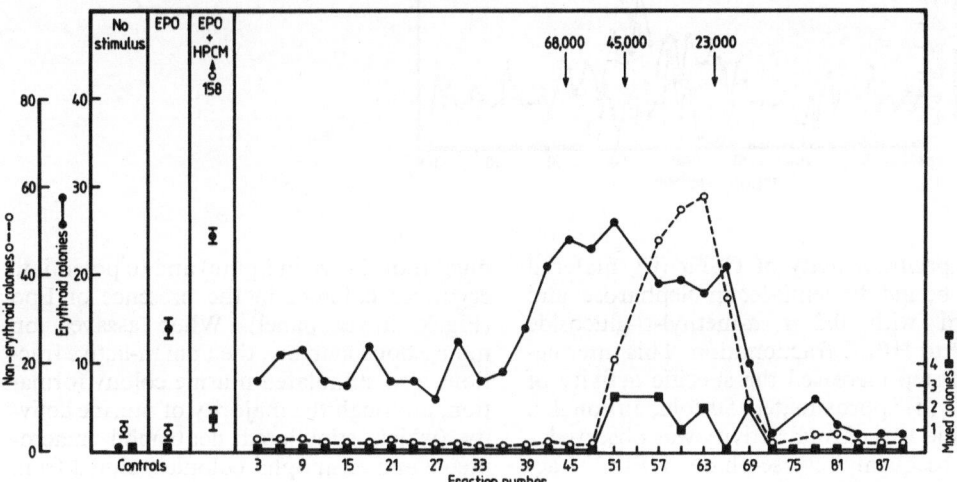

Fig. 2. Gel filtration chromatography. CSFα was loaded on an Ultrogel AcA44 column (2.6 × 100 cm) and eluted with phosphate buffered saline, 0.04 M, pH 7.4. *Arrows* denote the elution points of bovine serum albumin, ovalbumin and chymotrypsinogen. Colony number per 2 × 10⁵ low-density non-adherent human peripheral blood cells was determined after 14 days

potential colony formation and potentiated erythroid colony formation (Fig. 1).

Further fractionation of CSFα by gel filtration chromatography (LKB Ultrogel AcA44, 2.6 × 100 cm column; Fig. 2) separated an erythroid potentiating activity (EPA) with an apparent mol.wt. of 40–45 kD which stimulated no human colony formation alone but potentiated erythroid colony formation in the presence of Epo. This activity could be separated from a broad CSF peak [CSFα (ii)] with an apparent mol.wt. of 30 kD which had all the biological properties of CSFα. Depending on

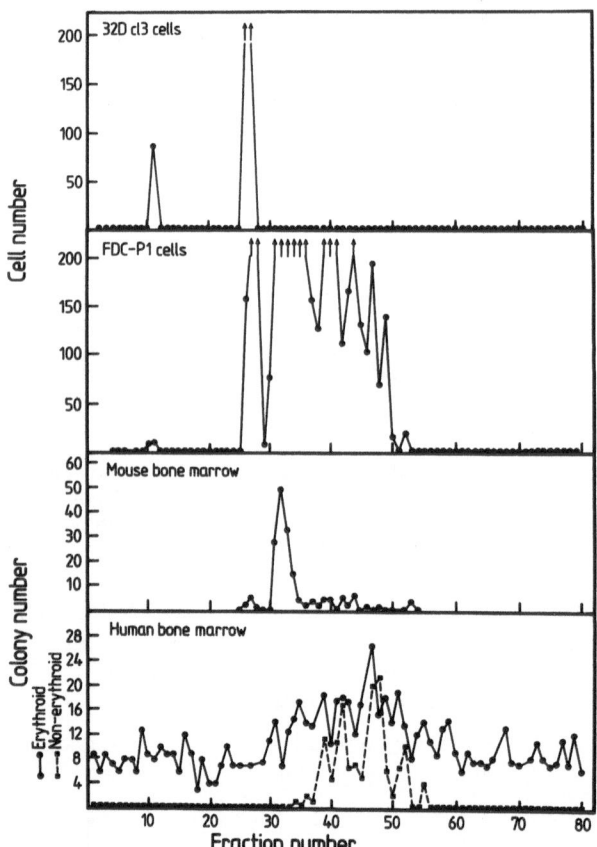

Fig. 3. Reverse-phase HPLC. Pooled fractions of CSFα (ii) were loaded onto a phenyl column (Waters). Bound proteins were eluted with two linear gradients of acetonitrile in 0.05% TFA. *Upper two panels:* fractions were assayed for the ability to stimulate the proliferation of 32D Cl.3 and FDC-P1 cells; *lower two panels:* the CSF activity of fractions was assayed on mouse bone marrow (5×10^4 cells/1 ml culture) and low-density non-adherent human bone marrow (3×10^4 cells/1 ml culture)

the specific activity of CSFα (ii), material was bound to lentil-lectin Sepharose and eluted with $0.2\ M$ α-methyl-D-glucoside prior to HPLC fractionation. This intermediate step increased the specific activity of CSFα (ii) approximately 50-fold, although a fivefold loss of total activity was observed.

Subsequent reverse-phase HPLC fractionation of CSFα (ii) was carried out using a Waters phenyl column and a two-stage linear gradient with a constant flow rate of 1 ml/min, first from 0% to 30% acetonitrile in 0.05% trifluoroacetic acid (TFA) over 10 min collecting 5-ml fractions, followed by a second linear gradient from 30% to 60% acetonitrile in 0.05% TFA over 60 min collecting 1-ml fractions. Multiple human-active peaks were detected eluting from the column between 38% and 46% acetonitrile (fractions 39 to 52), and all were able to stimulate neutrophil, macrophage, and eosinophil colonies as well as multipotential col-

onies (not shown in figure) and to potentiate erythroid colonies in the presence of Epo (Fig. 3, lower panel). When assayed on mouse bone marrow, the human-active fractions also stimulated murine colony formation, although the majority of murine activity (which stimulated neutrophil, macrophage and eosinophil colonies) eluted from the HPLC column prior to the human CSF peaks. Proliferation of FDC-P1 cells was supported by all fractions active on murine and human progenitors, while 32D Cl.3 cells responded only to a narrow band of fractions which also stimulated normal murine cells and FDC-P1 cells but not human cells.

To reduce carbohydrate heterogeneity, the same batch of CSFα (ii) was treated with neuraminidase [from *Clostridium perfringens* (Sigma) pH 5.0, 37 °C for 60 min] before HPLC fractionation. This treatment completely separated a murine CSF activity which also stimulated 32D Cl.3 cell proliferation from a human CSF activity which also stimulated FDC-P1 cells. However, neuraminidase treatment did not resolve the multiple peaks of activity observed in the human and FDC-P1 assays. Other deglycosylation agents may be useful in determining whether these peaks are related to a single CSF protein or are a result of multiple CSF activities not yet characterized.

C. Conclusion

Human recombinant GM-CSF (rHGM-CSF) has recently been tested on a variety of human target cells and murine cell lines [10], and, although possessing the same human repertoire as material fractionated from HPCM, rHGM-CSF at comparable doses does not stimulate proliferation of FDC-P1 cells. It is possible that native GM-CSF from a non-tumor source is heterogeneous and has a greater ability to interact with murine GM-CSF receptors present on FDC-P1 cells. Binding studies are now in progress to determine whether HPCM-derived fractions can compete with ^{125}I murine recombinant GM-CSF binding sites on FDC-P1 cells. The ability of monoclonal antibodies directed against rHGM-CSF to block the response of human progenitor cells to HPCM-derived fractions is also under investigation.

The nature of the activity which stimulated both 32D Cl.3 proliferation and murine colony formation is not clear. Based on purification and biological studies, it appears to be unrelated to G-CSF or M-CSF, since the molecule exhibited low hydrophobicity, had an apparent mol.wt. of 30 kD, and could stimulate murine granulocyte, macrophage and eosinophil colony formation. The role of this activity in human hemopoiesis is not yet clear, since alone or in combination with erythropoietin no stimulation of human progenitor cells could be demonstrated. However, the possibility still exists that it has a synergistic effect with other known CSFs in vitro. A recent report that IL-2 could stimulate 32D-clone 23 cells [11] suggested the possibility that the HPCM-derived 32D Cl.3 activity might be due to IL-2, although we were not able to stimulate the murine IL-2-dependent cell line CTLL with these fractions (less than 0.7 units IL-2/ml), and recombinant human IL-2 did not stimulate 32D Cl.3 cells (personal communication, Dr. A. Kelso).

These studies show that a normal human tissue, the placenta, contains hemopoiesis-stimulating activities similar to those recently purified from tumor cell lines and molecularly cloned. These include G-CSF, GM-CSF and EPA. In addition, the studies suggest that there may be multiple forms of activity with similarities to GM-CSF but also some activities with apparent specificity only for normal murine cells and murine factor-dependent cell lines.

Acknowledgements. This work was supported by the Royal Children's Hospital Research Foundation. The work at the Walter and Eliza Hall Institute was supported by the Carden Fellowship Fund of the Anti-Cancer Council of Victoria and The National Health and Medical Research Council, Canberra.

References

1. Souza LM et al. (1986) Science 232:61–65
2. Welte K et al. (1985) Proc Natl Acad Sci USA 82:1526–1530
3. Nagata S et al. (1986) Nature 319:415–418
4. Gasson JC et al. (1984) Science 226:1339–1342
5. Wang GG et al. (1985) Science 228:810–815
6. Westbrook CA et al. (1984) J Biol Chem 259:9992–9996
7. Gasson JC et al. (1985) Nature 315:768–771
8. Nicola NA et al. (1979) Blood 54:614–627
9. Nicola NA et al. (1985) Nature 314:625–628
10. Metcalf D et al. (1986) Blood 67:37–45
11. Warren HS et al. (1985) Lymphokine Res 4:195–204

Haematology and Blood Transfusion   Vol. 31
Modern Trends in Human Leukemia VII
Edited by Neth, Gallo, Greaves, and Kabisch
© Springer-Verlag Berlin Heidelberg 1987

Proliferative Effects of a Recombinant Human Granulocyte Colony-Stimulating Factor (rG-CSF) on Highly Enriched Hematopoietic Progenitor Cells

O. G. Ottmann[1], K. Welte[2], L. M. Souza[3], and M. A. S. Moore[1]

A. Introduction

Human multipotential and committed hematopoietic progenitor cells require the presence of specific glycoproteins, termed "colony-stimulating factors" (CSFs) for survival, clonal proliferation, and differentiation. Recently, a pluripotent G-CSF, constitutively produced by the human bladder carcinoma line 5637, has been purified to apparent homogeneity [1] and molecularly cloned with the complementary DNA copy of the gene expressed in *Escherichia coli* [2]. This factor induces terminal differentiation of the murine myelomonocytic cell line WE-HI3B(D$^+$), the human promyelocytic cell line HL60, and leukemic cells from patients with certain forms of ANLL [2, 3] and has been shown to stimulate the growth of day-7 granulocyte colonies, erythroid bursts (BFU-E), and multilineage colonies (CFU-GEMM) from human bone marrow [1–3]. Despite its similarity with murine G-CSF [4], the latter does not support the proliferation of BFU-E and CFU-GEMM [5], biological activities shared by murine IL3 and GM-CSF [6–8]. However, IL3 has not been reported to induce differentiation of leukemic cells [9], no significant homology was found between the deduced amino acid sequence for hG-CSF and those for murine IL3 [10, 11] and murine and human GM-CSF [12, 13], and specific binding of radiolabeled hG-CSF was inhibited by an excess of unlabeled

hG-CSF but not by hGM-CSF [2]. In these previous studies, accessory cell-mediated biological activities and direct effects on progenitor cells were not distinguished. To address these considerations, the effects of hG-CSF on accessory cell-free bone marrow populations highly enriched for hematopoietic progenitors were examined.

B. Methods

Low-density bone marrow separated by Ficoll-Hypaque density centrifugation was enriched 10- to 12-fold for progenitor cells by depletion of mature myeloid, monocytic, lymphoid, and erythroid cells using the mAbs Mol, MY8, MY3, N901, B4 (generously provided by J. Griffin, Boston), OKT4, OKT8, OKT11, and antiglycophorin by immunoadherence "panning" [14, 15] and complement-mediated cytotoxicity (LDAC-). By subsequent fluorescence-activated cell sorting, a nearly homogeneous blast population defined by low perpendicular and high forward light scatter (blast window) and expression of the HPCA-1 antigen (detected by the MY10 mAb), present on all hematopoietic progenitors [16], was isolated with a purity of 85%–95% and an overall plating efficiency of up to 30%. Alternatively to MY10, an anti-HLA-DR mAb (clone L243; both Abs a kind gift of N. Warner, Becton Dickinson) was used for positive selection of clonogenic cells [17]. DAD14 (d14) and DAY7 (d7) CFU-GM, BFU-E, and CFU-GEMM were assayed in agar and methylcellulose cultures respec-

[1] Laboratory of Developmental Hematopoiesis,
[2] Laboratory of Molecular Hematology, Memorial Sloan-Kettering Cancer Center, New York
[3] Amgen, Thousand Oaks, CA

tively. Erythropoietin (EPO) was added on d3 to eliminate background growth of BPA-independent, EPO-responsive BFU-E [18]. In cultures of MY10+ and HLA-DR+ populations no spontaneous colony formation was observed.

C. Results and Discussion

As shown in Table 1, 100–2000 units of recombinant G-CSF (specific activity approximately 1×10^8 units per mg protein) stimulate proliferation of CFU-GM in a dose-dependent manner and by direct action on MY10+ progenitor cells. Aggregates that had developed by day 7 were uniformly small, rarely exceeding 20–30 cells even at high concentrations of G-CSF, and purely granulocytic, containing mature neutrophils as demonstrated by esterase stains. No significant differences in either number or size of aggregates were observed when equivalent concentrations of recombinant and highly purified G-CSF were compared (data not shown), indicating that lack of glycosylation of the recombinant material does not adversely affect its biological activity. CFU-GM scored after 14 days were predominantly granulocytic (64%–75%); in addition, the formation of a small number of mixed granulocyte/macrophage colonies (4% at 250 U/ml, 10% at 2000 U/ml) and macrophage clusters of 6–20 cells (20%–30% of total aggregates in several experiments) was stimulated. In contrast, growth of eosinophil colonies was not supported, even by high concentrations of G-CSF, as judged by Congo red stains of agar cultures. These data are consistent with results obtained previously with murine G-CSF [5].

The capacity of rG-CSF to stimulate BFU-E and CFU-GEMM was examined in a highly sensitive BPA assay, using sequentially purified progenitor populations (LDAC- and sorted HLA-DR+, MY10+ blasts) as target cells. As shown in Fig. 1 for MY10+ cells, 50–2000 U/ml rG-CSF failed to stimulate CFU-GEMM or increase BFU-E formation above background levels. Identical results were obtained in numerous experiments irrespective of the target population used. Comparison of highly purified and recombinant G-CSF at both 1000 and 5000 U/ml confirmed that the absence of BFU-E- and CFU-GEMM-stimulating activity of rG-CSF is not a consequence of the lack of glycosylation. Readdition of autologous, unstimulated OKT4- and OKT8-positive lymphocytes, isolated by cell sorting with 98% purity, to cultures of MY10+ cells did not augment colony formation in either the absence or the presence of G-CSF (data not shown). These results are at variance with earlier studies [1–3], which employed target populations depleted of accessory cells by plastic adherence and E-rosetting, techniques that do not facilitate the degree of progenitor enrichment and accessory cell depletion achieved by the immunological techniques used in this study. It is conceivable that the stimulation of erythroid and multilineage colonies observed in those reports was mediated by an as yet unidentified accessory cell.

To assess whether or not G-CSF is able to facilitate the survival and or initial proliferation of BFU-E and CFU-GEMM, delayed addition experiments were carried out (Table 2). The almost complete loss of BPA-responsive BFU-E and of CFU-GEMM caused by delaying the addition of BPA till day 4 of culture is not abrogated by the continuous presence of G-CSF. This result differs slightly from that obtained with murine fetal liver cells, where G-CSF appeared to stimulate the initial proliferation of a subpopulation of multipotential and erythroid precursors [5].

Table 1. Stimulation by rhG-CSF of d7 and d14 CFU-GM from MY10+ bone marrow cells cultured in triplicate at 1000 cells/ml. Values (clusters: 4–50 cells; colonies: more than 50 cells) are expressed as mean±standard deviation calculated for 1×10^5 cells

rhG-CSF U/ml	CFU-GM (colonies/clusters)	
	Day 7	Day 14
0	0/0	0/0
100	0/2780 ± 490	1600 ± 400/1600 ± 330
250	0/4890 ± 570	2660 ± 530/1400 ± 70
500	0/5130 ± 176	2900 ± 70/1130 ± 130
2000	0/5380 ± 550	3470 ± 130/1130 ± 200

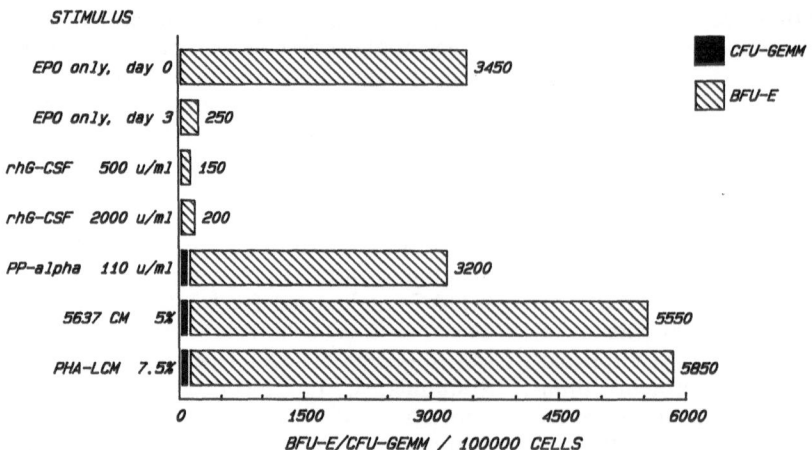

Fig. 1. Growth of BFU-E and CFU-GEMM in methylcellulose cultures of MY10+ cells cultured in duplicate at 1000 cells/ml. Comparison of rG-CSF with 5637 CM, PHA-LCM and PP-alpha (Pluripoietin-α), a GM-CSF-like activity purified from the bladder carcinoma line 5637 [20]. Recombinant EPO was added on day 3 of culture unless otherwise stated

Table 2. Delayed addition of burst-promoting activity (BPA) to methylcellulose cultures of enriched progenitor populations in the presence or absence of rhG-CSF. LDAC-, HLA-DR+, and MY10+ cells were plated at 1×10^4, 2.5×10^3, and 1×10^3 cells/ml respectively. 5637 CM was used as a source of BPA

Stimulus			Bone marrow fraction		
EPO	rhG-CSF	BPA	LD AC-	HLA-DR+	MY10+
Day of addition			Number of BFU-E/CFU-GEMM/10^5 cells		
3	–	–	90/ 0	40/ 0	350/ 0
3	–	0	700/10	1700/120	4800/420
3	0	–	160/ 0	200/ 0	200/ 0
3	–	4	210/ 0	180/ 0	300/ 0
3	0	0	140/ 0	0/ 0	400/ 0

In conclusion, it appears that the direct action of human G-CSF is restricted primarily to the granulocytic lineage, in which it supports the proliferation and differentiation of committed progenitors (d7 and d14 CFU-GM) and stimulates end-stage cells as determined by antibody-dependent cell-mediated cytotoxicity and induction of chemotactic peptide binding [2, 20].

Acknowledgement. The excellent technical assistance of Mrs. W. Wachter is gratefully acknowledged.

References

1. Welte K, Platzer E, Lu L, Gabrilove JL, Levi E, Mertelsmann R, Moore MAS (1985) Purification and biochemical characterization of human pluripotent hematopoietic colony-stimulating factor. Proc Natl Acad Sci USA 82:1526–1530

2. Souza LM, Boone TC, Gabrilove J, Lai PH, Zsebo KM, Murdock DC, Chazin VR, Bruszewski J, Lu H, Chen KK, Barendt J, Platzer E, Moore MAS, Mertelsmann R, Welte K (1986) Recombinant human granulocyte colony-stimulating factor: effects on normal

and leukemic myeloid cells. Science 232:61–65

3. Platzer E, Welte K, Gabrilove JL, Lu L, Harris P, Mertelsmann R, Moore MAS (1985) Biological activities of a human pluripotent hemopoietic colony-stimulating factor on normal and leukemic cells. J Exp Med 162:1788–1801

4. Nicola NA, Begley CG, Metcalf D (1985) Identification of the human analogue of a regulator that induces differentiation in murine leukaemic cells. Nature 314:625–628

5. Metcalf D, Nicola NA (1983) Proliferative effects of purified granulocyte colony-stimulating factor (G-CSF) on normal mouse hematopoietic cells. J Cell Physiol 116:198–206

6. Hapel AJ, Fung MC, Johnson RM, Young IG, Johnson G, Metcalf D (1985) Biologic properties of molecularly cloned and expressed murine interleukin-3. Blood 65:1453–1459

7. Suda J, Suda T, Kubota K, Ihle JN, Saito M, Miura Y (1986) Purified interleukin-3 and erythropoietin support the terminal differentiation of hemopoietic progenitors in serum-free culture. Blood 67:1002–1006

8. Sieff CA, Emerson SG, Donahue RE, Nathan DG, Wang EA, Wong GG, Clark SC (1985) Human recombinant granulocyte-macrophage colony-stimulating factor: a multilineage hematopoietin. Science 230:1171–1173

9. Ihle JN, Keller J, et al. (1983) Biologic properties of homogeneous interleukin-3. I. Demonstration of WEHI-3 growth factor activity, mast cell growth factor activity, P cell-stimulating factor activity, colony-stimulating factor activity, and histamine-producing cell-stimulating factor activity. J Immunol 131:282–287

10. Fung MC, Hapel AJ, Ymer S, Cohen DR, Johnson RM, Campbell HD, Young IG (1984) Molecular cloning of cDNA for murine interleukin-3. Nature 307:233–237

11. Yokota T, Lee F, Rennick D, Hall C, Arai N, Mosmann T, Nabel G, Cantor H, Arai K (1984) Isolation and characterization of a mouse cDNA clone that expresses mast-cell growth-factor activity in monkey cells. Proc Natl Acad Sci USA 81:1070

12. Gough NM, Gough J, Metcalf D, Kelso A, Grail D, Nicola NA, Burgess AW, Dunn AR (1984) Molecular cloning of cDNA encoding a murine hematopoietic growth regulator, granulocyte-macrophage colony-stimulating factor. Nature 309:763–767

13. Wong GG, Witek JS, Temple PA, Wilkens KM, Leary AC, Luxenberg DP, Jones SS, Brown EL, Kay RM, Orr EC, Shoemaker C, Golde DW, Kaufman RJ, Hewick RM, Wang EA, Clark SC (1985) Human GM-CSF: molecular cloning of the complementary DNA and purification of the natural and recombinant proteins. Science 228:810–815

14. Greenberg PL, Baker S, Link M, Minowada J (1985) Immunologic selection of hematopoietic progenitor cells utilizing antibody-mediated plate binding ("panning"). Blood 65:190–197

15. Levitt L, Kipps TJ, Engleman EG, Greenberg PL (1985) Human bone marrow and peripheral blood T-lymphocyte depletion: efficacy and effects of both T cells and monocytes on growth of human hematopoietic progenitors. Blood 65:663–679

16. Civin CI, Strauss LC, Brovall C, Fackler MJ, Schwartz JF, Shaper JS (1984) Antigenic analysis of hematopoiesis. III. A hematopoietic progenitor cell surface antigen defined by a monoclonal antibody raised against KG-1a cells. J Immunol 133:157–165

17. Beverly PCL, Linch D, Delia D (1980) Isolation of human hematopoietic progenitor cells using monoclonal antibodies. Nature 287:332–333

18. Sieff CA, Emerson SG, Mufson A, Gesner TG, Nathan DG (1986) Dependence of highly enriched human bone marrow progenitors on hemopoietic growth factors and their response to recombinant erythropoietin. J Clin Invest 77:74–81

19. Gabrilove JL, Welte K, Harris P, Platzer E, Lu L, Levi E, Mertelsmann R, Moore MAS (1986) Pluripoietin α: a second human hematopoietic colony-stimulating factor produced by the human bladder carcinoma cell line 5637. Proc Natl Acad Sci USA 83:2478–2482

20. Harris P, Ralph P, Gabrilove J, Welte K, Karmali R, Moore MAS (1985) Broad-spectrum induction by cytokine factors and limited induction by gamma interferon of differentiation in the human promyelocytic leukemia cell line HL60. Cancer Res 45:3090–3095

Haematology and Blood Transfusion   Vol. 31
Modern Trends in Human Leukemia VII
Edited by Neth, Gallo, Greaves, and Kabisch
© Springer-Verlag Berlin Heidelberg 1987

The *myc* Oncogene and Lymphoid Neoplasia: From Translocations to Transgenic Mice

S. Cory [1], A. W. Harris, W. Y. Langdon, W. S. Alexander, L. M. Corcoran, R. D. Palmiter, C. A. Pinkert, R. L. Brinster, and J. M. Adams

A. Introduction

The c-*myc* proto-oncogene encodes a nuclear phosphoprotein which probably plays a crucial role in growth control [4]. The protein has DNA-binding activity in vitro, but its function remains unknown. While avian retroviruses carrying the closely related v-*myc* sequence rapidly transform myeloid cells, the cellular *myc* gene has been strongly implicated in several types of lymphoid neoplasia. The fundamental mechanism releasing the oncogenic potential of c-*myc* is believed to be *deregulation* of its expression. Most chicken bursal lymphomas resulting from infection with avian leukosis virus, which does not itself bear an oncogene, carry a provirus near or within the c-*myc* gene [6]. About a quarter of T lymphomas with a retroviral aetiology also bear a c-*myc*-associated provirus [3]. Expression of the c-*myc* gene in these tumours is governed by the promotor and/or the enhancer in the viral long terminal repeat (LTR) [6, 13, 3]. In most plasmacytomas of the mouse and Burkitt lymphomas of man, a chromosome translocation couples the c-*myc* gene to the IgH constant region locus, presumably bringing c-*myc* under the control of factors that regulate heavy-chain expression [11, 8, 4].

B. Induction of B-Cell Neoplasia by a c-*myc* Gene Coupled to Immunoglobulin Enhancers

The evidence connecting deregulated *myc* expression with neoplasia was persuasive but remained circumstantial. Transgenic mice provided the means of testing the hypothesis directly. The results were dramatic: Transgenic mice carrying an essentially normal c-*myc* gene remained healthy, as did those with a *myc* gene devoid of its putative regulatory sequences [1]. However, mice bearing a cellular *myc* gene linked to the regulatory region within the LTR of the murine mammary tumour virus were found to have an increased susceptibility to mammary carcinomas [16]. Linkage to the SV40 promoter/enhancer also provoked tumours, but the incidence was relatively low [1]. In marked contrast, 13 or 14 of 15 primary transgenic animals bearing c-*myc* coupled to the heavy-chain enhancer (Eμ) developed lymphomas, as did six of 17 with c-*myc* linked to the kappa enhancer [1]. Thus c-*myc* is innoc·̇ous as a transgene in its "native state", or even ·̇fter removal of certain regulatory sequences. U... under the control of a strong exogenous regulatory element, however, it becomes a potent tumourigenic agent.

We have now made a detailed study of the disease induced by the Eμ-*myc* transgene (Harris et al., in preparation). Similar pathology was observed in several independent lines bred from different primary transgenic

---

[1] Royal Melbourne Hospital, Post Office, Melbourne, Victoria 3050, Australia

mice, so the chromosomal location of the transgene does not play a major role. One line was followed for five generations over 12 months, and 96% of the mice bearing the Eµ-*myc* locus succumbed to tumours before 6 months of age. In most cases, the disease pattern was a disseminated lymphoma involving most of the lymph nodes and often (but not always) the thymus. The lymphoma was usually accompanied by leukaemia. Some animals developed only a thymoma, or succumbed to a bowel obstruction probably caused by proliferation of tumour cells within the intestinal wall. The tumours grew rapidly, and most animals had to be killed within a month of exhibiting palpable inguinal lymph nodes. Transplantation tests established that the proliferating lymphoid cells were truly malignant. Indeed, injection of only 100 cells from one of the donors was sufficient to induce tumours in syngeneic recipients.

As expected, all the tumours exhibited relatively abundant transcription of the Eµ-*myc* transgene. Significantly, however, *no* normal c-*myc* transcripts could be detected [1], even after sensitive S1 analysis. Thus, the normal c-*myc* alleles had apparently been suppressed as a result of constitutive expression of the transgene. This result exactly parallels the situation found earlier in Burkitt's lymphomas and murine plasmacytomas, where expression was shown to be restricted to the translocated c-*myc* allele, the normal allele being essentially silent [2, 12]. The data favour the hypothesis [11, 14] that normal c-*myc* regulation operates via a negative feedback loop, possibly involving a repressor. The normal allele is presumed to be silenced via the protein produced by the rearranged allele, which is itself refractory to repression.

To identify which cell types had undergone transformation, about 50 different primary tumours were dissected from 20 mice and established in culture. All proved to be B lymphoid in origin, including those derived from thymic lymphomas. Thus, none displayed the T cell marker Thy 1, but all exhibited rearrangement of the J_H and/or Jκ loci and all expressed B-lineage-specific markers. While expecting to find B-cell neoplasia, we were somewhat surprised not to find any examples of T-cell or even mye-

loid tumours, because the IgH enhancer is thought to be active in at least some T and myeloid cells [7, 5].

The tumours represented several stages within the B differentiation lineage. About 40% were surface Ig-positive B cells, while the rest were pre-B cells of varying maturity having different combinations of IgH and κ rearrangements. While some were apparently stable, others continued to differentiate, either in vivo or in tissue culture. Thus, Eµ-*myc*-induced tumourigenesis does not totally prevent further differentiation.

C. Tumourigenicity Requires More than Deregulation of c-*myc*

Cancer has long been regarded as a multistep process. More recently, this concept has been represented in molecular terms as the need for collaboration between two (or more) oncogenes [9, 15]. It might be argued from the nearly invariant development of tumours by Eµ-*myc* mice that deregulation of c-*myc* is itself sufficient to cause cancer. However, this does not appear to be the case. Firstly, Eµ-*myc* tumours are clonal [1], even though all B-lineage cells express Eµ-*myc*. Secondly, the onset of tumours is highly variable and can occur as early as at 3 weeks of age and as late as at 6 months or more. Both these features argue that an additional change gives one cell a proliferative advantage over its fellows. Thirdly, and most compelling, in contrast to the tumour cells, the lymphoid cells from young animals which have not yet developed enlarged lymph nodes fail to induce tumours when injected in large numbers into syngeneic recipients [10]. Thus, even though the Eµ enhancer is turned on early in B-cell ontogeny, Eµ-*myc* mice exhibit a true pre-neoplastic phase.

D. Eµ-*myc* Promotes a Benign Polyclonal Expansion of Early B-Lineage Cells

Pre-lymphomatous Eµ-*myc* mice exhibit profoundly disturbed B-cell differentiation. We have analyzed this condition in some detail [10], because it provides a unique opportunity to discover the consequences of constitutive *myc* expression in "normal" cells. Cell surface marker analysis of foetal livers and the various lymphoid organs of young mice revealed a remarkable expansion of early B-lineage cells at the expense of mature B cells. The increase in pre-B cells is evident as early as at 18 days of gestation, and by 7 days after birth approximately half the cells in the bone marrow are pre-B cells, mostly the early Ly-5(B220)$^+$ ThB$^-$ type. In young adults, the expansion includes late pre-B cells and involves the spleen as well as the bone marrow. Overall, these animals exhibit a 4- to 5-fold increase in pre-B cell numbers and about a 30% reduction in sIg$^+$ B cells. Analysis of bone marrow DNA for J_H rearrangement established that the expansion is polyclonal and probably also includes a considerable number of pre-B cells which have not yet commenced J_H rearrangement.

The B-lineage cells in Eμ-*myc* mice differ remarkably in their size profile from those in normal mice. The small resting B cell and its immediate precursor, the small B220$^+$ ThB$^+$ pre-B cell, are absent from Eμ-*myc* mice, and all the B-lineage cells are large. Moreover, analysis of cellular DNA content suggests that at least one third of the pre-B and B cells are in cycle. We conclude that constitutive *myc* expression promotes and maintains B cells in cycle and may indeed preclude a G$_0$ state.

A notable consequence of Eμ-*myc* expression is the acquisition of the Ia surface antigen by many pre-B cells. Ia is normally found only on sIg$^+$ B cells, increasing after activation by mitogen or antigen plus growth factors. The significance of premature Ia expression is not clear, but it may indicate that enforced *myc* expression partially replaces the need for certain growth factors.

Clearly, Eμ-*myc* expression has affected both mitogenesis and differentiation within the B-cell lineage. To account for these results, we have proposed [10] that the level of c-*myc* expression is an important factor in setting the probability of self-renewal versus maturation during differentiation, with increased *myc* expression favouring self-renewal, as shown in Fig. 1.

In summary, constitutive *myc* expression strongly predisposes to malignancy. Its consequence for B-cell differentiation is to fa-

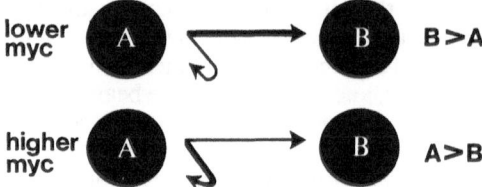

Fig. 1. A model for the role of c-*myc* in differentiation. The balance between self-renewal and maturation is set by the level of c-*myc* expression, with higher levels favouring self-renewal

vour self-renewal over maturation, and this results in a significant expansion of early cells. The increased proliferative potential presumably increases the probability of one cell within the population undergoing further change and becoming a fully malignant clone. It may be significant that the expanded population primarily comprises pre-B cells which actively undergo DNA rearrangement and which therefore may be more susceptible to genetic accident.

Acknowledgements. We thank Drs. D. Metcalf, B. Pike and T. E. Mandel for helpful discussions and M. Crawford, M. Trumbauer, L, Gibson and J. Mitchell for dedicated assistance. This work was supported in part by NIH grants CA-12421, HD-09172, HD-17321, the National Health and Medical Research Council (Canberra), the American Heart Association and the Drakensberg Trust. C.P. was a trainee on HD-07155.

References

1. Adams JM, Harris AW, Pinkert CA, Corcoran LM, Alexander WS, Cory S, Palmiter RD, Brinster RL (1985) Nature 318:533–538
2. Bern.. O, Cory S, Gerondakis S, Webb E, Adams JM (..83) EMBO J 2:2375–2383
3. Corcoran LM, Ad.. JM, Dunn AR, Cory S (1984) Cell 37:113–122
4. Cory S (1986) Adv Cancer Res 47:189–234
5. Grosschedl R, Weaver D, Baltimore D, Costantini F (1984) Cell 38:647–658
6. Hayward W, Neel BG, Astrin S (1981) Nature 290:475–480
7. Kemp DJ, Harris AW, Cory S, Adams JM (1980) Proc Natl Acad Sci USA 77:2876–2880
8. Klein G, Klein E (1985) Nature 315:190–195
9. Land H, Parada L, Weinberg R (1983) Nature 304:596–602

10. Langdon WY, Harris AW, Cory S, Adams JM (1986) Cell 47:11–18

11. Leder P, Battey J, Lenoir G, Moulding C, Murphy W, Potter H, Stewart T, Taub R (1983) Science 222:765–771

12. Nishikura K, ar-Rushdi A, Erikson J, Watt R, Rovera G, Croce CM (1983) Proc Natl Acad Sci USA 80:4822–4826

13. Payne GS, Bishop JM, Varmus HE (1982) Nature 295:209–214

14. Rabbitts TH, Forster A, Hamlyn P, Baer R (1984) Nature 309:592–597

15. Ruley HE (1983) Nature 304:503–607

16. Stewart TA, Pattengale PK, Leder P (1984) Cell 38:627–637

Haematology and Blood Transfusion   Vol. 31
Modern Trends in Human Leukemia VII
Edited by Neth, Gallo, Greaves, and Kabisch
© Springer-Verlag Berlin Heidelberg 1987

Cloning of Human Thymic Subcapsular Cortex Epithelial Cells by SV40 ori⁻ Transfection

S. Mizutani, S. M. Watt, and M. F. Greaves

A. Introduction

Critical steps in the early differentiation of T lymphocytes occur within the thymus. Bone-marrow derived cells migrating into this organ undergo extensive proliferation, clonal rearrangement of antigen receptor genes and an associated immunological "education" involving tolerance to self-antigens and positive selection for antigen recognition in association with self-MHC (Zinkernagel 1978; Haynes 1984; Rothenberg and Lugo 1985; Lo and Sprent 1986). The control of this complex process of commitment, expansion, clonal diversification, selection and maturation is not understood, but almost certainly involves selective interactions with distinct elements of the thymic stromal environment and diffusable regulators, thymic "hormones" or growth factors. The nonlymphoid stromal structure of thymic tissue consists of different types of epithelial cells derived from pharyngeal pouch endoderm or brachial cleft ectoderm, mesenchymal cells and bone-marrow derived histiocytes or interdigitating macrophages (Le Douarin et al. 1984; van de Wijngaert et al. 1984; Haynes 1984; Janossy et al. 1986).

Unravelling the interactions between developing T cells and microenvironmental components requires cell culture techniques similar to those established for bone marrow myelopoiesis (Dexter 1982) and methods for isolating and cloning individual stromal cell types.

Some success has been reported in culturing rodent and human thymic cells characterized as epithelial by desmosomes, tonofilaments, cytokeratins or membrane antigens and culture supernatants from such cells can regulate T-cell phenotype or immunological function (Itoh et al. 1981; Beardsley et al. 1983; Glimcher et al. 1984; Singer et al. 1985). However, cloned lines representing distinct subtypes of thymic epithelia have not so far been established.

The subcapsular epithelium of thymus has a distinctive structure and is probably the first site of interaction with migrating T-cell precursors (van de Wijngaert et al. 1984; Janossy et al. 1986; Haynes et al. 1984). We have sought to isolate and grow these epithelial cells by a combination of selective culture conditions and gene transfection techniques. We report here the successful establishment of two such cell lines which retain phenotypic properties of subcapsular epithelium and express some endocrine and growth-regulating functions.

B. Materials and Methods

I. Primary Epithelial Cell Culture

Thymic epithelial cells were derived from a 16-week-old human fetus obtained with the consent of the Ethics Committees of the Institute of Cancer Research and the Royal Marsden Hospital, London. Thymic tissue was minced and grown in a 25-cm² tissue culture flask in Dulbecco's modified Eagle's medium (DMEM; Gibco Biocult, Scotland),

Leukaemia Research Fund Centre, Institute of Cancer Research, London

supplemented with 5% (v/v) fetal calf serum (FCS; Sera Lab, England), 1.8×10^{-4} M adenine (Sigma, England), 5 µg/ml insulin (Sigma, England), 10^{-10} M cholera toxin (Sigma, England), 0.4 µg/ml hydrocortisone (Sigma, England) and 20 ng/ml epidermal growth factor (BRL). This AICHE-FCS medium was completely replaced each week.

II. Transfection of Primary Epithelial Cells

Epithelial enriched cultures were transfected 3 weeks after initiating their growth using calcium phosphate. Cells were transformed by cotransfection with the SV40 ori⁻ mutant 6-1 (Gluzman et al. 1980; Nagata et al. 1983) and PSV-2 neo. As controls, cells were either transfected with PSV-2 neo alone or were grown as primary epithelial cells as described above. One month after transfection, cells were selected with G418 (Gibco Biocult, Scotland) at a concentration of 1 µg/ml. The nontransfected cells were sensitive to these conditions and could not be maintained in culture for more than 4 weeks. Two colonies (SM1 and SM2) were obtained from the SV40 ori⁻ and PSV-2 neo cotransfected cultures and these reached confluence 3 weeks after transfection. These cells were passaged by trypsinization and replated at $1–2 \times 10^5$ cells per 25-cm² tissue culture flask.

C. Results and Discussion

I. Transformation of Thymic Epithelial Cells

Cells in the primary culture were morphologically heterogeneous and consisted of dense polygonal cell islands surrounded by spindle-shaped, elongated fibroblasts. Cytokeratin staining using the LE61 monoclonal antibody indicated that these cultures comprised 60%–70% epithelial cells. Cotransfection of such cells with SV40 ori⁻ and PSV-2 neo provided two transformed colonies, SM1 and SM2. SM2 cells appeared to be morphologically homogeneous, whereas

the SM1 consisted of two morphologically distinct cell types. The latter comprised small, elongated fibroblastoid cells and polygonal cells. SM1 cells were cloned by limiting dilution in the presence of a primary thymic stromal feeder layer which had been subjected to 5000 rads X-irradiation. Two weeks later two morphologically distinct subclones, SM1.1 and SM1.9, were selected by their G418 resistance. The former contained fibroblastoid-like cells, while the latter comprised the polygonal cells.

Both SM1 and SM2 cells had desmosomes and tonofilaments characteristic of epithelial cells (Fig. 1). The subclones SM-1 and SM1-9 also showed tonofilaments and desmosomes.

II. Immunocytochemical Characterization

Transfection of cells with SV40 ori⁻ was confirmed by the presence of nuclear large T antigen in the original SM1 and SM2 clones (Fig. 1; see Table 1 for summary). The epithelial nature of the original clones and of the SM1.1 and 1.9 subclones was shown by reactivity of intermediate filaments with cytokeratin antibodies (Lane 1982; Cooper et al. 1985; Chang 1986; see Fig. 1). Several monoclonal antibodies which had been characterized on thymic tissue sections (Haynes 1984; Janossy et al. 1986) were used to define the type of epithelial cells isolated (Table 1). Thy-1 human antibody reacted strongly with the original clones and the subclones as assessed by fluorescence microscopy and the FACS. Thy-1 has been shown previously to specifically identify the thymic subcapsular cortex epithelium (Ritter et al. 1981; Janossy et al. 1986). Thirty percent of cells in the original SM1 and SM2 clones were also positive for the A_2B_5 antigen, which is expressed on both the subcapsular cortex and medullary epithelia (Haynes et al. 1984). In addition, the RFD4 antibody, which recognizes the subcapsular cortex epithelium in pediatric thymus (Janossy et al. 1986) and the natural killer (NK) cell marker, Leu7, which occurs on the subcapsular cortex of the fetal thymus (Janossy et al. 1986) were found to react weakly with the isolated epithelial cells. These findings indicated that SM1 and SM2

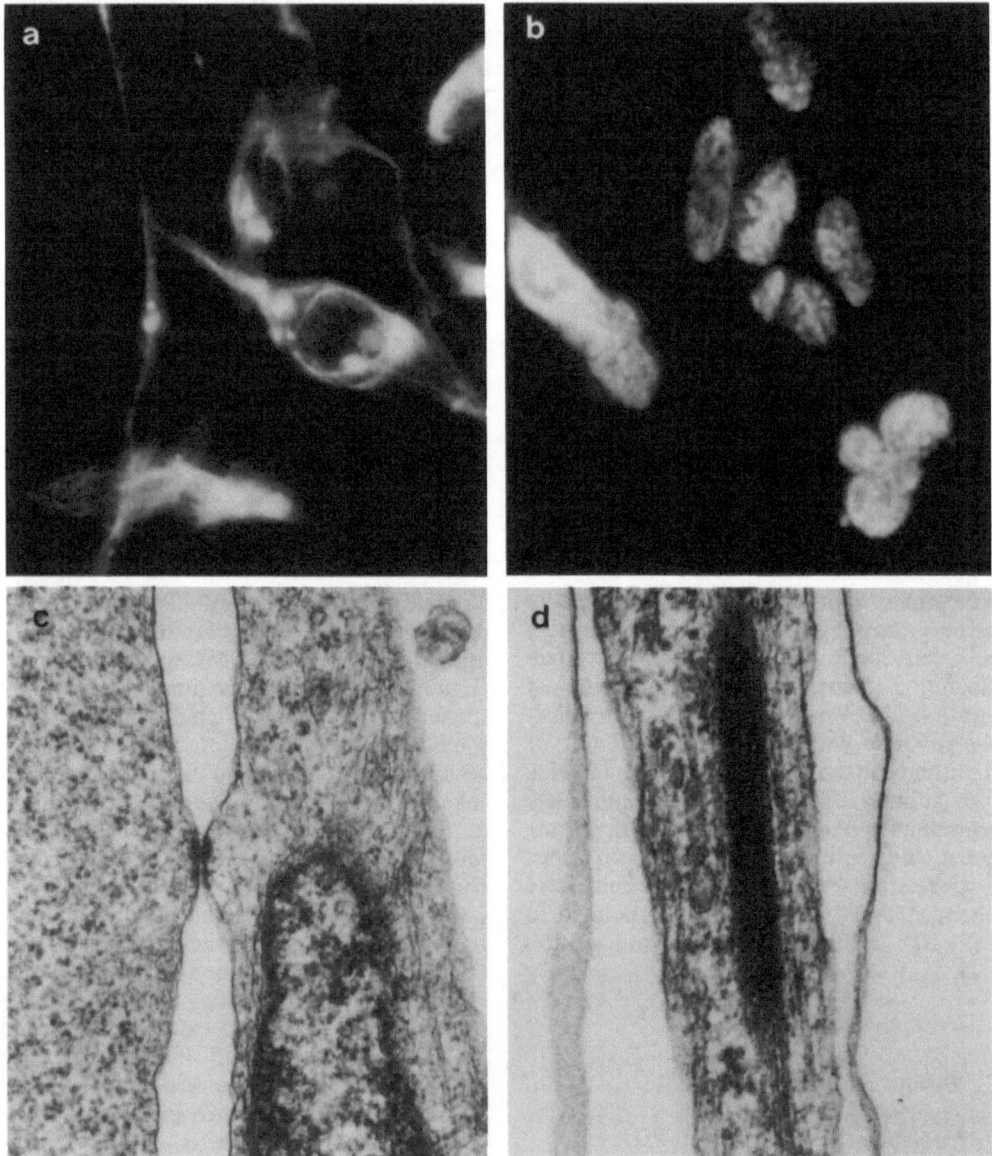

Fig. 1 a–d. Phenotypic characteristics of SV40-transformed human thymic subcapsular cells. **a** Immunofluorescent staining with monoclonal antibody (Le61) ω ~vtokeratin. **b** Immunofluorescent staining for nuclear SV40 large T antigen. **c** Desmosome. **d** Tonofilaments

were derived from subcapsular cortex epithelia and retained the antigenic phenotype characteristic of this tissue.

SV40 transformed subcapsular epithelial cells expressed HLA-AB determinants, but not HLA-DR, HLA-DQ, nor HLA-DP. Lymphoid cell markers which were defined by CD1, 2, 3, 4, 5, 7, 8, 10 specific monoclonal antibodies (Reinherz et al. 1986) could not be identified on any of the clones. There was also no reactivity with the 3.9 monoclonal antibody which recognizes thymic monocytes and interdigitating dendritic cells (Janossy et al. 1986).

Table 1. Phenotypic characterization of SV40 ori⁻ transformed thymic epithelial cells and their sublines

Clone	Positive cells (%)									
	Le61 Cyto-keratin[a]	SV40-T	Thy-1	A2B5	Chro-mo-granin	HLA-A, B	Trans-ferrin receptor	Vimen-tin	Leu7	RFD4
SM1	100	100	100	26	100	100	100	100	10	10
SM1-1	100	100	100	76						
SM1-9	100	100	100	83						
SM2	100	100	100	35	100	100	100	100	10	10

[a] Le61 recognizes a 40–45 daltons. Keratin components of intermediate filaments found predominantly in simple, nonstratified epithelia (Lane 1982; Cooper et al. 1985).
The clones did not react with antibodies to HLA-DR, CD1, CD2, CD3, CD4, CD5, CD7, CD8, CD10, Factor VIII, 3.9 (anti-monocyte), BI.3C5 (antihuman haemopoietic progenitor cell antigen, HPC-1), Desmin and HTLV-I P19.

III. Endocrine Characteristics of Subcapsular Cortex Epithelial Cells

The presence of chromogranin is thought to be indicative of endocrine function within the neuroendocrine system and has recently been identified in rat thymic epithelium (Hogue-Angeletti and Hickey 1985). Chromogranin was identifiable in the isolated clones SM1 and SM2 by an chromogranin monoclonal human antibody suggesting that these cells may have an endocrine function. There was no staining with antibodies to the thymic hormones thymopoietin and thymulin (FTS).

IV. Subcapsular Cortex Epithelial Cells Support Hemopoietic Cell Growth

It was of particular interest to know whether the SV40 transformed thymic epithelial cells could influence commitment to the T-cell lineage or induce the proliferation and differentiation of immature T cells. Fetal liver, a source of hemopoietic progenitors, was therefore cultured in methyl cellulose above irradiated or nonirradiated subcapsular cortex epithelial cells. Two types of colonies formed; one consisting of large tightly packed cells and the other comprising more diffuse colonies of smaller cells. Cytochemical staining revealed that both colony types contained nonspecific esterase (α-naphthyl butyrate esterase) and acid phosphatase positive cells. Morphologically, the more diffuse colonies contained small monocytes while the tightly packed colonies appeared to be activated macrophages. The monocyte-macrophage nature of these colonies was confirmed by positive staining of the cells with anti-3.9 and anti-HLA-DR monoclonal antibodies. None of the colonies tested contained either the intracellular TdT or T3δ markers characteristic of T-cell precursors (Furley et al. 1986). This culture system therefore did not support or induce early T-cell differentiation from fetal liver precursors, but rather induced macrophage development.

Thymic subcapsular epithelial cells probably have more than one function in T-cell development. Their physical location accords with a potential role in chemotaxis of bone marrow precursors and this possibility is being assessed with the clones described here. Our data suggest that these epithelial cells may also regulate the activity of immigrating or resident macrophages and thereby indirectly modulate the proliferation or selection of immature T cells. It is likely that thymic subcapsular epithelial cells are also involved in the activation of the dividing T lymphoblasts with which they are in intimate contact in situ (Janossy et al. 1986; Singer et al. 1986; Wekerle and Ketelson 1980). Further investigation of the functional activity of the SV40 transformed thymic epithelium cell lines is in progress.

Acknowledgements. We thank Drs. C. Marshall, H. Patterson and D. Toksoz for their advice and help concerning transfection procedures. Drs. Y. Gluzman and M. Fried for the SV40 ori⁻ DNA, Dr. R. Newbold for the PSV-2 neo plasmid, Drs. D. Lane, R. Hogue-Angeletti, N. Hogg, G. Janossy and B. Haynes for antibodies. We are grateful to L. Healy and L. Altass for technical assistance, to Mrs. J. Needham and Miss G. Parkins for typing the manuscript and to Dr. B. Haynes for providing advice and preprints prior to publication. This work is supported by the Leukaemia Research Fund of Great Britain

References

1. Beardsley TR, Pierschbacher M, Wetzel GD, Hays EF (1983) Induction of T-cell maturation by a cloned line of thymic epithelium (TEPI). Proc Natl Acad Sci USA 80:6005–6009
2. Chang SE (1986) In vitro transformation of human epithelial cells. Biochim Biophys Acta 823:161–194
3. Cooper D, Schermer A, Sun T-T (1985) Classification of human epithelia and their neoplasms using monoclonal antibodies to keratins: strategies, applications, and limitations. Lab Invest 52:243–254
4. Dexter TM (1982) Stromal cell associated haemopoiesis. J Cell Physiol [Suppl 1]:87
5. Furley AJ, Mizutani S, Weilbaecher K, Dhaliwal HS, Ford AM, Chan LC, Molgaard HV, Toyonaga B, Mak T, van den Elsen P, Gold D, Terhorst C, Greaves MF (1986) Developmentally regulated rearrangement and expression of genes encoding the T cell receptor-T3 complex. Cell 46:75–87
6. Glimcher LH, Kruisbeek AM, Paul WE, Green I (1983) Functional activity of a transformed thymic epithelial cell line. Scand J Immunol 17:1–11
7. Gluzman Y, Sambrook JF, Frisque RJ (1980) Proc Natl Acad Sci USA 77:3398–3902
8. Haynes BF, Scearce RM, Lobach DF, Hensley LL (1984) Phenotypic characterization and ontogeny of mesodermal-derived and endocrine epithelial components of the human thymic microenvironment. J Exp Med 159:1149–1168
9. Hogue Angeletti R, Hickey WF (1985) A neuroendocrine marker in tissues of the immune system. Science 230:89–90
10. Itoh T, Aizu S, Kasahara S, Mori T (1981) Establishment of a functioning epithelial cell line from the rat thymus. A cell line that induces the differentiation of rat bone marrow cells into T cell lineage. Biomed Res 2:11–19
11. Janossy G, Bofill M, Trejdosiewicz LK, Willcox HNA, Chilosi M (1986) Cellular differentiation of lymphoid subpopulations and their microenvironments in the human thymus. In: Muller-Hermelink HK (ed) Current topics in pathology, vol 75. Springer, Berlin Heidelberg, pp 89–125
12. Lane EB (1982) Monoclonal antibodies provide specific intramolecular markers for the study of epithelial tonofilament organization. J Cell Biol 92:665–673
13. Le Douarin NM, Dieterlen-Lievre F, Oliver PD (1984) Ontogeny of primary lymphoid organs and lymphoid stem cells. Am J Anat 170:261–299
14. Lo D, Sprent J (1986) Identity of cells that imprint H-2-restricted T-cell specificity in the thymus. Nature 319:672–675
15. Nagata Y, Diamond B, Bloom BR (1983) The generation of human monocyte/macrophage cell lines. Nature 306:597–599
16. Reinherz EL, Haynes BF, Nadler LM, Bernstein ID (ed) (1986) Human T lymphocytes (Leukocyte typing II, vol 1). Springer, New York
17. Ritter MA, Sauvage CA, Cotmore SF (1981) The human thymus microenvironment: in vivo identification of thymic nurse cells and other antigenically distinct subpopulations of epithelial cells. Immunology 44:439–446
18. Rothenberg E, Lugo JP (1985) Differentiation and cell division in the mammalian thymus. Develop Biol 112:1–17
19. Singer KH, Harden EA, Robertson AL, Lobach DF, Haynes BF (1985) In vitro growth and phenotypic characterization of mesodermal-derived and epithelial components of normal and abnormal human thymus. Human Immunol 13:161–176
20. van de Wijngaert FP, Kendall MD, Schuurman H. Rademakers LHPM, Kater L (1984) Heterogeneity of epithelial cells in the human thymus. An ultrastructural study. Cell Tissue Res 237:227–237
21. Wekerle H, Ketelson VP (1980) Thymic nurse cells – Ia bearing epithelium involved in T-lymphocyte differentiation. Nature 283:402–404

Haematology and Blood Transfusion Vol. 31
Modern Trends in Human Leukemia VII
Edited by Neth, Gallo, Greaves, and Kabisch
© Springer-Verlag Berlin Heidelberg 1987

v-H-*ras* Gene Reduces IL-3 Requirement in PB-3c Mastocytes In Vitro Followed by Autokrine Tumor Formation In Vivo

Asha P. K. Nair and Ch. Moroni

A. Introduction

The search for the physiological functions of proto-oncogenes has led to the notion that some code for products involved in control of mitosis as growth factor or growth factor receptor. This association of proto-oncogenes with mitotic control elements is consistent with the hypothesis that changes of various proto-oncogenes correlate with the multistep process of human carcinogesis, and there are numerous reports on specific proto-oncogene alterations in various human malignancies. What is not known, however, is the nature of the involvement of an altered proto-oncogene with the malignant process, i.e., the precise pathogenic role of the protein.

Of particular interest is the *ras* family of proto-oncogenes, H-, K-, and N-*ras,* which are activated by point mutations [1]. The ras-coded p21 proteins are located in the membrane, have a GTP-ase activity and show sequence homology to the G proteins, a family of proteins involved in the transmission of biological signals [2, 3]. It is thought that p21 proteins, by analogy with G proteins, mediate an external growth signal, by being associated with a specific growth receptor.

In acute myeloblastic leukemia (AML) cells one observes frequent activation of the N-*ras* gene [4–6]. As growth and differentiation of hematopoietic cells are controlled by a set of growth factors, it may be that in AML the activated N-*ras* gene exerts its putative pathogenic effect by being associated with the signal transmission of a growth factor necessary for myeloid cells.

To explore the role of *ras* genes on the growth regulation of hematopoietic cells, we have turned to a mouse model system. We report here that v-H-*ras* reduces the interleukin-III (IL-3) requirement of factor-dependent PB-3c mastocyte cells. Tumors derived from such cells grew in vitro without exogenous IL-3. In fact, we observed autokrine production of IL-3.

B. Material and Methods

I. Cells

PB-3c cells, a cloned line of normal, IL-3-dependent mouse mastocytes [7] were obtained from Dr. J.-F. Conscience. FDCP-1 cells [8], a myelomonocytic line of murine origin, requiring IL-3 or GM-CSF for growth were obtained through Dr. J. F. Delamarter. WEHI-3B cells, a myelomonocytic line producing IL-3 [9] were obtained from Dr. J.-F. Conscience. PB-3c and FDCP-1 cells were cultured in Iscove's modified Dulbecco medium (IMDM), supplemented with 50 μM β-mercapto-ethanol, 10% fetal calf serum, and IL-3 (see below).

II. Mitogenicity Assay

Cells were washed three times in IMDM lacking IL-3 and added to microtiter plates in 100-μl aliquots containing $2 \cdot 10^4$ cells. An IL-3 preparation (20 μl) was added to each

Friedrich Miescher-Institut, Postfach 2543, CH-4002 Basel, Switzerland well. Following 24 h incubation at 37 °C, 0.5 µCi of ³H-thymidine (25 Ci/nmol, Amersham, TRK 300) was added to each well. After 6 h, incorporation was determined by a filtration procedure and scintilation counting. When factor production by tumor cells was studied, the more sensitive FDCP-1 cells were used as targets, incubation in the presence of 20% tumor cell culture supernatant was carried on for 40 h, after which labelling was done for 8 h.

III. Antibody Inhibition of IL-3

An antibody preparation from rabbit serum directed against mouse IL-3 was generously provided by Dr. J. Ihle. Concentration was 30 ng/ml. For control, a rabbit anti-rat Ig preparation was used; 70 µl aliquots containing 20 µl mitogenic culture supernatant (from an A3-derived cell), 10 µl antibody preparation, and 40 µl IMDM were incubated for 2 h in microtiter plates. Then, $2 \cdot 10^4$ PB-3c cells in 50 µl were added. After 24 h incubation, ³H-thymidine incorporation was determined.

IV. Vector and Selection Procedure

Rash-1 cells were obtained from Dr. K. Marcu. They release a retroviral Zip vector [10] containing the v-H-*ras* gene inserted into the *Bam*H1 site and a gene for neomycin resistance. Supernatants from these cells transform NIH3T3 cells with a titer of $5 \cdot 10^3$ and transformed cells grow in the presence of G418 (data not shown).

To introduce the v-H-*ras* gene into PB-3c cells, $2 \cdot 10^6$ cells were incubated for 1 h in 2 ml rash-1 supernatant containing polybrene (16 µg/ml). Cells were spun and resuspended in growth medium. The next day, the selection for neomycin resistance was initiated by adding the drug G418. After about 3 weeks, infected PB-3c cells, but not control cells, contained viable cells growing in the presence of G418 at 1 mg/ml.

C. Results

In order to see whether introducing the v-H-*ras* gene into PB-3c cells would alter their

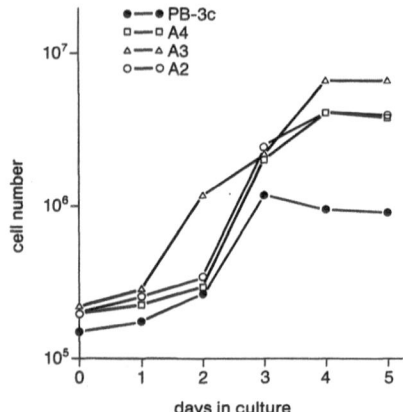

Fig. 1. Growth curve. Cells were cultured in the presence of IL-3 and numbers of cells were determined daily by Coulter counting

growth properties and/or IL-3 requirements, we infected these cells with a retroviral vector containing the v-H-*ras* gene and a gene for neomycin resistance as described in Methods. In this communication, we describe three infected cells, A2, A3, and A4. They express the *neo* gene, shown by growth in G418, and the v-H-*ras* gene, shown by elevated levels of p21 identified by immunoprecipitation with monoclonal antibody Y13-259 (data not shown).

Figure 1 shows the growth of A2, A3, and A4 compared with PB-3c. We observed an elevated saturation density of the infected cells, which showed a plateau at about $5 \cdot 10^6$ cells/ml, compared to PB-3c cells, which grew until 10^6/ml. This suggested that infected cells utilize IL-3 more efficiently and still grow when the factor becomes limiting. We therefore performed a titration of IL-3 on these cells. As can be seen in Fig. 2, the titration cur v_- ~f infected cells showed a shift to the right, indi...ing a 20-fold increased sensitivity to IL-3. Furthermore, infected cells, but not PB-3c cells, were able to grow at $^1/_{20}$ of the saturating concentration of IL-3 (data not shown).

We next wished to determine whether these cells would give rise to tumor formation following inoculation into syngeneic mice. As expected, PB-3c cells were nontumorigenic. Infected cells, in contrast, produced slowly growing tumors at the site of inoculation (Table 1). Most active were A3

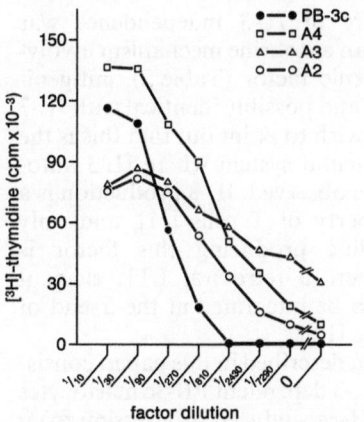

Fig. 2. Titration of IL-3. To 100-µl cultures containing $2 \cdot 10^4$ cells, 20 µl concentrated IL-3 preparation, diluted as indicated, was added. After 24 h, ^{3}H-thymidine incorporation during a 6-h pulse was determined. Values represent means of triplicate determinations

Table 1. Cumulative tumor incidence. Values show tumor incidence 5 months after subcutaneous inoculation into DBA/2 mice

Cell	No. of cells	Tumor/mice
PB-3c	10^6	0/5
	10^5	0/5
	10^4	0/5
A2	10^6	5/5
	10^5	4/5
	10^4	0/5
A3	10^6	5/5
	10^5	5/5
	10^4	5/5
A4	10^6	1/5
	10^5	0/5
	10^4	0/5

cells, where even 10^4 cells produced tumors in all mice inoculated.

To characterize these tumor cells further, we tried to establish them in culture. Generally, tumors, following surgical removal, yielded high numbers of cells which almost immediately took off in culture. To our surprise, their growth was now independent of IL-3 in all cases. Growth was observed also in the presence of G418, indicating that it was indeed the original cells which had be-

Table 2. Mitogenic activity of culture supernatant; 20-µl culture supernatants were assayed on FDCP-1 cells cultured in microtiter plates as described in the legend to Fig. 2

Culture	c.p.m. $\times 10^3$
–	0.2
A2D1	3.4
A2D5	2.3
A2D6	6.4
A2D7	12.7
A3D6	38.1
A3D7	98.0
A3D8	8.2
A4D1	6.4

come tumorigenic in vivo. We suspected that IL-3 independence might be the result of autoproduction of this factor by the tumor cells. We therefore tested supernatants from A2-, A3-, and A4-derived tumors for mitogenic activity. All cultures were positive (Table 2), however, to various degrees. The assay was performed on FDCP-1 cells, which are more sensitive to IL-3 than PB-3 cells, but the activity could also be demonstrated with PB-3 as target (data not shown). To see whether this activity was indeed IL-3, activity from a culture was preincubated with antibody to IL-3. Anti-IL-3, but not control antibody, was able to inhibit the mitogenic activity (Fig. 3).

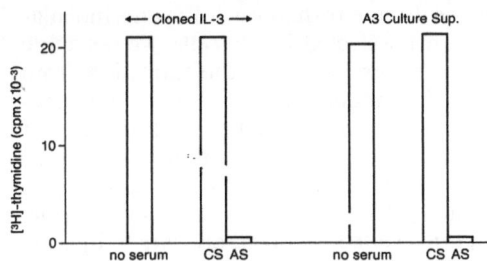

Fig. 3. Antibody inhibition. A mitogenic culture supernatant was incubated for 2 h with antibody and added to the cells. Cloned IL-3 (*left*) refers to recombinant *IL-3*, obtained from Dr. J. F. Delamarter, Biogen, and serves as positive control. A3 Culture Sup (*right*) denotes one of the A3-derived factor-independent lines. Mitogenic activity was determined as described in the legend to Fig. 1. *CS*, control antibody preparation; *AS*, anti-IL-3 preparation

D. Discussion

Introducing v-H-*ras* into IL-3 dependent PB-3c cells has allowed us to observe two phenomena. The first one is an altered growth behavior of v-H-*ras* containing cells, shown by a higher saturation density (Fig. 1). This is explainable by the increased response of these cells to limiting IL-3 concentration as shown in an IL-3 titration experiment (Fig. 2). As this effect on IL-3 utilization, observed immediately after selecting the cells with G418, correlates with increased p21 levels in these cells (data not shown) and is never found in cells selected with *neo* in the absence of v-H-*ras* (data not shown), we conclude that this effect is the result of the viral p21 protein. It may be that p21 acts as a G-like protein in association with a receptor for IL-3. But it may also be that v-H-p21 leads to an increase of number or affinity of the IL-3 receptor, or to the production of low levels of endogenous IL-3 in these cells which then could complement the exogenously added growth factor.

When infected cells were inoculated into syngeneic mice (Table 1), we observed tumor formation at the site of inoculation. It appears that the inoculated cells are not oncogenic per se but become so after going through at least one additional change. This conclusion is based on the observation that all tumors had become factor independent in vivo and remainded so following over 6 months of in vitro culturing. As we never observed tumor formation following inoculation of unselected PB-3c cells, we conclude that v-H-*ras* facilitates the transition from low IL-3 requirement to factor independence and tumorigenicity. The frequency of this transition is low, and differs amongst infected lines (compare tumor incidences in Table 1). Thus, v-H-*ras* plays a dual role. The early effect is direct, appears to operate in most if not all cells selected, affects IL-3 utilization, and is in its nature a premalignant change. Secondly, it conditions the cells, at some frequency, to proceed to a tumorigenic IL-3 independent phenotype.

The nature of IL-3 independence was found to be an autokrine mechanism involving a mitogenic factor (Table 2), antigenically related and possibly identical with IL-3 (Fig. 3). We wish to point out that this is the first experimental system where IL-3 autoproduction is observed. IL-3 production is a known property of T cells [11], and only non-T-cell line producing this factor is WEHI-3 where a retroviral LTR element was found to be integrated at the 5'-end of the *IL-3* gene [12].

The system described in this paper, consisting of the IL-3 dependent PB-3c mastocytes and their v-H-*ras*-induced progression from factor dependence, relaxed dependence to autokrine tumor growth represents a new and promising model to explore the multistep nature of carcinogenesis and the particular role of the *ras* oncogene.

References

1. Hall A (1984) In: Maclean N (ed) Oxford surveys on eukaryotic genes, vol 2. Oxford University Press, Oxford, pp 111–114
2. McGrath JP, Capon DJ, Goeddel DV, Levinson AD (1984) Nature (London) 310:644–649
3. Tanabe T, Nukada T, Nishikawa Y et al. (1985) Nature (London) 315:242–245
4. Gambke Ch, Singer E, Moroni Ch (1984) Nature (London) 307:476–478
5. Gambke Ch, Hall A, Moroni Ch (1985) Proc Natl Acad Sci USA 82:879–882
6. Bos JL, Toksoz D, Marshall CJ et al. (1985) Nature (London) 315:726–730
7. Ball PF, Conroy MC, Heusser CH, Davis JM, Conscience J-F (1983) Differentiation 24:74–78
8. Dexter TM, Garland J, Scott D, Scolnick E, Metcalf D (1980) J Exp Med 152:1036–1047
9. Warner NL, Moore MAS, Metcalf D (1969) INCI 43:963–???
10. Cepko CL, Roberts BE, Mulligan RC (1984) Cell 37:1053–1062
11. Ihle JN, Lee J, Rebar L (1981) J Immunol 127:2565–2570
12. Ymer S, Tucker WQJ, Sanderson CJ, Hapel AJ, Campbell HD, Young IG (1985) Nature 317:255–257

Haematology and Blood Transfusion   Vol. 31
Modern Trends in Human Leukemia VII
Edited by Neth, Gallo, Greaves, and Kabisch
© Springer-Verlag Berlin Heidelberg 1987

Modification of Oncogenicity of Tumour Cells by DNA-Mediated Gene Transfer

K. Hui and F. G. Grosveld

Major histocompatibility complex (MHC) class I antigens (termed H-2K, D and L in mice) are widely distributed on nearly all cell types and play an indispensable role in immunoregulation: lysis of neoplastic cells by cytotoxic T-lymphocytes depends on the expression of class I antigens. Therefore, it is of interest that certain tumours express decreased amounts of class I antigens. This may allow the tumours to escape immune surveillance *in vivo*.

The AKR leukaemia cell line K36, on which the H-2K^k antigen cannot be detected, is resistant to T-cell lysis and grows very easily in AKR mice. By expressing the

Institute of Molecular and Cell Biology, National University of Singapore, Kent Ridge, Singapore 0511

H-2K^k antigen in this tumour line following DNA-mediated gene transfer with a normal cloned *H-2K^k* gene, we demonstrated that the H-2K^k-positive transformed clones are rejected by AKR mice *in vivo* [1]. This is probably due to H-2K^k-restricted killing by cytotoxic T cells of the K36 tumour cells. However, since many tumour cells express MHC class I antigens, the lack of MHC-restricted cytotoxic T cells cannot be the sole explanation for the failure of hosts to abrogate tumour growth.

It has been reported that non-self class I antigens can be recognized as distinct targets by cytotoxic cells (allorecognition). We investigated in the work upon which this report is based the possibility of increasing the immunogenicity of tumour cells by expressing alloantigen on their cell surfaces following DNA-mediated gene transfer. We intro-

Table 1. Radioimmunoassay and tumour inducibility in AKR mice of H-2K^b-transfected K36 cells

Cell lines	Radiobinding with anti-H-2K^b monoclonal antibody (net I^{125} cpm)	Number of mice without tumour	
		Primary induction [a]	Secondary challenge [b]
K36	0	0/ 5	–
K^b-K36-2	360	10/10	0/10
K^b-K36-4	446	10/10	7/10
K^b-K36-6	386	10/10	6/10
K^b-K36-12	420	3/ 3	2/ 3
K^b-K36-13	460	2/ 2	0/ 2
K^b-K36-20	58	10/10	5/10

[a] 5×10^5 live K36 or K^b-K36-transformed clones were injected subcutaneously into AKR mice, and the number of mice without tumours was scored at the end of four weeks.
[b] Mice surviving after the primary challenge with the various K^b-K36-transformed clones were subsequently injected with 5×10^5 live K36 cells.

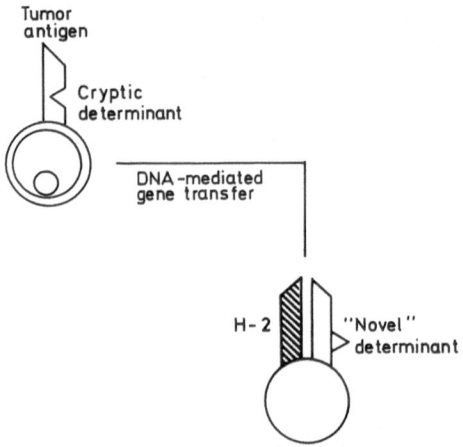

Fig. 1. Physical rearrangement of cell surface determinants

teresting to find that AKR mice immunized with some of these H-2K^b-transformed K36 clones are able to reject the original K36 tumour cells (Table 1). The induction of secondary immunity appears to be independent of the level of H-2K^b antigens expressed on these transformed clones (Table 1).

It is likely that during the process of DNA-mediated gene transfer with the *H-2K^b* cloned gene, some form of physical rearrangement of the cell membrane occurred and previously "cryptic (silent)" antigenic determinant(s) are exposed (Fig. 1). These previously weakly expressed antigenic determinant(s) are, in turn, being recognized and appear to be responsible for the secondary rejection of the original K36 tumour cells. The molecular and cellular mechanisms involved in the rejection of these transformed cells are now being studied.

duced the *H-2K^b* gene into K36 tumour cells (H-2^k) by DNA-mediated gene transfer. Transformed K36 clones which express a good level of the H-2K^b antigen are rejected (Table 1) by AKR (H-2^k) mice. It is also in-

Reference

1. Hui K, Grosveld F, Festenstein H (1984) Nature 311:750–752

Haematology and Blood Transfusion Vol. 31
Modern Trends in Human Leukemia VII
Edited by Neth, Gallo, Greaves, and Kabisch
© Springer-Verlag Berlin Heidelberg 1987

A Human Leukemic T-Cell Line Bears an Abnormal and Overexpressed c-myc Gene: Molecular and Functional Characterization of the Rearrangement *

D. Aghib[1], S. Ottolenghi[1], A. Guerrasio[2], A. Serra[2], C. Barletta[2], R. Dalla Favera[2], M. Rocchi[3], G. Saglio[2], and F. Gavosto[2]

Activation of the c-myc oncogene has been implicated in the pathogenesis of T-cell malignancies in species other than man [1–3]. In order to establish a possible involvement of this oncogene in human T-cell neoplasias, we investigated the c-myc structure in several primary T-cell tumors as well as in several leukemic T-cell lines. The Hut 78 line, derived from a Sezary syndrome patient, was found to have a c-myc rearrangement beginning immediately 3' to c-myc exon 3 [4]. The abnormal c-myc also appears to be duplicated compared to the normal allele. Chromosome analysis reveals that trisomy is the only cytogenetic anomaly involving chromosome 8, suggesting that the duplicated chromosome is the one carrying the abnormal c-myc and ruling out a Burkitt's type translocation event. This was also excluded by Southern blotting analysis, which showed a germ-line configuration of the heavy and light chain immunoglobulin genes. Similarly the involvement of the T-cell receptor α and β chain genes has been excluded. Compared to other human leukemic T-cell lines, the Hut 78 cells express a high

amount of c-myc transcript, suggesting that the 3' c-myc abnormality may cause a deregulation of the expression of the gene. The transmission of this c-myc anomaly through multiple cell passages and its duplication imply a possible relationship either with the leukemic process involving the Hut 78 cells or the maintenance of the abnormal phenotype in culture. In order to better characterize this c-myc anomaly, we have cloned in the 788 phage arms a genomic 13.8 kb Hind III fragment derived from the Hut 78 DNA, containing the entire c-myc gene and 4.5 kb of the 3' rearranged sequences. The latter are rich in human repetitive sequences, but a 1 kb EcoRI-Xba I fragment, useful as a probe, has been isolated.

By hybridization of this probe to a panel of human-hamster cell hybrids, the rearranged sequences may be located to either chromosome 2 or 8, while in situ hybridization confirms only the latter assignment. These data are compatible with the rearrangement in the Hut 78 cells being the product of either deletion of sequences 3' to the c-myc or an inversion linking originally distant sequences to c-myc. By genomic mapping of normal DNA, a 19 kb SacI fragment and a 16 kb BamHI, segments have been identified as the most useful to explore the structure of large DNA regions extending at both sides of this probe and, on this basis, we have investigated the possibility of rearrangements of this area in other T-cell leukemias and hematologic malignancies. Preliminary results show that two T-cell leukemias present abnormal SacI, but not BamHI fragments. Therefore, these data suggest that both cases bear rearrangements

* This work was supported by CNR-Rome "P.F. Oncologia" and by AIRC; A.D. is recipient of an AIRC fellowship
[1] Dipartimento di Genetica e di Biologia dei Microrganismi e Centro di Studio per la Patologia Cellulare del CNR, University of Milan; Dipartimento di Scienze Biomediche e di Oncologia Umana, University of Turin
[2] Department of Pathology and Kaplan Cancer Center New York University, School of Medicine, New York
[3] Ospedale Gaslini, Genova

having breakpoint positions similar to that present in the Hut 78 cell line.

Other 3' *c-myc* rearrangements in T-cell leukemias showing a t(8;14) translocation have been recently reported [5, 6]. In these cases a rearrangement with the genes coding for the TCR α chain has been demonstrated. Our study shows that a subset of T-cell leukemias may carry different *c-myc* abnormalities, arising from cytogenetically undetectable rearrangements within chromosome 8.

References

1. Payne GS, Bishop JM, Varmus HE (1982) Multiple arrangements of viral DNA and an activated host oncogene in bursal lymphomas. Nature 295:209–214
2. Neil JC, Hughes D, McFarlane R, Wilkie NM, Onions DE, Lees G, Jarrett O (1984) Transduction and rearrangement of the *myc* gene by feline leukemia virus in naturally occurring T-cell leukemias. Nature 308:814–820
3. Corcoran L, Adams J, Dunn A, Cory S (1984) Murine T lymphoma in which the cellular *myc* oncogene has been activated by retroviral insertion. Cell 37:113–122
4. Saglio G, Emanuel BS, Guerrasio A, Giubellino MC, Serra A, Lusso P, Rege Cambrin G, Mazza U, Malavasi F, Pegoraro L, Foa' R (1986) 3' *c-myc* rearrangement in a human leukemic T-cell line. Cancer Res 46:1413–1417
5. Mathieu-Mahul D, Caubet JF, Bernheim A, Mauchauffe' M, Palmer E, Berger R, Larsen CJ (1985) Molecular cloning of a DNA fragment from human chromosome 14 (14q11) involved in T-cell malignancies. EMBO J 4:3427–3433
6. Erikson J, Finger L, Sun L, ar-Rushdi A, Nishikura K, Minowada J, Finan J, Emanuel BS, Nowell PC, Croce CM (1986) Deregulation of *c-myc* by translocation of the α locus of the T-cell receptor in T-cell leukemias. Science 232:884–886

Haematology and Blood Transfusion   Vol. 31
Modern Trends in Human Leukemia VII
Edited by Neth, Gallo, Greaves, and Kabisch
© Springer-Verlag Berlin Heidelberg 1987

Association of the Heme-Controlled eIF-2α Kinase with Spectrin-Derived Peptides

G. Kramer, W. Kudlicki, S. Fullilove, and B. Hardesty

Translational control of mammalian protein synthesis frequently occurs at the level of peptide initiation. One control system in particular has been intensively studied during the last decade. It involves phosphorylation and dephosphorylation of the smallest subunit (α-subunit) of initiation factor 2, eIF-2. Two different substrate-specific protein kinases are recognized that can carry out this phosphorylation and thereby cause inhibition of protein synthesis. Both occur in inactive form in mammalian cells [1, 2]. One of the kinases is induced by interferon and activated by double-stranded RNA. The other is activated under conditions of heme deficiency and is known as the heme-controlled repressor (HCR) kinase. Our attention has been focused on the mechanism by which the latter enzyme is activated and regulated in rabbit reticulocytes and extracts of these cells. Although details of the mechanism are not known, we have evidence that spectrin and peptides derived from it by proteolysis are involved in its regulation [3]. Highly purified preparations of the kinase contain a prominent peptide of M_r 90000, a phosphopeptide of M_r 100000, and minor peptides of higher molecular weight. The M_r 90000 peptide was shown to react with monoclonal antibodies against spectrin, thus indicating that these peptides are structurally related. Other results led to the hypothesis that the M_r 90000 peptide is derived from the C-terminal end of β-spectrin by proteolysis [3]. Here we describe experiments extending our studies on the relationship of the M_r 90000 peptide to spectrin and the modulation of the HCR kinase activity by this peptide.

Monoclonal antibodies were raised against the highly purified M_r 90000 peptide. This peptide was separated from HCR activity and obtained in apparently homogeneous form by polyacrylamide gel electrophoresis run under nondenaturing conditions. The preparation had no HCR kinase activity. The purified peptide was injected directly into the spleen of a Balb/c mouse. After 4 days, the spleen was excised and the spleen cells were fused with myeloma cells. The resulting hybridomas were grown and assayed in an enzyme-linked immunosorbent assay (ELISA) [4]. Positive hybridomas were cloned; individual clones were grown and eventually used to produce ascites. Antibodies (IgM class for those used here) were partially purified by ammonium sulfate precipitation followed by chromatography on Sephacryl S300.

In Fig. 1, the antibodies raised against the M_r 90000 peptide are characterized. Peptides from an eIF-2α kinase preparation were separated on a denaturing polyacrylamide gel. Part of the gel was stained (Fig. 1 A, track 1). The other part was used for electrophoretic transfer of the peptides onto nitrocellulose which was then probed with the antibodies (Fig. 1 B). Subsequently, an antimouse second antibody linked to peroxidase was added. The reaction of the monoclonal antibodies with specific pep-

Clayton Foundation Biochemical Institute, Department of Chemistry, The University of Texas at Austin, Austin, Texas 78712, USA

* This research was supported in part by National Institutes of Health Grant CA16608 to B. Hardesty.

265

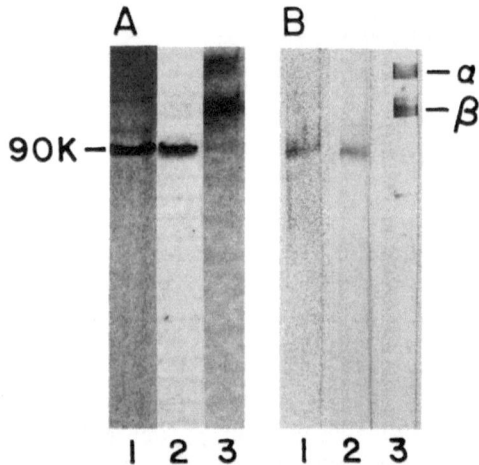

Fig. 1 A, B. Reaction of monoclonal antibodies with peptides of the eIF-2α kinase preparation and spectrin. Highly purified eIF-2α kinase (*track* 1), the isolated M_r 90 000 peptide (*track* 2), and spectrin (*track* 3) isolated from rabbit erythrocytes according to Ungewickell and Gratzer [5] were electrophoresed on 15% (*tracks* 1 and 2) or 7½% (*track* 3) polyacrylamide gels in sodium dodecylsulfate. **A** The separated peptides stained with silver (*track* 1) or Coomassie Blue (*tracks* 2 and 3). **B** Peptides stained with Biorad horseradish peroxidase substrate after the ELISA [4], using the monoclonal antibodies raised against the M_r 90 000 peptide

tides was visualized by applying a colored substrate for the peroxidase [3, 4], with the results shown in track 1. The M_r 90 000 peptide was visible after this ELISA procedure. For comparison, the purified M_r 90 000 peptide (track 2) and spectrin (track 3) were used as the antigen. There is evidence in the literature that monoclonal antibodies recognize both subunits of spectrin [6], and homology between both subunits has been demonstrated [7]. No reaction is seen when either the first or the second antibody is omitted, or when regulin [4] is substituted for spectrin. The data presented in Fig. 1 thus provide further evidence that the M_r 90 000 peptide of the eIF-2α kinase is related to spectrin. Interestingly, the same antibodies described above also recognize the prominent M_r 120 000 peptide found in a highly purified eIF-2α phosphatase fraction. This peptide has been detected by monoclonal antispectrin antibodies (Hardesty et al., this volume).

The monoclonal antibodies against the M_r 90 000 peptide characterized in Fig. 1 affect the activity of the eIF-2α kinase, thus indicating a regulatory function of the spectrin-derived peptide. Phosphorylation of eIF-2α is analyzed by polyacrylamide gel electrophoresis in sodium dodecylsulfate. An autoradiogram is prepared from the dried gel, the part of the gel containing the stained α-subunit is then cut, and its radioac-

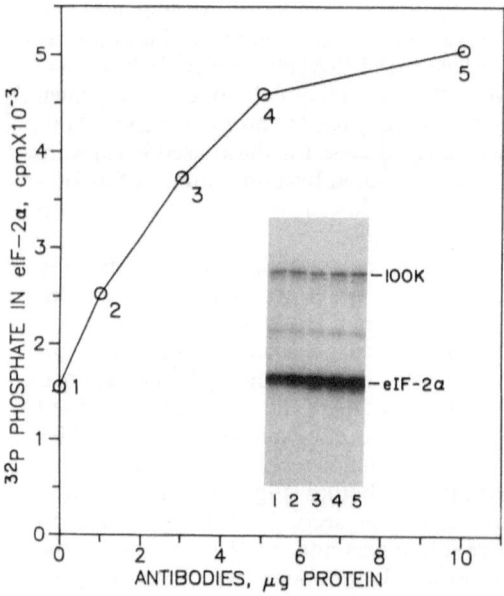

←

Fig. 2. Monoclonal antibodies against the M_r 90 000 peptide stimulate eIF-2α kinase activity. The enzyme (cf. 3; about 0.2 µg of protein) was preincubated with the indicated amount of the anti-M_r 90 000 antibodies for 30 min on ice before the phosphorylation reaction was carried out in the presence of about 5 µg eIF-2 and 0.1 mM $[\gamma^{-32}P]$ATP (about 2 Ci/mol). The reaction mixtures were analyzed on 15% polyacrylamide gels in sodium dodecylsulfate. The gel was stained with Coomassie Blue and an autoradiogram was prepared. The part of the gel corresponding to eIF-2α was then cut and its radioactivity determined by scintillation counting. The results from the incubations in the absence or presence of the antibodies are given. The *insert* represents the autoradiogram

tivity determined. Results thus obtained from the experiment with monoclonal antibodies are presented in Fig. 2. Preincubation of the eIF-2α kinase preparation with the anti-M_r 90 000 peptide antibodies causes an increase in enzyme activity. No such increase is seen when nonimmune mouse IgG or monoclonal antiregulin antibodies [4] are used (data not shown). These results appear to indicate that the HCR kinase is associated with a peptide derived from the β-subunit of spectrin which plays an important role in regulation of its enzymatic activity. Further implications of these findings are discussed in the chapter by Hardesty et al. in this volume.

References

1. Ochoa S (1983) Arch Biochem Biophys 233:325–349
2. Hardesty B, Kramer G, Kudlicki W, Chen S-C, Rose D, Zardeneta G, Fullilove S (1985) Adv Protein Phosphatases 1:235–257
3. Kudlicki W, Fullilove S, Kramer G, Hardesty B (1985) Proc Natl Acad Sci USA 82:5332–5336
4. Fullilove S, Wollny E, Stearns G, Chen S-C, Kramer G, Hardesty B (1984) J Biol Chem 259:2493–2500
5. Ungewickell E, Gratzer W (1978) Eur J Biochem 88:379–385
6. Kasturi K, Fleming J, Harrison P (1983) J Exp Cell Res 144:241–247
7. Speicher D (1986) J Cell Biochem 3:245–258

Haematology and Blood Transfusion Vol. 31
Modern Trends in Human Leukemia VII
Edited by Neth, Gallo, Greaves, and Kabisch
© Springer-Verlag Berlin Heidelberg 1987

Involvement of the Membrane Skeleton in the Regulation of the cAMP-Independent Protein Kinase and a Protein Phosphatase that Control Protein Synthesis

B. Hardesty, W. Kudlicki, S.-Ch. Chen, S. Fullilove, and G. Kramer

A. Introduction

The ultimate targets of transformational changes in cells are the sites in the nucleus and cytoplasm that affect transcriptional and translational control of protein synthesis. Products of a number of oncogenes appear to be analogues of proteins involved in the steps of transmembrane signalling (hormones or growth factors, receptors, G-type regulatory proteins, and tyrosine kinases), and some insight into the specific mechanism is emerging (for review see [1]). However, little is known of the mechanism by which a signal is transmitted from the inner surface of the plasma membrane to specific targets in the nucleus and cytoplasm. In at least some cases, changes in the activity of specific cyclic adenosine monophosphate (cAMP)-independent protein kinases and possibly phosphoprotein phosphatases appear to be involved. The counterpoised activities of these enzymes determine the phosphorylation level of their protein substrates.

Eukaryotic peptide initiation factor 2 (eIF-2) can be phosphorylated in its smallest subunit – α-subunit – by either of two different substrate-specific, cAMP-independent kinases (for review see [2, 3]). This phosphorylation blocks the release of guanosine

diphosphate (GDP) from eIF-2 by the GDP exchange factor [4, 5] and thereby prevents eIF-2 from functioning in peptide initiation. One kinase is induced by interferon and is activated by double-stranded RNA. It also appears to be involved in adenovirus-mediated control of host cell protein synthesis [6]. The other kinase is activated in reticulocytes under conditions of heme deficiency and is known as the heme-controlled repressor (HCR) (cf. [2, 3]). An eIF-2α kinase activated during heat shock of HeLa cells [7] was shown to be inhibited by antibodies against reticulocyte HCR [8]. Both kinases appear to phosphorylate the same serine residue(s) [9] in the N-terminal segment of eIF-2α [10, 11]. Here we describe the effect of the β-subunit of spectrin and peptides derived from it on the activity of the HCR protein kinase and protein phosphatase from rabbit reticulocytes that phosphorylate and dephosphorylate eIF-2α.

The isolation and characterization of these enzymes have proven to be particularly difficult. Both enzymes appear to be physically heterogeneous in size and may exist in inactive form in fresh cell extracts. Problems arise in the accurate quantitation of the enzymes (active and inactive forms) that are present in different cell fractions, particularly those containing membranes and the membrane skeleton. Although the details remain unclear, some insight into the basis for the physical heterogeneity and mechanism by which the enzymes are regulated is beginning to emerge.

Clayton Foundation Biochemical Institute, Department of Chemistry, The University of Texas at Austin, Austin, Texas 78712, USA

B. HCR Kinase

Although heterogeneous, as judged by polyacrylamide gel electrophoresis in sodium dodecyl sulfate (SDS), our highly purified preparations of the kinase (purified > 5000-fold on the basis of activity) contain a prominent M_r 90000 peptide (cf. Fig. 1) that does not have enzymatic activity by itself [12, 13]. Repeated attempts to isolate monoclonal hybridomas that would produce antibodies against the kinase resulted in antibodies that recognized this M_r 90000 peptide [13]. As shown in Fig. 1, these antibodies

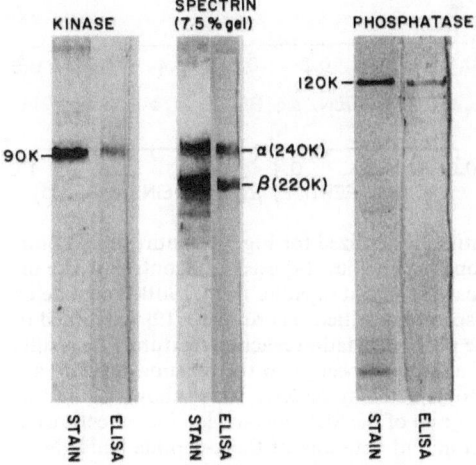

Fig. 1. Monoclonal antispectrin antibodies recognize both the M_r 90000 peptide of the eIF-2α kinase and the M_r 120000 peptide of the phosphoprotein phosphatase. Highly purified eIF-2α kinase or phosphatase was electrophoresed on 15% polyacrylamide gels in SDS. Part of the gel was stained with silver (ICN Rapid Ag Stain), the other part being electrophoretically transferred onto nitrocellulose which was then probed with the monoclonal antispectrin antibodies in an enzyme-linked immunosorbent assay (ELISA) (cf [14]). The antibodies used were of the IgM class and had been purified from ascites fluid by 0%–50% ammonium sulfate precipitation followed by chromatography on Sephacryl S300. Spectrin, isolated from rabbit erythrocytes according to [15], is shown for comparison. The spectrin subunits were separated on a 7½% polyacrylamide gel in SDS and then treated as described above, except that the first track is from a Coomassie-stained gel. 90K, 120K, 220K, and 240K denote the respective peptides of that size

also react with spectrin, the major protein component of the erythroid membrane skeleton. Without exception, of the considerable number of monoclonal antibody isolates we have tested, all those that recognize the M_r 90000 peptide also recognize β-spectrin (M_r 220000). Most of the monoclonal antibodies also recognize the M_r 240000 α-subunit of spectrin, as shown in Fig. 1. There is considerable sequence homology between the two spectrin subunits [16].

Similarity between the M_r 90000 peptide and β-spectrin is also indicated by phosphorylation with two protein kinases. The β-subunit of spectrin contains one threonine and three serine residues within a M_r 10000 region at the C-terminal end that can be phosphorylated [17]. In vitro, the catalytic subunit of the cAMP-dependent protein kinase and the cAMP-independent casein kinase II phosphorylate the β-subunit of spectrin. Both of these protein kinases also phosphorylate the M_r 90000 peptide [13]. Furthermore, a phosphorylated M_r 90000 peptide can be derived in vitro by proteolysis from phosphorylated β-spectrin [13]. Considered together, these results indicate that the M_r 90000 peptide is structurally related to a segment at the C-terminal end of β-spectrin and probably derived from it by proteolysis.

At the stage of purification of the kinase used for Fig. 1, the M_r 90000 peptide is the most abundant component in the preparation. However, traces of other spectrin peptides are present, and we have isolated fractions with high HCR kinase activity in which the most abundant component is one of several higher molecular weight spectrin fragments. Some of these fractions contain no M_r 90000 peptide. β-spectrin itself and the M_r 90000 fragment have been isolated and have no detectable kinase or phosphatase activity. The catalytic subunit of the kinase appears to be a M_r 95000 peptide that is associated with the spectrin fragments. Attempts to isolate active kinase free of all spectrin peptides have not been successful.

The enzymatic activity of the HCR kinase is markedly increased either by the antispectrin monoclonal antibodies that recognize the M_r 90000 peptide or by the M_r 90000 peptide itself, β-spectrin, and some of the spectrin peptides of intermediate size. The

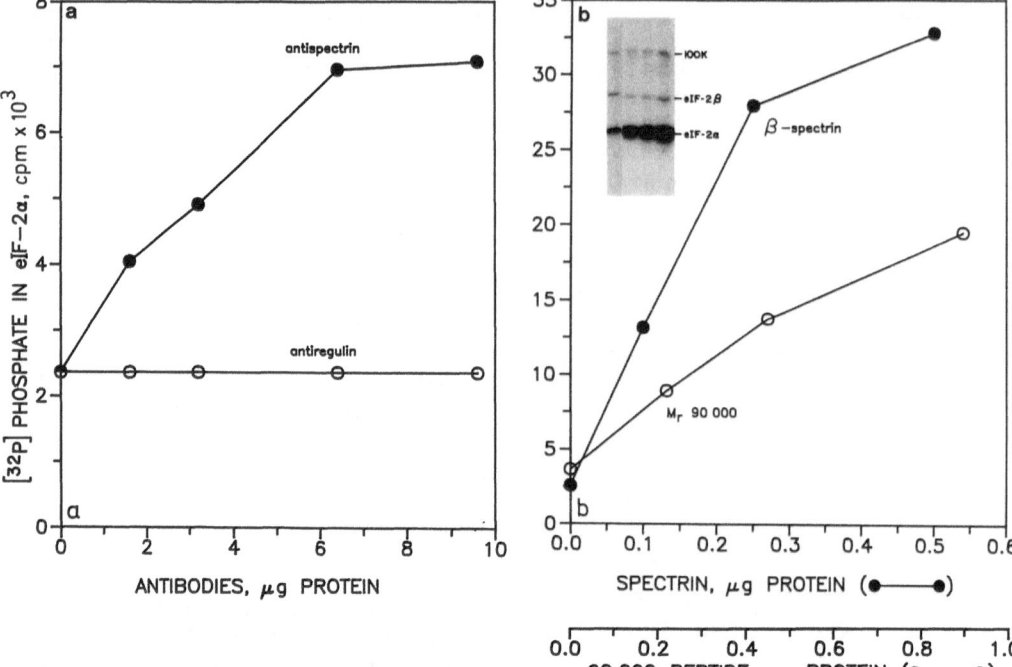

Fig. 2 a, b. Stimulation of HCR eIF-2α kinase activity by antispectrin monoclonal antibodies or by β-spectrin and M_r 90 000 peptide. About 0.2 μg of protein from the HCR kinase preparation was incubated with 5 μg of purified eIF-2 and 0.1 mM [γ^{32}P] adenosine triphosphate (2 Ci/mmol) under the conditions previously described [13]. The samples were electrophoresed in SDS on 15% polyacrylamide gels; the eIF-2α band was then excised and its radioactivity determined by liquid scintillation counting. **a** The HCR kinase preparation was preincubated for 30 min on ice with the indicated amount of the antispectrin monoclonal antibodies utilized for Fig. 1 or antiregulin monoclonal antibodies [14] used as a control. **b** The indicated amount of either the M_r 90 000 peptide or β-spectrin purified according to [19] was added to the phosphorylation reaction mixture. The results of adding β-spectrin to the reaction mixture are also depicted in the *inset*, which shows an autoradiogram of the SDS polyacrylamide gel before excision and counting of the α-peptide band. Note the large increase in eIF-2α phosphorylation, with little or no effect on the phosphorylation of eIF-2β or the M_r 100 000 phosphopeptide of the HCR kinase preparation

effect on eIF-2α phosphorylation of the antibodies used for Fig. 1 is shown in Fig. 2 a. The effect of the M_r 90 000 peptide and β-spectrin on enzymatic activity is shown in Fig. 2 b. The level of eIF-2α phosphorylation was determined by excising and counting the α-subunit from SDS polyacrylamide gels. The inset in Fig. 2 b shows an autoradiogram of such a gel. The mechanism by which kinase activity is increased is not clear.

C. Phosphoprotein Phosphatase

A Mn^{2+}-dependent protein phosphatase with high activity for dephosphorylation of eIF-2α was isolated from rabbit reticulocytes as part of our effort to characterize the components responsible for translational regulation of protein synthesis. The enzyme has many of the physical characteristics that are described above for the HCR kinase, ex-

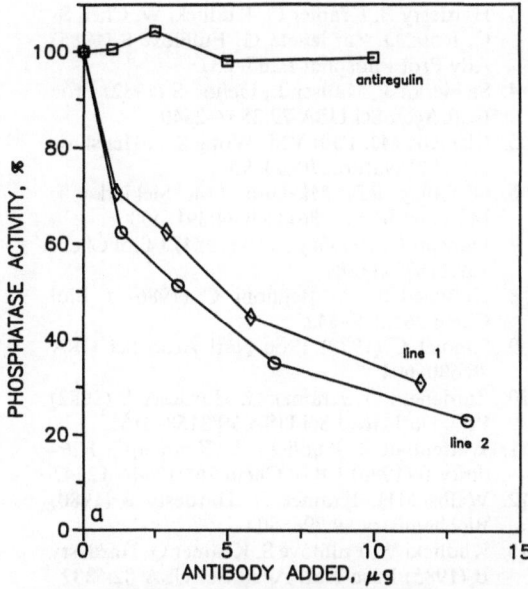

Fig. 3. Inhibition of protein phosphatase activity by antispectrin monoclonal antibodies. The phosphatase preparation (0.1 μg of protein) was incubated with [^{32}P]eIF-2(α-P) (about 46 pmol of [^{32}P]phosphate, 1 Ci/mmol). The dephosphorylation reaction was carried out in the presence of 0.25 mM Mn^{2+} and released phosphate determined as described previously [18]. 100 percent of enzyme activity equals the release of 5.0 pmol of [^{32}P]phosphate from the substrate in a 10-min dephosphorylation reaction. The enzyme preparation was preincubated for 1 h on ice with the indicated amount of monoclonal antibodies from three hybridoma lines. *Line 1* is that used in Fig. 1. *Line 2* is the monoclonal hybridoma isolate described by Kramer et al., this volume. Antiregulin monoclonal antibodies [14] were used as a control

cept that the most abundant component of highly purified preparations is a M_r 120 000 peptide (Fig. 1). Minor peptides of lower molecular weight are visible in the silver-stained track. Most monoclonal antibody isolates that react with β-spectrin and the M_r 90 000 peptide of the HCR kinase preparation also recognize the M_r 120 000 peptide, as exemplified in Fig. 1. However, in contrast to their effect on the HCR kinase, some of these monoclonal antibody isolates inhibit the enzymatic activity of the phosphatase, as indicated by the data in Fig. 3. Monoclonal antibodies from hybridoma

line 1 were those used for the data in Figs. 1 and 2. Monoclonal antibodies against regulin, a protein with physical properties somewhat similar to those of spectrin [14], have no effect on this protein phosphatase.

D. Discussion

The results described above indicate that both the HCR kinase and the phosphoprotein phosphatase interact with β-spectrin and peptides probably derived by proteolysis from its C-terminal region. The enzymatic activity of the kinase is increased by the interaction, whereas the activity of the phosphatase is decreased. Intact $(α, β)_2$ spectrin has no effect on the enzymatic activity of either the phosphatase or the kinase. It appears that proteolytic generation of the β-spectrin peptides in vivo would increase eIF-2α phosphorylation and reduce protein synthesis. The β-subunit itself has been shown to be a potent inhibitor of protein synthesis in the reticulocyte lysate system [19]. Association with β-spectrin and peptides derived from it appears to account for some of the physical properties of both the HCR kinase and the phosphoprotein phosphatase. In purified preparations both appear to be highly elongated structures, apparently reflecting their association with the spectrin peptides. In both cases the axial ratio was calculated from the Stokes' radius, measured by gel filtration chromatography, and from the sedimentation coefficient, measured by glycerol gradient centrifugation.

Spectrin [20, 21] is an unusually protease-sensitive 200 nm rod. The α- and β- subunits are aligned side to side to form heterodimers which associate head to head to form a tetrameric structure that is the major component of the two-dimensional network which is the membrane skeleton of mammalian erythrocytes. It is characteristic of erythroid cells; however, proteins with extensive structural homology to the β-subunit of spectrin occur in nonerythroid cells [22, 23]. Brain tissue contains an α, β-dimer [24] that appears to be structurally related to erythroid spectrin.

There is some indication that the C-terminal portion of the β-spectrin subunit may be related to certain other M_r 90 000 peptides found to be a component of steroid [25, 26] and glucocorticoid [27, 28] receptors, of the pp60^{src} complex [29] and the M_r 84000–90000 heat shock protein [30]. We have observed that monoclonal antibodies (obtained from Dr. David Toft, Mayo Clinic, Rocheser, Minnesota [26]) which recognize the M_r 90000 peptide of the progesterone receptor also recognize the β-subunit of spectrin (unpublished data). Toft and coworkers have demonstrated cross-reactivity of the progesterone-receptor-associated M_r 90000 peptide and the peptide of the same size that can form a cytosolic complex with pp60^{src} [31]. Also, the steroid receptor M_r 90000 peptide and a heat shock protein (M_r 90000) were shown to be very similar, if not identical, by peptide mapping [32].

The effects of heat shock and stress on protein synthesis in mammalian cells have been studied intensively. Heat shock causes a dramatic shut-off of protein synthesis followed by accumulation of several characteristic heat shock proteins, including the M_r 90000 peptide. The heat shock response has been attributed to an effect on the cytoskeleton [33, 34]. Alterations in the cytoskeleton organization that lead to release of β-spectrin or peptides derived from it may be involved in the inhibition of protein synthesis caused by heat shock. Several recent reports indicate that some oncogenes may affect the cytoskeleton. Aberrant cytoskeletal organization was observed in B-cell leukemia and hairy-cell leukemia [35]. The v-*fgr* oncogene of the Gardner-Rasheed strain of feline sarcoma virus encodes a 128-amino acid peptide from γ-actin [36], and the *onc D* gene from human colon carcinoma appears to code for a protein with a 221-amino acid sequence from nonmuscle tropomyosin [37].

Acknowledgments. This work was supported in part by Grant No. CA16608 to B.H. from the National Cancer Institute, National Institutes of Health.

References

1. Hunter T, Cooperman JA (1985) Annu Rev Biochem 54:897–930
2. Ochoa S (1983) Arch Biochem Biophys 223:325–349
3. Hardesty B, Kramer G, Kudlicki W, Chen S-C, Rose D, Zardeneta G, Fullilove S (1985) Adv Prot Phosphat I:235–257
4. Siekierka J, Mauser L, Ochoa S (1982) Proc Natl Acad Sci USA 79:2537–2540
5. Clemens MJ, Pain VM, Wong S-T, Henshaw E (1982) Nature 296:93–95
6. O'Malley RP, Mariano TM, Siekierka J, Mathews MB (1986) Cell 44:391–400
7. Duncan R, Hershey JWB (1984) J Biol Chem 259:11882–11889
8. DeBenedetti A, Baglioni C (1986) J Biol Chem 261:338–342
9. Samuel C (1979) Proc Natl Acad Sci USA 76:600–604
10. Zardeneta G, Kramer G, Hardesty B (1982) Proc Natl Acad Sci USA 79:3158–3161
11. Wettenhall R, Kudlicki W, Kramer G, Hardesty B (1986) J Biol Chem 261:12444–12447
12. Wallis MH, Kramer G, Hardesty B (1980) Biochemistry 19:798–804
13. Kudlicki W, Fullilove S, Kramer G, Hardesty B (1985) Proc Natl Acad Sci USA 82:5332–5336
14. Fullilove S, Wollny E, Stearns G, Chen S-C, Kramer G, Hardesty B (1984) J Biol Chem 259:2493–2500
15. Ungewickell E, Gratzer W (1978) Eur J Biochem 88:379–385
16. Speicher D (1986) J Cell Biochem 3:245–258
17. Harris HW, Lux SE (1980) J Biol Chem 255:11512–11520
18. Wollny E, Watkins K, Kramer G, Hardesty B (1984) J Biol Chem 259:2484–2492
19. Kudlicki W, Kramer G, Hardesty B (1986) FEBS Lett 200:271–274
20. Marchesi VT (1983) Blood 61:1–11
21. Bennett V (1985) Annu Rev Biochem 54:273–304
22. Lazarides E, Nelson WJ (1982) Cell 31:505–508
23. Nelson WJ, Lazarides E (1983) Proc Natl Acad Sci USA 80:363–367
24. Davis J, Bennett V (1983) J Biol Chem 258:7757–7766
25. Dougherty JJ, Puri RK, Toft DO (1984) J Biol Chem 259:8004–8009
26. Riehl RM, Sullivan WP, Vroman BT, Bauer VJ, Pearson GR, Toft DO (1985) Biochemistry 24:6586–6591
27. Housley PR, Sanchez ER, Westphal HM, Beato M, Pratt WB (1985) J Biol Chem 260:13810–13817
28. Mendel DB, Bodwell JE, Gametchu B, Harrison RW, Munck A (1986) J Biol Chem 261:3758–3763
29. Brugge J, Yonemoto W, Darrow D (1983) Mol Cell Biol 3:9–19
30. Sanchez ER, Toft DO, Schlesinger MJ, Pratt WB (1985) J Biol Chem 260:12398–12401

31. Schuh S, Yonemoto W, Brugge J, Bauer VJ, Riehl RM, Sullivan WP, Toft DO (1985) J Biol Chem 260:14292–14296

32. Catelli MG, Binart N, Jung-Testas I, Renoir JM, Baulieu EE, Feramisco JR, Welch WJ (1985) EMBO J 4:3131–3135

33. Van Bergen en Henegouwen P (1985) Dissertation, University of Utrecht

34. Tanguay RM (1983) Can J Biochem Cell Biol 61:387–394

35. Caligaris-Cappio F, Bergui L, Tesio L, Carbascio G, Tousco F, Marchisio PC (1986) Blood 67:233–239

36. Naharro G, Robbins K, Reddy E (1984) Science 223:63–65

37. Martin-Zanca D, Hughes S, Barbacid M (1986) Nature 319:743–748

Haematology and Blood Transfusion   Vol. 31
Modern Trends in Human Leukemia VII
Edited by Neth, Gallo, Greaves, and Kabisch
© Springer-Verlag Berlin Heidelberg 1987

Lineage Determination During Haemopoiesis

G. Brown [1], C. M. Bunce [1], J. M. Lord [1], P. E. Rose [2], and A. J. Howie [3]

"How do cells differentiate into one type or another? is one of the most fundamental questions in cell biology and is also pertinent to the problem of cell transformation, which may often involve progenitor cells [1] and derangement of developmental processes. Commitment of haemopoietic progenitor cells to differentiation along at least five distinct pathways during haemopoiesis continues throughout life, and the haemopoietic system provides an ideal model for studying the above problem. At present, it is not clear whether the haemopoietic stem cell can transform directly into a cell committed to differentiation along any one of five succeeding lines or whether this cell undergoes a series of binary decision-making steps throughout various cell cycles.

In a new model for the development of haemopoietic progenitor cells we have suggested that potentials for development along a pathway of differentiation are expressed individually, consecutively and in a particular order determined within the genome [2]. The model considers the fate of a haemopoietic stem cell which is induced to differentiate and gives rise to a cell(s) committed to decision-making that has lost its self-maintaining capacity. In the model, the committed progenitor cell first acquires a capacity for, and is then restricted to, mega-karyocyte differentiation. As this cell divides

it gives rise to cells able to develop towards megakaryocytes and to progress to the next stage of commitment to erythroid differentiation. This division process(es) may generate a cell(s) which is channelled towards megakaryopoiesis and a cell(s) which progresses to the next stage of commitment. Alternatively, progeny able to respond to inducers of megakaryopoiesis which fail to receive a signal for differentiation towards megakaryocytes progress to the next stage in the sequence of commitment during progenitor cell development. In this case, as the progenitor cell ages it loses the ability to respond to inducers of megakaryopoiesis as the potential for erythropoiesis is expressed. Subsequently and as above, in a genetically predetermined order, the potentials to respond to inducers of neutrophil, monocyte, B-cell and T-cell differentiation are expressed.

The notion that lineage potentials may be sequentially determined during haemopoiesis arises from studies of variant lines derived from the promyeloid cell line HL60 [2]. The variant cell lines were selected in medium containing 1.25% DMSO, which gives optimal induction of neutrophil differentiation within HL60 cultures. When cultured in 1.5%–2.0% DMSO, the lines show a variable capacity for differentiation induction into neutrophils. In contrast, when treated with inducers of monocyte differentiation, such as 12-0-tetradecanoylphorbol-13-acetate (TPA), the lines either differentiate like HL60 cells or fail to respond to a wide range of concentrations (4–50 nM TPA) of inducers of monocyte differentiation [2]. The variant lines are assumed to reflect the inher-

[1] Department of Immunology, University of Birmingham, Birmingham B15 2TJ, England
[2] Pathology Laboratory, Warwick CV34 5BJ, England
[3] Department of Pathology, University of Birmingham, Birmingham B15 2TJ, England

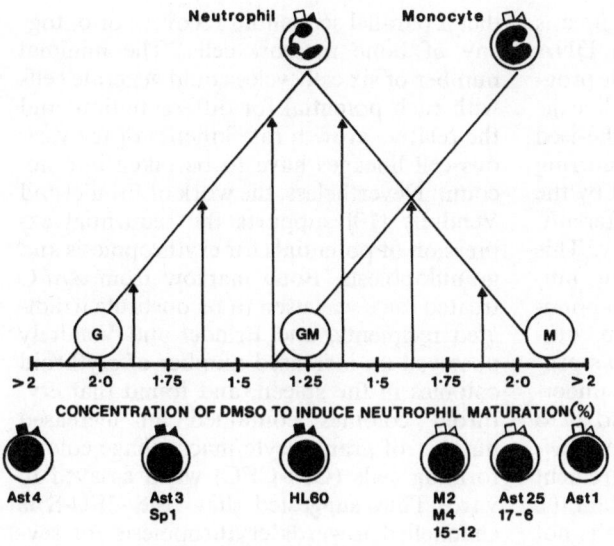

Neutrophil □▲   Monocyte □▲

G   GM   M

>2   2·0   1·75   1·5   1·25   1·5   1·75   2·0   >2

CONCENTRATION OF DMSO TO INDUCE NEUTROPHIL MATURATION(%)

Ast 4   Ast 3   HL60   M2   Ast 25   Ast 1
             Sp1   M4   17-6
                                      15-12

Fig. 1. Positions of variant cell lines derived from HL60 within a proposed developmental sequence. They are arranged in sequence as regards their responsiveness to inducer of neutrophil and monocyte differentiation and as to whether they express the AGF4.48 (▲) and AGF4.36 (■) myeloid antigens or fail to express these antigens (△, □)

ent heterogeneous responsiveness of HL60 cells to inducers of neutrophil and monocyte differentiation. As shown in Fig. 1, these data, together with analyses of surface antigen expression [2], suggest that the variant lines typify a developmental progression within HL60 cultures. During this process cells first acquire a capacity to be induced to differentiate terminally to neutrophils, as reflected by the concentrations of DMSO and other inducers required to induce differentiation. Subsequently, as this capacity for neutrophil differentiation is lost, cells acquire responsiveness to inducers of monocyte differentiation. Thus, variant lines unable to differentiate towards monocytes typify cells which have not yet undergone the differentiation step necessary to acquire the ability to respond to inducers of monocyte differentiation.

The hypothesis that sequential determination is not restricted only to granulocyte/macrophage commitment, but also applies to commitment to megakaryocyte, erythrocyte and neutrophil differentiation arises from consideration of the mature cell types produced in soft agar cultures by progenitor cells restricted to two differentiation pathways. Megakaryocyte/erythroid and erythroid/neutrophil progenitor cells, described in cultures of human and murine bone marrow cells [3], suggest close relationships between these lineages. Similarly, in the myelo-

dysplastic and myeloproliferative disorders, the combinations of megakaryocyte and erythroid, erythroid and granulocytic, megakarycytic, erythroid and granulocytic dysplastic or proliferating cells argue in favour of an ordered, close relationship between progenitor cells during their development [4]. A close relationship between the potentials for macrophage and B-cell differentiation is revealed by experiments in which macrophage-like sublines were isolated from cultures of the murine pre-B lymphoma ABLS8.1 after treatment with 5-azacytidine [5]. These experiments can be interpreted in a manner similar to the HL60 studies [2]. The close relationship between B and T progenitor cells is inferred from the findings that immunoglobulin heavy chain and T-cell receptor genes are partially rearranged in T- and pre-B-cell leukaemias respectively [6]. Commitment to T-cell differentiation is placed last in the developmental sequence. Interestingly, chronic T-cell malignancies such as mycosis fungoides and Sezary's syndrome never terminate in anything other than a proliferative T-cell malignancy. Furthermore, pre-B blast crises in patients with chronic granulocytic leukaemia can be readily explained by the proposed maturation sequence of progenitor cells.

The model, if valid, has important genetic implications. Since DNA is duplicated semiconservatively, sequential determination of

275

lineage potentials during haemopoiesis would allow the older of the two DNA strands to be retained by cells which progress through the various stages of lineage commitment [7]. The newly synthesised strand, together with any errors occurring during DNA replication, is collected by the daughter progenitor cells, which differentiates along a pre-determined pathway. This process lowers the risk of spontaneous mutation occurring in the progenitor cell population [7]. Most stem cells reside in an "out-of-cycle" Go state [1], and Lajtha has proposed that this is a period when cells undertake "slow DNA repair" processes so as to correct errors in the genome [1]. The previous considerations reduce the requirement for DNA screening in order to maintain the integrity of the genome. Thus, if Go is not essential for "genetic housekeeping" [1] this poses the problem of what happens during Go? In describing the model for progenitor cell development we proposed that during sequential determination cells rearrange genes pre-requisite for differentiation towards a particular cell type [2]. This process of DNA rearrangement may be pertinent to the Go state, and inappropriate gene recombination events provide an explanation for malignancy. The majority of stem cells and lymphocytes which rearrange genes with respect to receptor diversity reside in Go, and they represent "target" cells for most if not all haemopoietic malignancies [1].

Of particular interest is whether the proposed sequence of lineage commitment parallels the pattern of recovery of bone marrow cells following damage. Early in vivo studies of bone marrow recovery in irradiated guinea-pigs showed that the marrow first contained megakaryocytes; this was followed by a wave of erythropoiesis and subsequent recovery of neutrophils [8]. These data support the model proposed. However, the circumstances in which marrow damage is induced, to what extent various progenitor cell populations are affected, and species differences may considerably affect the pattern of recovery seen. In studies of marrow recovery in rats following X-irradiation and sublethal doses of alkylating agents there was no suggestion of sequential recovery of lineages [9]. The sequential determination model does not necessarily predict a parallel sequential recovery or ontogeny of bone marrow cells. The minimal number of six cell cycles could generate cells with each potential for differentiation, and the relative growth rate kinetics of the various cell lineages have to be taken into account. Nevertheless, the work of Frindel and Vendrely [10] supports the sequential expression of potentials for erythropoiesis and granulopoiesis. Bone marrow from Ara-C treated mice was used to reconstitute irradiated recipients, and Frindel and Vendrely observed an increased number of erythroid colonies in the spleen, and found that erythroid colonies contained an increased number of granulocyte/macrophage colony forming cells (GM-CFC) when assayed in vitro. They suggested that "the CFU-S is channelled towards erythropoiesis for several generations. After a certain number of cell divisions, the instruction' to differentiate towards erythropoiesis is lost and CFU-S differentiate in a normal stochastic manner. When the recipient mice were killed 9 or 10 days after marrow injection GM-CFC had not yet matured and were capable of giving rise to in vitro colonies."

If a sequential process of stem cell commitment is conservatively followed, the steps in the sequence would have been grafted on in the order in which the cells appear in phylogeny. Macrophage function (phagocytosis) is a primordial defense mechanism – lymphocytes evolved later, and the coagulation function of platelets may have originated prior to phagocytosis as a mechanism of defense. This pattern of evolution of immune functions can be equated with the proposed sequence. Similarly, it is conceivable that T-lymphocytes evolved later to assist B cells in their function and as a feedback control mechanism for driving and limiting the process of progenitor cell maturation [2].

Resolution of the problem of whether the haemopoietic stem cell is pluripotent in a strict sense is essential to our understanding of regulation of haemopoiesis and the origin and progression of malignant disease. Studies of the potentiality of progenitor cells in vivo or grown in soft agar investigate the outcome after several cell divisions, and therefore do not reveal the mechanism of differentiation processes. An approach to this problem is suggested by studies of variant HL60 cell lines. The lines, arranged in a sequence of development, suggest that potentials for granulocyte and monocyte differentiation are sequentially expressed. If this notion and the order of the variant cell lines are correct, then near-neighbour comparison of proteins of each of the lines by 2-D gel electrophoresis should verify the hypothesis. The model predicts that HL60 Ast 4 is similar to HL60 Ast 3 and less related to HL60 Ast 1 (see Fig. 1). This analysis should also identify proteins which are developmentally regulated in relation to cell commitment.

Acknowledgement. This work is supported by the Leukaemia Research Fund and the Medical Research Council (CMB).

References

1. Lajtha LG (1979) Differentiation 14:23–34
2. Brown G, Bunce CM, Guy GR (1985) Br J Cancer 52:681–686
3. Ogawa M, Porter PN, Nakahata T (1983) Blood 61:823–829
4. Brown G, Bunce CM, Rose PE, Howie AJ (1985) Lancet 8460:885
5. Boyd AW, Schrader JW (1982) Nature 297:691–693
6. Greaves MF, Chan LC, Furley AJW, Watt SM, Molgaard HV (1986) Blood 67:1–11
7. Cairns J (1975) Nature 255:197–200
8. Harris PF (1985) Lancet 8465:1240
9. Elson LA, Galton DAG, Till M (1958) Br J Haematol 4:355–374
10. Frindel E, Vendrely C (1982) External "manipulation" of pluripotent stem cells (CFU-S). Differentiation pathways: Role of Pluripoietins. In: Killman SV-AA, Cronkite EP, Muller-Berat CN (eds) Haemopoietic stem cells, characterisation, proliferation, regulation. Munksgaard, Copenhagen, pp 93–102

Haematology and Blood Transfusion Vol. 31
Modern Trends in Human Leukemia VII
Edited by Neth, Gallo, Greaves, and Kabisch
© Springer-Verlag Berlin Heidelberg 1987

Clinical Implications of Tumor Heterogeneity *

R. L. Schilsky [1]

Clinical oncologists have long recognized the great variability in the cellular morphology, natural history, and response to therapy of human tumors. Recent progress in molecular biology, biological chemistry, immunology, and other disciplines has now provided scientists with an array of new technologies that has allowed the study of neoplastic disease to go beyond morphologic and clinical description to examination of the malignant state at the cellular and molecular level. The availability of monoclonal antibodies, DNA hybridization techniques, hormone receptor assays, human tumor stem cell assays, and other methods now enables investigators to reveal, in greater detail than ever before, the great phenotypic and genotypic diversity present in most primary and metastatic tumors. Much of the information obtained thus far has been largely descriptive, cataloging the diversity in karyotypes, immune phenotypes, metastatic potential, drug sensitivity, and other cellular characteristics that commonly occurs in tumors that are seemingly identical morphologically.

The origin of tumor heterogeneity is less clearly understood, although the genetic instability inherent in the malignant state appears to be an important element in its generation and maintenance [1, 2]. Tumor het-erogeneity is a dynamic process, and changes in the composition of a neoplasm occur over a period of time in response to environmental selection pressures generated within the tumor (e.g., competition for nutrients), by the host's immune defense or imposed by the treating oncologist [3–5]. Indeed, tumors may be viewed as continually evolving within the host, with the treatment-resistant phenotype representing survival of the "fittest" malignant cells. This process is not random and uncontrolled, however, but is regulated in some way by interactions among the cellular subpopulations comprising the tumor such that rapid clonal diversification occurs under conditions of limited cellular diversity, thus ensuring the continued survival of the tumor in the face of varied therapeutic attempts.

Of considerable importance to clinical oncologists is the fact that much of this heterogeneity may be generated prior to clinical detection of the tumor. Even a 1-cm tumor mass contains at least a billion tumor cells, and the number of mitoses that a single cell must undergo to reach this volume will depend upon both the rate of cell growth and the rate of cell loss from the tumor mass. With the potential for genetic mutation to occur with each mitosis, it is not surprising that phenotypic diversity commonly occurs even in early-stage tumors.

An enormous challenge is thus presented to clinical oncologists from the perspective of assessing the "clinical relevance" of tumor heterogeneity and because of the need to develop new treatment strategies able to effectively eradicate multiple tumor subpopulations.

* Supported in part by a Junior Faculty Clinical Fellowship from the American Cancer Society.
[1] Associate Professor of Medicine and Associate Director, Joint Section of Hematology-Oncology, University of Chicago Pritzker School of Medicine and Michael Reese Hospital and Medical Center, Chicago, IL 60616, USA

The clinical importance of identifying tumor subpopulations is directly related to the impact such knowledge has on determining prognosis and making management decisions. Among the large-cell non-Hodgkin lymphomas, for example, histologic subtyping was initially reported to have a significant impact on treatment outcome and prognosis [6]. Patients with the blastic and pleomorphic pyroninophilic subtypes had a significantly worse prognosis than patients with the other histologic subtypes described. However, with the development of more aggressive and effective chemotherapy treatment regimens, differences in outcome for these histologic subtypes have disappeared [7]. Similarly, the use of monoclonal antibodies for immune phenotyping of non-Hodgkin's lymphomas has revealed a diversity not appreciated by standard morphologic analysis alone [8]. However, the therapeutic ramifications of detecting a particular immune phenotype on lymphoma cells are as yet unknown. Indeed, the overall effectiveness of combination chemotherapy in the treatment of diffuse large-cell lymphomas suggests that recognition of a particular immune phenotype in these diseases may not provide information of any practical importance. In other malignancies, however, such as childhood acute lymphoblastic leukemia (ALL), immune phenotype may well be an important determinant of prognosis and, to some extent, therapy [9], although further advances in ALL treatment are likely to diminish the importance of this prognostic factor as well. The clinical relevance of cellular heterogeneity to the prognosis and management of other tumors is presently unknown but can be assessed through well-designed clinical trials stratified prospectively for phenotypic variables. Clearly, the importance of phenotypic heterogeneity for some characteristics will diminish as therapy continues to improve.

The demonstration that tumor heterogeneity is a common phenomenon could easily create an air of pessimism among clinical oncologists. After all, it appears that tumors are infinitely adaptable, possessing the ability to metastasize widely prior to clinical detection and rapidly evolve new antigenic properties, hormone receptor levels, and patterns of drug resistance. Tumors, it seems, are always one step ahead of the treating physician. The alternative view, however, is that the recognition and understanding of tumor cell heterogeneity may in fact provide the foundation upon which successful new treatment strategies can be developed. One area of recent progress, for example, is the development of a new in vitro model for growing malignant cells as they exist in vivo. Traditional in vitro models rely on the growth of tumor cells in monolayer or suspension culture, conditions which rarely, if ever, re-create the growth of tumors in vivo. By contrast, multicellular spheroids approximate many characteristics of in vivo tumor growth, including three-dimensional intercellular contact, ranges in pH, oxygen tension, nutrient levels, and the ability to be grown in culture for weeks without trypsinization [10]. Yet spheroids can be grown under carefully controlled environmental conditions and may therefore provide a unique in vitro model of tumor cell heterogeneity. Indeed, this model has already been used successfully to explore the interactions between drug-sensitive and drug-resistant brain tumor cells [11]. Multicellular spheroids may well serve as a model of cellular heterogeneity of potential utility in drug sensitivity testing and screening for new agents. With such a system, new drugs could be selected for clinical trial on the basis of their activity in a screening system that more closely resembles tumor growth in vivo than those systems currently in use. The human tumor stem cell assay [12] and the development of drug-resistant human tumor cell lines offer other advantages over the traditional drug-screening systems and are currently being evaluated as experimental systems that could be employed in a more rational approach to screening for potential new cytotoxic agents.

While new drug development continues to be an important area of research, other more novel approaches to cancer treatment are being pursued in an effort to circumvent the problems created by tumor heterogeneity. Activated macrophages, for example, have been shown to selectively destroy tumor cells, while leaving normal cells intact [13]. In vitro, these cells are able to recognize and destroy many types of tumor cells, regardless of such cellular variables as metastatic potential and drug sensitivity. Lymphokine-activated killer (LAK) cells also exhibit the desirable property of nonspecifically killing tumor cells while leaving normal cells intact, a fact which suggests that they recognize a feature common to tumor cells that is not expressed by normal cells [14]. The possibility thus exists that in vivo activation of tumoricidal macrophages or LAK cells may be a useful therapeutic adjunct to conventional cytotoxic therapy. Ongoing clinical trials of LAK cells plus interleukin 2 may soon shed some light on this question.

The use of monoclonal antibodies to deliver radioisotopes or cellular toxins directly to the vicinity of a tumor mass may provide a more efficient system for the application of nonspecific cellular poisons in a tumor-specific way. The use of radioisotope antibody conjugates is particularly attractive since the energy emitted by the isotope may be sufficient to destroy those cells in the vicinity of the conjugate, even though antigenic heterogeneity may prevent the binding of the monoclonal antibody to each individual tumor cell.

Another novel approach to circumventing the problem of tumor heterogeneity lies in the use of agents capable of inducing tumor cell differentiation to a more "benign" phenotype. It has been postulated that drugs such as the polar solvents N, N-dimethylformamide and N-methylformamide could induce tumor cell maturation, limit the continued generation of tumor subpopulations, and thereby produce a more homogeneous tumor more likely to be eradicated with conventional treatments [15]. Interestingly, these agents have been shown to enhance the cytotoxic effects of alkylating agents [16] and ionizing radiation [17] in experimental systems. Clinical trials are currently in progress, and the results are awaited with great anticipation.

Though therapeutic approaches such as those discussed above hold great promise for the future, it is probable that conventional cytotoxic chemotherapy will continue to play a major role in cancer treatment. As such, a better understanding of the mechanisms by which drug resistance develops will enable the development of treatment stratagems to circumvent it. For some drugs, the biochemical mechanisms of resistance are well understood, and this knowledge has been applied to the development of drug analogs able to circumvent the resistant state. In the case of methotrexate (MTX), cellular resistance can develop owing to impaired membrane transport, increased content of dihydrofolate reductase (DHFR), altered affinity of DHFR, or impaired polyglutamylation [18]. There now exist methotrexate analogs able to overcome most of these potential mechanisms of resistance. Lipophilic diaminopyrimidine antifolates have been developed that are cytotoxic to transport-deficient MTX-resistant cells [19]; 2-amino-4-hydroxy-quinazoline antifolates have been synthesized that are able to inhibit thymidylate synthase directly, independently of DHFR content [20]; and a new trimethoxy quinazoline derivative of MTX – trimetrexate – which does not undergo polyglutamylation and is not cross-resistant with transport-deficient cells is currently undergoing clinical testing [21]. Thus, there now exist MTX analogs capable of overcoming essentially all known mechanisms of antifolate resistance. Combination chemotherapy with multiple antifolates has been effective in overcoming MTX resistance in vitro [22], and it is tempting to speculate that clinical chemotherapy with an antifolate combination might be effective as well. Indeed, recently reported studies in tumor-bearing animals indicate that the sequential use of MTX followed by trimetrexate is more effective than treatment with optimal doses of either drug alone [23].

Another strategy to overcome drug resistance that has received widespread attention is the use of calcium channel blockers and calmodulin inhibitors to enhance cellular sensitivity to anthracyclines, vinca alkaloids, and other drugs. Verapamil [24], trifluoperazine [25], and related drugs can successfully overcome doxorubicin resistance both in model systems and in drug-resistant human tumor cells [26]. Clinical studies are currently in progress to determine whether these drugs can be successfully used to circumvent resistance in patients with refractory tumors.

Understanding the heterogeneous nature of the malignant state serves only to emphasize the importance of one of the long-standing rubrics of the fight against cancer – early detection. Indeed, early detection and early application of effective therapy remain two of the most effective methods of limiting tumor cell heterogeneity and circumventing drug resistance. The mathematical model of drug resistance developed by Goldie and Coldman [27] suggests that resistance can develop rapidly, within only a few cell divisions; that alternation of non-cross-resistant regimens may be beneficial; and that chemotherapy must be given in high cytotoxic doses, lest its mutagenic potential actually contribute to the development of drug resistance. The application of intensive combination chemotherapy immediately following diagnosis and even prior to definitive local therapy may be the most effective method of eradicating micrometastases and producing long-term disease-free survival. Preoperative chemotherapy appears promising in head and neck cancer [28], osteogenic sarcoma [29], and even non-small-cell lung cancer [30], though many more years of follow-up are necessary before the final results are obtained. Nevertheless, these initial clinical trials should serve as the basis for the continued evaluation of primary chemotherapy in the management of solid tumors.

The time has come for clinical oncologists to look carefully at the evolving concepts of tumor biology, for from these concepts will come the clinical trials and treatment strategies of the future. The last decade has seen a tremendous increase in our knowledge of the extraordinary diversity of the malignant state. Armed with this knowledge, clinical oncologists can look forward to continued success in the development and application of new therapies likely to rapidly advance the state of the art of cancer treatment.

References

1. Nowell PC (1976) The clonal evolution of tumor cell populations. Science 194:23–28
2. Cifone MA, Fidler IJ (1981) Increasing metastatic potential is associated with increasing genetic instability of clones isolated from murine neoplasms. Proc Nat Acad Sci USA 78:6949–6952
3. Poste G, Doll J, Fidler IJ (1981) Interactions among clonal subpopulations affect stability of the metastatic phenotype in polyclonal populations of B16 melanoma cells. Proc Natl Acad Sci USA 78:6226–6230
4. Hill RP, Chambers AF, Ling V, Harris JF (1984) Dynamic heterogeneity: rapid generation of metastatic variants in mouse B16 melanoma cells. Science 244:998–1001
5. Poste G (1986) Pathogenesis of metastatic disease: implications for current therapy and for the development of new therapeutic strategies. Cancer Treat Rep 70:183–199
6. Strauchen JA, Young RC, DeVita VT, Anderson T, Fantone JC, Berard CW (1978) Clinical relevance of the histopathological subclassification of diffuse "histocytic" lymphoma. N Engl J Med 299:1382–1387
7. Fisher RI, Hubbard SM, DeVita VT, Berard CW, Wesley R, Cossman J, Young RC (1981) Factors predicting long term survival in diffuse mixed, histiocytic or undifferentiated lymphoma. Blood 58:45–51
8. Urba WJ, Longo DL (1985) Cytologic, immunologic and clinical diversity in non-Hodgkin's lymphoma: therapeutic implications. Semin Oncol 12:250–267
9. Kamps WA, Humphrey GB (1985) Heterogeneity of childhood acute lymphoblastic leukemia – impact on prognosis and therapy. Semin Oncol 12:268–280
10. Sutherland R, Carlson J, Durand R, Yuhas J (1981) Spheroids in cancer research. Cancer Res 41:2980–2984
11. Tofilon PJ, Buckley N, Deen DF (1984) Effect of cell-cell interactions on drug sensitivity and growth of drug-sensitive and resistant tumor cells in spheroids. Science 226:862–864
12. Shoemaker RH, Wolpert-DeFilippes MK, Kern DH, Lieber MM, Makuch RW, Melnick NR, Miller WT, Salmon SE, Simon RM, Venditti JM, Von Hoff DD (1985) Application of a human tumor colony forming assay to new drug screening. Cancer Res 45:2145–2153
13. Kleinerman ES, Erickson KL, Schroit AJ, Fogler WE, Fidler IJ (1983) Activation of tumoricidal properties in human blood monocytes by liposomes containing lipophilic muramyl tripeptide. Cancer Res 43:2010–2014
14. Rosenberg SA (1986) Adoptive immunotherapy of cancer using lymphokine activated killer cells and recombinant interleukin 2. In: DeVita VT, Hellman S, Rosenberg SA (eds) Important advances in oncology. Lippincott, Philadelphia, pp 55–91
15. Spremulli EN, Dexter DL (1984) Polar solvents: a new class of antineoplastic agents. J Clin Oncol 2:227–241
16. Harpur ES, Langdon SP, Fathalla SAK, Ishmael J (1986) The antitumor effect and toxicity of cis-platinum and N-methylformamide

in combination. Cancer Chemother Pharmacol 16:139–147

17. Leith JT, Lee ES, Vayer AJ, Dexter DL, Glicksman AS (1985) Enhancement of the responses of human colon adenocarcinoma cells to X-irradiation and cis-platinum by N-methylformamide. Int J Rad Oncol Biol Phys 11:1971–1976

18. Jolivet J, Cowan KH, Curt GA, Clendeninn NJ, Chabner BA (1983) The pharmacology and clinical use of methotrexate. N Engl J Med 309:1094–1104

19. Hill BT, Price CA (1980) DDMP. Cancer Treat Rev 7:95–112

20. Calvert AH, Jones TR, Dady PJ, Grzelakowska-Sztabert B, Paine RM, Taylor GA, Harrap KR (1983) Quinazoline antifolates with dual biochemical loci of action. Biochemical and biological studies directed towards overcoming methotrexate resistance. Europ J Cancer 16:713–722

21. Kamen BA, Eibel B, Cashmore A, Bertino JR (1984) Uptake and efficacy of trimetrexate, a non-classical antifolate in MTX resistant leukemia cells in vitro. Biochem Pharmacol 33:1697–1699

22. Diddens H, Neithammer D, Jackson RC (1983) Patterns of cross-resistance to the antifolate drugs trimetrexate, metoprine, homofolate and CB3717 in human lymphoma and osteo-sarcoma cells resistant to methotrexate. Cancer Res 43:5286–5292

23. Sobrero AF, Bertino JR (1986) Alternating trimetrexate with methotrexate delays the onset of resistance to antifolates in vitro and in vivo. Proc Am Assoc Cancer Res 27:269

24. Tsuruo T, Iida H, Tsukagoshi S, Sakurai Y (1982) Increased accumulation of vincristine and Adriamycin in drug resistant P388 tumor cells following incubation with calcium antagonists and calmodulin inhibitors. Cancer Res 42:4730–4733

25. Miller R, Bukowski RM, Ganapathi R, Budd GT, Purvis J (1984) Reversal of doxorubicin resistance by the addition of trifluoperazine. Clin Res 32:766A

26. Rogan AM, Hamilton TC, Young RC, Klecker RW, Ozols RF (1984) Reversal of adriamycin resistance by verapamil in human ovarian cancer. Science 224:994–996

27. Goldie JH, Coldman AJ (1984) The genetic origin of drug resistance in neoplasms: implications for systemic therapy. Cancer Res 44:3643–3653

28. Ensley JF, Kish JA, Jacobs J, Weaver A, Crissman J, Al-Sarraf M (1984) Incremental improvements in median survival associated with degree of response to adjuvant chemotherapy in patients with advanced squamous cell cancer of the head and neck. In: Jones SE, Salmon SE (eds) Adjuvant therapy of cancer IV. Grune and Stratton, Orlando, pp 117–126

29. Rosen G, Nirenberg A (1984) Chemotherapy for primary osteogenic sarcoma: Ten year evaluation and current status of prospective chemotherapy. In: Jones SE, Salmon SE (eds) Adjuvant therapy of cancer IV. Grune and Stratton, Orlando, pp 593–600

30. Bitran JD, Golomb HM, Hoffman PC, Albain K, Evans R, Little AG, Purl S, Skosey C (1986) Protochemotherapy in non-small cell lung carcinoma: an attempt to increase surgical resectability and survival. A preliminary report. Cancer 57:44–53

Haematology and Blood Transfusion   Vol. 31
Modern Trends in Human Leukemia VII
Edited by Neth, Gallo, Greaves, and Kabisch
© Springer-Verlag Berlin Heidelberg 1987

Tumour Cell Heterogeneity and the Biology of Metastasis

I. R. Hart[1]

The metastatic spread of malignant tumours remains as one of the most intractable problems in clinical oncology. Experimental analysis of this phenomenon is fuelled by the hope that a more complete understanding of the process will give rise to insights allowing the eventual development of novel and successful therapeutic interventions. The purpose of this paper is to provide a brief overview of the pathogenesis of tumour dissemination and to discuss the implications arising from an appreciation of the biological principles revealed by studies with experimental tumour systems. It is hoped that this paper will provide an introduction to supplement the work described by Dr. Feldman in a subsequent chapter.

Metastasis is a process consisting of a series of linked, sequential steps. An inability to complete any one of these steps effectively abrogates the whole process. Thus, in order to establish a secondary focus, malignant tumours must invade locally and penetrate small blood vessels or lymphatics. This step is thought to be achieved by a combination of mechanisms including breakdown of tissue architecture by pressure atrophy, the release of proteolytic enzymes which digest the cohesive framework of the extracellular matrix and active movement of single cells or sheets of cells into such areas of tissue damage [1]. Penetration of vascular channels must be followed by release of single cells or small emboli into the circulation and the survival of these neoplastic cells in the face of turbulence and trauma or the effects of such

specific and non-specific host immune effectors as natural killer (NK) cells, T lymphocytes, neutrophils and monocytes [2]. Having disseminated throughout the body metastatic cells must arrest and implant at distant sites, binding to areas of exposed basement membrane via specific attachment factors and cell surface receptors [3] or by direct penetration of endothelial cells [4]. Extravasation of cells into surrounding organ parenchyma is, presumably, accomplished by mechanisms much the same as those mediating initial invasion. Having reached the site of growth, tumour cells must establish and develop their own micro-environment; responding to local growth factors, releasing angiogenic factors to induce self-vascularisation and surviving host immune mechanisms to give rise to clinically obvious tumour deposits [5].

Given the highly complex nature of the process, it is perhaps not surprising that it is markedly inefficient [6]. Indeed, experimental analysis has shown that fewer than 0.1% of cells which gain access to the circulation may survive to form tumour deposits. This inefficiency posed the important question as to whether the survival observed was a consequence of random or selective events; that is do the eventual progenitors of secondary tumours result from the fortuitous survival of a few cells from the many shed into the blood or does it represent the selection of a pre-existent metastatic subpopulation from the parental tumour? Direct investigation of this possibility was reported by Fidler and Kripke [7] who used a modified Luria-Delbruck fluctuation analysis of clones, derived from single cells, to show that sub-popula-

---

[1] Imperial Cancer Research Laboratories, Lincoln's Inn Fields, London, WC2A 3PX, England

tions of metastatic cells pre-existed within the B16 melanoma. Subsequently several reports have described a similar degree of metastatic heterogeneity in a variety of rodent tumours [8–11].

A possible criticism of such demonstrations could be that they have all relied upon the use of transplantable tumours of rodent origin and the results obtained may not be applicable to human neoplasms. One obvious difficulty in any attempt to apply similar analytical procedures to human tumours lies in determining which animal can best be used to evaluate the degree of metastatic spread. The congenitally athymic nude mouse, which lacks significant numbers of T lymphocytes, would appear to be an ideal test animal in which to assess this parameter. Nude mice have been used frequently as recipients of human tumour xenografts, but while such implants commonly maintain their distinctive morphological and biochemical attributes they metastasize only rarely [12]. However, the situation with regard to the metastatic spread of established human tumour lines is much more equivocal and many lines have been shown to be capable of metastasizing readily in such recipients [13–15]. We have used this combination, the relevance of human material coupled with the ease of manipulation to be gained from established tissue culture lines, to determine whether human tumours manifest the degree of metastatic heterogeneity shown by rodent neoplasms.

The human melanoma line A375 was cloned by isolating discrete colonies growing in semisolid agar and individual lines were derived from these clones. The ability of the parental line and ten clonal lines to form lung tumour nodules in BALB/c nude mice was determined following i.v. injections. Four out of the ten clones examined differed significantly ($P < 0.005$) from the parental line with regard to their ability to form pulmonary tumour foci [16] indicating that this human line was no less heterogeneous for metastatic capacity than its murine counterparts. Recovery of cells from these lung nodules to form metastasis-derived lines followed by re-examination of their metastatic capacity demonstrated that these selected lines consistently were more metastatic than the starting population both in the i.v. ex-

perimental metastasis assay and in the more stringent spontaneous metastasis assay from a s.c. site [16]. We have interpreted these results as showing that human tumour spread in the nude mouse results from the preferential selection of metastatic subpopulations and have confirmed the generality of this observation using the human prostatic carcinoma line PC3 [17] and a further melanoma line DX-3 [18].

The source of metastatic heterogeneity (or in fact heterogeneity for any other phenotype) is not known. Should tumours have a multi-cellular origin [19], then the diversity found simply may be the reflection of differences between the progeny of several transformed cells. However, since most tumours appear to be unicellular in origin [20, 21] other mechanisms have had to be invoked to explain such multiformity. Nowell [22] proposed that acquired genetic lability and variability in neoplastic cells, when coupled with the intense selection pressure of growth in a responding host, led to the rapid emergence of new sublines with increased survival ability which was manifested as enhanced malignancy. A corollary of such a mechanism might be that variants of increasing metastatic capacity would be accompanied by increases in genetic instability and supportive evidence for such a possibility is provided by the work of Cifone and Fidler [23]. These authors showed that rates of mutation to ouabain and 6-thioguanine resistance were increased in variants of high metastatic activity when compared with mutation rates shown by variants of low metastatic activity isolated from the same neoplasm [23].

Irrespective of the exact forces driving tumours toward a more aggressive behavioural pattern, the finding of metastatic heterogeneity within tumours, coupled with the ability to select out more metastatic variants, has profound implications for experimental analysis of metastasis. Determination of the cellular properties that are important for expression of the malignant phenotype can now be achieved by using cell variants or lines of different biological behaviour isolated from the same tumour. Such an approach obviates the need to include control cells, which frequently are of doubtful validity, derived from unrelated tumour or normal tissue. The demonstration of a similar degree of metastatic heterogeneity in human tumour lines coupled with the ability to use the athymic nude mouse as a "selection vehicle" to pull out metastatic variants shows that similar investigations can now be conducted using human neoplasms.

References

1. Liotta L, Hart IR (eds) (1982) Tumor invasion and metastasis. Nijhoff, The Hague
2. Fidler IJ, Hart IR (1978) Host immunity in experimental metastasis. In: Castro JE (ed) Immunological aspects of cancer. MTP Press, Lancaster
3. Liotta LA, Rao CN, Barsky SH (1983) Tumor invasion and the extracellular matrix. Lab Invest 49:636–649
4. Roos E, Dingemans KP (1979) Mechanisms of metastasis. Biochim Biophys Acta 560:135–166
5. Fidler IJ, Gersten DM, Hart IR (1978) The biology of cancer invasion and metastasis. Adv Cancer Res 28:149–250
6. Weiss L (1985) Principles of metastasis. Academic, London
7. Fidler IJ, Kripke ML (1977) Metastasis results from pre-existing variant cells within a malignant tumor. Science 197:893–895
8. Dexter DK, Kowalski HM, Blazar BA, Fligiel Z, Fogel R, Heppner GH (1978) Heterogeneity of tumor cells from a single mouse mammary tumor. Cancer Res 38:3174–3178
9. Kripke ML, Gruys E, Fidler IJ (1978) Metastatic heterogeneity of cells from an ultraviolet-light-induced murine fibrosarcoma of recent origin. Cancer Res 38:2962–2967
10. Nicolson GL (1978) Experimental tumor metastasis: characteristics and organ specificity. Bioscience 28:441–446
11. Talmadge JE, Fidler IJ (1982) Enhanced metastatic potential of tumor cells harvested from spontaneous metastases of heterogeneous murine tumors. JNCI 69:975–980
12. Sharkey FE, Fogh J (1979) Metastasis of human tumors in athymic nude mice. Int J Cancer 24:733–738
13. Kyriazis AP, DiPersio M, Michael GJ, Pesie AJ, Stinnett JD (1978) Growth patterns and metastatic behaviour of human tumors growing in athymic mice. Cancer Res 38:3186–3190
14. Kyriazis AP, Kyriazis AA, McCombs WB, Kerejakes JA (1981) Biological behaviour of human malignant tumors growing in athymic mice. Cancer Res 41:3995–4000
15. Giovanella BC, Stehlin JS, Williams LJ (1974) Heterotransplantation of human malignant tumors in "nude" thymusless mice. II. Malignant tumors induced by injection of cell cultures derived from human solid tumors. JNCI 52:921–930
16. Kozlowski JM, Hart IR, Fidler IJ, Hanna N (1984) A human melanoma line heterogeneous with respect to metastatic capacity in athymic nude mice. JNCI 72:913–917
17. Kozlowski JM, Fidler IJ, Campbell D, Xu Z-L, Kaighn ME, Hart IR (1984) Metastatic behavior of human tumor cell lines grown in the nude mouse. Cancer Res 44:3522–3529
18. Ormerod EJ, Everett CA, Hart IR (1986) Enhanced experimental metastatic capacity of a human tumor line following treatment with 5-Azacytidine. Cancer Res 46:884–890
19. Reddy AL, Fialkow PJ (1979) Multicellular origin of fibrosarcomas in mice induced by the chemical carcinogen 3-methylcholanthrene. J Exp Med 150:878–883
20. Iannaccone PM, Gardner RL, Hans H (1978) The cellular origin of chemically-induced tumors. J Cell Sci 29:249–253
21. Fialkow PJ (1976) Clonal origin of human tumors. Biochim Biophys Acta 458:283–290
22. Nowell P (1976) The clonal evolution of tumor cell populations. Science 194:23–28
23. Cifone MA, Fidler IJ (1981) Increasing metastatic potential is associated with increasing genetic instability of clones isolated from murine neoplasms. Proc Natl Acad Sci USA 78:6949–6952

Haematology and Blood Transfusion   Vol. 31
Modern Trends in Human Leukemia VII
Edited by Neth, Gallo, Greaves, and Kabisch
© Springer-Verlag Berlin Heidelberg 1987

Cancer Clonality and Field Theory

G. T. Matioli[1]

A field theory [1] models malignancy as a state "added" to, and capable of interacting with, other normal states composing the field associated with any living cell. The theory may be downscaled from the (multi) cellular to the level of topologically disordered motions of chromatin and DNA strings occurring before or at interphase when chromatids are iteratively dilated in cells mitotically driven by a potential from special "source" cells. Clonal development of tumors might result from the extremely low efficiency with which the driving potential activates its corresponding gene(s) P in one (or exceedingly few) source-dependent cell. Most normal cells are assumed to have gene P "curled up" in some nonexpressed configuration in a segment j (say) within a lattice or plaquette unfolded from crumpled preimages during chromatid decondensation [11–13]. Through anharmonic, intermittent (generally frequency-incommensurable) stimulations from exogenous potential and after N mitoses, segment j might percolate in a rare cell into a less entangled chromatin phase, arbitrarily called "active or ballistic layer," where the probability for expressing P increases.

Chromatin loops are envisioned to reptate within a *finite* subvolume of the cell nucleus with snake-like, intermittent multicollisional motions [2], analogous to "string animals" described, for example, by Suzuki [3]. The kinematics of string subsections, including those of segment j imprinted by gene P, are

modeled thus by a "master" equation [3]:

$$\frac{\partial}{\partial t} P([x_j], t) = - \Sigma_j W_j([x_j]) P([x_j], t)$$

$$+ \Sigma_j W_j([x_j']) P([x_j'], t) ,$$

Therein, $P([X_j], t)$ may be roughly understood as the time-dependent probability for segment j to acquire a conformation optimal for expressing P out of $[X_j]$ configuring motions, and $W_j([X_j])$ as the transitional probability for segment j to percolate across the interphase "mass of string segments" during iterated chromatid unfoldings. Hence, the equation couples in one dimension two probabilities, none of them necessarily related to (point) mutations. These probabilities are: the distribution of conformational probabilities of gene P and the probability of percolative motions displacing P from its frustrated position. (Frustration may conceal local spins as epigenetic or topologic determinants of clonally directed site and tissue specific mutations.)

A solution of the above equation reads:

$$\langle X_j^2 \rangle_t \cong t^{D_f}$$

Exponent D_f relates to fractal and intermittently percolative motions iterated by segment j within the space-time (4D) mass of co-moving strings (a caged, monstrous Peano curve or Menger sponge). D_f is expected to fluctuate around values much less than unity [3, 4]. Therefore, even a long period (t) of mitotic activity is bound to yield a narrow spectrum of discommensured mo-

---

[1] USC Medical School, Los Angeles, California, USA

tions, thus reducing the probability that segment j will acquire a special conformation optimal for expressing P. Such a "unique"(?) conformation might occur most rarely within a population of cells, all initially stimulated and mitotically recruited by exogenous potential over extended times. The acquisition of autocatalytically synthesized potential is thus a rare event, expected to culminate clonally on top of the "Devil staircase" [5]. It is conjectured that all other mitosing cells dissipate exogenous potential in naive (nonexpressible) configurations of their chromatin segments, including j, with the exception of "almost" every other segment belonging to "ballistic or active layers" and imprinted by the genes of specific differentiation programs. The above conclusions are supported by the fact that only a small portion of the (human) genome encodes functionally active genes. The DNA bulk is often considered as a "useless ballast." However, by dynamic intermingling, such DNA traps many genes, including P, into innumerable entanglements greatly limiting changes in their (nonexpressible) conformations and accidental activation.

The complicated dynamics of disordered motions of concatenated strings within a finite space crowded by traps are being actively investigated. Additional information relevant to this paper is given in works on disordered-chaotic motions, Birkhoff signatures of tangles, classic-quantum multicollisional billiards, Krylov mixing, broken ergodicity, KAM (Kolmogoroff-Arnold-Moser) tori, their stability, Arnold's diffusion, etc. [6–10].

The very long, thin DNA is confined within finite nuclear subspaces. To fit into such small volumes, DNA must arrange many of its sections into looped configurations not too dissimilar, dynamically speaking, to the so-called KAM tori. While residing within such cages, gene P remains unexpressed because it is unable to modify its configuration and interact optimally with a suitable activating "matrix." Such a matrix may become available only at certain stages of differentiation. If so, the equation must include additional probabilities, none of them necessarily or sufficiently "mutational" in nature. These probabilities, coupled to those mentioned explicitly, fur-

ther reduce the chance of P activation in dividing cells. However, the form of the solution is not appreciably affected.

After N mitoses, caging tori might become genequaked or "messed up," with the result that in some cell gene P is repositioned into a new hierarchy of configurations. Two of these are particularly interesting. If P drifts into the so-called stochastic diffusion layer (Arnold's web) before cell terminal differentiation, there is an increased probability of its activation, if a matrix is available. In that case, a most "unlucky" cell becomes marginally or sufficiently autonomous for self-renewal. This is a prerequisite for the appearance of a new state (malignancy) among those states mapped in the "field" of a normal cell, absolutely dependent from local microenvironmental sources. Alternatively, if located ultrametrically in some residual and/or continuously re-forming insular trap near the boundary of Arnold's web, for example, gene P should remain forever silent.

In addition to immune surveillance, the permanent caging of gene P is thus an efficient mechanism against cancer development during a substantial part or even the entire life span of many individuals, in spite of constant or sporadic exposure to carcinogens and "mutagens."

Finally, there is valuable information to be collected by studying the cell genome in toto rather than by simply linear DNA sequencing, e.g., degree of lacunarity, unfolding of chromatids (spongy rods with zero or *negative* Gaussian curvature), and their quantal and asymmetric wobbles around fragile scaffold ($\pm$DNA) swivel points imposed by the bending energies of the nuclear envelope which contributes *positive* curvature during the cup-to-sphere transformation of the nucleus.

References

1. Matioli GT (1982) Annotation on stem cells and differentiation fields. Differentiation 21:139
2. De-Gennes P (1979) Scaling concepts in polymer physics. Cornell University Press, Ithaca
3. Suzuki M (1983) Brownian motion with geometrical restrictions. In: Yonezawa F, Ninomiya T (eds) Topological disorder in con-

densed matter. Springer, Berlin Heidelberg New York Tokyo (Springer series in solid-state sciences, vol 46)

4. Coniglio A, Stanley E (1984) Screening of deeply invaginated clusters and the critical behavior of the random superconducting network. Phys Rev Lett 52:1068

5. Mandelbrot BB (1983) The fractal geometry of nature. Freeman, San Francisco

6. Abraham RH (1985) Dynamics, vol 0–4. Sci Front Press

7. Percival I, Richards D (1985) Introduction to dynamics. Cambridge University Press, Cambridge

8. Krylov NS (1979) Raboty po obosnovaniiu statisticheskoi fiziki. Princeton University Press, Princeton

9. Lichtenberg AJ, Lieberman MA (1982) Regular and stochastic motion. Springer, Berlin Heidelberg New York

10. Zaslavsky GM (1985) Chaos in dynamic systems. Harwood, London

11. Rivier N (1987) Continuous random networks. From graphs to glasses. Adv Phys 36:95

12. Kantor Y, Kardar M, Nelson DR (1987) Tethered surfaces: Static and dynamics. Phys Rev A 35:3056

13. Coniglio A, Majid I, Stanley HE (1987) Conformation of a polymer chain at the "theta" point: Connection to the external perimeter of a percolation cluster. Phys Rev B 35:3617

Haematology and Blood Transfusion   Vol. 31
Modern Trends in Human Leukemia VII
Edited by Neth, Gallo, Greaves, and Kabisch
© Springer-Verlag Berlin Heidelberg 1987

Leukemia Progression: Role of Tissue Disorganization

Z. Grossman[1]

A. Introduction

Gene expression is not fixed or irreversible. Although under normal circumstances the pattern of gene expression of specialized cells is stable and heritable, it can be altered if the regulatory circuits between nucleus and cytoplasm are modified or disrupted [1]. Thus, changes in gene expression during cell development depend not only on the nucleus, but also on the cytoplasm which plays an essential role as signal transducer. The cytoplasm, in turn, is subject to modulation by extracellular factors and via membranal interactions. This leads to the concept of "phenotypic adaptability": the capacity of cells to change their patterns of gene expression in response to changes in the microenvironment. A role for DNA methylation in stabilizing epigenetically induced changes of gene expression has been proposed [2].

The following conceptions about cancer are widely accepted: (a) cancer is caused by discrete change, or changes, in the cell genome; and (b) a series of additional mutations, in the broad sense of the word, account for the progressive evolution of the tumor phenotypes – these mutations are due to the development of genetic instability in the transformed cells [3]. In particular, nonrandom chromosome alterations have been identified in myeloid and lymphoid leukemias and lymphomas. These alterations in turn are postulated to cause changes in the expression or regulation of proto-oncogenes

or other genes involved in the cell's growth and/or differentiation control. Duesberg [4] and others have questioned the validity and generality of this interpretation: it is not known whether these nonrandom chromosome changes are sufficient in themselves or even essential along with other changes for leukemogenesis; there is still no proof that activated proto-oncogenes are sufficient or even necessary to cause cancer.

On a more fundamental level, it has been argued that intracellular events cannot explain all of the changes involved in tumor progression in tissues where intercellular events regulate homeostasis [5–8]. Consistency with the concept of phenotypic adaptability, in particular, requires a more comprehensive approach. Such an approach will be outlined below, as a series of assumptions and propositions, with only a minimal reference to the supportive database (for more details and evidence, see [8–12]).

B. The Stem Cell Concept Revisited

Contrary to some theories, there is no obvious causal connection between division and differentiation-maturation at the single cell level. There is evidence in the lymphoid and hemopoietic systems and in other cell systems that differentiation can occur with or without mitosis and that the number of divisions that a cell performs at a given state of maturation is generally variable and subject to external regulation, in vivo and in vitro. Initiation of differentiation and entering into mitosis appear to be competing cellular events [13, 1]. Thus, there is no experimental

[1] Sackler Faculty of Medicine Tel Aviv University, Israel and Pittsburgh Cancer Institute, 230 Lothrop Street, Pittsburgh, PA 15213, USA

justification for the distinction between a self-renewal or stem cell division and an amplification division, which is regarded as an intrinsic part of a maturation process. Recognizable precursor cells do appear to divide and mature simultaneously under most conditions. However, this does not imply a constitutive relationship; it may reflect only a high rate of cycling, a high relative rate of maturation, and possibly an overlap between posttranscriptional and cell-cycle processes.

Assumption 1: The ratio between the probabilities of maturation and self-renewal for any mitotic cell is regulated by extracellular signals.

Corollary: Cells other than primitive pluripotential cells have a self-renewal potential, but their self-renewal activity is tightly regulated by inter-cell interactions.

Corollary: Competition may in principle take place not only among clones, but also within clones, i.e., among cells that belong to the same clone but are at different stages of maturation.

A number of models have been proposed on the basis of an externally regulated balance between cell division and cell differentiation-maturation [7]. A simplified possible scheme of the distinct regulatory steps in the stimulation of each cell is depicted in Fig. 1. R and A stand for "resting state" and "active state," respectively. S_1, S_2, and S_3 represent signals for initial activation, maturation, and replication, respectively. Each of these signals is partially constitutive (intracellular), partially generated (or modulated) by stromal cells, and partially elaborated by other hemopoietic cells. By definition, the latter component represents feedback. Each signal may be mediated by more than one factor or through direct intercellular interactions. There may be complete or partial overlap between the components of the different signals. Finally, the cellular origin, biochemical identity, and effects of these signals may vary according to the state of maturation of the target cell.

The dynamic aspect of hemopoiesis is provided by signals exchanged among hemopoietic cells. The feedback component need not be the main driving force, but it provides the "steering." The evidence is consistent

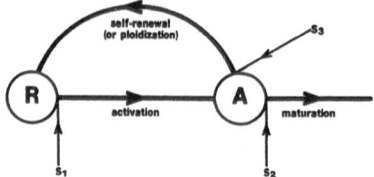

Fig. 1. Cell cycle associated levels of regulation

with the notion of internal feedback circuits, operating *within* the hemopoietic tissue, as well as with peripheral signals. The large overshooting in the numbers of CFU-S and other progenitors observed following marrow treatment by irradiation or by certain drugs and the long relaxation times and cycle times in cyclic hemopoiesis can be understood if there is a delay of several days along a regulatory loop. These patterns suggest that mature or maturing hemopoietic cells control the activity of earlier progenitors. Experimental evidence implicates granulocytes, monocytes, and lymphoid cells in this function.

Assumption 2: Maturation pressures on all progenitors and precursors increase with the size of the mature cell compartment.

In Fig. 2, Xi and Yi are resting and active cells in the i-th compartment, respectively $(i=1,...n)$; Z are mature cells. S represents the various signals indicated in Fig. 1, collectively. Although it is convenient to think of S as representing a set of factors, the feedback effects could be exerted more indirectly. Mature cells could modulate signals exchanged between progenitors or delivered to them by stromal cells. Alternatively, mature cells could interfere with autocatalytic proliferative signals exchanged among physically adjacent progenitors.

This minimal feedback model is based on the fact that differentiation in itself is growth-limiting. Differentiation out of a compartment decreases the population remaining within; no other inhibitory force is required. It has been assumed that differentiation pressures increase with the size of the system. The cells belonging to more primitive compartments are less sensitive to these pressures than their more differentiated progeny. Resistance to differentiation

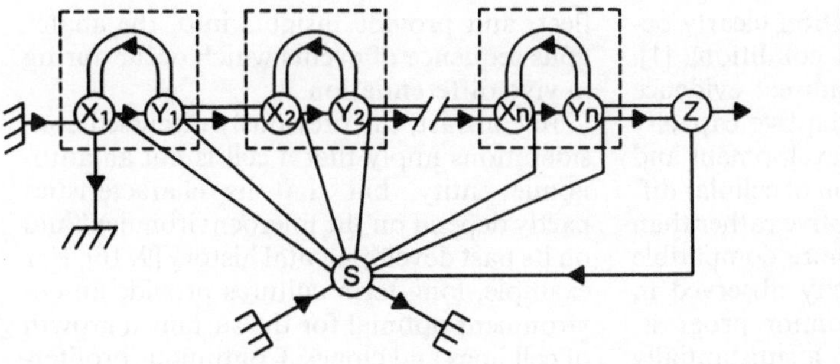

Fig. 2. "Balance-of-growth" model of hemopoiesis

pressures is a measure of the cell's self-renewal capacity. Thus, at steady-state the probabilities of self-renewal and differentiation in the earliest (most primitive) compartment are dynamically adjusted to be equal ($P = 0.5$ each). The "amplification" seen in the whole system results from renewal at probability smaller than 0.5 per activation event. It can rise to higher values when the steady state is perturbed following a change in peripheral demand, a tissue insult, or under culture conditions. Indeed, there is growing evidence that essentially normal cells of the committed progenitor phenotype can exhibit extensive self-renewal in vitro, in Dexter cultures or in suspension.

This scheme is largely nonspecific, embodying the view that the hemopoietic tissue functions as an integrated system rather than a set of cell lineages developing in parallel. This view is consistent with the data on growth factors active in cell culture which suggest that each of these factors effects a variety of progenitor cells at the earlier stages of differentiation and only later do lineage-specific effects become dominant (N.A. Nicola, this volume). The question, how do lineage-specific peripheral factors, such as erythropoietin or thrombopoietin, affect the production of cells of the respective lineages is discussed elsewhere [9, 10]. The scheme accounts for the fact that the response of recognizable precursor cells to changes in peripheral demand is more significant and occurs earlier than that of the colony-forming progenitors.

The rule that cells become more responsive to differentiation signals as they mature makes maturation an autocatalytic process. This, along with the feedback assumption, ensures both the stability and the flexibility

of the maturation hierarchy. It explains, for instance, why the slowly cycling primitive cells are not replaced as stem cells by their more active progeny. Certain changes in an early cell or in the tissue can weaken the differentiation feedback loop, leading eventually to leukemia.

C. "Differentiation" Revisited

"Differentiation" can be defined as inheritable changes in a cell's pattern of gene expression (not necessarily irreversible). "Maturation" is a particular step(s) of differentiation regularly observed within a cell lineage when the development of the cell is well-defined and predictable. "Adaptive differentiation" is differentiation which is guided to some extent by the cell's microenvironment.

Watching a differentiation sequence cannot tell us whether it is adaptive or not. It may owe its regularity to a constant set of constraints. Introducing modifications of the environment may lead to a modified phenotypic pattern in the developing cell population, possibly due to selection rather than adaptation. Thus, single-cell experiments are necessary to test whether reprogramming of cell differentiation can be effected in the absence of selection and to compare the early developmental steps of two daughter cells subject to different conditions. Metcalf et al. have shown that two different inducers, or different concentrations of the inducer, could push daughter cells of a CFU-C into the monocytic or into the granulocytic sublineage, respectively, and the effect appeared to be inductive, not selective [14]. Such experiments are scarce. Repro-

291

gramming of cell differentiation clearly occurs under highly artificial conditions [1]. There is a large body of indirect evidence supporting the notion of adaptive capacity of cells during embryonic development and into adult life. The conception of cellular differentiation as partially adaptive rather than rigidly preprogrammed is more compatible with the phenotypic plasticity observed in cultured cells and during tumor progress, when the cells are subject to a substantially modified environment for a prolonged period of time.

A programmatic approach implies "lineage fidelity" and discrete, intrinsically triggered determination (commitment) events. I prefer to see commitment as a manifestation of a gradually increasing bias for a given developmental fate. Such a bias is defined by the environment as well as by characteristics of the cell, e.g., by inducers in the environment and by the corresponding receptors on the membrane of the cell. Such commitment might be modulated or even reversed under different environmental conditions. In this light, it might be of interest to assess the fate of BFU-E under conditions of erythrocytosis induced by hypertransfusion, or that of the Meg-CFC shown to increase significantly in vivo, in some animals, without accompanying thrombocytosis [15].

Both their self-renewal capacity and pluripotency are aspects of stem cells' resistance to differentiation pressures. Because the build-up of differentiation bias is slow in these cells, competing small epigenetic modifications may switch on and off or fluctuate quantitatively. On the other hand, once a significant bias is attained and differentiation starts, the bias becomes self-enhancing and eventually irreversible within the same environment. This is equivalent to "commitment."

The concept of a "lineage" is based on the premise that the differentiation pathway of normal committed cells is fixed in advance under all conditions. This also provides the rationale for many in vitro experiments which aim to take a particular subpopulation of cells out of the complex physiological environment and place them into the simpler culture environment where they could be studied in detail. The assumption is that the events observed in vitro will accurately reflect, and provide insights into, the analogous sequence of events which occur during in vivo differentiation.

In contrast, the previously discussed considerations imply that a cell is not an autonomic entity, but that its characteristics partly depend on the microenvironment and on its past developmental history [9, 16]. For example, long-term cultures provide an environment optimal for the sustained growth of cell lines and clones. Continuous proliferation may lead not only to selection of particular subpopulations but also to adaptive phenotypic changes. In some cases, such adaptation leads these cells to specialize in self-replication. A set of genes associated with division maintains a high level of expression, possibly at the expense of other sets of genes, including perhaps those responsible for the karyotypic integrity of the cell's genome. This may lead to the accumulation of chromosomal aberrations.

In this scenario cell transformation in vitro is (a) secondary to the change in the microenvironment, and (b) described as a dynamic process in which changes in DNA sequence may follow irregular "differentiative" cellular changes (i.e., heritable changes in gene expression), which in turn follow reversible epigenic effects. The considerations in this section can be summarized by the following proposition:

Proposition 1: The phenotypic patterns of hemopoietic cells, including their profile of growth characteristics, are actively regulated by the same feedback interactions which control the numerical ratios among cells. (By "phenotypic pattern" I mean the coassociation of a given set of characteristics in the same cell.)

The stage is now set for proposing scenarios of leukemia progression in vivo.

D. The Origin of CML and the Blast Crisis

As mentioned earlier, it is their lower responsiveness to maturation pressures that endows the primitive cells with a growth advantage and stably couples them to the rest of the clone in Fig. 2, in spite of their slower cycling rate. These maturation pressures on all mitotic cells in the bone marrow are assumed to increase with the size of the mature cell compartment of that tissue.

Corollary: If the sensitivity to feedback of all the cells within a hemopoietic clone is reduced, the clone will expand in order to restore the (steady state) balance between self-renewal and differentiation.

It is convenient to define a common clonal measure of responsiveness, k, such that all cellular transition rate coefficients (or at least the maturation rates) are proportional to k, with $0 \leq k \leq 1$; k was named "inductivity." For normal clones $k = 1$; $k = 0$ at the limit of a complete maturation block; and cells in the intermediate range manifest different degrees of maturation arrest, in a quantitative sense.

Proposition 2. Chronic leukemia results from a reduced clonal inductivity (namely, from a partial maturation arrest).

The underlying biological mechanism could be direct (e.g., reduced numbers, or activity, of receptors for differentiation factors, or lower levels of transduction of the membranal signals) or indirect (e.g., increased numbers, or activity, of receptors for other growth factors, or impaired microenvironment). For specificity, and in line with the generally accepted interpretation, it may be supposed that a heritable change originated in an early transformed cell and propagated through the clone by proliferation and maturation of the original cell and its progeny.

What happens to normal hemopoietic cells in CML? The expansion of the leukemic clone is associated with increased maturation pressures which affect both leukemic and normal cells. At steady-state, the level of feedback control is adjusted to the reduced responsiveness of the leukemic stem cells, but is too high for normal stem cells. These are gradually induced to differentiate faster than they renew so that, in effect, normal clones become transitory.

If the feedback control mode of Fig. 2 (named "balance of growth") were the only means of controlling cell numbers, the number of mature cells at steady-state, Z_o, would be inversely related to the inductivity for $0 < k \leq 1$. In particular, for very small k, Z_o would be very large. However, for $k = 0$,

corresponding to a complete maturation block, $Z_o = 0$. This unacceptable singular behavior (in the mathematical sense) does not occur if cell density limitations are taken into account. Beyond a certain limit, increased cell density must have a negative effect on hemopoietic cell growth. This relatively nonspecific feedback suppression mode is normally secondary to the "balance of growth" mode, but becomes potentially significant in hyperplasia. Cell crowding conditions provide a selective pressure in favor of inherently fast-cycling cells; "blast cells" acquire a growth advantage over maturing cells and (slowly cycling) primitive progenitors (overriding the normal advantage of early progenitors – having stronger resistance to feedback maturation pressures).

Corollary: As the inductivity is reduced to small values, blast cells gain dominance.

Proposition 3. The blast crisis evolves from the chronic phase as a result of a progressive maturation arrest.

Note that a moderate maturation arrest accounts for the chronic phase. It is usually believed that quantitatively different types of cellular lesions are involved: while CML is associated with a proliferative abnormality, a "blast transformation" is postulated to cause "maturation block." In contrast, the present theory requires only one type of change in the function of the cell to explain both phases of the disease. The differences between CML and the blast crisis at the single-cell level may be only a quantitative one while the cell-population manifestations are drastically different. It is suggested that cell crowding, through its effect on the interactions between cells and between compartments, plays a causative role in the transition.

E. Leukemia Progression

While proposing to characterize the relevant cellular change of function – maturation arrest – and link its progression to the acquisition of malignancy, the hypothesis has yet to explain what drives this progression.

The concept of cancer progression, as defined by Foulds [3], refers to the develop-

293

ment of permanent, irreversible, qualitative, and heritable changes in one or more cellular characteristics. The central dogma in oncology is that these changes are due to the inherent genetic instability of the transformed cells, which in turn are manipulated by environmental selective pressures.

The present approach deviates from this dogma, or extends it, in two general aspects. First, it ascribes a deeper, more dynamic nature to the cell-environment relationship. If heritable – or at least recurrent – changes occur in somatic cells possessing extensive division capacity which affects their growth/differentiation characteristics, the tissue composition is bound to change. This in turn leads to additional cellular changes, and so on. The purpose of a more detailed analysis is to understand in quantitative terms the conditions under which the normally self-corrective, negative feedback relationship among cellular constituents may turn into a positive feedback circuit, whereby the different types of changes reinforce each other, leading to further disorganization [6, 8].

The second aspect is the suggestion that the acquisition of increased self-renewal capacity, or decreased sensitivity to maturation pressures, may reflect in the first place a *normal* adaptive capacity on the part of the transforming cells rather than aberrant genetic programs. In fact, the theoretical analysis cannot distinguish between a series of "small," frequent genetic events and a continuous (heritable) cellular change which is not associated with DNA-sequence modifications. The conditions under which the regulatory differentiation pressures are capable of preventing the accumulation of small karyotypic changes or of controlling a slow phenotypic variation may be quite similar. The difficulty to discriminate theoretically and experimentally between such genetic and epigenetic phenomena notwithstanding, it can be shown that a form of restricted adaptive variability of the cellular phenotype, beyond that which is usually implied by a "genetic program," is consistent with both the normal stability of the phenotypic patterns and their transformability in response to some perturbations. By assuming, in particular, that the growth characteristics of normal hemopoietic cells are subject to adaptive changes in both directions, and

not only to down-regulation of the self-renewal capacity with differentiation, it is possible to offer explanations for the progressive nature of chronic leukemia and preleukemia. Again, cell crowding may play a causative role in the transformation process, driving differentiation in the "wrong direction."

Assumption 3: Stimulation of cells to replicate tends to induce in them (slowly) an increased capacity for self-renewal (or equivalently, reduced sensitivity to differentiation signals). Stimulation to differentiate, or mature, has the opposite effect.

Some growth factors can regulate the expression and affinity of their own receptors. Several observations indicate that the capacity for self-renewal of hemopoietic cells can be up- or down-regulated by external influences (e.g., [17, 18]) and there is indirect evidence for a role for DNA methylation [19]. When populations identified by their capacity to form colonies under certain conditions are examined by other means, striking heterogeneities are uncovered [20].

With Assumption 3 incorporated into the scheme, proposition 3 can now be translated into a mathematical model corresponding to Fig. 2, but in which the inductivities are assumed to have constitutive (fixed) components as well as variable components [8, 12]. The latter may evolve (slowly) according to the actual self-renewal activity of the cells and to the cell densities. In Fig. 3, for example, the constitutive part is chosen to be 60% of the normal value, leading to a stable (chronic) hyperplasia and a stable steady state average for the variable part. The variability in the inductivity of the blast cells which was assumed here introduced only a small correction to their average inductivity as compared to a model with no such variability; this is because the rate of change in the inductivity of these cells is small in comparison to their turnover rate. However, further computer simulations of the model demonstrated the validity of the following proposition:

Proposition 4: Under conditions of excessive cell crowding, the stability both of the growth-characteristics' profile and of the numerical balance between compartments

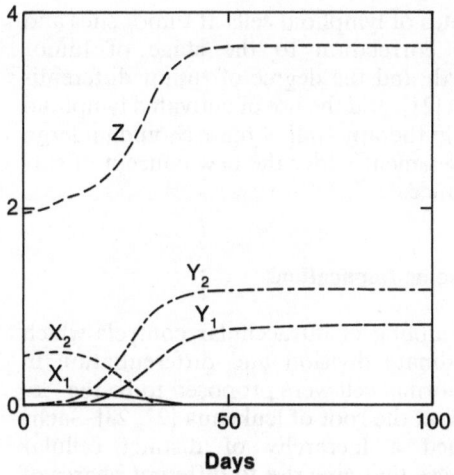

Fig. 3. Computer simulation of a simplified mathematical model corresponding to Fig. 2 with a variable inductivity for blast cells. For the stem cells, $k=0.6$ (normally, $k=1$). X_1 and X_2 are normal stem cell and blast cell numbers, respectively (in arbitrary units); Y_1 and Y_2 are leukemic stem cell and blast cell numbers; Z is the number of mature cells

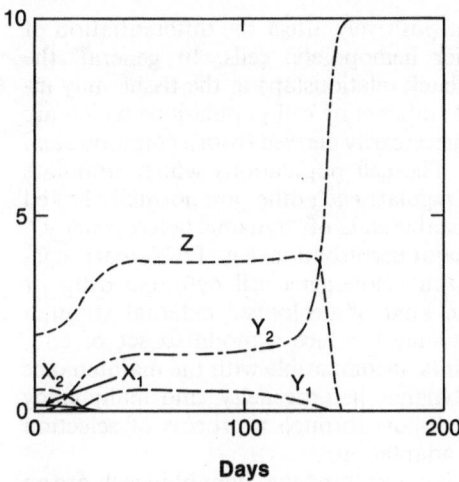

Fig. 4. Notations as in Fig. 3; $k=0.5$

may be reversed, with a consequent dominance of a transformed subpopulation manifesting a maximal maturation arrest.

In Fig. 4, the constitutive component of the inductivity is reduced to 50% of the normal value. A transient (chronic) state of hyperplasia emerges, but a self-driven process of selection and adaptation leads to a blast crisis 100 days later. The reversal of stability results from a failure of the feedback loop – because of cell crowding – to counteract downwards fluctuations in the inductivity with (transiently) increased numbers of mature cells which would enhance the maturation pressures and up-regulate the average inductivity [12]. This failure enables such downwards fluctuations to accumulate.

Proposition 5 (Summary): An initial heritable event in an early hemopoietic cell, generating a clone with partial maturation arrest, leads to CML. If the ensuing hyperplasia distorts the interpopulation balance within the dominant leukemic clone beyond a certain level, a snowball-like process of slipping control is initiated: the distortion feeds back onto the individual members of the clone, inducing further decline in the in-

ductivity and consequently more crowding and distortion (selection). This cascade of dynamic changes in the cells and in the tissue, which reinforce each other, leads to the blast cell dominance.

Alternative scenarios have also been proposed [8], corresponding perhaps to different pathogenic situations. In particular:

Proposition 6: Acute leukemia is a local version of the blast crisis. The whole process described above may take place in a small region of the bone marrow, and only later the dominant, transformed blast cells colonize other regions. In this case, the emergence of the acute phase is not preceded by a detectable (macroscopic) phase of chronic leukemia.

The conditions associated with the different routes of progression are not understood, but they could be related to quantitative factors that determine the order in which different cell compartments are eliminated in the course of the selection process: if the primitive leukemic progenitors are suppressed early in the process, cells that can migrate and colonize other niches may not become available until the blastic transformation is completed.

F. Dynamic Heterogeneity and "Immune Surveillance"

The leukemogenesis model described above assumed that cells in the mature compart-

295

ment positively affect the differentiation of earlier hemopoietic cells. In general, the feedback relationships in the tissue may include interacting cell populations which are not necessarily derived from a common stem cell. The cell populations which stimulate and regulate each other are normally linked in a stable state of "dynamic heterogeneity." A major perturbation, e.g., DNA rearrangement in a clonogenic cell, cytotoxic drug, or some kind of prolonged external stimulation, may produce a modified set of constraints, incompatible with the maintenance of dynamic heterogeneity, and malignancy may follow through a process of selection and adaptation.

It is conjectured that lymphoid cells are an important component of the regulatory cell population which generates maturation pressures in some tissue – in particular in the hemopoietic tissues. Since maintenance of these pressures is essential for the balance in the tissue, the conjecture defines a new mode of immune surveillance [11].

The old hypothesis of immune surveillance against cancer is based on two premises: (a) that transformed and normal cells generally have different antigenic qualities, and (b) that the immune system responds to the antigenically modified cells in essentially the same way as it responds to invasive microorganisms. Both premises have been questioned. Now it is suggested that a major function of lymphoid cells, in addition to their classical role as mediators of immune responses, is to assist in regulating the differentiation of a variety of normal cells. They mediate feedback interactions of the type attributed to Z in the leukemia model. The pertinent cognitive aspect of the immune systems in this capacity is recognition of self rather than recognition of foreign antigens. By forcing and steering the turnover of tissue cells, lymphoid cells do not permit accumulation of small irregular phenotypic and karyotypic changes in the tissue. Tumor escape from surveillance may be described as an escape from regulatory differentiation pressures.

The well-established association of neoplasia with various forms of immune deficiencies, the apparent enhancement of tumor "immunogenicity" as the expression of MHC antigens is increased, the role of in-

filtrates of lymphoid cells at tumor sites and their correlation to the stage of tumor growth and the degree of tumor differentiation [21], and the use of activated lymphoid cells in therapy – all of these should undergo reassessment under the new concept of surveillance.

G. Some Implications

Uncoupling of intracellular controls which coordinate division and differentiation in the normal cell were proposed to be the "lesion" at the root of leukemia [22, 23]. Sachs defined a hierarchy of distinct cellular changes that give rise to different phases of malignancy. While sharing with these hypotheses the concept that "arrest" is not an absolute bar to maturation, the present model associates the development of imbalance between proliferation and differentiation with uncoupling of cell subpopulations, and a progressive maturation arrest with changes in the tissue.

An animal model of transplantable leukemia [24] could serve to test these ideas. The theory predicts the possibility that blast crisis cells transplanted into healthy recipients may undergo differentiation in the host: the normal inductive forces in the host could be sufficient to induce differentiation of the partially responsive blasts and their leukemic progenitors. As the leukemic clone expands and gains dominance over the recipient hemopoietic cells a transient chronic phase may be expected to be followed by a blast crisis. Indeed, it was observed that a CML-like phase preceded the reemergence of blasts as the dominant population [24]. Chromosomal analysis is required to determine whether the mature cells at the chronic phase and the leukemic blasts belong to the same clone.

This interpretation suggests that even when reconstitution of the dominance of the normal cells is not possible (e.g., due to the depletion of the normal primitive progenitors), it may be possible to *recouple* the leukemic blast population to the rest of the leukemic clone [7] or, in other words, to restore the maturational heterogeneity. The feasibility of such a strategy depends on creating an appropriate cellular environment and providing, initially, the proper activation signals. Later on, a prolonged state of remission may be self-sustained, without therapy, if the steady state is stable (as in Fig. 3) or may require continuous intervention, at some level, if this is not the case. The period during which therapy is required may be finite if it is accompanied by adaptive cell normalization (in the model – increase in the heritable inductivity of the clonogenic cells). Due to the strong analogy drawn between the progression of acute leukemia from preleukemia and that of the blast crisis from CML, the same argument holds in principle for both diseases. As was noted [8, 12], in accord with the different respective scenarios offerred for the pathogenesis of these diseases, the dominance of blast cells in the blast crisis may be more complete and irreversible.

While chromosomal analysis in the guinea pig model has not yet been performed, new evidence in the human [25, 26] is relevant and intriguing. Recombinant DNA techniques were used to determine the origin of granulocytes in patients with acute nonlymphocytic leukemia, at presentation, in remission, and in relapse. The results provide evidence that leukemic blast cells can differentiate in vivo and that the same preleukemic clone has the potential to support normal hemopoiesis (in remission) or to allow the emergence of blastic leukemia (at presentation and in relapse). The interpretation of both the authors [25] and the editorial is that (a) leukemia arises from multiple genetic or epigenetic events, with early preleukemic stem cells coexisting with leukemic cells; (b) cytotoxic agents kill leukemic cells, but normal stem cell and preleukemic stem cells are resistant; (c) the preleukemic population can differentiate into mature elements. The experimental results, however, may be reinterpreted according to the present systemic approach. While in agreement with points (a) and (c) above, the new interpretation of the effect of the therapeutic agents is that they restore a closer-to-normal cellular environment which allows the recoupling of the blast cell compartment to the (previously suppressed) progenitor and mature cell compartments. This interpretation avoids the necessity to postulate a complete and highly selective elimination of leukemic blasts.

Whatever the fate of most of the original blasts is – cell death or forced terminal differentiation – the state of remission is stabilized, at least in part, by the imposed change of cellular organization. Discrimination between these interpretations using direct observations in human patients is difficult so that studies in animal models or in Dexter's cultures are required.

Another implication of the present approach is that, since the phenotypic patterns of the transforming cells during progression are assumed to reflect the degree of their adaptation to the changing tissue conditions, a careful monitoring of these patterns may turn out to be a more reliable prognostic tool than karyotypic analysis.

H. Concluding Remarks

A single type of change in the cell function is *sufficient* to account both for CML (or preleukemia) and for the progression into the blast crisis. The *minimal* number of "events" is one. Disorganization of the tissue plays a causal role in the process, beyond a selection for more aggressive clones.

Although the theory cannot discriminate between the accumulation of heritable epigenetic effects (i.e., changes in gene expression stabilized, e.g., by DNA methylation) versus that of small modifications in the DNA sequence, the first possibility is more attractive and constitutes the "minimal" interpretation consistent with the data. The "normalcy" of the transformation process, as an expression of essentially normal cellular phenotypic adaptability, is stressed. Genetic aberrations may contribute to the process, mainly at the later stages. Note that the accumulation of phenotypic changes occurred in a transitory cell population, not in stem cells, over a period much longer than the initial turnover time of this population. Accumulation of DNA modifications is more likely to take place within self-renewing cells.

Killing or changing the behavior of all the bad cells directly might not be feasible. The present approach stresses the need for the understanding of the "dynamic heterogeneity" in the tissue in order to restore it or prevent its disruption in the early stages of carcinogenesis or in remission.

As was recently stressed[1], current paradigms have a heavy impact on research in the field of carcinogenesis; there is a need to reevaluate the strengths and weaknesses of the presently fashionable paradigms.

References

1. Blau HM et al. (1985) Science 23:758–766
2. Razin A, Cedar LH (1984) Int Rev Cytol 92:159–185
3. Foulds L (1969) Neoplastic development. Academic Press, New York
4. Duesberg PH (1985) Science 228:669–677
5. Smithers DW (1962) Lancet:493–499
6. Rubin H (1985) Cancer Res 45:2935–2942
7. Grossman Z (1984) In: Avula XJR (ed) Mathematical modeling in science and technology. Pergamon, New York, pp 933–938
8. Grossman Z (1986) EMBO J 5:671–677
9. Grossman Z (1986) Leuk Res 10:937–950
10. Grossman Z, Levine RF (1986) In: Levine RF et al. (eds) Megakaryocyte development and function. Liss, New York, pp 51–69

11. Grossman Z, Herberman RB (1986) Immunol Today 7:128–131
12. Grossman Z (1986) Math Modeling 7:1255–1268
13. Bennett DC (1983) Cell 34:445–453
14. Metcalf D (1980) Proc Natl Acad Sci USA 77:5327–5330
15. Levin J (1986) In: Levine RF et al. (eds) Megakaryocyte development and function. Liss, New York, pp 157–177
16. Grossman Z, Herberman RB (1986) Cancer Res 46:2651–2658
17. Spooncer E, Boettiger D, Dexter TM (1984) Nature 310:228–230
18. Chang LJ-A, McCulloch EA (1981) Blood 57:361–367
19. Motoji T et al. (1985) Blood 65:894–901
20. McCulloch EA, Smith LJ, Minden MD (1982) Cancer Surv 1:279–298
21. Ioachim HL (1976) JNCI 57:465–475
22. Greaves MF (1979) In: Boelsma E, Rümke P (eds) Tumor markers. Elsevier, Amsterdam, pp 201–211
23. Sachs L (1980) Proc Natl Acad Sci USA 77:6152–6156
24. Evans WH, Miller DA (1982) Leuk Res 6:819–825
25. Fearon ER et al. (1986) N Engl J Med 315:15–23
26. Fearon ER et al. (1986) N Engl J Med 315:56–57

---

[1] Announcement of the International Conference on Theories of Carcinogenesis, Oslo, August 1986

Haematology and Blood Transfusion Vol. 31
Modern Trends in Human Leukemia VII
Edited by Neth, Gallo, Greaves, and Kabisch
© Springer-Verlag Berlin Heidelberg 1987

The Nucleoskeleton: Active Site of Transcription and Replication

D. A. Jackson and P. R. Cook

A. Introduction

Nuclei and chromatin are rarely studied at a physiological salt concentration since they aggregate so readily [16]. As a result, they are generally studied in the presence of "stabilizing" divalent cations under hyper- or hypotonic conditions. Such conditions are unsatisfactory for several reasons. The "stabilizing" cations activate nucleases, destroying template integrity and supercoiling, and unphysiological salt concentrations may introduce artefacts. It has been suggested that structures called variously the nuclear matrix, cage or scaffold, are the site of replication and transcription [8], but they are not seen in the micrographs of "genes in action" obtained by Miller and colleagues using hypotonic conditions [15, 14]. These powerful images resembling Christmas trees are interpreted in terms of a mobile polymerase which processes along the DNA and is unat-

Sir William Dunn School of Pathology, University of Oxford, South Parks Road, Oxford, OX1 3RE, England

tached to any larger structure. Such models are now included in most standard textbooks [1]. As a result, we have two paradoxical views of DNA function: in the one, the skeletal substructure is the essential active site; in the other, it is not required and may not even exist.

We have described a method for isolating chromatin using a physiological salt concentration. Living cells are encapsulated in agarose microbeads. The bead pores are large enough to allow free exchange of protein as large as 1.5×10^8 daltons but not of chromosomal DNA [3, 9]. Therefore, when encapsulated cells are immersed in Triton X-100 at a physiological salt concentration, most cytoplasmic proteins and RNA diffuse out through the pores to leave encapsulated chromatin. If cells are lysed in the presence of EDTA, the resulting DNA remains intact. The procedure yields essentially a preparation of encapsulated nuclei (Fig. 1). However, these nuclei differ from their unencapsulated counterparts in that they contain unbroken DNA and can be manipulated freely. The chromatin within the bead is well pro-

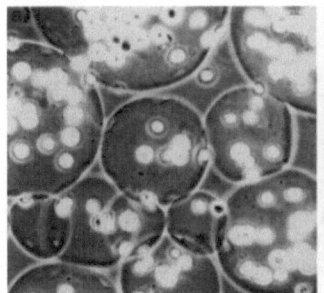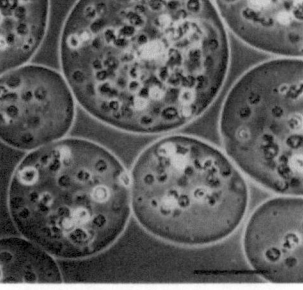

Fig. 1. Phase contrast micrographs of 0.5% agarose beads containing HeLa cells before (**a**) and after (**b**) lysis. *Bar* = 100 µm. (From Jackson and Cook [10])

tected from aggregation and shearing but is nevertheless completely accessible to enzymes and other probes used in modern molecular biology.

I. Two Models for Transcription

Two extremely different views of how transcription might occur are presented in Fig. 2. The essential difference is the participation of a larger nuclear substructure in the active site of the transcription complex. They can be distinguished by fragmenting the chromatin with an endonuclease and removing any unattached chromatin by electrophoresis. If view B is correct, then the transcription complex will remain associated with the larger structure and so trapped in the bead; if view A is correct, it should escape from the bead on electrophoresis [10].

The encapsulated nuclei contain a very active RNA polymerase which is sensitive to α-amanatin, a specific inhibitor of RNA polymerase II, and which synthesizes RNA at a rate roughly equivalent to that found in

Table 1. Active transcription complexes cannot be removed electrophoretically from beads following treatment with *Eco*RI and RNase (from Jackson and Cook [10])

Treatment	% Remaining		
	DNA	RNA[a]	Polymerase
Control	100	100	100
*Eco*RI	30	100	85
RNase	100	< 5	86
*Eco*RI and RNase	27	< 5	70

After various treatments, the incorporation of [^{32}P] UTP into RNA in 30 min was expressed as a percentage of the control.
[a] RNA remaining after pulse-labelling cells for 2.5 min with [^{3}H] uridine.

vivo. *Eco*RI digestion reduces both the initial rate of RNA synthesis and the total amount of RNA made to ~60% of the control (Fig. 3, curves 1 and 2), presumably because the template is truncated. Removing 75% of the chromatin by electrophoresis reduces the activity no further (Fig. 3,

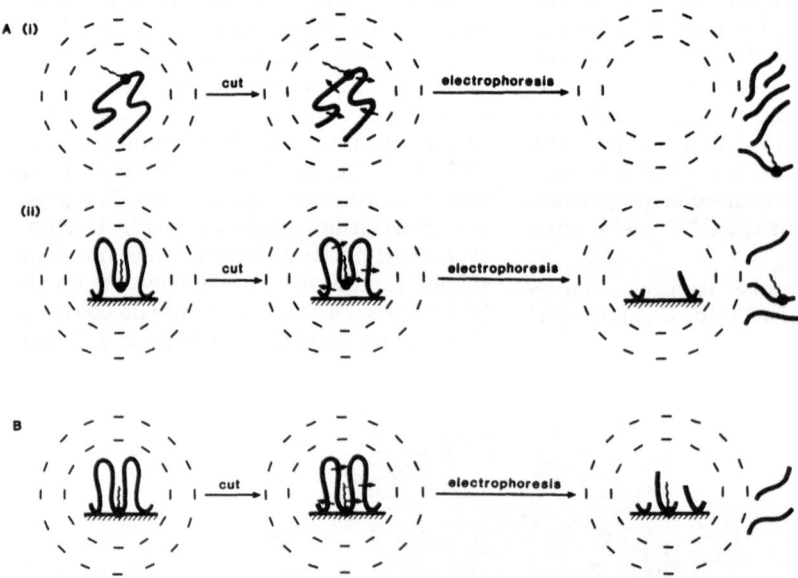

Fig. 2. Two models for transcription. **A,** RNA polymerase (●) processes along the DNA (−) synthesizing a nascent transcript (∼). **B,** Transcripts are generated as DNA moves past a polymerase associated with the nuclear skeleton (*hatched* area). After cutting DNA with an endonuclease (*arrow*) and electrophoresis, the transcribed sequence, nascent RNA and polymerase should be retained within the bead (*broken circles*) in B but not A. (From Jackson and Cook) [10])

300

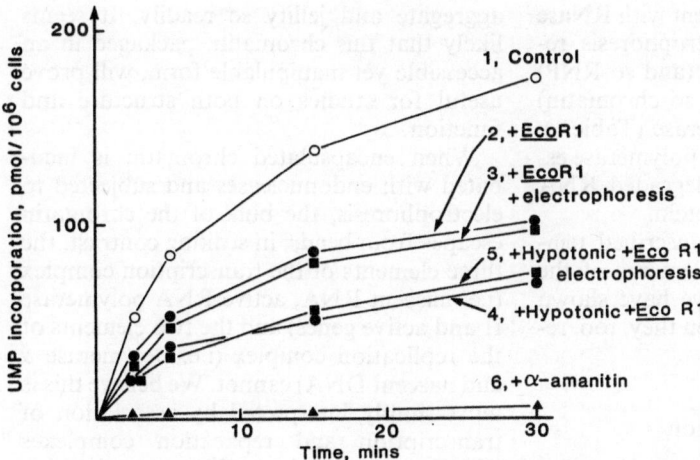

Fig. 3. *Eco*RI treatment and electrophoresis do not remove active RNA polymerase. Cells were labelled overnight with [³H]thymidine, encapsulated, lysed and washed. Sample *1*, beads were kept on ice; sample *2*, incubated with *Eco*RI and then kept on ice; sample *3*, incubated with *Eco*RI, subjected to electrophoresis; sample *4*, as 2, with hypotonic treatment preceding *Eco*RI digestion; sample *5*, as 3, with hypotonic treatment preced-

ing *Eco*RI digestion. The samples were then incubated with [³²P]UTP and appropriate cofactors for various lengths of time and the amount of label incorporated into RNA was determined; 100% of the ³H initially present was recovered in samples 1, 2 and 4, 25% in sample 3 and 20% in sample 5. In a parallel experiment, beads were also incubated with 10 μg/ml α-amanitin (sample *6*). (From Jackson and Cook [10])

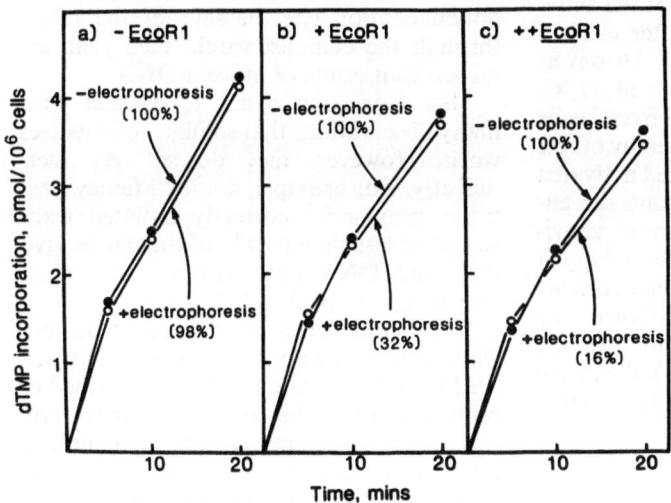

Fig. 4. The replication complex is closely associated with the nucleoskeleton. Cells labelled for 24 h with [³H] thymidine were encapsulated and lysed, and beads were washed. MgCl₂ was added and samples incubated with (*a*) 0, (*b*) 1000 and (*c*) 5000 units/ml *Eco*RI. Half of each set of beads was subjected to electrophoresis in isotonic buffer.

After recovering beads, the rate of incorporation of [³²P] dTTP into DNA was determined. The amount of [³H] in equal volumes of each sample was determined and expressed as a percentage (*brackets*) of the sample in (a) that had not been treated with *Eco*RI or subjected to electrophoresis. (From Jackson and Cook [11])

curve 3). A combined treatment with RNase and *Eco*RI, followed by electrophoresis, removes >95% nascent RNA (and so RNP) and 73% of the DNA (and so chromatin) but only 30% of the polymerase (Table 1). Clearly, little – if any – active polymerase escapes with the chromatin, degraded RNA and associated ribonucleoprotein.

Nascent RNA and the transcribed template constitute two other elements of the transcription complex and we have shown that following *Eco*RI digestion they, too, resist electroelution [10].

II. Two Models for Replication

Replication might also involve attached or unattached polymerases [11]. Encapsulated nuclei contain a DNA polymerase α which is found only in S-phase cells and which is not stimulated by added "activated" templates, preferring the endogenous chromatin; most importantly, it is extremely efficient. For example, under the suboptimal concentration of dTTP that we use here, the initial rate of incorporation is 9% of that in vivo; under more optimal concentrations it exceeds 75%. It is relatively stable at 4 °C and resists electroelution, with about 90% of the activity being recovered in beads after electrophoresis for 5 h in isotonic buffer. However, this activity is relatively unstable at 37 °C, becoming soluble, able to escape from beads and more like the activities studied by others (e.g. it is now stimulated by added activated templates or by nicking or cutting the endogenous template). These aberrant activities easily obscure the authentic activity if broken templates are available. *Eco*RI treatment of encapsulated nuclei followed by electroelution removed up to 84% of the chromatin but no activity (Fig. 4); the active polymerizing complex also resists electroelution.

B. Discussion

Some of the experiments described here involve several enzyme digestions or assays in physiological salt concentrations, treatment with detergents and electrophoresis overnight – manipulations that would be impossible using free nuclei or chromatin which aggregate and jellify so readily. It seems likely that this chromatin, packaged in an accessible yet manipulable form, will prove useful for studies on both structure and function.

When encapsulated chromatin is incubated with endonucleases and subjected to electrophoresis, the bulk of the chromatin escapes from beads; in striking contrast, the three elements of the transcription complex (i.e. nascent RNA, active RNA polymerase II and active genes) and the two elements of the replication complex (i.e. polymerase α and nascent DNA) cannot. We believe this is most simply interpreted by association of transcription and replication complexes with the nucleoskeleton. This naturally begs the question: To what is the complex attached? As nascent transcripts, DNA, and active genes are closely associated with the nuclear cage [5–7] and matrix [17], it seems likely that these structures isolated in $2M$ NaCl are intimately related to it. We use the term "nucleoskeleton" to describe the analogous structure found under isotonic conditions and envisage it as one part of the active site of the transcription and replication complex, organizing the template in three-dimensional space into close proximity to the polymerization site. Passage of the DNA through the complex would then yield attached transcripts or nascent DNA.

This suggestion seems to conflict with many observations that soluble polymerases work. However, they do so very inefficiently. For example, crude "Manley" extracts polymerize correctly initiated transcripts at less than 0.01% of the rate in vivo [13], and DNA polymerases also initiate very inefficiently [2, 12].

If the polymerase is tethered to the nucleoskeleton, then only genes closely associated with this skeleton will be transcribed or replicated: those that are remote from it will not. Then it becomes easy to imagine how selective attachment of genes to the nucleoskeleton might underlie selective gene activity during development or oncogenesis. Indeed, gross detachment correlated with total inactivation of the avian erythrocyte nucleus [4] and the attachment of infecting viral sequences, the ovalbumin gene and viral oncogenes with their expression [5, 7, 17].

302

Acknowledgements. We thank the Cancer Research Campaign for support, and the editors of the E.M.B.O. J. for permission to reprint the figures.

References

1. Alberts B, Bray D, Lewis J, Raff M, Roberts K, Watson JD (1983) Molecular biology of the cell. Garland, New York
2. Ariga H, Sugano S (1983) J Virol 48:481–491
3. Cook PR (1984) EMBO J 3:1837–1842
4. Cook PR, Brazell IA (1976) J Cell Sci 22:287–302
5. Cook PR, Lang J, Hayday A, Lania L, Fried M, Chiswell DJ, Wyke JA (1982) EMBO J 1:447–452
6. Jackson DA, McCready SJ, Cook PR (1981) Nature 292:552–555
7. Jackson DA, Caton AJ, McCready SJ, Cook PR (1982) Nature 296:366–368
8. Jackson DA, McCready SJ, Cook PR (1984) J Cell Sci Suppl 1:59–79
9. Jackson DA, Cook PR (1985) EMBO J 4:913–918
10. Jackson DA, Cook PR (1985) EMBO J 4:919–925
11. Jackson DA, Cook PR (1986) EMBO J 5:1403–1410
12. Li JJ, Kelly TJ (1984) Proc Natl Acad Sci USA 81:6973–6977
13. Manley JL, Fire A, Cano A, Sharp PA, Gefter ML (1980) Proc Natl Acad Sci USA 77:3855–3859
14. McKnight SL, Miller OL (1979) Cell 17:551–563
15. Miller OL, Beattie BR (1969) Science 164:955–957
16. Ohlenbusch HH, Olivera BM, Tuan D, Davidson N (1967) J Mol Biol 25:299–315
17. Robinson SI, Nelkin BD, Vogelstein B (1982) Cell 28:99–106

Immunology

Haematology and Blood Transfusion   Vol. 31
Modern Trends in Human Leukemia VII
Edited by Neth, Gallo, Greaves, and Kabisch
© Springer-Verlag Berlin Heidelberg 1987

Henry Kaplan Award for H. J. Stauss

N. A. Mitchison[1]

The award was made for the poster describing the work of Dr. Hans Stauss in the laboratory of Professor Hans Schreiber in Chicago on the grounds that it solves, or at least goes a long way towards solving, a longstanding enigma in tumour immunology, namely, the nature of the tumour-specific transplantation antigens on ultraviolet-induced tumours. This is a problem of great general interest because of the unusually strong potency of these antigens and also be-

[1] Department of Biology, Medawar Building, University College London, Gower Street, London WC1E 6BT

cause of their analogy with the antigens of human skin cancer. In this connection, it should be remembered that skin cancer is one of the few forms of human neoplasm that is under strong immune surveillance, as judged from the elevated incidence of these cancers in immunosuppressed individuals. Indeed, Harald Zur Hausen at this meeting discussed these cancers and their antigens in the context of papilloma virus infection. The judges liked Dr. Stauss' work for its use of a judicious combination of classical transplantation techniques and modern molecular biology. In addition, the poster itself was masterly.

Haematology and Blood Transfusion   Vol. 31
Modern Trends in Human Leukemia VII
Edited by Neth, Gallo, Greaves, and Kabisch
© Springer-Verlag Berlin Heidelberg 1987

Identification of a Gene Encoding a Tumor-Specific Antigen that Causes Tumor Rejection

H. J. Stauss [1]. M. A. Fink, B. Starr, and H. Schreiber [2]

A. Introduction

Transplantation experiments have clearly demonstrated the existence of unique (individual) tumor-specific antigens on cancers induced by physical or chemical carcinogens. These antigens often induce a tumor-specific immune response upon immunization with a tumor which protects the host against a subsequent challenge with the same tumor, but not against a challenge with any other independently induced tumor [1]. Unique antigens were observed even when the tumors were induced with the same carcinogen in the same organ system in the same strain of mice [2]. This finding of unique tumor specificity raises questions about the mechanism by which these tumor-specific antigens are generated. The critical questions regarding such unique tumor-specific antigens are their composition, genetic origin, and possible role as target antigens for the immune system. However, the identification of tumor-specific antigens that cause tumor rejection has proven to be extremely difficult in the past. Serological probes with unique tumor specificity are difficult to obtain [3], and the serologically recognized antigens may not be the target for tumor rejection [4] that is primarily T-cell mediated [5].

We used UV-induced tumors of mice for studying the nature of tumor-specific antigens for the following reasons: (a) the unique tumor-specific rejection antigens on UV-induced tumors are stronger than those on chemically induced tumors, in that UV-induced tumors often regress after transplantation into normal mice even without prior immunization; (b) several of the tumor-specific rejection antigens on one such UV-induced regressor tumor, called 1591-RE, have been defined by cytolytic T-cell clones; (c) monoclonal antibodies with unique specificity for this UV-induced regressor tumor have been generated which reacted with novel MHC class I molecules on this tumor; and (d) the genes encoding the antibody-recognized novel class I molecules have been cloned and identified by transfection. We describe here the relationship between the novel MHC class I molecules encoded by the cloned genes and the rejection antigens of the 1591 tumor. Recently, we found that one of the novel 1591 class I genes encodes an antigen that causes immunological tumor rejection in normal mice [6]. Transfection of this novel class I gene into a 1591 progressor tumor variant leads to the rejection of the gene-transfected progressor tumor, demonstrating that a single gene can revert the progressive growth behavior and establish the regressor phenotype characteristic of the parental 1591-RE tumor.

[1] Supported by a Fellowship of the National Cancer Cytology Center and a Fellowship of the Deutsche Forschungsgemeinschaft
[2] Supported by Grants PO1 CA-19266, RO1 CA-22677 and RO1 CA-37156 from the National Cancer Institute
Department of Pathology, University of Chicago, Chicago, IL 60637, USA

B. Results

The 1591 tumor contains three novel class I genes designated 216, 166, and 149 which account for the abnormal reactivity of the tumor cells with MHC class I-specific monoclonal antibodies [7]. The gene 216 encodes an antigen that is selectively recognized by the 1591 tumor-specific antibody CP28 [8]. The molecules encoded by the genes 149 and 166 cross-react with monoclonal antibodies specific for allogeneic MHC class I antigens. Together, the three 1591 class I genes 216, 166, and 149 can account for all the novel MHC class I determinants expressed by

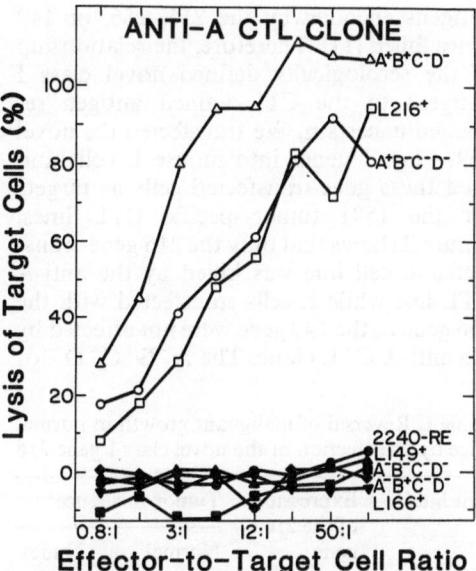

Fig. 2. The 1591 class I gene 216 encodes the antigen that is recognized by the tumor-specific anti-A CTL clone. This T-cell clone defines the A antigen on the 1591 tumor as rejection antigen because it selects in vitro from the parental regressor tumor for antigen loss variants that grow progressively in normal mice. The two 1591 regressor tumors with the phenotype $(A^+B^+C^-D^-)$ and $(A^+B^-C^-D^-)$, and the 216 gene-transfected L cells are lysed by this CTL clone. L cells transfected with the 1591 class I genes 149 or 166 or the A^- variants of the 1591 tumor or an unrelated UV-induced C3H tumor (2240-RE) are not lysed in a 4.5-h ^{51}Cr release assay. (A, B, C, and D are CTL defined 1591 tumor-specific antigens) (Reproduced from Ref. 6)

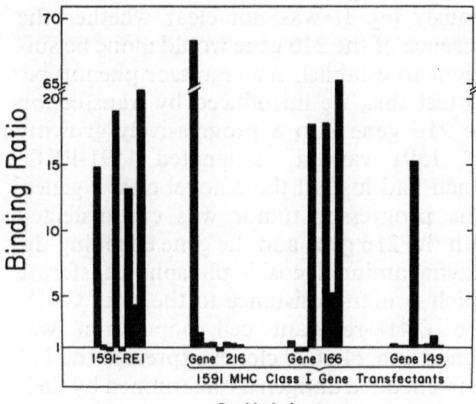

Cell Lines

Fig. 1. The 1591 class I genes 216, 166, and 149 account for all the novel MHC class I determinants that are expressed by the parental 1591-RE tumor. Furthermore, the novel class I gene 216 selectively encodes for the antigen reactive with the syngeneic tumor-specific monoclonal antibody CP28. Shown is the binding of nine MHC class I-specific monoclonal antibodies to the parental 1591 tumor (1591-RE1) or to mouse L cells transfected with the 1591 class I genes 216, 166, and 149, respectively. Untransfected L cells do not react with any of the nine monoclonal antibodies (not shown). The fluorescence-activated cell sorter, FACS IVB, was used to determine the indirect fluorescence listed as binding ration, i.e., fluorescence of the cells stained with the first (anti-MHC class I) and second (fluoresceinated goat anti-mouse) antibody over the fluorescence of the cells stained with the second antibody alone. The bars (left to right) indicate the binding of the antibodies CP28, 34-2-12 (D^d), 34-5-8 (D^d), 28-14-8 (L^dD^b,q), 34-4-20 (L^dD^d), 30-5-7 ($L^dD^qL^qL^b$), 23-5-21 ($D^bD^dD^s$,q,p), and CP3F4 to the tested cells (Reproduced from Ref. 6 with permission of the editors)

1591 tumor cells (Fig. 1). In addition, the 1591-RE1 tumor expresses multiple independent CTL-defined antigens [9] each of which can independently cause tumor rejection. In the first part of our study, we determined whether any of the three novel MHC class I genes (216, 166, or 149) encoded the antigen recognized by anti-A CTL. We have shown previously that tumor variants selected for the loss of the anti-A CTL-defined antigen are no longer rejected by normal mice [10] implicating a close linkage between (or even identity of) the A antigen and the antigen leading to tumor rejection. However, careful attempts to block A antigen-specific CTL clones with antibodies specific for any one of the three novel class I MHC antigens encoded by the 216, 166, or 149 genes failed [11]. Therefore, the relationship of the serologically defined novel class I antigens to the CTL-defined antigen remained uncertain. We transfected the novel 1591 class I genes into mouse L cells and used these gene-transfected cells as targets for the 1591 tumor-specific CTL lines. Figure 2 shows that only the 216 gene-transfected L cell line was killed by the anti-A CTL line while L cells transfected with the 166 gene or the 149 gene were not affected by the anti-A CTL clone. The $A^-B^+C^-D^-$ or

the $A^-B^-C^-D^-$ variants of the 1591 were not killed. As expected, however, the $A^+B^-C^-D^-$ variant of 1591 was killed by the anti-A CTL, as was the $A^+B^+C^-D^-$ parental 1591-RE regressor tumor line. Anti-B, anti-C, or anti-D CTL did not kill any of the L cells transfected with the novel MHC class I genes (not shown). Together, our data clearly indicate that the 216 gene-encoded novel class I antigen is recognized by both the CP28 monoclonal antibody (Fig. 1) as well as the anti-A CTL clone (Fig. 2).

We have shown previously that all the in vivo- or in vitro-derived progressor variants of the 1591-RE tumor had lost all three novel class I genes 216, 166, and 149 simultaneously [6]. It was not clear whether the presence of the 216 gene would alone be sufficient to establish the regressor phenotype. To test this, we introduced by transfection the 216 gene into a progressively growing A^- 1591 variant, designated 1591-PRO, which had lost all three novel class I genes. This progressor tumor was cotransfected with the 216 gene and the gene encoding the enzyme aminoglycoside phosphotransferase which confers resistance to the drug G418. The G418-resistant cell population was cloned and 24 of 77 clones expressed the 216 gene-encoded antigen as determined by their reactivity with the CP28 antibody. Two 216 genes expressing, A antigen-positive clones, designated $TR216^+.1$ and $TR216^+.2$, and two negative clones, designated $TR216^-.3$

Table 1. Reversal of malignant growth in normal mice by transfection of the novel class I gene 216

Cell line[a]	Expression of the 216 gene product[b]	Tumor incidence[c]	
		Normal mice	Nude mice
1591-PRO TR216$^+$1	+	1/5[d]	2/2
1591-PRO TR216$^+$1	+	0/5	2/2
Total		1/10 (10%)	
1591-PRO TR216$^-$3	−	5/5	2/2
1591-PRO TR216$^-$4	−	4/5	2/2
Total		9/10 (90%)	
1591-PRO TR216.1 reisolate[d]	−	5/5 (100%)	ND
1591-PRO	−	8/10 (80%)	ND
1591-RE	+	0/10 (0%)	2/2

[a] A clone of the progressor tumor, 1591-PRO was transfected with the 216 gene and the neomycin-resistant gene. The G418 drug-resistant cell population was cloned and two clones which expressed the 216 gene-encoded antigen (1591-PRO TR216$^+$1 and 1591-PRO TR216$^+$2) and two clones which did not express the 216 gene-encoded antigen (1591-PRO TR216$^-$3 and 1591-PRO TR216$^-$4) were used to challenge five normal mice or two nude mice with tumor fragments containing $> 10^8$ tumor cells.
[b] Expression of the 216 gene product was determined by FACS IVB analysis using the monoclonal antibody CP28 that specifically recognized this gene product and a fluoresceinated second antibody. Cell lines designated positive for expression of the 216 gene product stained at least two times above background (binding ratio > 2), while all cell lines designated negative for 216 gene

expression stained less than 1.5-fold above background (binding ratio < 1.5).
[c] Number of mice with progressively growing tumors/number of mice challenged. Mice receiving the 216$^-$ clones died within approximately 6 weeks due to the large tumor burden. The mice that were challenged with the 216$^+$ transfectants did not develop tumors even after 4 months, except for one mouse that grew out an antigen loss variant approximately 2.5 weeks after injection. All cell lines used in this experiment readily formed tumors in nude mice.
[d] One of the mice injected with the transfected 1591-PRO TR216$^+$1 cell line developed a progressively growing tumor that was reisolated (designated 1591-PRO TR216.1 reisolate) and reanalyzed for expression of the 216 gene by FACS IVB (Fig. 3) and for tumor incidence in normal mice. (Reproduced from Ref. 6)

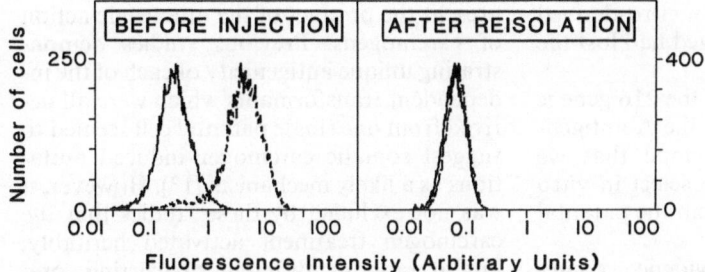

Fig. 3. Loss of expression of the transfected 216 gene in a reisolated 1591-PR0 tumor that grew progressively despite transfection with the 216 gene. The 216 gene-transfected tumors analyzed are the same as those used for the experiments described in Table 1. The *first panel* shows the histogram of the 1591-PR0 TR216$^+$.1 cell line and the *second panel* shows the histogram of the 1591-PR0 TR216.1 reisolate. Cells were incubated with the monoclonal antibody CP28 followed by incubation with fluerescein-coupled goat anti-mouse immunoglobulin antibodies (‒‒) or incubated with only the goat anti-mouse immunoglobulin (—). Ten thousand cells were analyzed with the FACS IVB. (Reproduced from Ref. 6)

and TR216$^-$.4, which were G418 resistant but did not express the 216 gene-encoded antigen were analyzed further. Cells of these four clones were injected into nude mice and fragments of the growing tumors were used to challenge normal animals. The use of tumor fragments grown in nude mice ensured that the cloned transfectants were still capable of growing as a malignant tumor in nude mice. Table 1 shows that the 216 gene expressing TR216$^+$.1 clone grew out in only one of five animals and the 216 gene expressing TR216$^+$.2 clone was rejected in all animals despite the fact that the mice were challenged with a large tumor dose ($>10^8$ cells). In contrast, the clones TR216$^-$.3 and TR216$^-$.4 which do not express the 216 gene-encoded antigen grew in five of five and four of five mice, respectively, and all these mice died of progressive tumor growth. The single tumor which grew out in one of the animals that were challenged with the 216 gene expressing TR216$^+$.1 clone was readapted to culture and analyzed for the expression of the 216 gene-encoded antigen with the fluorescence-activated cell sorter. All cells of the reisolate were negative for the 216 antigen, indicating that the cells either lost the transfected 216 gene or that its expression was prevented by some other mechanism. This variant that did not express the 216 gene-encoded antigen was injected into five normal animals and tumor growth resulted in all the mice (Table 1). Together,

these data indicate that the stable expression of the 216 gene-encoded antigen is sufficient to change the phenotype of a progressor tumor so that it is rejected by the normal animal. Furthermore, the loss of the expression of this 216 antigen in transfected tumor cells allows these cells to regain the progressor phenotype characteristic of the untransfected parental progressor tumor.

C. Discussion

Many years ago, studies clearly demonstrated that tumor-specific antigens that are distinct (unique) for each individual tumor can lead to a complete immunological destruction of experimental cancers. However, the molecules eliciting (and being the target of) these immune responses have remained obscure. We have cloned and analyzed the genes encoding novel class I molecules expressed by a UV-induced murine skin tumor, designated 1591, to determine their role in the immunobiology of tumor rejection and tumor progression. Several lines of evidence clearly indicate that one of these genes, called gene 216, encodes an antigen that elicits 1591 tumor-specific rejection and is the target molecule of tumor rejection:

1. The 216 gene-encoded antigen must be lost before the tumor can grow progressively in a normal immunocompetent mouse. Southern blot analysis showed

311

that all of the in vivo- or in vitro-derived progressor variants analyzed had lost the 216 gene [6].

2. The molecule encoded by the 216 gene is specifically recognized by the A antigen-specific cytolytic T-cell clone that we have previously shown to select in vitro for progressor variants from the parental regressor tumor cell line.

3. The most conclusive evidence comes from the fact that transfection of the 216 gene into progressively growing 1591 tumor variants leads to the expression of the 216 gene-encoded antigen on the tumor and to complete rejection of all cells expressing this antigen. Thus, the progressor tumor reverted to the parental regressor phenotype following transfection.

Unique tumor-specific transplantation antigens are antigenically distinct for independently induced tumors. These different antigens may, therefore, be encoded either by numerous different unrelated genes or by a single gene which underwent multiple different mutational changes. Alternatively, these antigens might be encoded by the members of a gene family such as the immunoglobulin genes, the T-cell receptor genes, the MHC class I and class II genes, or the genes of the multiple retroviral proviruses which are present in the murine genome. Some of these gene families are known to contain the coding information for a large variety of distinct molecules and could therefore account for the observed remarkable antigenic polymorphism among tumor-specific transplantation antigens. It is interesting to notice that even a single malignant cell can express multiple unique tumor-specific antigens as has been shown for the tumor P815 [12] or 1591-RE [9]. To determine whether these antigens are encoded by a family of related genes or by multiple unrelated genes, it is necessary to analyze more tumors and to identify molecularly and genetically more unique tumor-specific transplantation antigens.

Another important and still unresolved question regarding the origin of unique tumor-specific antigens is whether the genes encoding such antigens are preexisting in the genome or whether these genes appear as the result of somatic mutation and as such re-present the product of the mutagenic action of carcinogens. Previous studies demonstrating unique antigenicity of each of the independent transformants which were all derived from one single parental cell seemed to suggest somatic carcinogen-induced mutations as a likely mechanism [13]. However, it was not excluded by these studies that the carcinogen treatment activated heritably, but at random, different preexisting, previously silent genes. Such a mechanism could also account for the observed immunogenicity of tumors in the autochthonous host [2]. In order to determine whether somatic mutations are involved in the malignant transformation and in the generation of tumor-specific antigens, we are presently searching for genetic changes in tumor cells which are not present in normal cells of the same individual.

References

1. Prehn RT, Main JM (1957) Immunity to methylcholanthrene-induced sarcomas. JNCI 18:769
2. Klein G, Sjogren HO, Klein E, Hellstrom KE (1960) Demonstration of resistance against methylcholanthrene-induced sarcomas in the primary autochthonous host. Cancer Res 20:1561
3. Old LJ (1982) Cancer immunology: the search for specificity. Natl Cancer Inst Monogr 60:193
4. Davey GC, Currie GA, Alexander P (1979) A serologically detected tumor-specific membrane antigen of murine lymphomas which is not the target for syngeneic graft rejection. Br J Cancer 40:168
5. Rouse BT, Roellinghoff M, Warner NL (1972) Anti-0 serum-induced suppression of cellular transfer of tumor-specific immunity to a syngeneic plasma cell tumor. Nature (New Biol) 238:116
6. Stauss HJ, Van Waes C, Fink MA, Starr B, Schreiber H (1986) Identification of a unique tumor antigen as rejection antigen by molecular cloning and gene transfer. J Exp Med 164:1516
7. Stauss HJ, Linsk R, Fischer A, Banasiak D, Haberman A, Clark I, Forman J, McMillan M, Schreiber H, Goodenow RS (1986) Isolation of the MHC genes encoding the tumor-specific class I antigens expressed on a murine fibrosarcoma. J Immunogenet 13:101–111

8. Philipps C, McMillan M, Flood PM, Murphy DB, Forman J, Lancki D, Womack JE, Goodenow RS, Schreiber H (1985) Identification of a unique tumor-specific antigen as a novel class I major histocompatibility molecule. Proc Natl Acad Sci USA 82:5140

9. Wortzel RD, Philipps C, Schreiber H (1983) Multiple tumor-specific antigens expressed on a single tumor cell. Nature (Lond) 304:165

10. Wortzel RD, Urban JL, Schreiber H (1984) Malignant growth in the normal host after variant selection in vitro with cytolytic T cell lines. Proc Natl Acad Sci USA 81:2186

11. Philipps C, Stauss HJ, Wortzel RD, Schreiber H (1986) A novel MHC class I molecule as tumor-specific antigen: correlation between the antibody-defined and the CTL-defined target structure. J Immunogenet 13:93

12. Uyttenhove C, Maryanski J, Boon T (1983) Escape of mouse mastocytoma P815 after nearly complete rejection is due to antigen-loss variants rather than immunosuppression. J Exp Med 157:1040

13. Embleton MJ, Heidelberger C (1972) Antigenicity of clones of mouse prostate cells transformed in vitro. Int J Cancer 9:8

Haematology and Blood Transfusion   Vol. 31
Modern Trends in Human Leukemia VII
Edited by Neth, Gallo, Greaves, and Kabisch
© Springer-Verlag Berlin Heidelberg 1987

Formation of a Hybrid *bcl*-2/Immunoglobulin Transcript as a Result of t(14;18) Chromosomal Translocation

M. L. Cleary and J. Sklar

A. Introduction

Specific chromosomal changes are consistently associated with several morphologically or histologically distinct forms of cancer [1]. In a few hematolymphoid malignancies, chromosomal translocations are known to occur near or within the cytologic loci for cellular homologues of retroviral-encoded oncogenes [2]. For example, both the c-*abl* and c-*myc* proto-oncogenes are targets for interchromosomal translocations in chronic myelogous leukemia and Burkitt's lymphoma, respectively [3, 4]. Recent molecular studies have elucidated the structural consequences that chromosomal translocations have upon these cellular proto-oncogenes [5–7]. However, most of the recurring chromosomal translocations which have been described, particularly in hematolymphoid malignancies, do not result in structural alterations of cellular homologues for known retroviral oncogenes. Presumably these cytogenetic abnormalities affect cellular genes which have not been transduced by retroviruses and therefore remain largely undefined. One approach toward isolation and characterization of these candidate human proto-oncogenes is to clone from appropriate tumors chromosomal transloca-

tion breakpoints. The breakpoint DNAs can then be used to identify closely linked transcriptional units for further study.

A particularly common translocation is the reciprocal t(14;18) translocation that occurs in at least 85%–90% of human follicular lymphomas [8]. We and others have shown that the points of crossover on chromosome 14 for these translocations always occur within or directly adjacent to an Ig heavy chain joining region [9–11]. The molecular features of t(14;18) crossovers suggested that these interchromosomal translocations result from errors in V-D-J joining during B-cell differentiation. Clustering of t(14;18) chromosomal breakpoints also occurs on chromosome 18, adjacent to or within a previously undefined transcriptional unit. The term *bcl*-2 was proposed for this potentially new human proto-oncogene [12], which may be involved in the pathogenesis of human follicular lymphomas. We describe here the structural characterization of the *bcl*-2 gene and its mRNA product. Our data show that the proposed *bcl*-2 protein shares significant homology with a hypothetical Epstein-Barr virus (EBV) protein. We also show that most t(14;18) translocations disrupt the *bcl*-2 gene, creating a hybrid *bcl*-2/IgH transcriptional unit. The results indicate that the molecular mechanism of most t(14;18) translocations is a regulatory alteration of the expression of the *bcl*-2 gene.

B. Structure of the *bcl*-2 Gene, RNA, and Predicted Protein

A variety of hematolymphoid cell lines were screened for expression of *bcl*-2 mRNA, us-

Laboratory of Experimental Oncology, Stanford University Medical Center, Stanford, California 94305. This work was supported by grants CA 38621, CA 34233, and CA 42971 from the National Institutes of Health, IM32Z from the American Cancer Society, and a grant from the Lucille P. Markey Charitable Trust. M.L.C. is a scholar of the Lucille P. Markey Charitable Trust

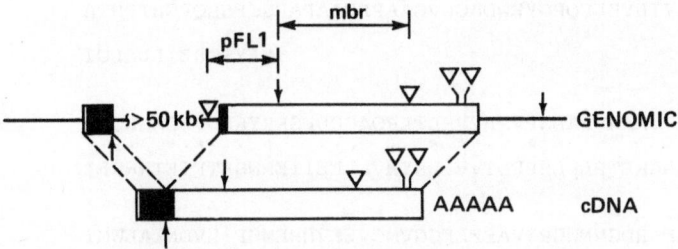

Fig. 1. Physical maps of the *bcl*-2 gene and its mRNA transcript. The physical structure determined for the configuration of the *bcl*-2 gene is shown along with a map of the *bcl*-2 mRNA predicted by the nucleotide sequence [14]. The gene consists of two exons separated by more than 50 kb of intervening sequence as determined by restriction enzyme mapping studies and nucleotide sequence determinations. The genomic locations of the pFL-1 hybridization probe and the t(14;18) major breakpoint cluster region (*mbr*) are denoted with *brackets*. Restriction enzyme cutting sites are as follows: *Bam*H1(↑), *Eco*R1(↓), and *Hin*dIII(∇)

ing a 1.5 kb fragment of chromosome 18 DNA (pFL-1) derived from a cloned t(14;18) breakpoint [9]. The results indicated that the normal transcription product of the *bcl*-2 gene, at least in B-lineage cell lines, was a 6.0 kb mRNA and that the B-cell precursor cell line SUP-B2 derived from a common acute lymphoblastic leukemia [13] expressed reasonably high levels of this mRNA. A lambda gt10 cDNA library was constructed using poly(A)⁺ RNA from SUP-B2, and hybridizing phages were identified and purified using the pFL-1 chromosome 18 DNA probe. Analysis of phage DNA inserts showed that overlapping cDNA had been obtained comprising a total of 6 kb (as shown in Fig. 1). Nucleotide sequence determinations showed that the largest open reading frame initiated at the first ATG codon at the 5′ end of the cDNA [14]. The reading frame initiated by this codon terminated 717 nucleotides downstream at the first in-phase stop codon, followed thereafter by multiple stop codons in all three reading frames. The sequence predicted the unusual structure for the *bcl*-2 mRNA shown in Fig. 1, which consisted of a short open reading frame at the 5′ end followed by a long 3′ untranslated region.

The nucleotide sequence predicted a 239 amino acid polypeptide as the putative product of the *bcl*-2 gene, whose sequence is shown in Fig. 2. When this sequence was compared with those currently contained in the NBRF protein database, significant homology was observed with the Epstein-Barr virus (EBV) protein BHRF1, a hypothetical protein corresponding to an open reading frame in the EBV genome [15]. A computer, generated alignment of the two sequences is shown in Fig. 2. There is 25% identity between the two sequences over a 149 amino acid overlap, which increases substantially if conservative amino acid replacements are considered to be identical. The findings indicate that the predicted *bcl*-2 polypeptide is evolutionarily related to the hypothetical BHRF1 protein.

The *bcl*-2 cDNAs were used to determine the genomic configuration of *bcl*-2 DNA. The results indicated that a major portion of the *bcl*-2 cDNA was contained within a single large exon, which overlapped with the pFL-1 hybridization probe, as shown in Fig. 1. Nucleotide sequence determinations confirmed that all but the 5′ 614 nucleotides of the cDNA were contained within this single large exon. The 5′ 614 nucleotides of the *bcl*-2 cDNA are encoded greater than 50 kb away, as determined by restriction mapping studies. This distance may be considerably larger since DNA was not isolated spanning the entire linkage. The structure of the genomic DNA showed that the major t(14;18) breakpoint cluster region (*mbr*) containing most t(14;18) translocations was located within the gene, in the middle of the large exon containing the 3′ untranslated region of the *bcl*-2 mRNA. The nucleotide sequences of several previously described

315

```
  1'      MAHAGRTGYDNREIVMKYIHYKLSQRGYEWDAGDVGAAPPGAAPAPGIFSSQPGHTPHTA

  1"                                                         MAYSTREILLALCI


 61'      ASRDPVARTSPLQTPAAPGAAAGPALSPVPPVVHLTLRQAGDDFSRRYRRDFAEMSRQLR
                             ***  .** *   .    ... *  . .*.*  ...
 15"      RDSRVHGNGTLHPVLELAARETPLRLSPEDTVV-LRYHVLLEEIIERNSETFTETWNRFI


121'      LTPFTARGRFATVVEELF-RDGVNWGRIVAFFEFGGVMCVESVNREMSP-LVDNIALWMT
           .  .   *...*  *.* *... .  **  .*.....   *   .. .*  *  .....
 74"      THTEHVDLDFNSVFLEIFHRGDPSLGRALAWMAWCMHACRTLCCNQSTPYYVVDLSVRGM


179'      EYLNRHLHTWIQDNGGWDAFVELYGPSMRPLFDFSWLSLKTLLSLALVGACITLGAYLGHK
           . *...**...***.... *. *.  ***  . . *.*.*.   *   *
134"      LEASEGLDGWIHQQGGWSTLIEDNIPGSRR---FSWTLFLAGLTLSLLVICSYLFISRGRH
```

Fig. 2. Alignment of the predicted *bcl*-2 and BHRF1 amino acid sequences. The predicted amino acid sequences for the *bcl*-2 protein and the hypothetical EBV protein BHRF1 are shown following alignment for maximum homology determined by the program DFASTP [19]. *Asterisks* denote identical amino acids and *dots* indicate conservative replacements shared by the two sequences. The single letter amino acid designations are according to Dayhoff [20]. *Numbers* denote residue positions for *bcl*-2 (*prime*) and BHRF1 (*double prime*)

t(14;18) breakpoints were compared with the nucleotide sequences determined for the *bcl*-2 genomic DNA and cDNA; this comparison showed that seven t(14;18) crossovers occurred within 500 nucleotides of each other in the 3' untranslated segment of the *bcl*-2 gene. These data indicate that the majority of t(14;18) translocations divide the *bcl*-2 gene within the middle of a *bcl*-2 exon.

C. Structure of the Translocated *bcl*-2 Gene and mRNA

We determined the genomic configuration of the translocated *bcl*-2 gene in the SU-DHL-4 cell line [16], which contains a t(14;18) translocation, by means of genomic Southern blot hybridizations. The results indicated that the *bcl*-2 gene was split by t(14;18) and the 3' half of the gene was lost from the translocated allele. The results showed a head-to-tail juxtaposition of the truncated *bcl*-2 gene with an Ig heavy chain gene, as shown in Fig. 3. For the *bcl*-2 gene, the point of crossover was within the exon containing the 3' untranslated portion; on chromosome 14 the point of crossover was at joining region J4. The results indicated that in the SU-DHL-4 cell line, following

t(14;18) translocation, a hybrid *bcl*-2/IgH transcriptional unit was created.

To investigate the structure of *bcl*-2 mRNA in cells containing the t(14;18) translocation, Northern blot hybridization analyses were carried out on poly(A)$^+$ RNA isolated from the SU-DHL-4 cell line. When a 5' *bcl*-2 cDNA fragment was used as a probe, two abnormally sized RNAs of 5.8 and 3.8 kb were detected in SU-DHL-4 cells (Fig. 4). However, when the same RNA preparation was hybridized with a 3' cDNA probe, no transcripts were detected in SU-DHL-4, confirming that the translocation in this cell line prematurely truncates the *bcl*-2 mRNA. Since karyotype analyses and Southern blot hybridizations of this cell line indicated that a normal chromosome 18 was present, the lack of a detectable 6 kb mRNA with the 3' probe also indicated that the nontranslocated *bcl*-2 allele in SU-DHL-4 was silent. Both the 5.8 and 3.8 kb abnormally sized *bcl*-2 transcripts in this cell line also hybridized to a gamma heavy chain probe, suggesting that two hybrid *bcl*-2/Ig transcripts were produced by t(14;18) translocation.

To confirm that the abnormal transcripts actually encoded hybrid *bcl*-2/Ig mRNAs, a cDNA library was constructed from SU-DHL-4 mRNA, and overlapping cDNAs representative of the 5.8 kb transcript were

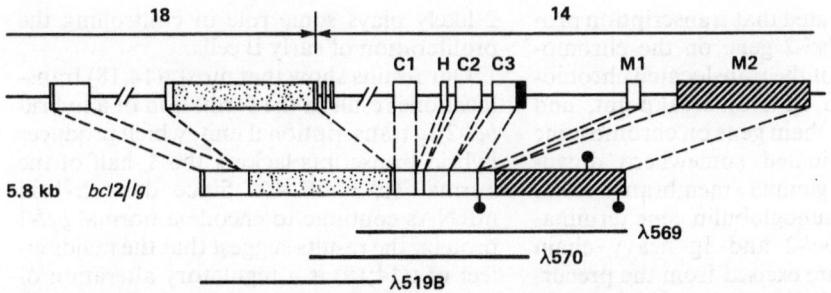

Fig. 3. Schematic diagram of the translocated *bcl*-2 gene and its 5.8 kb hybrid transcription product synthesized in the SU-DHL-4 cell line. A schematic physical map of the fused *bcl*-2 and immunoglobulin Cγ heavy chain genes in SU-DHL-4 based on Southern blotting experiments is shown. The structure of the 5.8 kb hybrid *bcl*-2/IgH mRNA transcribed from the fused genes is shown immediately below the configuration of the genes with necessary processing events indicated. Three overlapping cDNA clones isolated from SU-DHL-4 which together contain the entire 5.8 kb hybrid transcript are shown below the schematic. Open reading frames and 5' untranslated regions for both *bcl*-2 and Cγ are represented by *open boxes*. The *bcl*-2 3' untranslated region is shown as a *stippled box*. The Ig Cγ^m 3' untranslated region is represented as a *crosshatched box* and that for Ig Cγ^s as a *solid box*. Restriction enzyme cutting sites: SmaI (◆ and SacII (●)

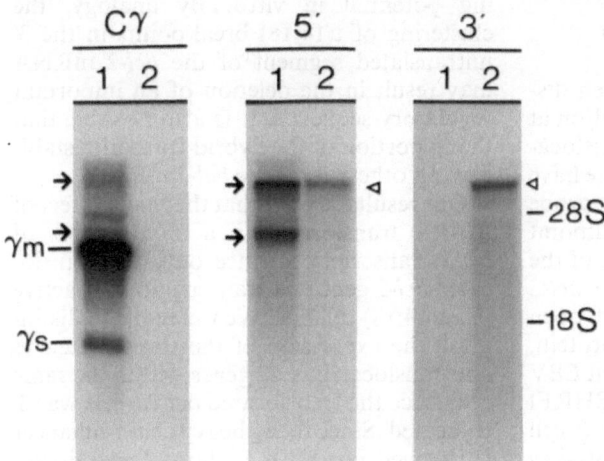

Fig. 4. Autoradiograms of Northern blots analyzing *bcl*-2- and immunoglobulin-homologous transcripts in the B-lineage cell lines SU-DHL-4 and SUP-B2. Three micrograms of poly(A⁺) RNA from cell lines SU-DHL-4 (*lanes 1*) and SUP-B2 (*lanes 2*) were fractionated through formaldehyde/0.8% agarose gel. Following transfer to nylon membranes, the immobilized, paired RNAs were hybridized separately with a 5' *bcl*-2 cDNA fragment, a 3' *bcl*-2 cDNA fragment, and a human γ4 Ig constant region probe. The 6.0 kb *bcl*-2 mRNA detected in SUP-B2 is denoted with a *triangle;* the two abnormal 5.8 and 3.8 kb *bcl*-2 mRNAs detected in SU-DHL-4 are denoted with *arrows*, as are the Cγ-homologous mRNAs of identical size observed in this cell line

purified and characterized. Nucleotide sequence analyses showed that this abnormal RNA consisted of the 5' approximate half of the *bcl*-2 mRNA fused to a decapitated Ig heavy chain mRNA, as shown in Fig. 3. A translation termination codon in the *bcl*-2 3' untranslated segment adjacent to the point of fusion is in phase with the gamma heavy chain translational reading frame, thus preventing production of a chimeric Ig protein. The sequence and restriction mapping results for the hybrid *bcl*-2/Ig transcript from this cell line indicated that transcription proceeds from the *bcl*-2 gene on the chromosome 18 portion of the translocated chromosome, across the t(14;18) breakpoint, and into the Ig heavy chain gene on chromosome 14, to be terminated somewhere downstream of the gamma membrane RNA exons, at an immunoglobulin gene termination site. The *bcl*-2 and Ig heavy chain mRNA introns are excised from the precursor in a manner similar to that which occurs during processing of normal *bcl*-2 and heavy chain mRNAs, respectively. However, the point of t(14;18) crossover, where sequences of the *bcl*-2 3' untranslated segment join an Ig J_H segment, is not spliced out of the hybrid mRNA. The 3.8-kb hybrid transcript most likely results from differential processing of the immunoglobulin portion at the 3' end of the hybrid *bcl*-2/Ig precursor.

D. Molecular Mechanisms of t(14;18)

The *bcl*-2 transcriptional unit has been discovered solely by virtue of its localization at the site of frequent chromosomal translocations in human B-cell malignancies. We have now used a chromosome 18 DNA probe flanking the major t(14;18) breakpoint cluster region to isolate cDNA copies of the normal transcription product of the *bcl*-2 gene. The *bcl*-2 mRNA contains an open reading frame for a 26 kilodalton protein, which is distantly related to a predicted EBV protein. It is not clear whether the BHRF1 protein participates in EBV-induced B-cell immortalization; however, recent studies have identified a BHRF1 protein in EBV-infected cells and suggest it is a highly abundant immediate early viral protein (Pearson and Kieff, personal communication). Purely structural analyses of the *bcl*-2 sequence do not suggest a specific subcellular role for the *bcl*-2 protein. Since there is no apparent transmembrane hydrophobic segment, it is unlikely to span the nuclear or plasma membrane. It also does not share homology with the conserved domains of all known protein kinases. It is likely that, since the *bcl*-2 gene is the frequent target of chromosomal translocations in developing B cells, and its protein product shares significant homology with a probable regulatory viral protein, *bcl*-

2 likely plays some role in controlling the proliferation of early B cells.

Our results show that most t(14;18) translocations result in the formation of a hybrid *bcl*-2/Ig transcriptional unit, which produces hybrid transcripts lacking the 3' half of the normal *bcl*-2 mRNA. Since these hybrid mRNAs continue to encode a normal *bcl*-2 protein, the results suggest that the major effect of t(14;18) is a regulatory alteration of *bcl*-2 expression. Part of this regulatory alteration may be posttranscriptional, since the hybrid transcripts lack the 3' half of the normal *bcl*-2 mRNA. There is precedent for activation of cellular proto-oncogene expression due to alterations of the 3' untranslated portions of the mRNA, as described by Meijlink et al. for the c-*fos* gene [17]. Deletion of a 67 nucleotide A-T rich region from the 3' untranslated segment of the c-*fos* mRNA is sufficient to activate its transforming potential in vitro. By analogy, the clustering of t(14;18) breakpoints in the 3' untranslated segment of the *bcl*-2 mRNA may result in the deletion of an important regulatory sequence. It is also possible that the Ig portion of the hybrid transcript stabilizes an otherwise labile *bcl*-2 mRNA.

Our results suggest that the major effect of t(14;18) translocation is a *cis* alteration of *bcl*-2 transcription, since only the translocated *bcl*-2 gene was transcriptionally active in a t(14;18) cell line. We were able to distinguish the expression of the translocated vs nontranslocated *bcl*-2 genes within the same cell, since the translocated *bcl*-2 allele was 3' truncated. Since the Ig heavy chain enhancer is retained on the $14q^+$ homologue downstream of the *bcl*-2 portion within the hybrid transcriptional unit following t(14;18), it may play a role in *cis* alteration of *bcl*-2 gene expression. However, our results indicate that the 5' end of the *bcl*-2 gene is at least 50 kb away from the point of t(14;18) crossover, requiring that the enhancer exert its effect on the *bcl*-2 promoter over a considerable distance. It is also possible that other dominant cis-acting long-range properties of the Ig heavy chain locus affect *bcl*-2 gene expression similar to the deregulation of c-*myc* gene expression in Burkitt's lymphoma.

The mechanism for alteration of *bcl*-2 expression presented here applies for most t(14;18) translocations since two-thirds of all crossovers occur within the major breakpoint cluster region (*mbr*). However, approximately one-third of t(14;18) breakpoints cluster at another site on chromosome 18 which has not been linked within 20–30 kb of the *bcl*-2 transcriptional unit [18]. It is possible therefore that there are additional mechanisms for activation of *bcl*-2 or, alternatively, there is a second gene at 18q32 whose expression can be altered by t(14;18).

References

1. Sandberg AA (ed) (1980) The chromosomes in human cancer and leukemia. Elsevier/North-Holland, Amsterdam
2. Yunis JJ (1983) The chromosomal basis of human neoplasia. Science 221:227–236
3. deKlein A, Geurts van Kessel A, Grosveld G, Bartram CR, Hagemeijer A, Bootsma D, Spurr NK, Heisterkamp N, Groffen J, Stephenson JR (1982) A cellular oncogene is translocated to the Philadelphia chromosome in chronic myelocytic leukemia. Nature 300:765–767
4. Varmus ME (1984) The molecular genetics of cellular oncogenes. Annu Rev Genet 18:553–612
5. Gale RP, Canaani E (1984) An 8-kilobase *abl* RNA transcript in chronic myelogenous leukemia. Proc Natl Acad Sci USA 81:5648–5652
6. Shtivelman E, Lifshitz B, Gale RP, Canaani E (1985) Fused transcript of *abl* and *bcr* genes in chronic myelogenous leukemia. Nature 315:550–554
7. Leder P, Battey J, Lenoir G, Moulding C, Murphy W, Potter H, Stewart T, Taub R (1983) Translocations among antibody genes in human cancer. Science 222:765–771
8. Yunis JJ, Oken MM, Kaplan ME, Ensrud KM, Howe RR, Theologides A (1982) Distinctive chromosomal abnormalities in histologic subtypes of non-Hodgkin's lymphomas. N Engl J Med 307:1231–1236
9. Cleary ML, Sklar J (1985) Nucleotide sequence of a t(14;18) chromosomal breakpoint in follicular lymphoma and demonstration of a breakpoint cluster region near a transcriptionally active locus on chromosome 18. Proc Natl Acad Sci USA 82:7439–7443
10. Bakhshi A, Jensen JP, Goldman P, Wright JJ, McBride OW, Epstein AL, Korsmeyer SJ (1985) Cloning the chromosomal breakpoint of t(14;18) human lymphomas: clustering around J_H on chromosome 14 and near a transcriptional unit on 18. Cell 41:899–906
11. Tsujimoto Y, Gorham J, Cossman J, Jaffe E, Croce CM (1985) The t(14;18) chromosome translocations involved in B-cell neoplasms result from mistakes in VDJ joining. Science 229:1390–1393
12. Tsujimoto Y, Finger LR, Yunis J, Nowell PC, Croce CM (1984) Cloning of the chromosome breakpoint of neoplastic B cells with the t(14;18) chromosome translocation. Science 226:1097–1099
13. Smith SD, Uyeki EM, Lowman JT (1978) Colony formation in vitro by leukemic cells in acute lymphoblastic leukemia (ALL). Blood 52:712–718
14. Cleary ML, Smith SD, Sklar J (1986) Cloning and structural analysis of cDNAs for *bcl*-2 and a hybrid *bcl*-2/immunoglobulin transcript resulting from t(14;18) chromosomal translocation. Cell 47:19–28
15. Baer B, Bankier AT, Biggin MD, Deininger PL, Farrell PJ, Gibson TJ, Hatfull G, Hudson GS, Satchwell SC, Seguin C, Tuffnell PS, Barrell BG (1984) DNA sequence and expression of the B95-8 Epstein-Barr virus genome. Nature 310:207–211
16. Epstein AL, Levy R, Kim H, Henle W, Henle G, Kaplan HS (1978) Biology of the human malignant lymphomas. IV. Functional characterization of ten histiocytic lymphoma cell lines. Cancer 42:2379–2391
17. Meijlink F, Curran T, Miller AD, Verma IM (1985) Removal of a 67-base-pair sequence in the noncoding region of proto-oncogene *fos* converts it to a transforming gene. Proc Natl Acad Sci USA 82:4987–4991
18. Cleary ML, Galili N, Sklar J (1986) Detection of a second t(14;18) breakpoint cluster region in follicular lymphomas. J Exp Med 164:315–320
19. Lipman DJ, Pearson WR (1985) Rapid and sensitive protein similarity searches. Science 227:1435–1441
20. Dayhoff M (1978) Atlas of protein sequence and structure, vol 5, Suppl 3. National Biomedical Research Foundation, Silver Spring, Maryland, USA

Haematology and Blood Transfusion   Vol. 31
Modern Trends in Human Leukemia VII
Edited by Neth, Gallo, Greaves, and Kabisch
© Springer-Verlag Berlin Heidelberg 1987

Involvement of the D Segment (DQ_{52}) Nearest to the J_H Region in Immunoglobulin Gene Rearrangements of Lymphoid-Cell Precursors

S. Mizutani, T. M. Ford, L. M. Wiedemann, L. C. Chan, A. J. W. Furley, M. F. Greaves, and H. V. Molgaard

A. Introduction

The specific antigen recognition molecules expressed by B and T lymphocytes, the immunoglobulins (Ig) and the T-cell receptor for antigen (TCR) are coded for by genes which are assembled in an ordered series of somatic DNA recombination events during lymphocyte differentiation. In B lymphocytes the heavy chain gene of the Ig molecule (IgH) is the first to be assembled and this occurs by two successive DNA rearrangements in which first a diversity segment (D) and then a variable gene segment (V) are joined, usually by a process of intrachromosomal deletion, to a joining segment (J) to form a complete variable region sequence (for a review, see Alt et al. 1986). A similar sequence of DNA recombinations leads to the assembly of variable region sequences from V, D and J gene segments in the TCR genes (for a recent review, see Kronenberg et al. 1986).

The initial gene rearrangement events are not entirely lineage restricted. About half of mouse T-cell lines, hybridomas and thymomas have IgH rearrangements (Forster et al. 1980; Cory et al. 1980; Kurosawa et al. 1981; Zuniga et al. 1982). IgH gene rearrangements in T lineage cells and TCR (β, γ) gene rearrangements in B lineage cells have been reported in 10%–30% of human lymphoid neoplasms (Pelicci et al. 1985; Rabbitts et al. 1985; Tawa et al. 1985; Greaves et al. 1986). These "cross-lineage" rearrangements appear to be nonfunctional and incomplete with no involvement of V regions.

In order to better understand the nature of these DNA alterations and their possible significance for lymphoid lineage commitment we have analysed the IgH gene rearrangements occurring in a group of human T-cell leukaemias and T-cell lines with precursor phenotypes and a similar group of B lineage leukaemias. These studies indicate that immature T cells frequently undergo an unusual type of DJ rearrangement of the IgH gene and that this rearrangement is only seen in B cells with the most primitive immunophenotypes. A detailed account of these studies is reported elsewhere (Mizutani et al. 1986).

B. Methods

Leukaemic blood cells from untreated patients were isolated and immunophenotyped with a panel of monoclonal antibodies as described previously (Greaves et al. 1982; Furley et al. 1986).

DNA isolation and restriction enzyme analysis was carried out essentially as previously described (Ford et al. 1983), except that the DNA probes were radiolabelled by the random primer method (Feinberg and Vogelstein 1984).

The J gene probes used are shown in Fig. 1. Probe D was excised from λ CH 28-6 (Ravetch et al. 1981; a kind gift from P. Leder) and subcloned in a plasmid vector. Probes A, B, C and E were excised from fragment D. Probe C was subcloned and re-excised before use. Probe F derives from

Leukaemia Research Fund Centre, Institute of Cancer Research, London

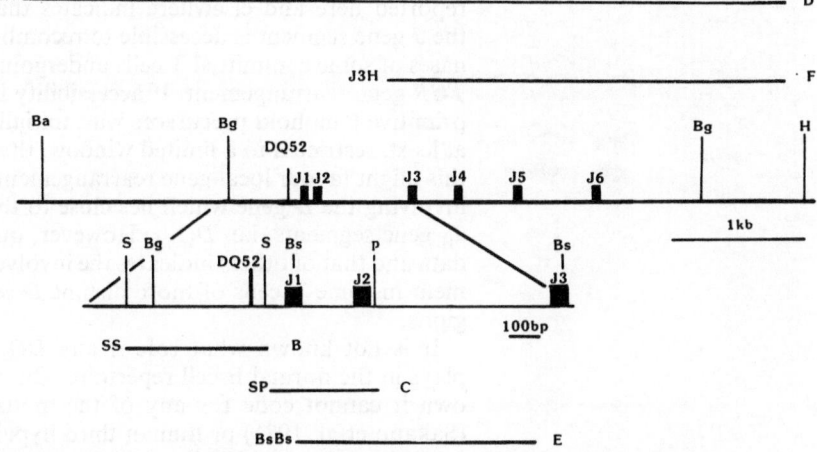

BaBg ———————————————— A

BaH ———————————————————————————— D

J3H ——————————————— · F

Ba   Bg   Bg   H
           DQ52
           J1 J2   J3   J4   J5   J6
                                                       1 kb

S   Bg   S Bs   p   Bs
   DQ52 | | |
             J1   J2   J3
                         100bp

SS ——————————— B

SP ———————— C

BsBs ———————— E

Fig. 1. Map of the human J_H gene region showing the restriction enzyme sites used to generate the DNA probes. *Ba*, *Bam*HI; *Bg*, *Bgl*II; *Bs*, *Bst*EII; *H*, *Hin*dIII; *S*, *Sma*I; *P*, *Pst*I. The restriction sites used to excise the probes are shown beside each probe. The 5′ end of fragment F terminates at J_3 in a *Bam*HI site created during the cloning of the genomic DNA (Rabbitts et al. 1981). This map is based on the published map and sequence of the *J* gene region (Ravetch et al. 1981). The restriction enzyme sites for *Eco*RI and one of the *Bam*HI and *Hin*dIII sites used in the gene rearrangement studies lie outside the region shown

C76R51 (Rabbitts et al. 1981; a kind gift from Dr. T. Rabbitts).

In order to analyse the *J* gene rearrangements, we isolated a series of DNA fragments from the *J* gene region as shown in Fig. 1. These DNA probes allowed us to identify gene rearrangement and to test whether it was accompanied by deletion of sequences 5′ to and within the *J* gene region as would be expected if rearrangement had occurred by intrachromosomal deletion. The *J* gene rearrangements were analysed with these probes using Southern transfers of DNA from the leukaemias digested with restriction enzymes which cut outside the *J* gene region.

I. Immature T Cell Leukaemias

In order to identify *IgH* J_H gene rearrangements in T-cell leukaemia DNAs, we first used the complete *J* region probe, D in Fig. 1. Since rearrangement usually involves the loss of DNA 5′ to the *J* regions, we next probed the Southern transfers with fragment A (see Fig. 1). DNA from nine T-cell leukaemias and 21 B-cell lineage leukaemias was tested in this way. Figure 2 shows the results of this procedure. The T-ALL DNA shown (Fig. 2 I) has clearly retained sequences 5′ to J. DNA from five other T-cell leukaemic cells gave a similar result (Table 1). The rearranged allele retaining fragment A (cf. Fig. 1) shows a small decrease in size of 1–2 kb from the unrearranged fragment size irrespective of the restriction enzyme used. This suggested that these rearrangements resulted from small deletions within or close to the *J* gene segments. This was confirmed using probes C and E (see Fig. 1) which reveal that sequences between J_1 and J_3 have been deleted. These rearrangements are therefore consistent with DQ_{52} joining to J_3 or *J* segments 3′ to J_3. Two T-ALLs did not retain 5′ J in their rearranged μ gene and one (JM) had an unusual rearrangement probably involving DQ_{52}, but with no detectable deletion at all.

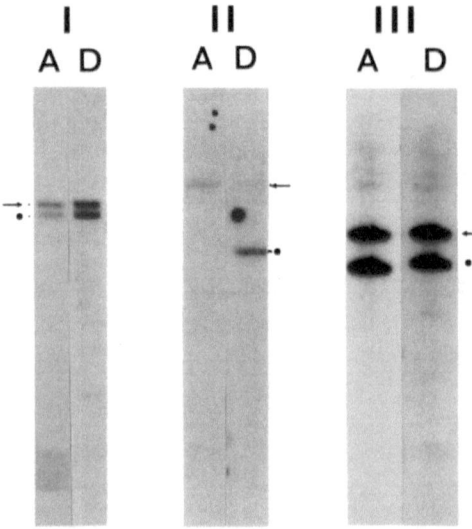

Fig. 2 I–III. J_H gene rearrangement and retention of 5' to J sequences in some lymphoid precursor leukaemias. **I.** DNA from a T-ALL digested with *Bam*HI. **II.** DNA from common (B cell precursor) ALL digested with *Eco*RI. **III.** DNA from null (early B cell precursor) All digested with *Hind*III. *A.* Detected with probe A (see Fig. 1). *D.* Detected with probe D (see Fig. 1). Note retention of rearranged band/5' J in samples **I** and **III**, but not **II**. →, germ line position, ○, rearranged allele

No retention of the 5' J fragment was observed in DNA from ten common ALL B-cell precursor leukaemias (Fig. 2 II); however, DNA from three out of ten null ALL which have a more immature B-precursor phenotype appear to have undergone the same rearrangement involving DQ_{52} as seen in T cells (Fig. 2 III; Table 1).

The occurrence of very similar recombination signal sequences – the conserved heptamer and nanomer sequences (for a review, see Alt et al. 1986) in the V, D and J gene segments in both the Ig genes and the TCR genes suggests that both sets of genes make use of common enzymes during rearrangement. This has further been established by the ability of AMuLV transformed pre-B cell lines to rearrange an introduced $TCR\ \beta$ gene (Yancopoulos et al. 1986). The endogenous $TCR\ \beta$ gene in the AMuLV transformed line was not rearranged, suggesting that control of gene rearrangement in lymphocyte development is mediated by accessi-

bility in cells where the recombinases are active. The occurrence of bigenotypic (IgH/TCR) rearrangements in immature T cells as reported here and elsewhere indicates that the J gene segment is accessible to recombinases of some committed T cells undergoing TCR gene rearrangement. If accessibility in primitive lymphoid precursors was, initially at least, restricted to a limited window, then this might favour local gene rearrangements involving the D gene which lies close to the J_H gene segments, i.e. DQ_{52}. However, our data and that of others indicates the involvement in some T cells of more distant D regions.

It is not known what role if any DQ_{52} plays in the normal B-cell repertoire. On its own it cannot code for any of the mouse (Sakano et al. 1981) or human third hypervariable regions which have been reported on. It is found rearranged in the mouse myeloma QUPC52 (Sakano et al. 1981) and may also be present at the 3' end of the third hy-

Table 1. Summary of J region rearrangements in the T and B lineage leukaemic cells

Leukaemias	Numbers tested	Numbers showing retention of 5' region (DQ_{52}) in at least one allele
T Lineage (T-ALL)	9[a]	6[b]
B Lineage[c]		
Null ALL[d]	10	3
Common ALL	10	0
Mature B	1	0

[a] Selected from a larger group of T-ALL investigated; 15 others tested had no IgH rearrangements (Furley et al. 1986; Greaves et al. 1986). Of the nine, three were cell lines, the remainder were diagnostic samples from untreated patients.
[b] One T-ALL (the cell line JM) had undergone a different type of nondeletional recombination involving insertion or inversion of DNA near the J locus, but the breakpoint appears to be at or close to DQ_{52} (see Mizutani et al. 1986, for details).
[c] All diagnostic samples except one common ALL cell line (Nalm-6) and one mature B cell line (B85).
[d] Reactive with the pan B monoclonal antibody B4 (CD19; Nadler et al. 1984), but not expressing the common ALL (gp100/CD10) associated antigen (Greaves et al. 1981).

322

pervariable region in the expressed allele of a human CLL (Ravetch et al. 1981); in this latter case it may be part of a *VDDJ* rearrangement.

It is possible that DQ_{52} to *J* joins occur in normal B cells as a relatively common early or primary rearrangement event (reflecting limited accessibility) to be masked by later *D* to *J* or *D* to *DJ* rearrangements. This accords with the observation that the only three B lineage leukaemias (out of 21 tested) found to have J rearrangement with no deletion of the 5' *J* region were in the subgroup with the most immature B lineage phenotypes (null ALL, see Table I). An analysis of *J* gene rearrangement in AMuLV transformed B-cell precursors also revealed a few examples of events which could be due to DQ_{52} to *J* rearrangement (Alt et al. 1981).

Further studies involving DNAase I sensitivity and hypersensitive site analysis are in progress to further investigate the possibility that the DQ_{52}-*J* region of the *IgH* gene might become preferentially accessible as a consequence of early events underlying commitment of the lymphoid lineages.

References

1. Alt FW, Blackwell TK, DePinho RA, Reth MG, Yancopoulos GD (1986) Immunol Rev 89:5–30
2. Cory S, Adams JM, Kemp DJ (1980) Proc Natl Acad Sci USA 77:4943–4947
3. Fedderson RM, van Ness BG (1985) Proc Natl Acad Sci USA 82:4793–4797
4. Feinberg AP, Vogelstein B (1984) Analyt Biochem 137:266–267
5. Ford AM, Molgaard HV, Greaves MF, Gould HJ (1983) EMBO J 2:997–1001
6. Forster A, Hobart M, Hergartner H, Rabbitts TH (1980) Nature 286:897–899
7. Furley AJ, Mizutani S, Weilbaecher K, Dhaliwal HS, Ford AM, Chan LC, Molgaard HV, Toyonaga B, Mak T, van den Elsen P, Gold D, Terhorst C, Greaves MF (1986) Cell 46:75–87
8. Greaves MF, Delia D, Newman R, Vodinelich L (1982) Monoclonal antibodies in clinical medicine. Academic Press, London, pp 129–165
9. Greaves MF, Janossy G, Peto J, Kay H (1981) Br J Haematol 48:179–197
10. Greaves MF, Mizutani S, Furley AJW, Sutherland DR, Chan LC, Ford AM, Molgaard HV (1986) In: Hoffbrand AV (ed) Clinics in haematology, vol 15. WB Sanders pp 621–639
11. Kronenberg M, Siu G, Hood L, Shatri N (1986) Annu Rev Immunol 4:529–591
12. Kurosawa Y, von Boehmer H, Haas W, Sakaro H, Trauncher A, Tonegawa S (1981) Nature 290:565–570
13. Mizutani S, Ford AM, Wiedemann LM, Chan LC, Furley AJW, Greaves MF, Molgaard HV (1986) EMBO J 5:3467–3473
14. Nadler LM, Korsmeyer SJ, Anderson KC, Boyd AW, Slaughenhoupt B, Park E, Jensen J, Coral F, Mayer RJ, Sallan SE, Ritz J, Schlossman SF (1984) J Clin Invest 74:332–340
15. Pelicci P, Knowles DM, Dalla Favera R (1985) J Exp Med 162:1015–1024
16. Rabbitts TH, Stinson A, Forster A, Foroni L, Luzatto L, Catovsky D, Hammerstrom L, Smith CIE, Jones D, Karpes A, Minowada J, Taylor AMR (1985) EMBO J 4:2217–2224
17. Rabbitts TH, Forster AR, Milstein CP (1981) Nucleic Acids Res 9:4509–4524
18. Ravetch JV, Siebenlist V, Korsmeyer S, Waldmann TA, Leder P (1981) Cell 27:583–591
19. Sakano H, Kurosawa Y, Weigert M, Tonegawa S (1981) Nature 290:582–585
20. Tawa A, Hozumi N, Minden M, Mak TW, Gelfand EW (1985) N Engl J Med 313:1033–1037
21. Yancopoulos GD, Blackwell TK, Suh H, Hood L, Alt FW (1986) Cell 44:251–259
22. Zuniga MC, D'Eustachio P, Ruddle NH (1982) Proc Natl Acad Sci USA 79:3015–3019

Haematology and Blood Transfusion Vol. 31
Modern Trends in Human Leukemia VII
Edited by Neth, Gallo, Greaves, and Kabisch
© Springer-Verlag Berlin Heidelberg 1987

Pattern Recognition Among T-Cell Epitopes

J. B. Rothbard [1], A. Townsend [2], M. Edwards [3], and W. Taylor [3]

A. Introduction

T cells recognize protein antigens by mechanisms qualitatively different from those used by B cells. B cells are capable of binding antigens via their surface immunoglobulins, as in other well-understood ligand-receptor interactions. In contrast, T cells are unable to bind antigen in the absence of the major histocompatibility class I or class II gene products [1]. The details of this possible tertiary interaction are still poorly understood. One puzzling feature of the contrasting recognition processes is that the antigen receptor on T cells exhibits great structural similarity with immunoglobulins [2, 3].

One possible resolution of this apparent contradiction is the proposal that the form of the antigen which the two populations of lymphocytes see is different. Recent work from a number of laboratories has revealed that B cells recognize protein antigens with their native conformation intact, while the majority of T cells recognize protein antigens with their native conformation disrupted [4, 5]. The most lucid demonstration supporting this generalization was the experiment by Watts and McConnell, who successfully stimulated an ovalbumin specific T-helper clone with a peptide corresponding to a region of the protein and the correct class II antigen anchored in a lipid monolayer. The intact protein in its native conformation was completely ineffective [6]. Work in other laboratories examining other T-cell clones has revealed that both enzymatically derived peptides and synthetic peptides are excellent stimulators of helper and cytolytic T cells.

The interaction between antigen, T-cell receptor and class II proteins was first extensively studied by Heber-Katz and Schwartz, who used cytochrome-specific helper clones [7, 8]. The region of the molecule which stimulated their clones was the linear region corresponding to residues 88–103. This C-terminal helical region of the protein stimulated the clones as well as the intact protein. By examining the cross-reaction between their cytochrome-specific clones and cytochromes from other species they concluded that residues between 98 and 103 were necessary for the specificity. However, these residues alone were insufficient for stimulation. Longer peptides were necessary for maximum stimulation of their clones. The authors concluded that the longer peptides could stabilize a preferred conformation, in this case a helix, and could therefore bind the receptor with higher affinity. Various modifications to the sequence provided additional support for this concept.

Concurrently with this work, Berzofsky [9] and Livingstone et al. [10] were analysing the T-cell epitopes within myoglobin. In this molecule as well, the epitopes seen by T cells were located within linear regions of the protein sequence composing helical regions. The ovalbumin epitope previously mentioned could not be unequivocally designated as helical because its X-ray structure was not known; however, it was composed

[1] Imperial Cancer Research Fund, Lincoln's Inn Fields, London WC2A 3PX, England
[2] John Radcliffe Hospital, Oxford, England
[3] Birkbeck College, London, England

of residues which could easily be modeled to be an amphipathic helix.

In compiling these and the other epitopes known at the time, Berzofsky postulated that T cells interact with amphipathic regions of protein antigens [11]. A large number of the epitopes he examined can adopt a conformation with separate polar and non-polar faces. In his model, the T-cell receptor would interact with one facade, while the class II or class I molecule would interact with the other. The analysis he used was that of Eisenberg, who used vector analysis to generate moments of inertia (in this case, moments of hydrophobicity) to quantitate the amphipathic character of a region of protein sequence [12].

In this paper, we have analysed 30 T-cell epitopes and have discovered a pattern that is present in 29. The pattern is present in the linear sequence and does not require the region to adopt a particular conformation. Using the known epitopes as a data base, we have generated a template for predicting T-cell epitopes in other protein sequences and have predicted a likely region within the sequence of the nucleoprotein of influenza. This region was synthesized and shown to be the principal region seen by cytotoxic T cells isolated from CBA mice. We believe that this simple motif can be of general use for prediction and is an interesting model on which experiments analysing the interaction of T cells and proteins can be based.

B. Methods

Analyses of the hydrophic moment for the peptides and proteins were made as described by Eisenberg [12]. The protrusion indices were calculated as described by Thornton et al. [13]. Sequence alignments and generation of templates were carried out by methods created by Thornton and Taylor [14]. Synthesis of peptides was done by standard Merrifield techniques [15] on an Applied Biosystems 430A peptide synthesizer [16]. T-cell lines were isolated from CBA mice and maintained in vitro as described [17]. A standard procedure was used for ^{51}Cr release assay [16] and the transfected NP target cells were prepared as previously described [18].

C. Results, Analyses and Discussion

The known helper and cytotoxic T-cell epitopes composing the database of this analysis are shown in Table 1. They are a combination of human and murine epitopes which have been either published or communicated to us.

We were dissatisfied, for several reasons, with Delisi and Berzofsky's generalization that T-cell epitopes are localized to regions of proteins that are amphipathic, particularly amphipathic helices. The first was that any generalization is only as accurate as its database. In this case, the number of epitopes examined was small, and the particular type of protein from which many of the epitopes were derived was not representative of all protein structures. The proteins exclusively composed of α-helices were over-represented. Secondly, as published, the correlation with amphipathic character was purely qualitative. Using the vector analysis of Eisenberg, discrete values are generated for linear regions of sequence. If their correlation is correct, the highest values should be recognized most often. Such a correlation is not seen (see below). When the angle used in generating the vectors of hydrophobicity is restrained at 100° (that consistent with standard α-helix of 3.6 residues per turn), only approximately 60%–75% of epitopes are consistent with the correlation. By varying the angle, and consequently increasing the areas of the protein that are possible, the correlation does improve. When analysed critically, the correlation simply implies that all areas of globular proteins are possible T-cell epitopes, with the exception of loops and turns – the prominent sites for B-cell recognition [13, 34, 35].

To examine this possibility, we plotted both the known linear B-cell epitopes and T-cell epitopes on to the protrusion index profile for myoglobin and lysozyme. As can be vividly seen, the B-cell epitopes map to highly exposed areas, whereas the areas preferentially recognized by T cells are poorly exposed (Fig. 1 a, b).

If proteolytic events are involved in antigen processing in order for T cells to recognize protein antigens, the most sterically available sites would be preferentially cleaved by enzymes for the same reasons

Table 1. Compilation of reported T-cell epitopes

Position				1	2	3	4	5	6	7	8	9											Reference
SPERM WHALE MYOGLOBIN 69–78				L	T	A	L	G	A	I	L	K	K										[10]
SPERM WHALE MYOGLOBIN 106–118				E	F	I	S	E	A	I	I	H	V	L	H	S	R						[9]
SPERM WHALE MYOGLOBIN 110–121				A	I	I	H	V	L	F	R	K	D	I	A	A	K						[10]
SPERM WHALE MYOGLOBIN 132–145				N	K	A	L	E	L	F	R	K	D	I	A	A	K						[9]
INSULIN B-CHAIN 5–16			H	L	C	G	S	H	L	V	E	A	L										[19]
CYTOCHROME PIGEON 93–104			K	S	E	R	V	D	L	I	A	Y	L	K	D	A	T	S	K				[7]
CYTOCHROME BOVINE 13–25				K	C	A	Q	H	T	V	E	K	G	G	K	H	K						[20]
OVALBUMIN 323–329			S	I	S	Q	A	V	H	A	A	H	A	E	I	N	E	A	G	R			[21]
FLU NUCLEOPROTEIN (34/68) 335–349		I	A	A	F	E	D	L	R	V	L	S	F	I	R	G							[16]
FLU NUCLEOPROTEIN (1968) 365–379		I	A	S	M	E	N	M	D	A	M	E	S	S	T	L							[16]
FLU NUCLEOPROTEIN (1934) 365–379			A	S	M	E	N	M	E	T	M	E	S	S	T	L							[16]
FLU NUCLEOPROTEIN (34/68) 50–63			S	D	Y	E	G	R	L	I	Q	N	S	L	T	I							[22]
FLU HAEMAGGLUTININ PR/8 111–120				F	E	R	F	E	I	F	P	K	E										[23]
FLU HAEMAGGLUTININ A/TEXAS/1/77 115–128			S	S	G	T	L	E	F	I	N	E	G	F	N	W							[24]
FLU HAEMAGGLUTININ PR8/34 302–313				C	P	K	Y	V	R	S	A	K	L	R	M								[24]
FLU HAEMAGGLUTININ A/NT/60/68 302–313				C	P	K	Y	V	K	Q	N	T	L	K	L								[24]
FLU HAEMAGGLUTININ A/TEXAS/1/77 311–324				Q	N	T	L	K	L	A	T	G	M	R	M	V							[24]
RAT MYELIN BASIC PROTEIN 5–20		P	S	K	Q	R	H	G	S	K	Y	L	A	T	A								[25]
RAGWEED ALLERGEN Ra3 51–65	E	V	W	R	E	E	A	Y	H	A	C	D	I	K	D								[26]
RAGWEED ALLERGEN Ra 51–65																							[26]
HUMAN AChR GAMMA 125–147				K	S	Y	C	E	I	I	V	T	H	F	P	F	D	Q	Q	N	C		[27]
HEN EGG LYSOZYME 34–45	F	E	S	N	F	N	T	E	A	T	N	R											[28]
HEN EGG LYSOZYME 46–61	N	T	D	G	S	T	D	Y	G	I	L	Q	I	N	S	R							[29]
HEN EGG LYSOZYME 78–93	I	P	C	S	A	L	L	S	S	D	I	T	A	S	V	N							[30]
HERPES GLYCOPROTEIN D 8–23				S	L	K	M	A	D	P	N	R	F	R	G	K	D	L	P				[31]
STAPH. NUCLEASE 61–80	G	L	A	Y	I	Y	A	D	D	G	K	M	V	N	A	K	K	I	E	V	E	F D	[32]
STAPH. NUCLEASE 86–100		Y	I	Y	A	D	D	G	K	M	V	N	E	A	L	V	R						[32]
STAPH. NUCLEASE 91–105		Y	I	Y	A	D	G	K	M	V	N	E	A	L	V	R							[32]
VP1 FOOT-MOUTH VIRUS 141–160	R	G	D	L	Q	V	L	A	Q	K	V	A	R	T	L	P							[33]

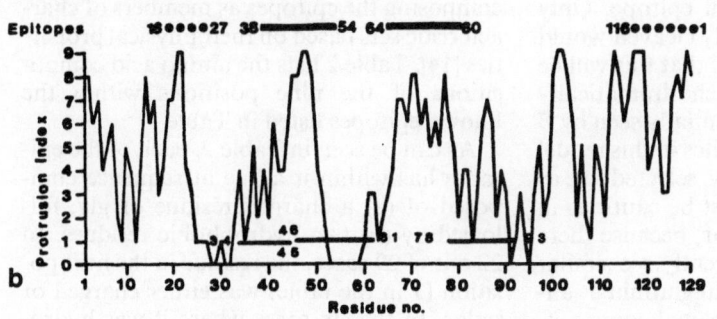

LYSOZYME – HEN EGG

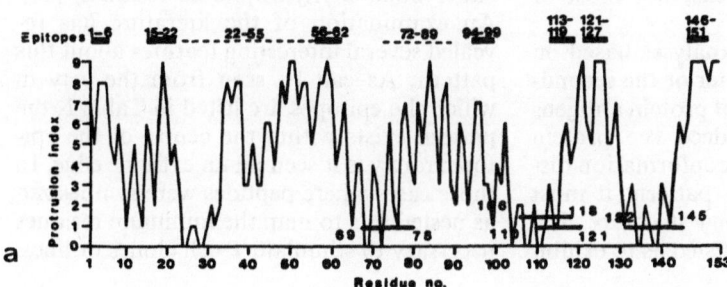

MYOGLOBIN – SPERM WHALE

Fig. 1 a, b. Known B-cell epitopes (*upper bars,* **a, b**) and T-cell epitopes (*lower bars,* **a, b**) plotted on protrusion index profile [13] of myoglobin and lysozyme

Table 2. Amino acid compositions of different positions within defined T-cell epitopes

Position	
1	3A 2L 3F Y W 2T 6E K H 2N Q S 2C G 12 phobic 8 charged 6 polar 1 gly
2	6A 2I Y 3T 4D E 3R 3N 2S 2C 2G P 12 phobic 8 charged 7 polar 3 gly and pro
3	2V 6L I T F 2Y 2M E K H 4S 2Q C 3G 2P 15 phobic 3 charged 6 polar 5 gly and pro
4	3D 8E 9K 5H 3R 2G *28 charged* *2 gly*
5	7A 3V 5L 5I 2T F 3Y 4M *30 hydrophobic*
6	4A 7V 5L 6I 2T 2F Y C 2M *29 hydrophobic* 1 polar
7	3A V L I T 3D 5E K 3H 3R 4N 2Q S P 6 phobic *15 charged* *7 polar* 1 pro
8	3A 2I F Y 3T 2E 4K H R S 2N Q P 2G 10 phobic 8 charged 4 polar 3 pro and gly
9	4A 2V 3L 2I M D 2E 2K H R 3S C 2G 12 phobic 7 charged 4 polar 2 gly

that they are seen by B cells. Consequently, these regions would no longer be intact and could not compose a T-cell epitope. Only those areas not preferentially cleaved would be possible epitopes. We feel that this will be an important pattern which dramatically differs from the sites preferentially seen by B cells. Obviously, the T-cell sites in this model are negatively, not positively, selected for, as are the B-cell sites. We must be cautious in carrying this concept too far, because there are T-cell clones that apparently see similar areas of the influenza haemagglutinin as antibodies (D. B. Thomas, personal communication). A useful model is to view the two groups of epitopes as composing two sets that have overlapping areas, but most of each set is unique.

A major concern with analyses based on either amphipathic character or the secondary and tertiary structure of protein antigens is that if T cells do indeed see protein antigens with their native conformation disrupted, then if there is a pattern, it must manifest itself in the *primary* structure. The epitopes in Table 1 are so listed as to exhibit the pattern we have discerned. This pattern was determined by examining the residues composing the epitopes as members of characteristic sets based on their physical properties [14]. Table 2 lists the amino acid compositions of the nine positions within the known epitopes listed in Table 1.

As can be seen in Table 2, each of the epitopes has within it a line at sequence composed of (a) a charged residue or gly, followed by (b) two hydrophobic residues. In 22 out of 29 cases, the residue in the next position (7 in the table) was either charged or polar. In the six cases where it was hydrophobic, all had a polar residue in the next position (tyrosine and threonine can act as either polar or hydrophobic residues) [14]. An examination of the literature has revealed several interesting features about this pattern. As can be seen from the way in which the epitopes are listed in Table 1, the pattern exists within the centre of the epitope; rarely is it seen on an extreme edge. In those cases where peptides were synthesized as nested sets to map the minimum residues necessary to stimulate T-cell clones or lines,

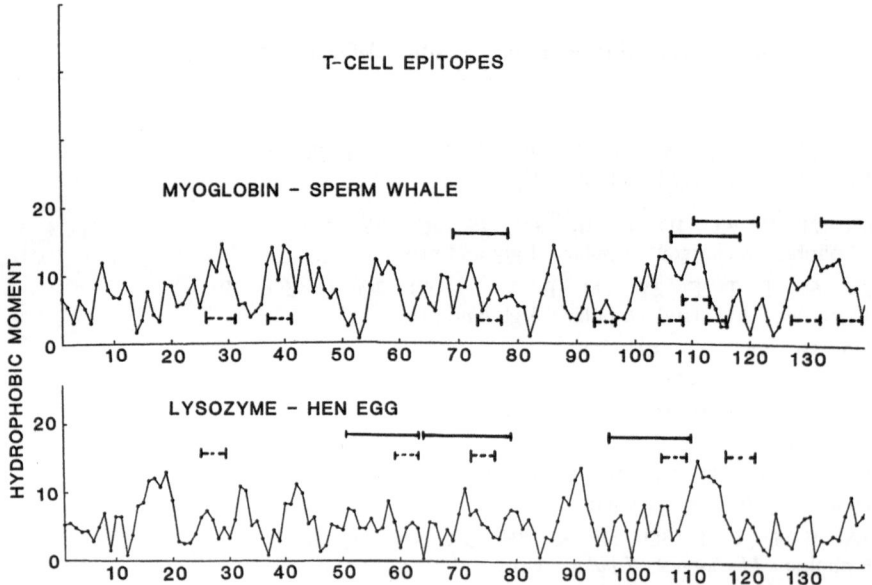

Fig. 2. Hydrophobic moments calculated for sperm whale myoglobin and hen egg lysozyme, plotted against their residue number [12]. The window size was 6 residues and the angle was 100° (hen egg lysozyme sequence contained the leader of 19 amino acids). Known T-cell epitopes are marked with *solid bars,* while predicted areas containing the pattern of charged or gly, hydrophobic, hydrophobic are marked with *broken bars*

never has a peptide lacking residues composing this pattern been able to stimulate.

In three cases, the pattern exists in two separate areas of a known epitope (ragweed, influenza, haemagglutinin and myoglobin), and we believe that they constitute two overlapping but distinct epitopes which could explain differences in the fine specificities of the clones stimulated by the large peptide. In order to examine both how often this pattern occurs in proteins and how well it correlates with known epitopes, we generated a template for the pattern, using the known compositions of amino acids at the nine sites listed in Tables 1 and 2. We imposed the further restriction that all areas demarcated had to have a charged residue or glycine at position four and hydrophobic residues at positions five and six. The sites predicted for myoglobin and lysozyme are shown in Fig. 2.

As can be seen, many of the T-cell epitopes map to regions with high hydrophobic moments; however, they do not simply correlate with the areas with highest values. In fact, much of both molecules has high (8)

amphipathicity. The pattern described in this report is limited to well-defined regions (9 in myoglobin and 5 in lysozyme) that correlate well with the known epitopes. As previously mentioned, there are separate patterns for the two overlapping epitopes in region 110 in myoglobin. This is illuminating, but it is not a stringent test of the model, because the template used was created from known epitopes. A more useful test is its ability to predict previously unknown epitopes.

The system chosen for analysis was the recognition of influenza nucleoprotein by murine cytotoxic T cells resulting from an infection with intact virus. Previous work in our laboratory has demonstrated that the principal region recognized by the strain of mice lies within the first 77 residues. Figure 3 shows the known (16) and the predicted sites of T-cell recognition in two areas of the protein. On the basis of the pattern described, we synthesized a peptide corresponding to residues 50–63. When used in the chromium release assay, it acted as a substitute for the intact virus, the intact protein and the de-

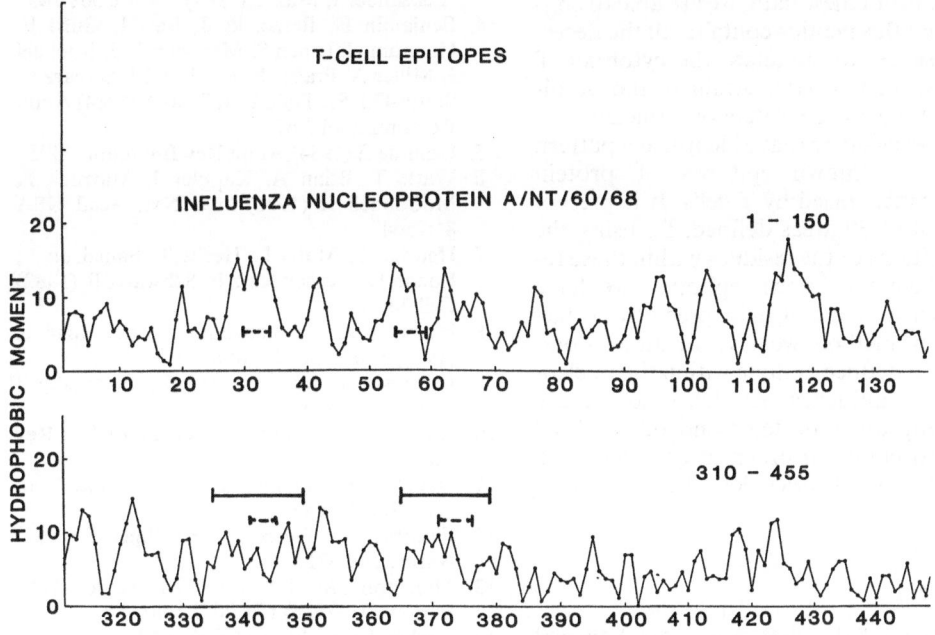

Fig. 3. The plot of hydrophobic moments against residue number of two regions of influenza nucleoprotein. The known epitopes are delineated with *solid bars;* the areas containing the predicted pattern of charged or glycine, hydrophobic, hydrophobic are delineated with *broken bars*

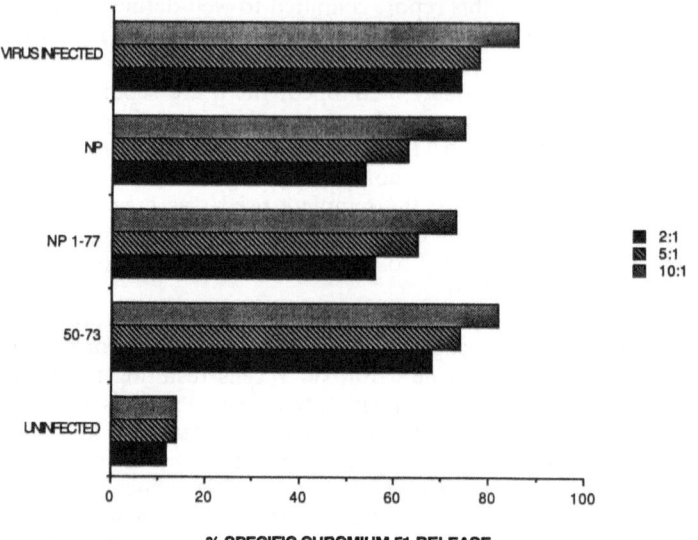

SPECIFICITY OF CTL LINES FROM CBA MICE

% SPECIFIC CHROMIUM 51 RELEASE

Fig. 4. Results of lysis of chromium-labelled target 2 cells (H-2^k) infected with virus, transfected with intact nucleoprotein (*NP*) or a fragment of NP, 1– 77, or simply pulsed with peptide corresponding to residues 50–73 as described [16]

leted protein corresponding to residues 1–77 (Fig. 4). From these data, we are able to conclude that this peptide contains all the necessary residues to stimulate the cytotoxic T lymphocytes from this strain of mouse directed at the nucleoprotein of influenza.

In conclusion, we have identified a pattern within the known epitopes of protein antigens recognized by T cells. It is present in 29 out of 30 areas defined. By using the compositions of the residues within these regions from the known epitopes, we have constructed a template with predictive value. Using this method, we have identified a previously undefined epitope within the nucleoprotein of influenza. At this time, we are examining other proteins and other T-cell lines and clones in order to confirm or to contradict the theories described in this report.

References

1. Schwartz RH (1985) Annu Rev Immunol 3:237
2. Hendrick S, Nielson E, Kavaler J, Cohen D, Davis MM (1984) Nature 308:153
3. Yanagi Y, Yoskikai Y, Leggett K, Clark S, Aleksander I, Mak T (1984) Nature 308:145
4. Benjamin D, Berzofsky J, East I, Gurd F, Hannum C, Leach S, Morgoliash E, Michael J, Miller A, Prager E, Reichlin M, Sercarz E, Smith-Gill SJ, Todd P, Wilson A (1984) Annu Rev Immunol 2:67
5. Unanue E (1984) Annu Rev Immunol 2:395
6. Watts T, Brian A, Kappler J, Marrack P, McConnell H (1985) Proc Natl Acad USA 81:7564
7. Hedrick S, Matis L, Hecht T, Samelson L, Longo D, Herber-Katz E, Schwartz R (1982) Cell 30:141
8. Herber-Katz E, Hansburg D, Schwartz R (1983) J Mol Cell Immunol 1:3
9. Berkower I, Buckenmeyer G, Berzofsky J (1986) J Immun
10. Livingstone A, Fathman CG (1986) Ann Rev Immunol 5:477
11. DeLisi C, Berzofsky J (1985) Proc Natl Acad Sci USA 82:7048
12. Eisenberg D, Weiss R, Terwilliger T (1982) Nature 299:371
13. Thornton JM, Edwards MS, Taylor WR, Barlow DJ (1986) EMBO J 5:409
14. Taylor WR (1986) J Mol Biol 188:233
15. Erickson B, Merrifield B (1976) The proteins, vol 2, 3rd edn. Academic, New York, pp 257–493

16. Townsend A, Rothbard J, Gotch F, Bahadut G, Wraith D, McMichael AJ (1986) Cell 44:959

17. Townsend A, Skehel J (1984) J Exp Med 160:552

18. Townsend A, McMichael A, Carter N, Huddleston J, Brownlee G (1984) Cell 39:13

19. Thomas JW, Danho W, Bullesbach E, Fohles J, Rosenthal A (1981) J Immunol 126:1095

20. Corradin GP, Juillerat M, Vita C, Ehgers H (1983) Mol Immunol 20:763

21. Watts T, Gariepy J, Schoolnik G, McConnell H (1986) Proc Natl Acad Sci USA 82:5480

22. Townsend A, Rothbard J (unpublished results)

23. Hackett C, Dietzschold B, Gerhard W, Ghrist B, Knorr R, Gillessen D, Melchers F (1983) J Exp Med 158:294

24. Lamb J, Green N (1983) Immunology 50:659

25. Zamvil S, Mitchell D, Moore A, Kitamura K, Steinman L, Rothbard J (1986) Nature 324:258

26. Ku isaki J, Atassi H, Atassi M (1986) Eur J Immunol 16:236

27. Lennon V, McCormick D, Lambert E, Griesmann G, Atassi M (1985) Proc Natl Acad Sci USA 82:8805

28. Allen P, Strydon D, Unanue E (1984) Proc Natl Acad Sci USA 81:2489

29. Allen P, Matsueda G, Haber E, Unanue E (1986) Proc Natl Acad Sci·USA 83:4509

30. Manca F, Clarke J, Miller A, Sercarz E, Shastri N (1984) J Immun 133:2075

31. Heber-Katz E, Hollosi M, Dietzschold B, Hudecz F, Fasman G (1986) J Immunol 135:1385

32. John Smith (private communication)

33. Francis MJ, Fry CM, Rowlands D, Brown F, Bittle J, Houghton R, Lerner R (1985) J Gen Virol 66:2347

34. Westof E, Altschuh D, Moras D, Bloomer A, Mondragon A, Klug A, van Regenmortel M (1984) Nature 311:123

35. Tainer J, Getzoff E, Alexander H, Houghton R, Olsen A, Lerner R, Hendrickson W (1984) Nature 312:127

Haematology and Blood Transfusion Vol. 31
Modern Trends in Human Leukemia VII
Edited by Neth, Gallo, Greaves, and Kabisch
© Springer-Verlag Berlin Heidelberg 1987

Regulation of *Ig* Gene Expression in Murine B-Lymphocytes *

A. Schimpl, U. Chen-Bettecken, and E. Wecker

A. Introduction

B cells at different stages of maturation exhibit distinct patterns of *Ig* gene transcription. Most of the information we have about those patterns is derived from tumour systems. Using B myelomas as models for pre-B cells, B lymphomas for early B cells and plasmacytomes as analogues of fully differentiated plasma cells, several groups have reported that the rate of transcription across the heavy-chain locus differs only slightly in these various lines and that the steady-state levels of heavy-chain mRNA are predominantly regulated by post-transcriptional events [7, 8]. In contrast, Yuan and Tucker (1984) [14], who investigated the heavy-chain transcription in resting normal B cells and in B cells stimulated with LPS for 4 days, described an eight- to tenfold increase in the rate of transcription. This increase is smaller than that observed in the amount of steady-state μ-specific mRNA upon LPS stimulation.

B. Stimulation of μ and κ Transcription After LPS Stimulation

To evaluate the relative contributions of transcriptional and post-transcriptional regulation of both H and L chains at various times in normal B-cell development, we studied B cells activated either by LPS alone or by LPS together with anti-*Ig* antibodies. The latter model system was chosen in order to gain some understanding of the events which might take place in situations in which the Ag receptor is occupied by the relevant antigen. Heavy- and light-chain transcription was studied by nuclear run on assays, and the transcription rates were related to the amounts of steady-state mRNA for the κ chain and for the membrane and secreted forms of the μ chain.

Our data showed that after LPS stimulation of normal B cells, the amounts of both μ and κ are regulated at the level of transcription [4]. Transcriptional activation is accompanied by μ_m–μ_s transition. The increase in the transcription rates (30- to 60-fold) quite faithfully reflects the increase in steady-state μ and κ mRNA (30- to 100-fold); delta expression, on the other hand, seems to be negatively regulated at the post-transcriptional level. This is inferred from the observation that although transcription across the delta locus did not terminate after stimulation, no mature mRNA was detectable.

C. Post-transcriptional Regulation of μ and κ Expression in Cells Co-stimulated with LPS and anti-*Ig* Antibodies

While LPS stimulation of B cells thus clearly leads to high levels of *Ig*-relevant mRNA, stimulation with anti-μ or anti-κ alone, which induces proliferation, has no such ef-

* This work was supported by the Sonderforschungsbereich 105 of the Deutsche Forschungsgemeinschaft and by the Fonds der Chemie.
Institut für Virologie und Immunbiologie der Universität Würzburg

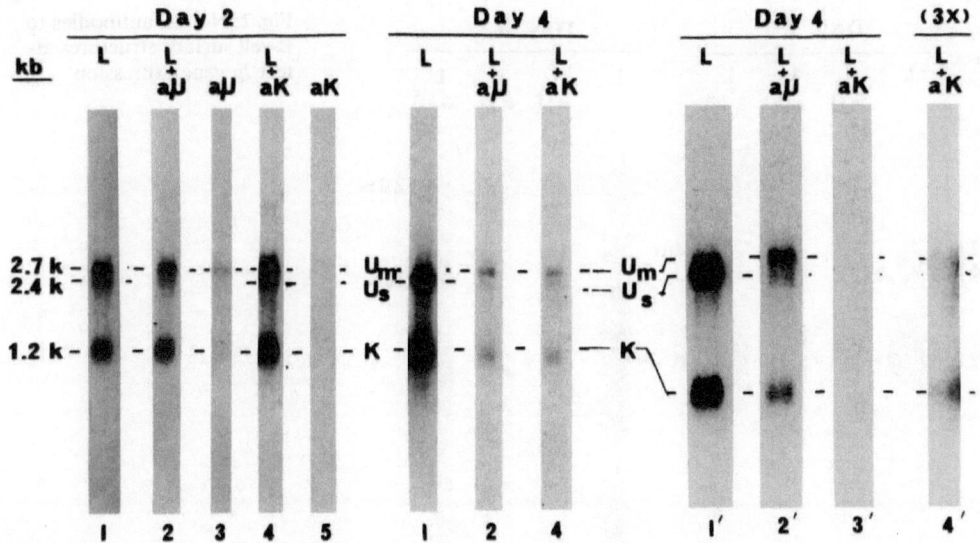

Fig. 1. Co-stimulation of B cells with anti-μ/anti-κ and LPS leads to profound effects on H- and L- chain mRNAs. For cell preparations and RNA analyses see [3]

fect. Indeed, it has been found that co-stim-ulation of normal B cells with LPS and F(ab')$_2$ fragments of antibodies to μ and κ decreases LPS-induced *Ig* secretion while high levels of proliferation are maintained [1, 3].

We studied the effect of co-stimulation of LPS and anti-receptor antibodies on the steady-state mRNA levels for μ and κ (Fig. 1). It was possible to draw the follow-ing conclusions: (a) anti-μ or anti-κ treat-ment by itself does not lead to mRNA levels higher than those observed in resting cells (resting cells not shown) even though, under the conditions used in the experiment, the cells incorporate thymidine and have been shown to undergo at least one cell cycle. (b) LPS plus anti-μ treatment leads to increased μ_m and κ mRNA levels on day 2, compara-ble to those observed with LPS alone, but to no μ_s mRNA, which makes up approxi-mately 50% of the total μ mRNA detected in LPS-stimulated cells at that time. LPS plus anti-κ-treated cells on day 2 show high levels of both μ_m/μ_s and κ mRNAs. (c) In either case, on day 4, μ_s, μ_m and κ mRNA levels are very low in all doubly treated cells, while B cells stimulated with LPS alone show the μ and κ levels characteristic of that state of B-cell development [10, 3]. Treatment with

anti-μ or anti-κ F(ab')$_2$ fragments affects the mRNA levels of both chains, i.e. even those not directly recognized by the antibody. Non-*Ig*-related gene expression such as *H-2* is not affected (data in [3]).

Using nuclear run-on assays, we were able to show that the loss of μ and κ mRNAs is due not to cessation of transcription but mostly to post-transcriptional events which affect stability and/or processing of the H- and L-chain RNA [3].

Not all antibodies to B-cell surface struc-tures affect *Ig* gene expression equally. Figure 2 shows that antibodies to the delta chain of the *Ig* receptor and to *I-A* do not af-fect LPS-induced mRNA levels to the same extent as anti-μ or anti-κ. When RNA was analysed on day 2, LPS plus anti-I-A-stimu-lated cells exhibited an mRNA pattern iden-tical to that observed with LPS alone. Anal-ysis on day 4 again showed co-stimulation with anti-I-A to have little or no effect. Co-stimulation with anti-delta does lead to a certain reduction in μ-specific mRNA. Tran-sition to μ_s is somewhat delayed (see day 4 as compared to LPS controls), but not pre-vented. Since these experiments were per-formed with total resting splenic B cells, the weaker suppression by anti-delta might be due to the fact that only 30%–50% of these

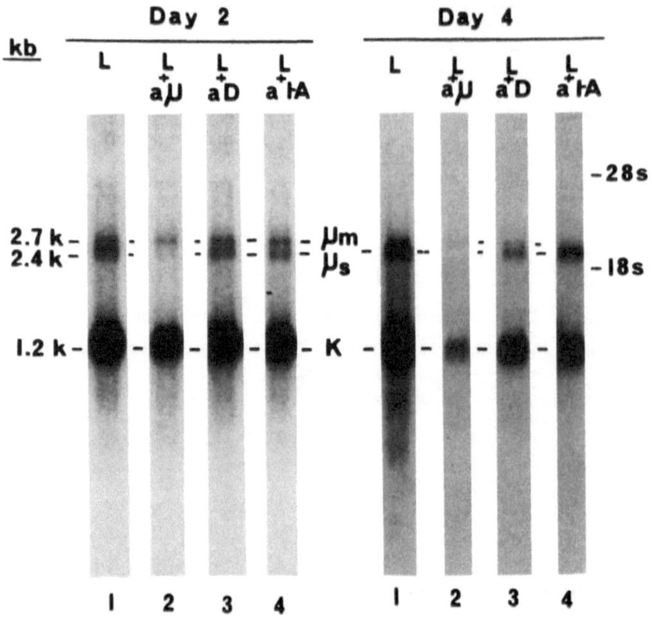

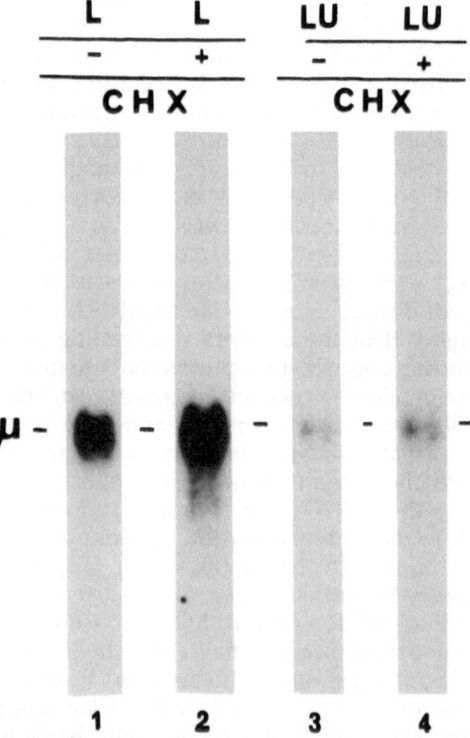

Fig. 2. Not all antibodies to B-cell surface structures affect *Ig* gene expression

cells carry delta on the surface and that the delta-negative cells can be stimulated by LPS. If this is so, the data also imply that only cells directly interacting with anti-*Ig* antibodies exhibit downregulation of *Ig* expression; this argues against an indirect effect mediated by some unknown suppressor mechanism.

D. Post-transcriptional Downregulation Induced by anti-μ Antibodies Cannot be Reversed by Cycloheximide

Recently, several systems have been described in which mRNA levels are post-transcriptionally regulated. In several of these systems, e.g. *c-myc* [5], *c-fos* [11] and *Il-2* [6], cycloheximid can stabilize mRNA levels without affecting transcription [6]. In the pre-B-like 70Z cells, cycloheximide treatment has in addition been shown to increase κ gene transcription [13]. We therefore attempted to influence or stabilize μ-mRNA levels in LPS plus anti-μ co-stimulated cells. Figure 3 shows that contrary to the systems described above, cycloheximide has very little, if any, effect. This would suggest that the mechanism of post-transcriptional con-

Fig. 3. Lack of mRNA stabilization after treatment of single or doubly stimulated cells with cycloheximide. *L*, LPS; *LU*, LPS + anti-μ

trol operative in the LPS plus anti-μ system is different from that observed with c-*myc*, c-*fos* and *Il-2*.

E. Signals Which May Mediate Anti-*Ig*-Induced Downregulation

Binding and cross-linking of anti-μ and anti-κ to the Ag receptor leads to receptor shedding and endocytosis. It also leads to activation of the phosphatidyl-inositol pathway, resulting in inositol triphosphate and diacylglycerol formation, and thus in the mobilization of intracellular Ca^{2+} and the activation of protein kinase C [2]. To investigate whether the endocytosed antibodies or the signal induced by them are responsible for *Ig*-mRNA downregulation, we replaced the receptor-specific antibodies with phorbol esters and the Ca-ionophore ionomycin in the co-stimulation with LPS. Table 1 shows that this treatment closely mimics that of antibody treatment with respect to both sustained proliferation and inhibition of *Ig* secretion, at least up to day 3–4 of culture. If these observations can be substantiated by molecular analysis of gene transcription and mRNA accumulation, they would suggest that endocytosis of the antibodies to the receptors is not obligatory. However, these experiments do not rule out the possibility that the endocytosed receptor itself might medi-

ate the negative effect, since treatment of B cells with ionomycin and phorbol esters leads to rapid disappearance of IgM from the surface (data not shown).

F. Possible Relevance of *Ig*-RNA Downregulation for B-Cell Physiology

Continued proliferation of B cells with concomitant downregulation of *Ig* gene expression might be valuable for the generation of memory cells. Downregulation of *Ig* secretion prevents the cells from reaching the end-stage of plasma cells, while continued proliferation might allow for the events leading to *Ig* class switch to take place. To investigate this possibility we established hybridomas from B cells either stimulated with LPS alone or with LPS plus anti-μ F(ab')$_2$. The two types of cells were fused on days 4 and 5 after stimulation; hybridomas were established and analysed for the Ig class formed. Table 2 shows the results. They indicate that both LPS and LPS plus anti-μ stimulated cells give rise to *Ig*-secreting hybridomas, i.e. anti-μ-induced inhibition of *Ig* secretion is reversible. The data also show that fusion on day 5 leads to hybridomas producing *Igs* other than IgM and that these occur more frequently in the doubly stimulated cells than in those stimulated by LPS alone. The hybridomas obtained after LPS plus anti-Ig stimulation might lead to a valuable insight into the mechanism of the class switch which in normal B cells, in addition to other signals, may be favoured by a transient post-transcriptional downregulation of *Ig* gene expression such as has been found in the model system described here.

Table 1. Inhibition of *Ig* secretion in B cells stimulated with LPS and phorbolmyristate acetate plus ionomycin

Treatment of cells	cpm/5 × 10⁴	PFC/5 × 10⁴
Med	794	18
LPS	15041	2000
LPS+PMA +ionomycin	19330	36
PMA+ionomycin	11774	25

Resting splenic B cells were isolated and stimulated with either LPS (10 µg) or phorbolmyristate acetate (5 ng) plus ionomycin (0.5 µM), or with a combination of both reagents. Cultures were pulsed with 0.25 µCi of ³H-thymidine for 16 h on day 3 or assayed for polyclonal Ig secretion on day 4, using a modified reverse plaque assay [12]. PFC, plaque-forming cells.

Table 2. IgG-producing hybridomas from LPS or LPS + µF(ab')$_2$-stimulated B cells

Day of fusion	LPS	LPS + µF (ab')$_2$
4	0/24	0/12
5	4/70	12/60

Resting B cells were isolated and activated as described in [3]. On the days indicated, hybridomas were established [9].

335

References

1. Andersson Y, Bullock WW, Melchers F (1974) Eur J Immunol 4:715–722
2. Bijsterbosch MK, Meade CJ, Turner GA, Klaus GGB (1985) Cell 41:999–1006
3. Chen-Bettecken U, Wecker E, Schimpl A (1985) Proc Natl Acad Sci USA 82:7384–7388
4. Chen-Bettecken U, Wecker E, Schimpl A (1987) Immunobiol 174:162–176
5. Dani CH, Blanchard JM, Piechaczyk M, Sabouty S, Marty L, Chanteur P (1984) Proc Natl Acad Sci USA 81:7046–7050
6. Efrat S, Kaempfer R (1984) Proc Natl Acad Sci USA 81:2601–2605
7. Gerster T, Picard D, Schaffner W (1986) Cell 45:45–52
8. Grosschedl R, Baltimore D (1985) Cell 41:885–897
9. Köhler G, Milstein C (1975) Nature 256:495–497
10. Lamson G, Koshland ME (1984) J Exp Med 160:877–892
11. Mitchell RL, Zokas L, Schreiber RD, Verma IM (1985) Cell 40:209–217
12. Molinaro GA, Maron E, Eby WC, Dray S (1975) Eur J Immunol 5:771–774
13. Wall R, Briskin M, Carter C, Govan H, Taylor A, Kincade P (1986) Proc Natl Acad Sci USA 83:295–299
14. Yuan D, Tucker PW (1984) J Exp Med 160:564–583

Haematology and Blood Transfusion   Vol. 31
Modern Trends in Human Leukemia VII
Edited by Neth, Gallo, Greaves, and Kabisch
© Springer-Verlag Berlin Heidelberg 1987

Isolation, Biochemical Analysis, and *N*-Terminal Amino Acid Sequence of a Cell Surface Glycoprotein that Binds to the "Erythrocyte Receptor" of T-Lymphocytes *

T. Hünig, R. Mitnacht, G. Tiefenthaler, and F. Lottspeich

A. Introduction

Recent findings have provided strong evidence in support of a functional role of the "erythrocyte receptor" of human T-lymphocytes in T-cell activation. Thus, binding of appropriate ligands (erythrocytes or monoclonal antibodies) to the CD2 molecule, as this receptor is now called, can either block (Palacios and Martinez-Maza 1982; Martin et al. 1983; Krensky et al. 1983) or stimulate (Larsson et al. 1978; Meuer et al. 1984) T-cell proliferation and expression of T-cell function. We have previously suggested that CD2 is a cell interaction molecule, the natural ligand of which is expressed on cells with which T-lymphocytes interact during immune responses (Hünig 1985, 1986). Since the CD2 molecule had previously been characterized by the T11 antigen(s), we have named this ligand T11 target structure or T11TS. In our search for T11TS, we have assumed that the molecule recognized by CD2 on white blood cells during the cellular interactions involved in T-cell activation is identical to the one recognized on autologous and xenogeneic red cells in E-rosette formation. Consequently, a monoclonal antibody (mAb) to sheep red blood cells (SRBC) was selected that completely blocks the attachment of SRBC to either human or sheep T-lymphocytes (Hünig 1985). This mAb detects a cell surface glycoprotein of about 42 k MW which is, as we had postulated, expressed on both red and white blood cells (Hünig 1986). Furthermore, this anti-T11TS mAb inhibits the mixed lymphocyte reaction between outbred sheep, thus suggesting an involvement of T11TS in T-cell activation (Hünig 1986). Here we report some biochemical properties of T11TS, including its N-terminal amino acid sequence.

B. Materials and Methods

The E-rosette inhibition assay has been described (Hünig 1985). Affinity purification of T11TS from detergent lysates of SRBC was performed with mAb L180/1 (anti-T11TS) coupled to glutaraldehyde-activated glass beads. Preparative sodium dodecyl sulfate (SDS)-polyacrylamide gel electrophoresis (PAGE) was performed using slab gels of 12% acrylamide content. Trace-labeled T11TS was identified by autoradiography and electroeluted according to Goding (Goding 1984). Purified T11TS was radioiodinated employing immobilized lactoperoxidase. The N-terminal amino acid sequence was determined on an Applied Biosystems gas-phase sequencer.

C. Results

Figure 1 illustrates the complete inhibition of SRBC binding to human T cells by Fab fragments of mAb L180/1 (anti-T11TS). The specificity and concentration dependence of this effect has been studied and described in detail (Hünig 1985).

* Supported by the Bundesministerium für Forschung und Technologie and the Zentrum für Gentechnologie e.V.

337

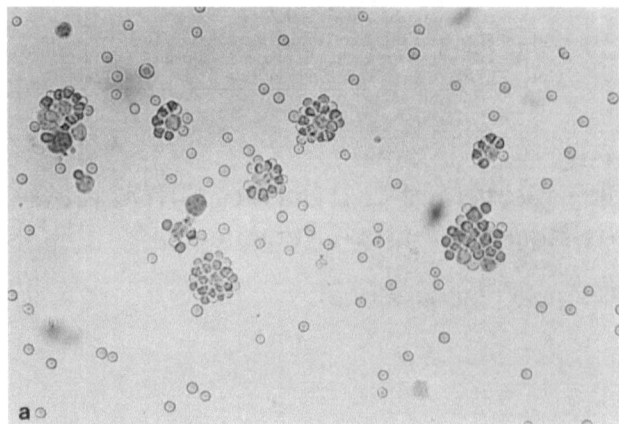

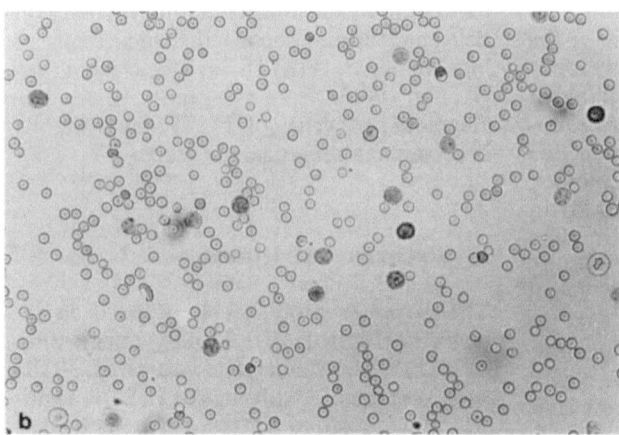

Fig. 1 a, b. Inhibition of rosette formation between SRBC and human T-lymphocytes by mAb L180/1. Nylon-wool-passed human PBL were incubated with SRBC in the absence (*panel a*) in the presence (*panel b*) of 5 µg/ml of purified Fab fragments of mAb L180/1

In order to obtain further information on the structure of T11TS, we purified the molecule to homogeneity. This was achieved in a two-step procedure using affinity chromatography on mAb L180/1 coupled to glass beads and preparative SDS-PAGE (Fig. 2). A sample of the purified material was radioiodinated and digested with endoglycosidase F, an enzyme that specifically removes N-glycosidically linked carbohydrate side chains (Fig. 3). From the intermediary products observed before the end product of about 32 k apparent MW is obtained, one can conclude that T11TS contains either three N-linked carbohydrate chains of roughly even size or two side chains of different size. From the absence of galactos-

amine observed during amino acid analysis (data not shown), it can be concluded that T11TS contains no O-glycosidically linked carbohydrate. In addition, a sample of radioiodinated T11TS was subjected to isoelectric focusing (Fig. 4). T11TS is an acidic membrane glycoprotein with a pI of 4.5.

The first 27 N-terminal amino acids of T11TS were determined by gas-phase microsequencing. The sequence is: FSQDIY GAMNGS(?)VTFYVSESQ PFTEIM. A search of the protein database from the Protein Identification Resource (George et al. 1985) has indicated that we are dealing with a previously unsequenced molecule with no obvious homologies of the sequenced portion of T11TS to known protein sequences.

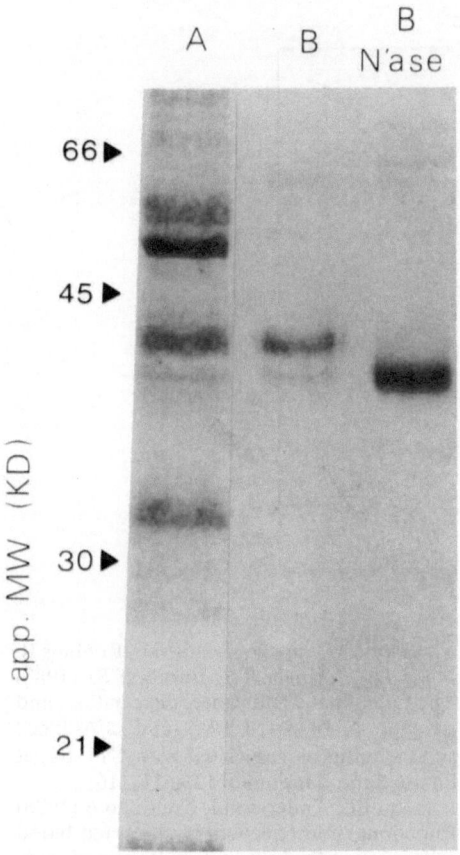

Fig. 2. Purification of T11TS. Detergent-solubilized SRBC were passed over a mAb L180/1 affinity column. In the high-salt eluate (*A*), the band at 42 k was identified as T11TS by trace labelling and autoradiography (data not shown). *B*, T11TS after electroelution from preparative slab gel of material A. *B N'ase*, material B pretreated with neuraminidase to reveal possible contaminants comigrating with T11TS. Coomassie blue stain of SDS-PAGE (12% acrylamide, reduced)

This sequence and several short stretches of sequence determined from internal peptides of T11TS provide the basis for our current efforts to isolate the T11TS gene.

D. Conclusions

The present report and our published work show that a previously undefined glycoprotein expressed on sheep red and white blood cells is recognized by the E receptor in rosette formation. This molecule is a good candidate for the hypothetical cell interaction molecule that binds to the CD2 structure during cellular interactions of T-lymphocytes with cells of the immune system. The latter point will be difficult to prove in the sheep system. However, the known binding of human erythrocytes to human T cells via CD2 (Scheffel et al. 1982; Hünig 1985) is a strong indication that a human homolog of T11TS must exist. Indeed, recent experiments by Springer and colleagues have identified this human ligand of CD2 as the lymphocyte function-associated (LFA)-3 molecule (Selvaraj et al. 1987).

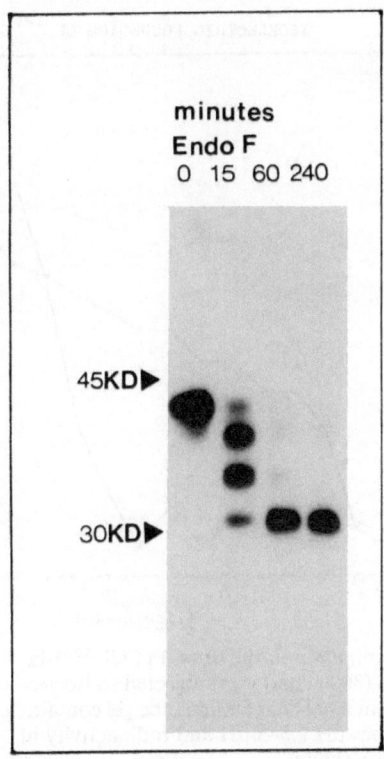

Fig. 3. Endoglycosidase F digestion of T11TS. ^{125}I-labeled purified T11TS was treated with 2U endoF for the number of times indicated, subjected to SDS-PAGE (12% acrylamide, reduced), and autoradiographed

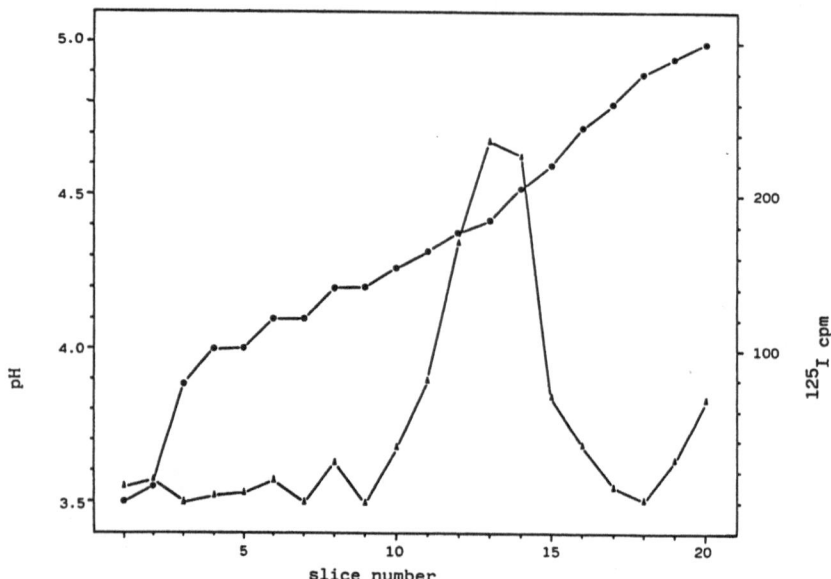

Fig. 4. Determination of the pI of T11TS. ^{125}I-labeled T11TS (3000 cpm) was subjected to isoelectric focusing in a polyacrylamide tube gel containing ampholines pH 2.5–5 pH and radioactivity in serial slices are shown

Acknowledgements. We thank Dr. M. Lohoff for his collection of anti-SRBC mAbs from which the anti-T11TS mAb was isolated and Dr. E. Winnacker for his support.

References

1. George DG, Orcutt BC, Dayhoff MO, Barker WC (1985) PIR report REL-0185, version 2.0. National Biomedical Research Foundation, Georgetown University Medical Center, Washington
2. Goding JW (1984) A simple and efficient device for electrophoretic elution of proteins from SDS-polyacrylamide gels. Annu Rev Walter and Eliza Hall Inst 1983–1984:49–50
3. Hünig T (1985) The cell surface molecule recognized by the erythrocyte receptor of T lymphocytes. Identification and characterization using a monoclonal antibody. J Exp Med 162:890–901
4. Hünig T (1986) The ligand of the erythrocyte receptor of T-lymphocytes: expression on white blood cells and possible involvement in T-cell activation. J Immunol 136:2103–2108
5. Krensky AM, Sanchez-Madrid F, Robbins E, Nagy JA, Springer TA, Burakoff SJ (1983) The functional significance, distribution, and structure of LFA-1, LFA-2, and LFA-3: cell surface antigens associated with CTL-target interactions. J Immunol 131:611–616
6. Larsson EL, Andersson J, Coutinho A (1978) Functional consequences of sheep red blood cell rosetting for human T-cells: gain of reactivity to mitogenic factors. Eur J Immunol 8:693–696
7. Martin PJ, Longton G, Ledbetter JA, Neumann W, Braun MP, Beatty PG, Hansen JA (1983) Identification and functional characterization of two distinct epitopes on the human T-cell surface protein tp50. J Immunol 131:180–185
8. Meuer SC, Hussey RE, Fabbi M, Fox D, Acuto O, Fitzgerald KA, Hodgdon JC, Protentis JP, Schlossman SF, Reinherz EL (1984) An alternative pathway of T-cell activation: a functional role for the 50 KD sheep erythrocyte receptor protein. Cell 36:897–906
9. Palacios R, Martinez-Maza O (1982) Is the E-receptor on human T-lymphocytes a "negative signal receptor"? J Immunol 129:2479–2485
10. Scheffel JW, Swartz SJ (1982) Inhibition of autologous rosette formation by monoclonal antibody to the sheep erythrocyte receptor. J Immunol 128:1930–1932
11. Selvaraj P, Plunkett ML, Dustin ME, Sanders ME, Shaw S, Springer TA (1987) The t-lymphocyte glycoprotein CD2 binds the cell surface ligand LFA-3. Nature 326:400–402

Haematology and Blood Transfusion   Vol. 31
Modern Trends in Human Leukemia VII
Edited by Neth, Gallo, Greaves, and Kabisch
© Springer-Verlag Berlin Heidelberg 1987

The Regulation of T-Cell Proliferation:
A Role for Protein Kinase C

D. A. Cantrell, A. A. Davies, W. Verbi, and M. J. Crumpton

A. Introduction

T-lymphocyte proliferation is regulated by the T-cell growth factor interleukin 2 (IL-2) which exerts its biological effects through an interaction with high-affinity specific IL-2 receptors [1–3]. Quiescent T-lymphocytes neither produce IL-2 nor express IL-2 receptors [2, 4]. However, following immune stimulation there is transcriptional activation of both the IL-2 and IL-2 receptor genes which results in IL-2 synthesis and IL-2 receptor expression [5–7]. T-cell proliferation can then proceed via an autocrine pathway in which the population secretes and responds to its own growth factor.

Recently there have been considerable advances in our understanding of the signals that initiate IL-2 production and IL-2 receptor expression. In particular, the T-cell membrane structures involved in antigen recognition and the associated immune activation have been identified. The T-cell antigen receptor is an idiotypic disulphide-linked heterodimer (Ti) comprising two glycosylated polypeptides (α and β) of M_r 50 000 and 43 000 respectively [8–11]. Ti is associated noncovalently on the cell surface with the invariant T3 antigen [8, 12]. T3 consists of three chains [13, 14] – two glycosylated polypeptides of M_r 26 000 and 21 000 (γ and δ) respectively and one non-N-glycosylated peptide of M_r 19 000 (ε) – and is generally considered to be involved in the intracellular transduction of the signals that initiate

Cell Surface Biochemistry, Imperial Cancer Research Laboratories, Lincoln's Inn Fields, London, UK

T-cell growth [15, 16]. The nature of these intracellular signals has not been defined although it has been proposed that the T3/Ti complex is linked to a phosphodiesterase that metabolizes phosphatidylinositol and generates two potential intracellular signals, inositol triphosphate and diacylglycerol [17]. Inositol triphosphate is thought to mobilize intracellular calcium and thus elevate intracellular Ca^{2+} concentrations whereas diacylglycerol has been linked to activation of a calcium/phospholipid dependent kinase, protein kinase C [18]. In this respect, calcium ionophores which elevate intracellular Ca^{2+} concentrations and phorbol esters which stimulate protein kinase C can mimic the effect of immune activation and initiate T-cell proliferation via the IL-2 system [19].

An interesting feature of the T cell is that IL-2 production and IL-2 receptor expression are both transient [4–7]. For example, the polyclonal activation of T-lymphocytes induces a short phase (3–4 days) of autocrine proliferation followed by a prolonged phase (10–14 days) in which the cells are responsive to an exogenous supply of IL-2 [4]. These proliferative characteristics reflect the fact that initially there is induction of both IL-2 production and IL-2 receptor expression which then drives T-cell proliferation in an autocrine system. IL-2 production is switched off rapidly, which is why autocrine proliferation ceases, whereas IL-2 receptor expression and hence IL-2 responsiveness declines more slowly over the 10–14 day period. These unique characteristics of the T-cell proliferative system have focused obvious questions as to the molecular events that determine the transient nature of IL-2 production and IL-2 receptor expression, since these ensure the homeostasis of the T-cell proliferative response.

In the present report we have used phorbol esters to explore the role of protein kinase C in the regulation of T-cell proliferation. Our data show that protein kinase C may have a dual role in the T cell since activation of protein kinase C can deliver positive signals crucial for the initiation of IL-2 production and IL-2 receptor expression. As well, activation of protein kinase C can deliver negative signals to the T cell and induce unresponsiveness with respect to the initiation of T-cell proliferation via triggering of the T3/T cell antigen receptor complex. Consequently protein kinase C may determine the transient nature of the T-cell growth response.

B. The Role of Protein Kinase C as a Positive Growth-Regulatory Signal in the T Cell

Quiescent T-lymphocytes can be activated by monoclonal antibodies that recognize the T3 antigen and trigger the T3/T-cell antigen receptor complex [20–22]. For optimal induction of T-cell proliferation there is an obligate requirement for monocytes/macrophages as accessory cells. This monocyte requirement can be substituted by phorbol esters which activate protein kinase C. As well, T3/Ti triggering can be substituted by calcium ionophores which increase the concentration of cytoplasmic free calcium [23].

To compare the effect of these stimuli, either singly or in combination, on the induction of IL-2 production and IL-2 receptor expression, we examined the initiation of T-cell growth in the presence or absence of exogenous IL-2. The induction of autocrine T-cell proliferation requires optimal induction of both IL-2 receptor expression and IL-2 production. However when IL-2 is nonlimiting (e.g. provided exogenously in excess) the T-cell proliferative response is a direct measure of the cellular density of high-affinity IL-2 receptors. Consequently, a comparison of the signals is necessary to induce autocrine T-cell proliferation versus IL-2 responsiveness allows a rapid comparison of the

signals that induce IL-2 receptor expression and IL-2 production. For such studies we have chosen to examine the secondary stimulation of T-lymphocytes that have been arrested in the G_0/G_1 stage of the cell cycle by prior activation and clonal expansion in IL-2. After 10–14 days of culture such cells assume the phenotype of a quiescent T-cell population and have the advantage of giving a synchronous response to activation [4]. Additionally it is possible to obtain large numbers (10^9) of T cells with no contaminating accessory cells present.

The data in Fig. 1 are derived from an experiment in which quiescent T-lymphocytes were exposed to various combinations of the anti-T3 antibody OKT3, phorbol 12,13 dibutyrate (Pdbu), the calcium ionophore, ionomycin, and IL-2. A combination of OKT3 plus Pdbu (Fig. 1 a, c) or ionomycin plus Pdbu (Fig. 1 b, c) could stimulate autocrine T-cell proliferation whereas the various stimuli given singly or the combination of OKT3 plus ionomycin were ineffective. In contrast, a single stimulation with Pdbu or OKT3 could induce IL-2 responsiveness (Fig. 1 a, c); ionomycin had no effect. These results suggest that a single stimulus of T3/Ti triggering or activation of protein kinase C by Pdbu is sufficient to induce IL-2 receptor expression and hence IL-2 responsiveness. In contrast, a combined stimulus of T3/Ti triggering plus protein kinase C activation or calcium ionophore plus protein kinase C activation is necessary to ensure both IL-2 receptor expression and IL-2 production and hence allow an autocrine proliferative response.

C. The Role of Protein Kinase C as a Negative Growth-Regulatory Signal in the T Cell

Activation of protein kinase C by Pdbu induces T cells to become responsive to IL-2 (Fig. 1 c). However, Pdbu-activated T cells are refractory to proliferative signals delivered via the T3/Ti complex by anti-T3 antibodies (Fig. 2). Since Pdbu-activated T cells can respond to IL-2 (Fig. 1 c), it is probable that the lack of a growth response to anti-T3 reflects an inhibition of T3/Ti-in-

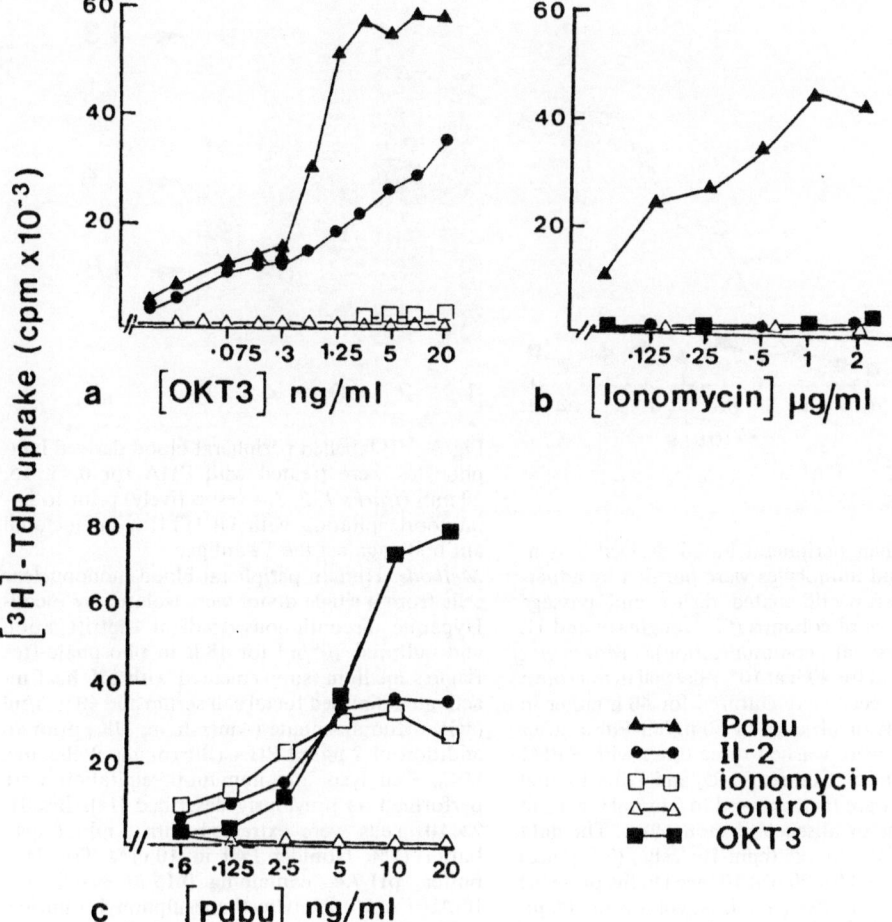

Fig. 1 a–c. Human T cells were prepared as described previously [4, 26]. Briefly, peripheral blood derived T cells were activated polyclonally by incubation for 72 h in RPMI 1640 supplemented with 10% FCS and 1 ng/ml OKT3 (Ortho Pharmaceuticals). Cells were maintained during activation at 37 °C in a humidified 5% CO_2/air incubator. Thereafter cells were maintained at 10^5–10^6/ml in the presence of 1 unit/ml recombinant IL-2 for 10–14 days, after which the cells became quiescent and did not produce IL-2 or express IL-2 receptors. For restimulation 10^5 cells/well were cultured for 48 h in microtest II plates in a final volume of 200 μl in the presence of the activating signals described below. Tritiated thymidine (^{3}H-TdR) incorporation (0.5 μCi/ml) was monitored over a 4-h period as an estimate of DNA synthesis. Data are shown as ^{3}H-TdR uptake (cpm/10^5 cells). **a** Cells were exposed to various concentrations of OKT3 (0–20 ng/ml) alone (△–△) or in the presence of 5 ng/ml Pdbu (▲–▲), 1 unit/ml IL-2 (●–●), or 0.5 μg/ml ionomycin (□–□). **b** Cells were exposed to various concentrations of ionomycin (0–4 μg/ml) either alone (△–△) or in the presence of 5 ng/ml OKT3 (■–■), 1 unit/ml IL-2 (●–●), or 5 ng/ml Pdbu (▲–▲). **c** Cells were exposed to various concentrations of Pdbu (0–50 ng/ml) either alone (△–△) or in the presence of 5 ng/ml OKT3 (■–■), 1 unit/ml IL-2 (●–●), or 0.5 μg/ml ionomycin (□–□)

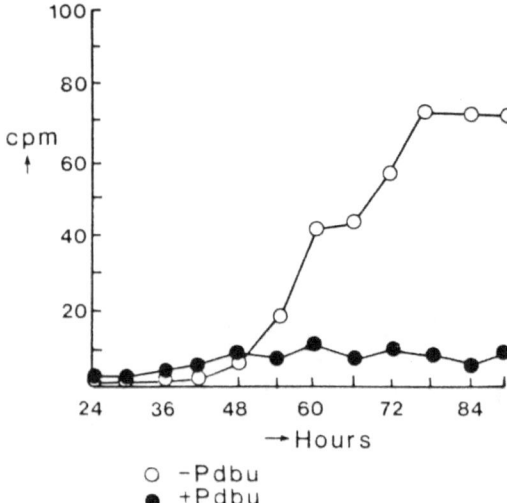

O —Pdbu
● +Pdbu

Fig. 2. Human peripheral blood derived T-lymphocytes and monocytes were purified by adherence to fibronectin-coated dishes and passage over nylon wool columns (G. Dougherty and H. Hogg, personal communication). Monocytes were cultured for 40 h at 10^4 cells/well in microtest II plates. T cells were cultured for 40 h either in the presence or absence of 50 ng/ml Pdbu, after which cells were washed three times with RPMI 1640/10% FCS. Control (o–o) and Pdbu-treated cells (●–●) were then exposed to 5 ng/ml OKT3 in the presence or absence of monocytes. The data show ^{3}H-TdR uptake (cpm/10^5 cells) (2-h pulse) in cells cultured for 90 h at 10^5/well in the presence of 10^4 monocytes/well in a final volume of 200 µl. No detectable ^{3}H-TdR uptake was detected in T cells exposed to OKT3 in the absence of monocytes or in T cells cultured with monocytes alone

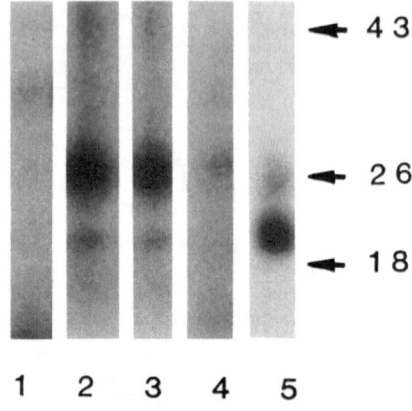

Fig. 3. ^{32}P-labelled peripheral blood derived lymphocytes were treated with PHA for 0, 5, 15, 40 min (*tracks 1, 2, 3, 4* respectively) prior to immunoprecipitation with UCHT1, a monoclonal antibody against the T3 antigen.

Methods: Human peripheral blood mononuclear cells from a single donor were isolated by Ficoll-Hypaque discontinuous gradient centrifugation and cultured 10^6/ml for 18 h in phosphate-free Eagle's medium, supplemented with 5% heat inactivated dialysed foetal calf serum and 40 µCi/ml (^{32}P)-orthophosphate (Amersham, UK) prior to addition of 2 µg/ml PHA (Burroughs Wellcome, UK). Cell lysis and immunoprecipitation were performed as previously described [14]. Briefly, 2×10^7 cells were extracted with 1 ml of lysis buffer (1% Nonidet P40 in 10 mM Tris HCl buffer, pH 7.4, containing 0.15 M NaCl, 1% BSA, 1 mM phenylmethanesulphonyl fluoride, 1 mM EDTA and 50 mM NaF) for 10 min at 4 °C. After centrifuging for 195 000 gmin, lysates were precleared with fixed *Staphylococcus aureus* organisms and rabbit anti-(mouse immunoglobulin). Precleared lysate (1 ml) was precipitated with 5–10 µg of monoclonal antibody UCHT1 [16], covalently coupled to Sepharose 4B beads (Pharmacia Fine Chemicals). Immunoprecipitates were washed sequentially with lysis buffer containing (a) 0.65 M NaCl, (b) lysis buffer plus 0.1% SDS, and (c) 0.1% Nonidet P40 in 10 mM Tris HCl, pH 7.4, and then analyzed by SDS-PAGE on a 12% gel run under reducing conditions

duced IL-2 production. It is noteworthy that previous studies have shown that phorbol esters can inhibit antigen-mediated proliferative and cytolytic responses [24, 25]. It thus seems likely that there is an intracellular signalling pathway between the phorbol ester target, protein kinase C, and the T3/T cell antigen receptor complex. Exposure to phorbol esters down-regulates the surface expression of T3/Ti [26, 27]. However, the lack of response to anti-T3 antibodies in phorbol ester treated cells is not necessarily due to down-regulation of T3/Ti since, when phorbol esters are removed, T3 levels recover rapidly (within 2–3 h) (unpublished data). The alternative possibility is that ex-

posure to phorbol esters inactivates the transmembrane signalling functions of T3/Ti.

This functional inhibition could be due to the effects of phorbol esters on protein kinase C expression since treatment with phorbol esters greatly reduces cellular levels of protein kinase C (unpublished data). Nevertheless, protein kinase C is not totally removed by exposure to phorbol esters; thus the possibility exists that the T3/Ti signalling system is inactivated by some other mechanism. One potential mechanism for inactivation is protein kinase C mediated phosphorylation of T3. Phorbol esters induce phosphorylation of the γ subunit of T3 [26]. As well, similar phosphorylation of the T3 γ chain occurs in T cells activated with antigen (data not shown) or a polyclonal activator such as PHA. Thus the data in Fig. 3 show that PHA induces phosphorylation of a M_r 26 000 T3 polypeptide that has been identified as the T3 γ chain. It is of interest therefore that T3 phosphorylation is a common feature of T-cell activation with those stimuli that have been shown to down-regulate the surface expression and/or functions of T3/Ti.

D. Discussion

We have used phorbol esters to activate protein kinase C in order to evaluate the role of this kinase in the regulation of T-cell proliferation. We have provided evidence that protein kinase C can deliver positive growth-regulatory signals in the T-cell and initiate IL-2 receptor expression and hence IL-2 responsiveness. As well, stimulation of protein kinase C can induce IL-2 production if a concomitant signal elevating intracellular Ca^{2+} levels is provided. This second stimulus can be generated by a calcium ionophore or by triggering of the T3/Ti complex with anti-T3 antibodies.

A single stimulus with an anti-T3 antibody can initiate IL-2 receptor expression but not IL-2 production. It is not known whether protein kinase C has an intermediate role in this latter signalling system or whether some unidentified pathway is important. A single stimulus with anti-T3 has been shown to induce phosphatidylinositol metabolism and inositol triphosphate release which then generates a Ca^{2+} signal. Nevertheless, elevation of intracellular Ca^{2+} levels is not sufficient to induce IL-2 receptor expression since calcium ionophores were ineffective in this respect. The metabolism of phosphatidylinositol would also generate diacylglycerol which could activate protein kinase C and thus initiate IL-2 receptor expression. However, if T3/Ti triggering delivers the dual signals of Ca^{2+} and protein kinase C activation, there is the discrepancy regarding why this does not result in IL-2 production unless an additional signal such as phorbol ester is also present. One explanation may reside in the predicted differences in the kinetics of protein kinase C activation in response to phorbol esters or endogenous diacylglycerol production. The latter pathway would give a transient activation of protein kinase C whereas phorbol esters would be expected to give prolonged stimulation.

Consequently we would propose that there are two major differences with respect to the signal requirements for induction of the IL-2 and IL-2 receptor genes. Firstly, induction of IL-2 production requires both a Ca^{2+} signal and protein kinase C activation whereas induction of Il-2 receptors requires only protein kinase C activation. Secondly, a transient activation of protein kinase C may be sufficient to induce IL-2 receptor expression whereas a more prolonged stimulation is necessary to ensure Il-2 production. To test this model it will be necessary to establish directly whether a single stimulus of T3/Ti triggering can activate protein kinase C.

Activation of protein kinase C can also deliver a negative signal to T cells, since phorbol esters can down-regulate the surface expression and functions of T3/Ti molecules and inhibit antigen-regulated functions such as cytotoxicity and proliferation. The molecular basis for this regulation may be protein kinase C mediated phosphorylation of the T3 γ chain. There are other examples of receptor functions controlled by phosphorylation/dephosphorylation. For example, desensitisation of α and β adrenergic receptors is associated with their phosphorylation [28, 29]. There is also an interesting parallel in the fibroblasts in which protein kinase C regulates the surface expression and functions of the epidermal growth factor receptor via phosphorylation/dephosphorylation [30–33].

In summary, we would propose a model in which protein kinase C has a dual role in the regulation of T-cell proliferation. Immune stimulation of T cells via the T3/T cell antigen receptor complex results in activation of protein kinase C, which then functions as a positive signal in the induction of the IL-2/IL-2 receptor genes and may be a critical component of the intracellular mechanisms that regulate IL-2 production and IL-2 receptor expression via T3/Ti. Protein kinase C activation also initiates a negative feedback pathway that terminates the functions of the T3/T-cell antigen receptor complex and may therefore be relevant to the molecular events that determine the transient nature of the T-cell proliferative response. This model is based on the assumption that the biological response to phorbol esters is due solely to the effects of phorbol esters on protein kinase C. Moreover, there is also the assumption that pharmacological activation of protein kinase C with phorbol esters will have effects similar to physiological activation of the kinase. However, it must not be ruled out that phorbol esters can have direct effects on alternative signalling systems, and in this respect it is noteworthy that there are indications of a family of molecules structurally related to protein kinase C [34, 35]. These might also be cellular targets for phorbol esters and may have a role as intracellular signals in the T cell.

References

1. Smith KA (1980) Immun Rev 41:337
2. Robb R, Munck A, Smith KA (1981) J Exp Med 154:1455
3. Cantrell DA, Smith KA (1984) Science 224:1313
4. Cantrell DA, Smith KA (1983) J Exp Med 158:1895
5. Efrat S, Pilo S, Kaempfer R (1982) Nature 297:236
6. Leonard WJ, Kronke M, Peffer NJ, Depper JM, Greene WC (1985) Proc Natl Acad Sci USA 82:6281
7. Grabstein K, Dower S, Gillis S, Urdal D, Larsen AJ (1986) Immunol 136:4503
8. Meuer SC, Fitzgerald KA, Hussey RE, Hodgdon JC, Schlossman SF, Reinherz EL (1983) J Exp Med 157:707
9. Acuto O, Hussey RE, Fitzgerald KA, Protentis S, Meuer SC, Schlossman SF, Reinherz EL (1983) Cell 34:717
10. Meuer SC, Cooper DA, Hodgdon JC, Hussey RE, Fitzgerald KA, Schlossman SF, Reinherz EL (1983) Science 222:1239
11. Meuer SC, Acuto O, Hussey RE, Hodgdon JC, Fitzgerald KA, Schlossman SF, Reinherz EL (1983) Nature 303:808
12. Brenner MB, Trowbridge JS, Strominger JL (1985) Cell 40:183
13. Kannelopoulus JM, Wigglesworth NM, Owen MJ, Crumpton MJ (1983) Embo J 2:1807
14. Borst J, Alexander S, Elder J, Terhorst C (1983) J Biol Chem 258:5135
15. Oettgen HC, Terhorst C, Cantley LC, Roscoff PM (1985) Cell 40:583
16. Roscoff PM, Cantley LW (1983) J Biol Chem 260:14053
17. Imboden JB, Stobo JO (1985) J Exp Med 161:446
18. Berridge MJ (1984) Biochem J 220:345
19. Truneh A, Albert F, Golstein P, Schmitt Verhulot (1985) Nature 313:318
20. Van Wauve JP, De Mey JR, Goosens JG (1980) J Immunol 124:2708
21. Burns GF, Boyd AW, Beverley PCL (1982) J Immunol 129:1451
22. Reinherz EL, Meuer SC, Fitzgerald KA, Hussey RE, Levine H, Schlossman S (1982) Cell 30:735
23. Weiss A, Wiskocil RL, Stobo JD (1984) J Immunol 133:123
24. Ando I, Hariri G, Wallace D, Beverley P (1983) Euro J Immunol 15:196
25. Delia D, Greaves MF, Newman M, Sutherland DR, Minowada J, Kung P, Goldstein G (1982) Int J Cancer 29:23
26. Cantrell DA, Davies AA, Crumpton MJ (1985) Proc Natl Acad Sci USA 82:8158
27. Davies AA, Cantrell DA, Crumpton MJ (1985) Biosciences 5:867
28. Sibley DR, Strasser RH, Caron MG, Lefkowitz RJ (1985) J Biol Chem 260:3883
29. Huganir RL, Delcour AH, Greengard P, Hess G (1986) Nature 321:774
30. Shoyab M, Daharao JE, Todaro GT (1979) Nature (London) 279:387
31. Cochet C, Gill GN, Meisenhelder J, Cooper JA, Hunter T (1984) J Biol Chem 259:2553
32. Iwashita S, Fox CF (1984) J Biol Chem 259:2559
33. Davis RJ, Czech MP (1985) Proc Natl Acad Sci USA 82:1974
34. Parker PJ, Coussens L, Totty N, Rhee L, Young S, Chen E, Stabel S, Waterfield MD, Ullrich A (1986) Science 233:853
35. Coussens L, Parker PJ, Rhee L, Yang-Feng TL, Chen E, Waterfield MD, Francke U, Ullrich A (1986) Science 233:859

Haematology and Blood Transfusion   Vol. 31
Modern Trends in Human Leukemia VII
Edited by Neth, Gallo, Greaves, and Kabisch
© Springer-Verlag Berlin Heidelberg 1987

Activation of Natural Killer Function Through the T11/E Rosette Receptor *

R. E. Schmidt [1], S. F. Schlossman [2], E. L. Reinherz [2], and J. Ritz [2]

Natural killer (NK) cells have been identified as a population of circulating lymphocytes capable of mediating direct cytotoxicity against a variety of target cells without prior immunization. There is now considerable experimental evidence to suggest that this lymphocyte subpopulation is capable of immune surveillance against tumor cells in vivo and that NK cells may exert important regulatory functions within the immune system [1, 2, 6, 24, 25]. In recent years it has become evident that NK cells themselves can be regulated through interaction with various lymphokines such as interferon and interleukin 2 (IL-2) [5, 7, 13, 22, 26, 27]. In the present studies, we demonstrate that the cytotoxic function of NK cells can be markedly enhanced through activation of the receptor for sheep erythrocytes (T11/E rosette receptor) and that this enhancement is comparable to that observed following IL-2 activation.

The T11/E rosette receptor antigen has been shown to be a pathway for antigen-independent activation of peripheral blood T lymphocytes [12] and is expressed on thymocytes, T cells and NK cells [3, 9, 14]. Three different epitopes on the T11 antigen have been defined. Activation through the T11

complex is independent of expression of T-cell receptor for antigen and has been found to occur with immature thymocytes as well as with T3 negative NK clones [18]. In addition, it has been demonstrated that cellular activation with anti-T11$_2$ and anti-T11$_3$ monoclonal antibodies induces MHC-independent killing by cytolytic T-cell clones as well as cytotoxicity of NK clones against otherwise resistant targets [23].

In the present studies, we examined whether the cytotoxicity of purified peripheral blood NK cells could be activated via the T11/E rosette receptor and compared these effects to those observed following IL-2 activation. Human NK cells were purified from peripheral blood by immunofluorescent flow cytometric cell sorting of NKH1 positive cells [8, 17]. NKH1 has previously been demonstrated to be a pan-NK cell antigen expressed by cells that morphologically appear as large granular lymphocytes and which comprise approximately 12% of peripheral blood mononuclear cells (PBMC). All cells in peripheral blood with NK activity express NKH1$^+$ but this antigen is not expressed by T cells, B cells, monocytes or granulocytes [8, 17]. When PBMC are separated into NKH1$^+$ and NKH1$^-$ fractions (Fig. 1 A) all of the natural cytotoxicity against a standard NK target cell, K562, is contained within the NKH1$^+$ population. Following 18 h incubation with recombinant IL-2 (Fig. 1 B), the NK activity of unseparated PBMC is significantly enhanced, but cytotoxicity remains confined to the NKH1$^+$ subset. Results shown in Fig. 1 C demonstrate that enhancement of cytotoxicity can also be seen follow-

* Supported by NIH grant CH 34183. J.R. is a scholar of the Leukemia Society of America
[1] Abt. Immunologie und Transfusionsmedizin, Zentrum Innere Medizin und Dermatologie, Medizinische Hochschule Hannover, Postfach 61 01 80, D-3000 Hannover 61, FRG
[2] Division of Tumor Immunology, Dana-Farber Cancer Institute and Department of Medicine, Harvard Medical School, Boston, MA 02115, USA

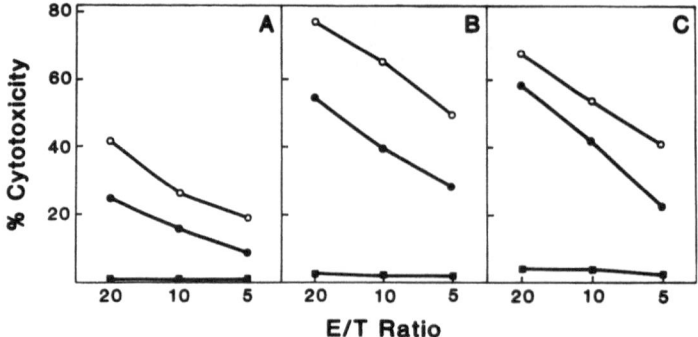

Fig. 1. NK activity of PBMC (●—●), NKH1⁺ (○—○), and NKH1⁻ (□—□) cells were measured against K562 target cells after incubation with either media (*panel A*), purified recombinant IL-2 (*rIL-2*) (*panel B*), or T11₂/₃ monoclonal antibodies (*panel C*). Cytotoxicity assays were performed according to a standard chromium release method previously described [8, 19]. All experiments were done in triplicate using V bottom microtiter plates. Medium was RPMI 1640 + 5% pooled human AB serum and 1% penicillin streptomycin. Assays were performed at various effector/target (E/T) ratios using between 3000 and 5000 K562 target cells/well

ing 18 h incubation with anti-T11₂/₃ monoclonal antibodies. Moreover, the triggering of peripheral blood NK cells with anti-T11₂/₃ antibodies is as effective as with rIL-2 and is also restricted to NKH1⁺ cells.

To directly examine the effect of anti-T11 monoclonal antibodies on effector-target cell binding, we evaluated the ability of activated effector cells to form cell conjugates with K562 targets. As shown in Table 1, preincubation of NKH1⁺ cells with either anti-T11₂/₃ or IL-2 significantly enhances conjugate formation. This effect is stronger for anti-T11₂/₃ than for IL-2 triggering. In-

terestingly, conjugate formation is also induced in NKH1⁻ cells when activated through the T11 pathway, although these cells are not able to mediate direct cytotoxicity. In contrast, IL-2 does not induce the formation of conjugates in the NKH1⁻ population. Blocking studies using anti-LFA-1 antibody (data not shown) suggest that the T11-induced enhancement of cytotoxicity is at least in part due to an increased binding of effectors to target cells that is mediated through LFA-1 antigen [23].

To test whether T11 activation of NKH1⁺ cells would induce cytotoxicity

Table 1. Effector: target cell conjugates induced by anti-T11₂/₃ and recombinant IL-2

Time[a]	NKH1⁺ cells			NKH1⁻ cells		
	Media	Anti-T11₂/₃	rIL-2	Media	Anti-T11₂/₃	rIL-2
20′	10[b]	50	44	4	88	0
60′	10	68	52	8	94	8
120′	32	72	46	6	96	2

[a] Following 18 h incubation, effector cells were incubated with K562 target cells (20/1; E/T ratio) for 20, 60, or 120 min at 37° C prior to enumeration of conjugates.
[b] Each value represents percent K562 target cells forming conjugates of at least one effector cell.
Peripheral blood mononuclear cells were separated into NKH1⁺ and NKH1⁻ populations by immunofluorescent cell sorting and subsequently incubated with either media, anti-T11₂ and anti-T11₃ monoclonal antibodies (1:250 final ascites dilution) or recombinant IL-2 (1000 U/ml) for 18 h at 37° C.

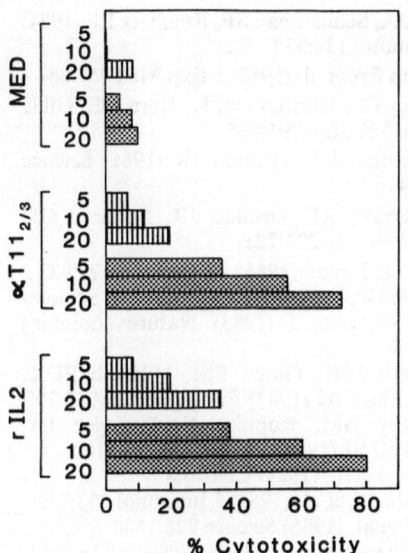

Fig. 2. Cytotoxic activity of PBMC (|||) and purified NKH1$^+$ (::::) cells against the NK-resistant Burkitt lymphoma line Daudi. Assays were performed after 18 h incubation with media, T11$_{2/3}$ antibodies, or *rIL-2*. Methods for purification of NKH1$^+$ cells and cytotoxicity assays are as described for Fig. 1

against "NK-resistant" tumor cells, we performed similar experiments using Daudi Burkitt's lymphoma cells as targets. As shown in Fig. 2, PBMC and resting NKH1$^+$ cells exhibit very little killing activity against Daudi cells. However, when purified NKH1$^+$ cells were stimulated with T11$_{2/3}$ antibodies, significant cytotoxicity against Daudi was induced. Similar results were observed after activation with purified recombinant IL-2 and with both methods of activation, this enhancement was found only within the NKH1$^+$ population. T11-induced enhancement of cytotoxicity was also found against other tumor lines (data not shown).

In summary, this study demonstrates that the cytotoxicity of purified NKH1$^+$ peripheral blood NK cells can be significantly enhanced via the T11/E rosette receptor pathway. The extent of NK enhancement after an 18-h incubation period is quite similar to the effects seen following IL-2 activation. Moreover, our data indicate that activation

using either IL-2 or monoclonal T11$_{2/3}$ antibodies induces cytotoxicity against so-called NK-resistant target cells. The cell separation studies done in conjunction with in vitro activation consistently demonstrate, that cytotoxicity is contained exclusively within the NKH1$^+$ cell fraction.

Although IL-2 and T11 activation lead to similar degrees of enhancement of cytotoxicity, there are differences in the effects of IL-2 and anti-T11 which suggest that distinct cellular mechanisms may be involved. One major difference is the enhancement of conjugate formation in the NKH1$^-$ population that can be induced by anti-T11 but not by IL-2 (Table 1). It is also known that 1 h incubation with IL-2 is sufficient for enhancement of cytotoxicity [15], whereas the effects of anti-T11 antibodies require at least 6–8 h stimulation before significant enhancement can be detected (data not shown). The effects of these two activators on cloned NK and CTL effectors have also shown disparate results since only anti-T11 is able to induce killing of resistant targets by cultured cell lines [8, 17, 19]. In addition, it has been observed that IL-2 induces proliferation as well as cytotoxicity of NKH1$^+$ purified NK cells, whereas anti-T11$_{2/3}$ antibodies do not induce in vitro proliferation of these cells (data not shown).

Since it is known that T11$_{2/3}$ activation results in rapid expression of IL-2 receptor, it is possible that IL-2 may also play a significant role in the functional effects seen following stimulation with anti-T11$_{2/3}$. In this regard, the addition of both IL-2 and anti-T11$_{2/3}$ antibodies does not enhance the maximal activation of NK activity seen following either stimulus alone (data not shown). Further studies will be necessary to explore the different roles and potential mechanisms of interaction between IL-2 and T11 activation in the regulation of NK activity.

Another important issue addressed by the present studies is the identification of those cells capable of mediating cytotoxicity following in vitro activation. Other investigators have previously demonstrated that some cells in normal peripheral blood can be induced to spontaneously kill a variety of target cells following incubation with various lymphokines and clinical studies utilizing in vitro activated cytotoxic cells in patients with metastatic cancer have recently been reported [15, 16]. These cells have been termed lymphokine activated killer (LAK) cells [4] under the assumption that they are different from both T cells and NK cells. The results presented in this report consistently demonstrate that spontaneous cytotoxicity against a variety of target cells is exclusively contained within the NKH1[+] population of PBMC. In vitro activation by either IL-2 or anti-T11$_{2/3}$ results in marked enhancement of cytotoxicity against NK-sensitive targets as well as simultaneous induction of cytotoxicity against previously NK-resistant targets. However, with both stimulated and unstimulated effector cells, enhanced cytotoxicity remains confined to the NKH1[+] population which only represents a small fraction (approximately 12%) of PBMC. These studies therefore strongly suggest that LAK is a direct result of the activation and proliferation of NKH1[+] natural killer cells and argues against a separate lineage derivation of these cells [20]. In contrast, our studies support the view that the LAK phenomenon primarily reflects the functional effects of various lymphokines on the regulation of NK activity in vivo.

References

1. Abruzzo LV, Rowley DA (1984) Science 222:581
2. Degliantoni et al. (1985) J Exp Med 162:1512
3. Fox DA, Schlossman SF, Reinherz EL (1984) J Immunol 134:330
4. Grimm EA et al. (1983) J Exp Med 157:884
5. Henney CS, Kuribayashi K, Kern DE, Gillis S (1981) Nature 291:335
6. Herberman RB, Ortaldo JR (1981) Science 214:24
7. Herberman RB, Ortaldo JR, Bonnard GD (1979) Nature 227:221
8. Hercend T et al. (1985) J Clin Invest 75:932
9. Hercend T, Reinherz EL, Meuer SC, Schlossman SF, Ritz J (1983) Nature (London) 301:158
10. Hildreth JEK, Gotch FM, Hildreth PDK, McMichael AJ (1983) Eur J Immunol 13:202
11. Krensky AM, Robbins E, Springer TA, Burakoff SJ (1984) J Immunol 132:2180
12. Meuer S et al. (1984) Cell 36:897
13. Ortaldo JR et al. (1984) J Immunol 133:779
14. Ritz J et al. (1985) Science 228:1540
15. Rosenberg SA et al. (1984) Science 223:1412
16. Rosenberg SA et al. (1985) N Engl J Med 313:1485
17. Schmidt RE, Hercend T, Schlossman SF, Ritz J (1985) Klin Wochenschr 63:1189
18. Schmidt RE et al. (1985) J Immunol 135:672
19. Schmidt RE et al. (1985) Nature 318:289
20. Shivela M (1985) Scand J Immunol 22:479
21. Siliciano R, Pratt J, Schmidt RE, Ritz J, Reinherz EL (1985) Nature 317:428
22. Smith KA (1980) Immunol Rev 51:337
23. Springer T et al. (1982) Immunol Rev 68:171
24. Tilden AB et al. (1983) J Immunol 130:1171
25. Trinchieri G, Perussia B (1984) Lab Invest 50:489
26. Trinchieri G et al. (1984) J Exp Med 146:1299
27. Trinchieri G, Santoli D, Dee RR, Knowles BB (1978) J Exp Med 147:1299

Haematology and Blood Transfusion   Vol. 31
Modern Trends in Human Leukemia VII
Edited by Neth, Gallo, Greaves, and Kabisch
© Springer-Verlag Berlin Heidelberg 1987

Tumor Necrosis Factor:
A Potent Mediator of Macrophage-Dependent Tumor-Cell Killing *

J. L. Urban [1], J. L. Rothstein [2], M. H. Shephard [3], and H. Schreiber [2]

A. Introduction

Macrophages (Mϕ) can be activated to show highly selective cytotoxicity toward malignant cells in vitro [6, 8, 9, 13, 14] and there is some evidence that they may destroy neoplastic cells in vivo [1]. The importance of activated Mϕ (aMϕ) in controlling tumor growth in vivo has been further implicated in experiments involving murine ultraviolet light (UV)-induced tumors, which are highly immunogenic regressor tumors [10] sensitive to Mϕ in vitro [22]. Variants of these tumors demonstrating progressive growth in the normal host were found to invariably express an increased resistance to aMϕ [22]. Furthermore, exposure of regressor tumor cells to aMϕ in vitro also resulted in selection for Mϕ-resistant cancer cells which displayed an increased early growth potential in vivo [22]. More recently we have utilized these tumor variants resistant to aMϕ to explore the mechanism by which aMϕ induce tumor cell destruction [23]. Our results suggest a major role for tumor necrosis factor type α (TNF-α) in Mϕ-mediated tumor cell killing in vitro and in vivo [23].

* This work was supported by grants CA-22677, CA-19266, CA-37156, 5-T32 AI-07090, and 5-T32 GMO-7281 from the National Institutes of Health
[1] Division of Biology, California Institute of Technology, Pasadena, CA 91125
[2] La Rabida-University of Chicago Institute, Department of Pathology, University of Chicago, Chicago, IL 60649
[3] Genentech Inc., Department of Pharmacological Sciences, South San Francisco, CA 94080

B. Methods

Mϕ were peritoneal exudate cells obtained from thioglycollate-primed C3H/HeN (MTV$^-$) mice, activated in vitro for 6 h with lipopolysaccharide and lymphokine and used as effectors in a 16-h ^{51}Cr release assay, a 72-h ^{51}Cr postlabelling assay, or a 72-h [^{3}H]-thymidine release assay as described [22, 23]. C3H/HeN (MTV$^-$) mice were obtained from the National Cancer Institute, Frederick Cancer Research Facility. The UV-induced tumors 1591-RE and 2240-RE were induced in these mice by M. L. Kripke [10]. Human recombinant (r) TNF-α [18], B-cell lymphotoxin (TNF-β) [7], murine rTNF-α [19], polyclonal rabbit antibody to murine rTNF-α, and monoclonal antibody to human rTNF-α were produced at Genentech (South San Francisco, CA). Recombinant murine interleukin 1 (IL-1) [12] was kindly provided by Hoffman-LaRoche.

C. Results

Mϕ are known to secrete a number of different cytotoxic substances, including interleukin 1 (IL-1) [16], reactive oxygen intermediates, such as hydrogen peroxide [15] and TNF-α [5, 18, 21]. To test each of these as potential mediators of Mϕ-dependent tumor cytotoxicity, we analyzed each for preferential killing of the 1591 parent tumor over several of its Mϕ-resistant variants. Figure 1 shows that of these substances, only human rTNF-α demonstrated selective killing of the parent tumor over Mϕ-resistant variants isolated in vitro (panel d) or in

351

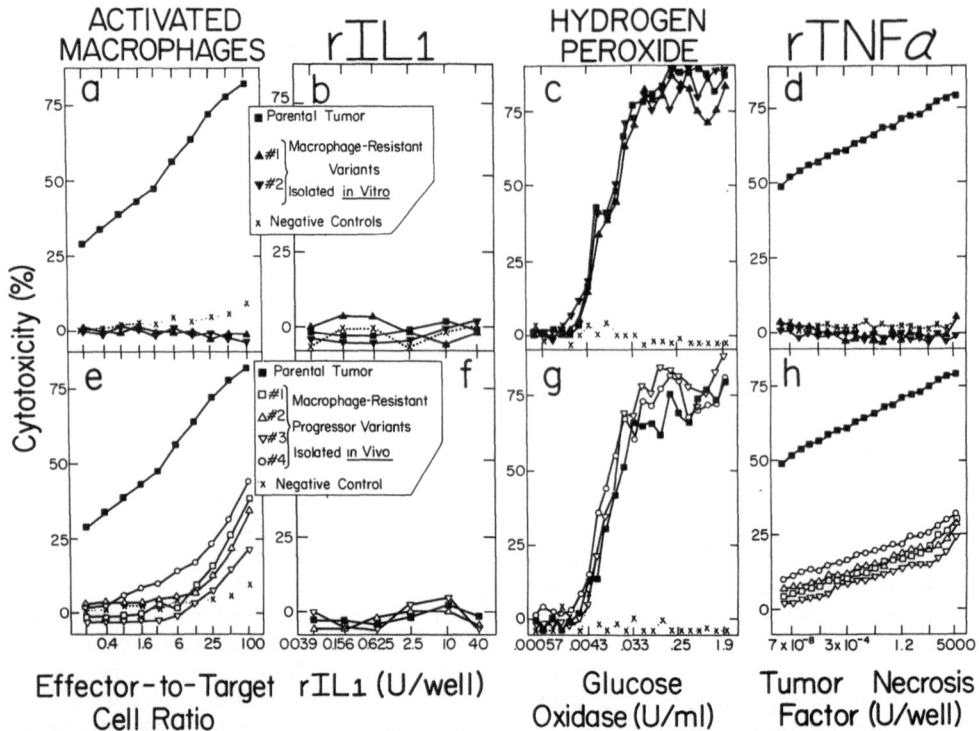

Fig. 1 a–h. Sensitivity of Mφ-resistant 1591 tumor variants to soluble mediators of cytotoxicity. Results utilizing Mφ-resistant variants selected in vitro are shown in **a–d** and results with variants selected in vivo are shown in **e–h**. Mφ were activated as described [23] and used as effectors in a 16 h ^{51}Cr release assay (**a** and **e**); 10T1/2 fibroblasts were used as negative controls. Murine rIL-1 was quantified using a thymocyte proliferation assay [12] with heat-inactivated IL-1 used as a negative control. Hydrogen peroxide was generated using glucose oxidase [15] with 1 unit defined as the generation of 1 μmol H_2O_2 per min. Catalase added at 40 units/well served as the negative control. Susceptibility to human rTNF-α was analyzed in a 72 h ^{51}Cr postlabelling assay [22]. The negative control consisted of preincubation with monoclonal anti-TNF-α antibody at 1.85 μg/ml for 16 h. The data represent pooled values from three separate experiments with the SEM for each point indicated as ≤10% of the value of each point shown [23]

vivo (panel h). This closely mimicked the action of aMφ themselves on these targets (Fig. 1, panels a, e). Furthermore, the effects of human rTNF-α on 1591 were completely neutralized by preincubation with a monoclonal antibody directed against human rTNF-α (Fig. 2 d, negative control). The resistance of the variants to aMφ and human rTNF-α was selective in that the variants were fully sensitive to the effects of osmotic lysis, natural killer cells, and cytolytic T cells [23].

To confirm the linkage between resistance to human rTNF-α and resistance to aMφ, two human rTNF-α-resistant 1591 cell lines were selected and tested for resistance to aMφ. Figure 2a shows that these human rTNF-α-resistant variants were substantially more resistant to aMφ than was the parental 1591 tumor. The small residual sensitivity of the variants to aMφ was completely abrogated by selecting with murine rather than with human rTNF-α (Fig. 2a). Additional evidence to suggest that the observed cytotoxic effects of aMφ and TNF-α follow identical pathways is given in Fig. 2b. Increasing concentrations of a polyclonal antibody that neutralizes murine rTNF-α inhibited aMφ killing of 1591 in a dose-dependent fashion, whereas incubation of aMφ with preim-

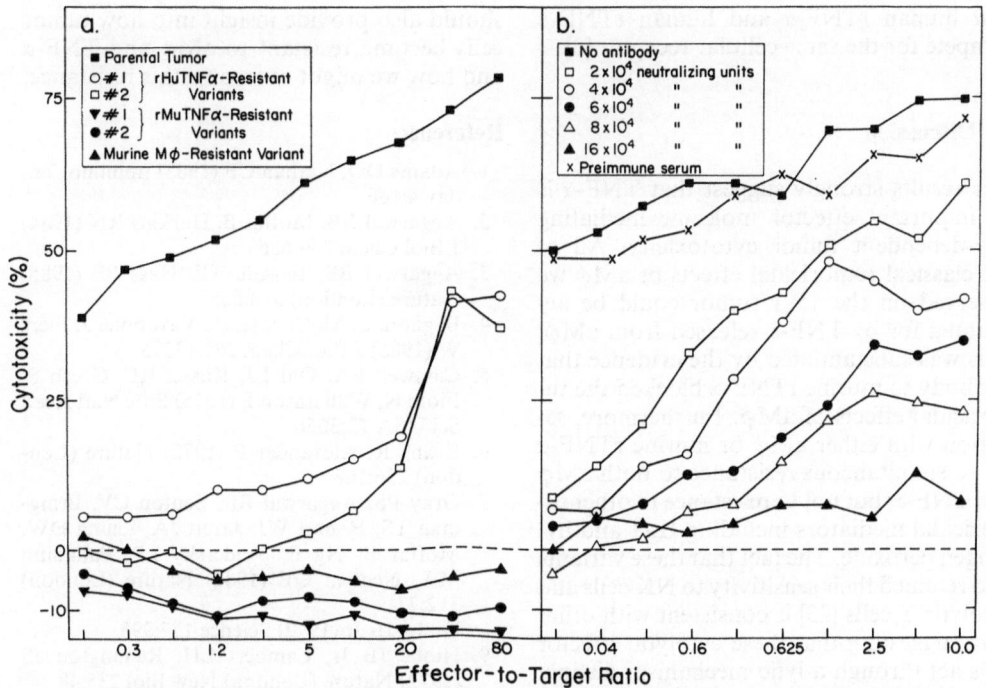

Fig. 2. a Complete resistance of the variants selected with murine rTNF-α to the cytolytic effects of aMφ. Variants selected with human rTNF-α show only partial resistance. **b** Neutralization of Mφ-mediated tumor cytotoxicity using rabbit polyclonal antibody against murine rTNF-α. Data represent the pooled results from two experiments using a modified ⁵¹Cr release assay [22, 23]

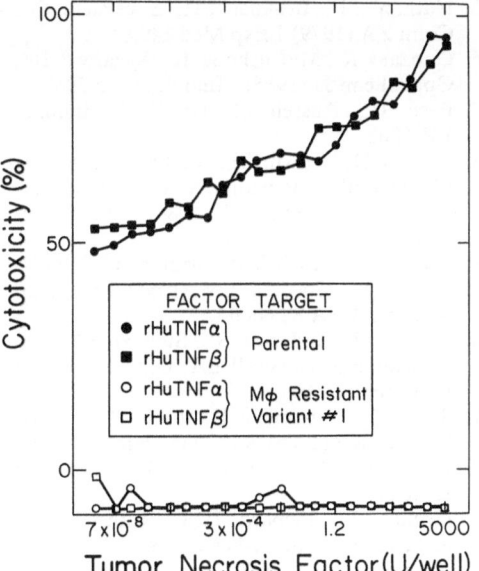

Tumor Necrosis Factor (U/well)

mune serum resulted in a cytotoxic response similar to that of aMφ alone.

Human TNF-β is a cytotoxic protein whose sequence is about 30% homologous to human TNF-α [2]. Figure 3 shows that human TNF-β was identical to human TNF-α in exerting a potent selective cytotoxic effect on the parental 1591 tumor over the 1591 Mφ-resistant variant. This result raises the possibility that TNF-α and TNF-β employ common effector pathways, a suggestion consistent with other data indicating

Fig. 3. Resistance of the Mφ-selected 1591 tumor variant to the cytotoxic effects of human rTNF-α and human rTNF-β. The parental 1591 tumor cells are equally sensitive to both recombinant proteins in a 72 h ⁵¹Cr postlabelling assay. The data represent pooled values from two separate experiments [23]

that human rTNF-α and human rTNF-β compete for the same cellular receptor [3].

D. Discussion

Our results strongly suggest that TNF-α is an important effector molecule mediating Mϕ-dependent tumor cytotoxicity. All of the classical tumoricidal effects of aMϕ we observed on the 1591 tumor could be accounted for by TNF-α released from aMϕ. This was substantiated by the evidence that antibody to murine rTNF-α blocked the tumoricidal effects of aMϕ. Furthermore, selection with either aMϕ or murine rTNF-α led to simultaneous resistance to both aMϕ and TNF-α, but not to resistance to other tumoricidal mediators including IL-1 and hydrogen peroxide. The fact that these variants also retained their sensitivity to NK cells and cytolytic T cells [23] is consistent with other data suggesting that these cytolytic effector cells act through a lytic mechanism distinct from that of aMϕ [1].

Mϕ-resistant tumor variants isolated in vitro have been shown to display enhanced growth in the normal host [22], but the role of aMϕ in destroying or inhibiting nascent tumor cell growth is not fully understood. Furthermore, the precise mechanism by which TNF-α from aMϕ reaches the target cell remains unknown. In vivo, cell-to-cell contact may be required to prevent rapid diffusion and to assure a sufficiently high local concentration of TNF-α in the narrow space between the aMϕ and the bound target cell, while in vitro contact may only be required for less sensitive target cells.

The variants we have derived from selection with either aMϕ or rTNF-α retain their phenotype through prolonged passage in vivo or in vitro and it is clear that the resistance is heritable and may, therefore, have a genetic basis. Whether resistance to TNF-α may be associated with a decrease in the number of TNF receptors on the tumor cells has been investigated [4, 11, 20]. The variants we have described provide a new tool with which to dissect the precise mechanism of Mϕ-mediated cytotoxicity and to uncover the molecular and genetic mechanisms of malignant transformation leading to susceptibility to aMϕ. A study of these variants

should also provide insight into how tumor cells become resistant to aMϕ and TNF-α and how we might overcome this resistance.

References

1. Adams DO, Nathan CF (1983) Immunol Today 4:166
2. Aggarwal BB, Moffat B, Harkins RN (1984) J Biol Chem 259:686
3. Aggarwal BB, Eessalu TE, Hass PE (1985) Nature (London) 318:665
4. Baglioni C, McCandless S, Vavermier J, Fiers W (1985) J Biol Chem 260:13395
5. Carswell EA, Old LJ, Kassel RL, Green S, Fiore N, Williamson B (1975) Proc Natl Acad Sci USA 72:3666
6. Evans R, Alexander P (1972) Nature (London) 236:168
7. Gray PS, Aggarwal BB, Benton CV, Bringman TS, Henzel WJ, Jarett JA, Leung DW, Moffat B, Ng P, Svedersky LP, Palladino MA, Nedwin GE (1984) Nature (London) 312:721
8. Hibbs JB Jr (1972) Science 177:998
9. Hibbs JB Jr, Lambert LH, Remington JS (1972) Nature (London) New Biol 235:48
10. Kripke ML (1981) Adv Cancer Res 34:69
11. Kull FC Jr, Jacobs S, Cuatrecasas P (1985) Proc Natl Acad Sci USA 82:5756
12. Lomedico PT, Gubler U, Hellmann CP, Dukovich M, Giri JG, Pan YE, Collier RS, Chua AO, Mizel SB (1984) Nature (London) 312:458
13. Meltzer MS (1981) J Immunol 127:179
14. Nathan CF, Karnovsky ML, David JR (1971) J Exp Med 133:1356
15. Nathan CF, Brukner LH, Silverstein SC, Cohn ZA (1979) J Exp Med 149:84
16. Onozaki K, Matsushima K, Aggarwal BB, Oppenheim JJ (1985) J Immunol 135:3962
17. Pace JL, Russell SE (1981) J Immunol 126:1863
18. Pennica D, Nedwin GE, Hayflick JS, Seeburg PH, Derynk R, Palladino MA, Kohr WJ, Aggarwal BB, Goeddel DV (1984) Nature (London) 312:724
19. Pennica D, Hayflick JS, Bringman TS, Palladino MA, Goeddel DV (1985) Proc Natl Acad Sci USA 82:6060
20. Rubin BR, Anderson SL, Sullivan SA, Williamson BD, Carswell EA, Old LJ (1985) J Exp Med 162:1099
21. Shirai T, Yamaguchi H, Ito H, Todd CW, Wallace RB (1985) Nature (London) 313:803
22. Urban JL, Schreiber H (1983) J Exp Med 157:642
23. Urban JL, Shepard HM, Rothstein JL, Sugarman BJ, Schreiber H (1986) Proc Natl Acad Sci USA 83:5233

Haematology and Blood Transfusion Vol. 31
Modern Trends in Human Leukemia VII
Edited by Neth, Gallo, Greaves, and Kabisch
© Springer-Verlag Berlin Heidelberg 1987

Organ-Associated Macrophage Precursor Cells as Effector Cells Against Tumor Targets and Microorganisms

M.-L. Lohmann-Matthes, T. Decker, and M. Baccarini

A. Introduction

In the past 10 years much attention has been paid to the phenomenon of natural resistance as a first line of defense against tumors and microorganisms. Such natural resistance can be attributed to a certain degree to resting and activated macrophages [1, 2]. The most widely discussed natural effector cell has, however, been the so-called natural killer (NK) cell. Based on their morphological features, NK cells could be classified either as medium-sized lymphocytes [3] or as immature macrophage precursor cells. These two cell types are, in fact, morphologically indistinguishable. We previously presented evidence [4–9] that the NK compartment consists, at least in part, of cells in the early differentiation stages of macrophages. Nonadherent and nonphagocytic macrophage precursor cells can be obtained from in vitro liquid cultures of mouse bone marrow. These cells exert NK-like activity against YAC-1 cells, but leave P815 cells totally unaffected [4, 5]. The same cells behave as potent effector cells in ADCC against tumor targets [4]. Along this line the same cell type was isolated from human peripheral blood of healthy donors [10], indicating for the first time that such immature cells of the macrophage lineage reside also outside the bone marrow. In the present short review we summarize our recent data indicating that the same cell type can be isolated from the spleen of normal mice and that it can easily

and efficiently be induced into organs like the spleen and liver under recruitment or inflammatory conditions [7–9]. As an extension of the previously described NK-like anti-YAC activity, we were able to attribute to this same cell type strong microbicidal activity against *Candida albicans* and *Leishmania enriettii* [6–9]. Since macrophages as a lineage are represented early in phylogenesis and successfully mediated natural resistance and protection long before the specific immune system evolved, their influence on the evolution and development of the specific immune system could be much more pronounced than evidenced at the present moment.

B. Materials and Methods

All materials and methods have been described in detail [6–9].

C. Results

Macrophage precursors were isolated either from erythrocyte-depleted splenocytes or from liver nonparenchymal cells, after destruction of the hepatocytes by enzymatic treatment. Spleen cells and liver nonparenchymal cells were filtered through nylon-wool columns in order to eliminate all adherent cells. The eluted cells were then applied to a discontinuous Percoll gradient (a slight modification of the gradient described by Timonen and Saksela [11]). By means of this gradient a cell fraction highly enriched for NK activity, and essentially free of small

Department of Immunobiology, Fraunhofer Institute of Toxicology and Aerosol Research, Nikolai-Fuchs-Str. 1, D-3000 Hannover 61, FRG

Table 1. Effect of separation by means of specific antimacrophage antibody-mediated rosetting on the candidacidal and tumoricidal activity of Percoll fraction 40.8–45.3 derived from normal nonadherent splenocytes as compared to its proliferating ability in the presence or absence of CSF-1

Effector cells	Candidacidal activity[a]	Natural killer activity[b]	[^{3}H]dThd uptake (mean cpm)[c]	
			Without CSF-1[d]	With CSF-1
Fr. 40.8–45.3	42.6	40.2	3328	19730
F4/80$^-$	26.1*	26.4	474	5905
F4/80$^+$	59.4*	42.3	2333	27543.7

[a] Candidacidal activity was determined in a 12-h colony forming unit inhibition assay at the effector:target ratio 10:1.
[b] Natural killer activity is expressed as % specific ^{51}Cr release from radiolabeled YAC-1 target cells at the e:t ratio 25:1 in a 12-h assay.
[c] [^{3}H]dthd (1 µCi/well) was added, after 3 days of cultivation, 18 h before terminating the assay.
[d] L-929 fibroblast-conditioned medium was added at the concentration of 20% as a source of CSF-1.
Data are the means of triplicate samples. Standard errors, usually <3%, have for clarity been omitted.
* $P < 0.01$, according to Student's t-test.

Table 2. Effect of separation by means of specific antimacrophage antibody-mediated rosetting on the candidacidal, tumoricidal and CSF-1 dependent proliferating ability of Percoll fraction 40.8–45.3 derived from nonadeherent splenocytes from cyclophosphamide pretreated mice (Cy 150 mg/kg, 12 days before the assay)

Effector cells	Candidacidal activity[a]	Natural killer activity[b]	[^{3}H] dThd uptake (mean cpm)[c]	
			Without CSF-1[d]	With CSF-1
Fr. 40.8–45.3	36.64	38.4	763	61250
F4/80$^-$	15.8*	22.2*	819	15650
F4/80$^+$	52*	40.9	1003	77234

[a] Candidacidal activity was determined in a 12-h colony forming unit inhibition assay at the effector:target ratio 5:1.
[b] Natural killer activity is expressed as % specific ^{51}Cr release from radiolabeled YAC-1 target cells at the e:t ratio 12.5:1 in a 12-h assay.
[c] [^{3}H]dthd (1 µCi/well) was added, after 3 days of cultivation, 18 h before terminating the assay.
[d] L-929 fibroblast-conditioned medium was added at the concentration of 20% as a source of CSF-1.
Data are the means of triplicate samples. Standard errors, usually <3%, have for clarity been omitted.
* $P < 0.01$, according to Student's t-test.

lymphocytes and granulocytes was gathered [6, 7]. These cells were further separated by an indirect rosetting technique [7–9] on the basis of the expression of the macrophage specific surface marker F4/80 [12]. The cells sorted by this procedure are further referred to as F4/80 negative and F4/80 positive cells.

Data obtained with normal spleen cells separated as described are summarized in Table 1. Data obtained with cells from spleen under recruitment conditions (mice treated with cyclophosphamide 12 days before the assay [7]) are presented in Table 2, and data concerning inflammatory liver cells (mice treated with MVE-2 3 days before the assay [8]) are documented in Table 3. All tables show NK activity and candidacidal activity of the cells as well as their ability to incorporate ^{3}H-thymidin ([^{3}H]dThd) in response to the macrophage-specific growth factor CSF-1. All F4/80 positive fractions gave rise to large macrophage colonies in soft agar. This fraction obviously consisted

Table 3. Effect of separation by means of specific antimacrophage anti-body-mediated rosetting on the candidacidal, tumoricidal, and CSF-1 dependent proliferating ability of Percoll fraction 40.8–45.3 derived from liver non-parenchimal cells obtained from MVE-2 pretreated mice (MVE-2 25 mg/kg, 3 days before the assay)

Effector cells	Candidacidal activity[a]	Natural killer activity[b]	[3H]dThd uptake (mean cpm)[c]	
			Without CSF-1[d]	With CSF-1
Fr.40.8–45.3	29.44	30.3	2994	219143
F4/80⁻	6.1*	39.9*	1499	4304
F4/80⁺	44.2*	24.0	3741	33499

[a] Candidacidal activity was determined in a 12-h colony forming unit inhibition assay at the effector: target ratio 2.5:1.
[b] Natural killer activity is expressed as % specific ^{51}Cr release from radiolabeled YAC-1 target cells at the e:t ratio 12.5:1 in a 12-h assay.
[c] [3H]dthd (1 μCi/well) was added, after 3 days of cultivation, 18 h before terminating the assay.
[d] L-929 fibroblast-conditioned medium was added at the concentration of 20% as a source of CSF-1.
Data are the means of triplicate samples. Standard errors, usually <3%, have for clarity been omitted.
* $P<0.01$, according to Student's t-test.

of cells of the macrophage lineage in various differentiation stages, since the response to CSF-1 was heterogeneous. Some cells matured within 24–48 h to typical macrophages without forming colonies whereas others developed small clusters and soon matured to macrophages. Some of the cells also gave rise to large macrophage colonies in response to CSF-1. No cell death was observed in the F4/80 positive fraction under these culture conditions. When the F4/80 negative fraction was cultivated the same way, no early maturation to macrophages could be scored. Colonies developed with a lag phase of about 3–5 days compared to the F4/80 positive fraction. Thus, precursor cells committed to the macrophage lineage are apparently present in the F4/80 negative fraction. These cells are, however, too immature at the time of separation to be recognized by F4/80.

All three tables show that candidacidal activity and NK-like activity as well as proliferation in response to CSF-1 are attributes of the F4/80 positive fractions. Since the F4/80 positive fraction represents a virtually homogeneous population of cells of the macrophage lineage, these data prove the presence, in both organs, of functionally active macrophage precursors. These cells were characterised as nonadherent and non-phagocytic, possessed (like NK cells) a low buoyant density, expressed macrophage-specific surface antigens, and actively respond to CSF-1 with proliferation. In the spleen this cell type has been defined as a constituent of the normal, noninduced organ.

D. Discussion

NK cells are potent tumoricidal effectors, whose lineage has been a matter of discussion for years. NK cells have been described as lymphocytes, based on their morphology and on their inability to phagocytose and adhere. The surface antigens described up to now did not help in assigning these cells to one or the other lineage, since NK cells share surface antigens with lymphocytes [13–15] as well as with cells of the monocyte/macrophage lineage [16–18] and with granulocytes [16, 17]. Evidence for a T-cell nature of NK cells came mostly from IL-2 dependent cytotoxic T-cell clones which, after long in vitro culture, were found to be able to destroy NK targets [19]. These clones, however, have lost their specificity and most probably are not related to any of the in vivo occurring cell types. Freshly isolated NK cells do not express a T-cell receptor [20]. These data substantiate the view that NK cells and T cells are not closely related. A separate lineage has also been proposed for NK cells [21].

Our data demonstrate that a significant part of the the NK activity under normal as well as under inflammatory conditions is exerted by cells belonging to the macrophage lineage. These cells were positively sorted on the basis of the highly lineage-specific macrophage marker F4/80 and proved to be capable of exerting NK and candidacidal activity and of responding to the lineage-specific factor CSF-1 with proliferation and maturation. The nature of the effectors present in the F4/80 negative fraction is an object of current investigation. Cells in the early stages of macrophage differentiation are present in this fraction, as demonstrated by response to CSF-1 stimulation, but as yet it has not been possible to rule out the contribution of another, unrelated cell type.

Another major implication of our work is the possible in vivo role of macrophage precursors. The presence of this cell type in the spleen and liver of normal mice and its inducibility in large amounts upon inflammation suggest that macrophage precursors can actively contribute in vivo to natural resistance. Data describing the contribution of these cells to the resistance against a systemic *Candida albicans* infection in immunomodulated mice have recently been published [22, 7].

The cells belonging to the macrophage lineage derive, according to a current theory [23], exclusively from the bone marrow compartment. Recent investigations performed in our lab, however, strongly point to the existence of an extramedullary generation of macrophage precursors taking place in the spleen and in the liver. In the light of the unexpectedly widespread importance of these cells the advantage represented by several independent sources able to supply macrophage precursors upon induction is obvious.

References

1. Keller R (1978) Macrophage-mediated natural cytotoxicity against various target cells. In: Nelson D (ed) Immunobiology of the macrophage. Academic, New York, p 487
2. Lohmann-Matthes ML, Kolb B, Meerpohl HG (1978) Susceptibility of malignant and normal target cells to the cytotoxic action of bone marrow macrophages activated in vitro with the macrophage cytotoxic factor (MCF). Cell Immunol 41:231
3. Kumagai K, Itoh K, Suzuki R, Hinuma S, Saitoh F (1982) Studies on murine large granular lymphocytes. I. Identification as effector cells in NK and K cytotoxicities. J Immunol 129:2788
4. Domzig W, Lohmann-Matthes ML (1979) Antibody-dependent cellular cytotoxicity against tumor cells II. The promonocyte identified as effector cell. Eur J Immunol 9:267
5. Lohmann-Matthes ML, Domzig W, Roder J (1979) Promonocytes have the characteristics of natural killer cells. J Immunol 123:1883
6. Baccarini M, Bistoni F, Lohmann-Matthes ML (1985) In vitro natural cell-mediated cytotoxicity against *C. albicans:* macrophage precursors as effector cells. J Immunol 134:2658
7. Baccarini M, Bistoni F, Lohmann-Matthes ML (1986) Organ-associated macrophage precursor activity: isolation of candidacidal and tumoricidal effectors from the spleen of cyclophosphamide-treated mice. J Immunol 136:837
8. Decker T, Baccarini M, Lohmann-Matthes ML (1986) Liver-associated macrophage precursors as natural cytotoxic effectors against *Candida albicans* and YAC-1 cells. Eur J Immunol 16:693
9. Baccarini M, Kiderlen AF, Decker T, Lohmann-Matthes ML (1986) Functional heterogeneity of murine macrophage precursors from spleen and bone marrow. Cell Immunol 101:339
10. Lohmann-Matthes ML, Zähringer M (1981) Zerstörung von Tumorzellen durch Makrophagen-Vorstufen bei Maus und Mensch. Blut 42:283
11. Timonen T, Saksela E (1980) Isolation of human natural killer cells by density gradient centrifugation. J Immunol Methods 36:285
12. Lee SH, Starkey PM, Gordon S (1985) Quantitative analysis of total macrophage content in adult mouse tissues: immunochemical studies with antibody F4/80. J Exp Med 161:475
13. Herberman RE, Nunn ME, HOlden HT (1978) Low density of Thy 1 antigen on mouse effector cells mediating natural cytotoxicity against tumor cells. J Immunol 121:304
14. Koo GC, Jacobsen JB, Hämmerling GJ, Hämmerling U (1980) Antigenic profile of murine natural killer cells. J Immunol 125:1003
15. Beck BW, Gillis S, Henney CS (1982) Display of the neutral glycolipid ganglio-N-tetraosylceramide (asialo GM1) on cells of the natural killer and T lineages. Transplantation 33:118

16. Holmberg LA, Springer TA, Ault KA (1981) Natural killer activity in peritoneal exudates of mice infected with *Listeria monocytogenes:* characterisation of natural killer cells by using monoclonal rat-anti murine macrophage antibody (M1/70). J Immunol 121:1792

17. Scheid MP, Triglia D (1979) Further description of the Ly 5 system. Immunogenetics 9:423

18. Sun D, Lohmann-Matthes ML (1982) Cells with natural killer activity are eliminated by treatment with monoclonal specific anti-macrophage antibodies plus complement. In: Herberman RB (ed) NK and other natural effector cells. Academic, New York, p 243

19. Brooks CG (1983) Reversible induction of natural killer cell activity in cloned murine cytotoxic cell lines. Nature 305:155

20. Young H, Ortaldo JR, Herberman RB, Reynolds CW (1986) Analysis of T cell receptor in purified rat and human large granular lymphocytes (LGL): lack of a functional 1.3 Kb β-chain mRNA. J Immunol 136:2701

21. Hackett J Jr, Bennett M, Kumar V (1985) Origin and differentiation of natural killer cells. I. Characteristics of a transplantable NK cell precursor. J Immunol 134:3731

22. Baccarini M, Bistoni F, Puccetti P, Garaci E (1983) Natural cell-mediated cytotoxicity against *Candida albicans* induced by cyclophosphamide: nature of the in vitro cytotoxic effector. Infect Immun 42:19

23. Van Furth R, Cohn ZA (1968) The origin and kinetics of mononuclear phagocytes. J Exp Med 128:415

Haematology and Blood Transfusion Vol. 31
Modern Trends in Human Leukemia VII
Edited by Neth, Gallo, Greaves, and Kabisch
© Springer-Verlag Berlin Heidelberg 1987

Immune Functions and Hematopoietic Progenitor Cell Activity in Plasmacytoma-Bearing Mice Cured by Melphalan

D. Douer, O. Sagi, E. Sahar, and I. P. Witz

A. Introduction

The incidence of secondary acute myeloid leukemia is higher in multiple myeloma (MM) than that predicted for normal persons. The etiology and pathogenesis of this leukemia is unclear, but it is commonly attributed to a leukemogenic effect of melphalan. The risk for secondary leukemia seems to be greater in MM than in other categories of cancer patients receiving similar drugs, and it is difficult to ascribe the high incidence of AML in MM to treatment alone. Host factors related to the primary malignancy might also be involved in the progression of a transformed but premalignant cell to clinical leukemia. Several immune effector mechanisms operating during the leukemia latency period were postulated to mediate surveillance of potentially malignant cells. We studied the immune profile of a mouse model bearing a transplanted plasmacytoma that was cured by melphalan for 1 year after tumor eradication and cessation of therapy. In melphalan-treated MM patients deficient immunity might be caused by the primary tumor per se or by the drug. We therefore assayed the same parameters in normal mice, without plasmacytoma, given melphalan in the same way. Marrow myeloid progenitor cell (CFU-C) growth was also studied. We were able to discriminate

Department of Microbiology and the Moise and Frida Eskenasy Institute for Cancer Research, Department of Biotechnology, the George S. Wise Faculty of Life Sciences, and the Institute of Hematology, Sheba Medical Center, Sackler Faculty of Medicine, Tel-Aviv University, Israel

between long-term changes of immune and hematopoietic systems caused by melphalan from those related to the occurrence of the tumor in the past.

B. Experimental Setup

On a day marked as zero, 1000 MOPC-315 plasmacytoma cells are inoculated intramuscularly to BALB/C mice. A growing tumor forms locally, causing the death of all untreated mice by day 50. Mouse groups studied were (a) *group T+M:* mice with plasmacytoma treated on day 14, when the tumor size was 0.5×0.9 cm, with 250 µg melphalan and again with 400 µg melphalan on day 24. The tumor disappeared and did not recur either locally or systemically during the entire study period; (b) *group M:* normal mice that were not inoculated with plasmacytoma cells but were treated with melphalan in the same way; (c) *untreated normal controls.* Survival rates on day 50 for mouse groups T+M and M were similar (86% and 92% respectively).

C. Results and Discussion

At monthly intervals for 1 year, nine to twelve mice from each group were assayed for a number of splenic immune parameters and marrow CFU-C growth (results at days 50 and 200 are depicted in Table 1). Life table analysis shows that the 1-year survival for group M was 33%, for group T+M 73%. In normal mice (group M), shortly

Table 1. Immune and hematopoietic functions of mice without (group M) or with (group T+M) plasmacytoma, treated with melphalan

Parameter	Day 50		Day 200	
	M	T+M	M	T+M
Allogeneic MLR	66	44	100	40
Thy1.2 + cells	76	46	95	60
IL-2 production	82	67	130	75
NK activity	31	108	90	60
Asialo GM1 + cells	0	0	111	104
sIg+ cells	50	0	108	132
CFU-C colonies	121	78	57	60

Results are expressed as percentage of the value of each parameter in normal untreated control mice. Day zero was the day of MOPC-315-cell inoculation.

after treatment with melphalan, the numbers of T (Thy1.2+) cells, NK (asialo GM1+) cells and B (sIg+) cells as well as T-cell function (allogeneic MLR), IL-2 production, and NK activity were all reduced. All these immune parameters recovered spontaneously by 3–4 months after treatment and remained whithin the normal range during the rest of the study. In plasmacytoma-bearing mice treated with melphalan (group T+M) similar reduced immunity was found shortly after treatment. However, mouse group T+M continued to manifest long-lasting cellular immune defects. They showed a significant reduction in T-cell number compared with group M and untreated controls, a capacity to proliferate in response to alloantigens, and IL-2 production up to 1 year after cessation of therapy. The number of NK cells was normal but their activity was slightly reduced. These data indicate that a short and intensive course of melphalan given to normal mice causes only transient immune deficiency shortly after treatment. However, plasmacytoma-bearing mice that receive melphalan develop long-term cellular immune deficiency, which is not due to melphalan alone. Interestingly, following a transient reduction, the splenic B-cell number in group T+M recovered and remained persistently higher than that in untreated controls and group M. Comparison with MOPC-315 cells ruled out the possibility that the B cells in group T+M were residual plasmacytoma cells. Contrary to immune parameters, the marrow CFU-C colony growth was persistently reduced in both the T+M and the M mouse group following treatment with melphalan.

Taken together, the data indicate that the presence of malignancy in the past played a role in the development of long-lasting immune deficiency, especially in T-cell number and function. On the other hand, melphalan per se causes long-lasting damage to a hematopoietic progenitor cell. We suggest that this mouse model may be useful for studying the role of immune aberrations related to the primary plasmacytoma in the development of overt leukemia from a hematopoietic stem cell, altered and maybe transformed by melphalan.

Haematology and Blood Transfusion   Vol. 31
Modern Trends in Human Leukemia VII
Edited by Neth, Gallo, Greaves, and Kabisch
© Springer-Verlag Berlin Heidelberg 1987

Recombinant Vaccinia Viruses as Live Vaccines

G. L. Smith [1]

A. Summary

Recombinant vaccinia viruses can be constructed that express foreign antigens. These viruses retain their infectivity and synthesise the foreign gene product in tissue culture and in vaccinated animals. Following vaccination, specific antibody and cell-mediated immune responses are generated against the foreign protein and in several cases these have protected the animal against subsequent challenge with the corresponding pathogen. The potential use of recombinant vaccinia viruses as medical or veterinary vaccines is discussed.

B. Introduction

Vaccinia virus is the world's oldest vaccine and was successfully used to immunise against and eradicate smallpox. This immunisation campaign remains the most successful ever conducted, and its success derives from a number of factors. The vaccine was cheap, stable and plentiful and the disease was acute, easily identifiable and had no animal reservoir. In addition, the World Health Organisation (WHO) was fully committed to the eradication campaign and vigorously pursued this goal. The last naturally occurring case of smallpox was in Somalia in 1977.

Since that time, interest in vaccinia virus has diminished, but it has remained a subject of active research due to its possession of a number of interesting biological properties (Moss 1985). The virus has a large, complex virion structure and a double-stranded DNA genome of 185 000 base pairs. Unlike most DNA viruses, which replicate in the nucleus of infected cells, vaccinia virus (the prototype orthopoxvirus) replicates in the cytoplasm. To enable the virus to do this, it possesses a complete transcriptional enzyme system that is able to transcribe the virus genome into functional mRNAs. The virus-coded RNA polymerase does not transcribe genes normally recognised by the host RNA polymerase II, and the promoters recognised by the vaccinia RNA polymerase are structurally and functionally distinct from those of the host cell and other viruses.

An increased understanding of the molecular biology of vaccinia virus together with the advent of recombinant DNA technology enabled vaccinia virus to be used as a cloning and expression vector. Following the expression of the first foreign genes in vaccinia in 1982, there has been an explosion of interest in recombinant vaccinia viruses. The construction of recombinant vaccinia viruses has recently been reviewed (Mackett and Smith 1986) and so it will only be briefly described here. The unique nature of the virus promoters and presence of the virus-coded RNA polymerase required that vaccinia promoters be used to drive expression of foreign genes in vaccinia virus. So the first step in construction of a recombinant virus is to link the foreign protein-coding sequences to a vaccinia promoter. This gene is

[1] Department of Pathology, University of Cambridge, Tennis Court Road, Cambridge CB2 1QP, UK

then inserted into the vaccinia genome by homologous recombination in cells infected with wild type (WT) vaccinia virus and transfected with a plasmid containing the foreign gene. To facilitate this process, the plasmid also contains vaccinia virus DNA, flanking the foreign gene, that is taken from a nonessential locus of the virus genome. Within the transfected cells, homologous recombination results in insertion of the foreign gene into the position of the virus genome specified by the flanking vaccinia DNA. Several such loci have been identified (Panicali and Paoletti 1982) but the most widely used one is the vaccinia thymidine kinase (TK) gene, since this permits genetic selection of the recombinant viruses as TK⁻ mutants (Mackett et al. 1982, 1984). Other methods of selecting the recombinant viruses have been used such as DNA:DNA hybridisation (Panicali and Paoletti 1982), expression of selectable genetic markers (Mackett et al. 1982; Franke et al. 1985), or expression of enzymes which permit visual detection of recombinants due to conversion of chromogenic substrate (Chakrabarti et al. 1985). A variety of plasmid vectors have been constructed for the cloning of foreign genes into vaccinia (Mackett et al. 1984; Boyle et al. 1985; Chakrabarti et al. 1985).

C. Expression of Foreign Antigens

Many foreign genes have been expressed in recombinant vaccinia viruses and so far none have proved toxic to the virus replication. Since vaccinia replicates in the cytoplasm and does not splice its mRNAs, only cDNAs or genes without introns may be expressed. Correct DNA engineering, to ensure utilisation of the translational start and stop codons of the foreign gene, results in the foreign protein being of the predicted size. Additionally, posttranslational modifications such as glycosylation, proteolytic cleavage and carboxylation also occur within the vaccinia-infected cells. The foreign gene products have been indistinguishable antigenically from the authentic antigen.

The time and level of expression depend upon the type of vaccinia promoter chosen. These are either early (before virus DNA replication commences), late (after DNA replication commences) or early and late. Promoters from genes of all three types have been used for expression of foreign genes. A commonly used promoter is one taken from a gene that maps within the inverted terminal repetition of the virus genome, which is expressed throughout the virus replicative cycle and which codes for a protein of 7500 daltons (Mackett et al. 1984).

D. Immunisation of Animals

Recombinant vaccinia viruses expressing a variety of foreign antigens, particularly eukaryotic viral glycoproteins, have been used to immunise experimental animals. Following dermal inoculation a local vaccinial lesion appears, which heals in 2–3 weeks. During this time no viraemia has been found (Smith et al. 1983a) and the virus does not establish latent or persistent infections. Both antibody and cell-mediated immune responses against the foreign antigen have been subsequently detected. For instance, a recombinant expressing the influenza virus haemagglutinin (HA) produced antibody in vaccinated rabbits that was able to neutralise influenza virus infectivity in vitro (Panicali et al. 1983; Smith et al. 1983b). This recombinant virus also induced murine cytotoxic T lymphocytes (CTL) that recognised the influenza HA in a major histocompatibility complex (MHC) class I restricted manner (Bennink et al. 1984, 1986).

The ability of the recombinant viruses to stimulate specific immune responses is obviously important for the potential use of these viruses as live vaccines. However, there are also other scientific applications. For instance, the virus may be used to raise specific antisera against the foreign gene product. Such antisera may be useful in characterising the corresponding antigen within its normal environment, and for determining if the antigen has potential use in future vaccines (Cranage et al. 1986). The recombinant viruses are also useful for the study of antigen recognition by CTL. This is possible because (a) the recombinant virus can be used to make target cells against which effector CTL can be tested in cytotoxicity assays and (b) the recombinant virus can itself prime animals for a CTL response against the foreign gene product. Experiments of these types have demonstrated that several influenza virus antigens, previously considered to be intracellular, can be recognised by class I MHC antigen-restricted CTL in a manner cross-reactive among different influenza A virus subtypes (Yewdell et al. 1985).

E. Protection of Vaccinated Animals Against Challenge with Pathogens

Experimental animals vaccinated with recombinant vaccinia viruses have been protected against several pathogenic eukaryotic viruses including influenza, hepatitis B, rabies, herpes simplex, vesicular stomatitis and respiratory syncytial virus. As a specific example, experiments involving the hepatitis B virus surface antigen are described in more detail.

Hepatitis B virus (HBV) remains a serious global health problem, with approximately 200 million chronic carriers of the disease. The virus infection has been associated with several pathological conditions including liver cirrhosis, fulminant hepatitis and primary hepatocellular carcinoma, one of the most common male cancers. A subunit vaccine against HBV has been developed and licensed. The vaccine is composed of the surface antigen of the virus (HBsAg) and is purified from the plasma of chronically infected patients, where it can circulate at high concentrations. Although effective, this vaccine is expensive and available in insufficient quantities to meet the enormous global demand. Cloning and sequencing of the HBV genome identified the gene coding for HBsAg and permitted its expression in a variety of vector systems. This is providing an alternative and potentially greater source of the antigen, which may lead to a cheaper and more universally available vaccine.

As another approach to the development of new HBV vaccines, the HBsAg gene was expressed in recombinant vaccinia virus (Smith et al. 1983a; Paoletti et al. 1984). Since the recombinant virus would simultaneously synthesise the HBsAg and present it to the immune system of the vaccinated host, no expensive protein purification would be necessary. Initial experiments demonstrated that the HBsAg was excreted from cells infected with the recombinant virus and that it had biochemical and immunological properties indistinguishable from authentic HBsAg. Rabbits vaccinated with the recombinant virus produced antibodies against HBsAg (anti-HBs) at levels far greater than those necessary to confer protection against HBV in humans. However, due to the restricted tropism of HBV, protection experiments can only be done in primates (usually chimpanzees). Accordingly, two chimpanzees were vaccinated with the recombinant virus and another animal immunised with WT vaccinia. Disappointingly, the animals failed to produce anti-HBs. Nonetheless, when challenged with HBV by intravenous injection 14 weeks later, there was a dramatic difference between the WT- and recombinant-vaccinated animals (Moss et al. 1984). The control animal developed a typical acute HBV infection with antigenaemia, biochemical evidence of liver disease and subsequently anti-HBs and antibodies against the virus core antigen (anti-c). In contrast, the two animals vaccinated with the recombinant vaccinia virus had no antigenaemia or liver disease but rapidly produced high levels of anti-HBs. Subsequently they both also produced low levels of anti-c, indicating that a HBV infection had been initiated. The animals had been antigenically primed following the original vaccination and had produced anti-HBs following re-exposure to the antigen when challenged with HBV.

Although the animals were not completely protected from HBV infection, the single vaccination had protected them against liver disease following severe challenge with HBV. The vaccine might be improved to provide complete protection in a number of ways. First, by using a stronger vaccinia virus promoter, larger amounts of HBsAg would be produced that might induce a strong primary antibody response. Secondly, HBsAg is a mixture of three polypeptides called S, MS and LS, and the first recombinant vaccinia virus expressed only the S form. All share the same 226 carboxyl terminal amino acids, but MS and LS have an additional 55 and 174 amino terminal amino acids, respectively. Recently an epitope on the LS molecule has been identified which acts as a receptor binding site for hepatocytes. Antibody to this epitope might be expected to block virus attachment to the target organ in vivo; accordingly, a vaccinia recombinant that expresses the LS protein was constructed. In vaccinated rabbits, antibodies are produced which recognise a synthetic peptide specific for LS (Cheng et al. 1986). The ability of such a recombinant virus to protect chimpanzees is under evaluation.

F. Discussion

These experiments demonstrate the potential use of recombinant vaccinia viruses as new vaccines against HBV. As mentioned already, vaccinia recombinants have also protected animals against several other pathogenic viruses, and specific immune responses against AIDS virus antigens and malarial antigens have been demonstrated. Although there are numerous advantages to using vaccinia recombinants as a means of delivering vaccine antigens to the immune system (see below), there are also potential problems. First, vaccination against smallpox with vaccinia carried with it a small but finite risk of postvaccinial complications. Although these were acceptable in the face of life-threatening smallpox, they became of greater concern as smallpox disappeared, and the risk from vaccination eventually outweighed any possible benefit. If recombinant vaccinia viruses are to be reintroduced as a vaccinating agent, safer, more attenuated strains of the virus are desirable. Fortunately, recombinant DNA technology permits the deletion of vaccinia genes as well as insertion of foreign genes. As the genes responsible for vaccinia pathogenicity are identified, these may be specifically deleted to construct safer vaccine strains; already some success has been achieved towards this goal (Buller et al. 1985). A second potential problem with reuse of vaccinia as a vaccine is the existing immunity to vaccinia in a large proportion of the world's population. However, since smallpox vaccination has been discontinued for 10 years or more, an ever growing population of nonimmune children exists. Vaccination against most infectious diseases is carried out during childhood. Re-vaccination can also be successful, as demonstrated by the accidental vaccination of a human with a recombinant vaccinia virus. Despite the vaccinee having previously had a smallpox vaccination, a good antibody response to the foreign gene was evoked.

The advantages of live recombinant vaccinia virus vaccines include (1) the ability to stimulate both antibody and cell-mediated immune responses, (2) the capacity for large amounts of foreign DNA encoding multiple foreign antigens (Smith and Moss 1983; Perkus et al. 1985), (3) the low cost of the vaccine to manufacture and administer, (4) the vaccine stability without refrigeration, and (5) the wide host range permitting application in veterinary and human medicine.

If vaccinia is to be reused in humans, efficacy will need to be demonstrated initially in limited clinical trials. Probably these would take place in populations where the advantages from successful vaccination against a particular disease far outweigh the worst conceivable rate of vaccine-associated complications. Life-threatening diseases such as AIDS, malaria or hepatitis B would seem to provide such a scenario in certain populations.

Acknowledgments. I would like to thank Professor Neth for his kind invitation to attend this symposium and Mary Wright for typing the manuscript.

References

1. Bennink JR, Yewdell JW, Smith GL, Moller C, Moss B (1984) Recombinant vaccinia virus primes and stimulates influenza virus haemagglutinin-specific cytotoxic T lymphocytes. Nature 311:578–579
2. Bennink JR, Yewdell JW, Smith GL, Moss B (1986) Recognition of cloned influenza virus haemagglutinin gene products by cytotoxic T lymphocytes. J Virol 57:786–791
3. Boyle DB, Couper BEH, Both GW (1985) Multiple-cloning-site plasmids for the rapid construction of recombinant poxviruses. Gene 35:169–177
4. Buller RML, Smith GL, Cremer K, Notkins AL, Moss B (1985) Decreased virulence of recombinant vaccinia virus expression vectors is associated with a thymidine kinase-negative phenotype. Nature 317:813–815
5. Chakrabarti S, Brechling K, Moss B (1985) Vaccinia virus expression vector: co-ex-

pression of β-galactosidase provides visual screening of recombinant virus plaques. Mol Cell Biol 5:3403–3409

6. Cheng KC, Smith GL, Moss B (1986) Hepatitis B virus large surface protein is not secreted but is immunogenic when selectively expressed by recombinant vaccinia virus. J Virol 60:337–344

7. Cranage MP, Kouzardies T, Bankier AT, Satchwell S, Weston K, Tomlinson P, Barrell B, Hart H, Bell SE, Minson AC, Smith GL (1986) Identification of the human cytomegalovirus glycoprotein B gene and induction of neutralising antibodies via its expression in recombinant vaccinia virus. EMBO J 5:3057–3063

8. Franke CA, Rice CM, Strauss JH, Hruby DE (1985) Neomycin resistance as a dominant selectable marker for selection and isolation of vaccinia virus recombinants. Mol Cell Biol 5:1918–1924

9. Mackett M, Smith GL (1986) Recombinant vaccinia viruses. J General Virol 67:2067–2082

10. Mackett M, Smith GL, Moss B (1982) Vaccinia virus: a selectable eukaryotic cloning and expression vector. Proc Natl Acad Sci USA 79:7415–7419

11. Mackett M, Smith GL, Moss B (1984) General method for production and selection of infectious vaccinia virus recombinants expressing foreign genes. J Virol 49:857–864

12. Moss B, Smith GL, Gerin JL, Purcell RH (1984) Live recombinant vaccinia virus protects chimpanzees against hepatitis B. Nature 311:67–69

13. Moss B (1985) Replication of poxviruses. In: Fields BN, Chanock RM, Roizman B (eds) Virology. Raven, New York, pp 658–703

14. Panicali D, Paoletti E (1982) Construction of poxviruses as cloning vectors: insertion of the thymidine kinase from herpes simplex virus into the DNA of infectious vaccinia virus. Proc Natl Acad Sci USA 79:4927–4931

15. Panicali D, Davis SW, Weinberg RL, Paoletti E (1983) Construction of live vaccines by using genetically engineered poxviruses: biological activity of recombinant vaccinia virus expressing influenza virus haemagglutinin. Proc Natl Acad Sci USA 80:5364–5368

16. Paoletti E, Lipinskas BR, Samsanoff C, Mercer S, Panicali D (1984) Construction of live vaccines using genetically engineered poxviruses: biological activity of vaccinia virus recombinants expressing the hepatitis B virus surface antigen and the herpes simplex virus glycoprotein D. Proc Natl Acad Sci USA 81:193–197

17. Perkus ME, Piccini A, Lipinskas BR, Paoletti E (1985) Recombinant vaccinia virus: immunization against multiple pathogens. Science 229:981–984

18. Smith GL, Moss B (1983) Infectious poxvirus vectors have capacity for at least 25,000 base pairs of foreign DNA. Gene 25:21–28

19. Smith GL, Mackett M, Moss B (1983a) Infectious vaccinia virus recombinants that express hepatitis B virus surface antigen. Nature 302:490–495

20. Smith GL, Murphy BR, Moss B (1983b) Construction and characterization of an infectious vaccinia virus recombinant that expresses the influenza virus haemagglutinin gene and induces resistance to influenza infection in hamsters. Proc Natl Acad Sci USA 80:7155–7159

21. Yewdell JW, Bennink JR, Smith GL, Moss B (1985) Influenza A virus nucleoprotein is a major target antigen for cross-reactive anti-influenza A virus cytotoxic T lymphocytes. Proc Natl Acad Sci USA 82:1785–1789

Haematology and Blood Transfusion Vol. 31
Modern Trends in Human Leukemia VII
Edited by Neth, Gallo, Greaves, and Kabisch
© Springer-Verlag Berlin Heidelberg 1987

Use of Fluorescence-Activated Cell Sorting to Select Hybrid Hybridomas Producing Bispecific Monoclonal Antibodies

L. Karawajew, B. Micheel, O. Behrsing, M. Gaestel, and G. Pasternak

A. Introduction

Antibodies containing two different antigen-binding sites were prepared for the first time in 1961 by Nisonoff and Rivers [1] by dissociating two different antibodies and reassociating the mixture of half molecules. But this method of chemical recombination has some disadvantages because it results in protein denaturation and therefore loss of antibody activity.

The production of bispecific antibodies by hybrid cells containing the antibody genes for expressing two different antibodies is, therefore, regarded as a more reliable method. Such hybrid cells are produced by fusing selection medium-sensitive antibody-producing parental cell lines and isolating the fused cells by means of the corresponding selection media [2, 3].

This paper describes a method of selecting bispecific antibody-producing hybrid hybridomas by using a fluorescence-activated cell sorter. This method avoids the labor-intensive production of selection medium-sensitive mutants of the parental cell lines which is substituted by labeling the cell lines by two different fluorescent markers [4].

B. Experimental Set-up and Results

Two mouse hybridoma cell lines producing monoclonal antibodies to human alpha-fetoprotein (AFP; [5]) and horseradish peroxidase (HRP; [6]) were used for the experi-

---

Central Institute of Molecular Biology, Academy of Sciences of the GDR, 1115 Berlin-Buch, GDR

ments. Cells of these lines were labeled by fluorescein isothiocyanate (FITC; 0.5 µg/ml) or tetramethyl rhodamin isothiocyanate (TRITC; 1.5 µg/ml) and then fused by using polyethylene glycol (PEG) according to the standard fusion method [7]. After cultivating the mixture for 4 h the cells were analyzed by a fluorescence-activated cell sorter (FACS III, Becton Dickinson, Sunnyvale, USA), and the fused hybrid hybridomas were sorted out which gave a double (green and red) fluorescence.

The sorted cells were immediately cloned in microtitration plates and 2 weeks later grown clones were checked for the production of bispecific antibodies with anti-AFP/anti-HRP activity. A solid-phase immunoassay was used with the following incubation steps: purified AFP, phosphate-buffered saline containing 10% calf serum, culture fluid to be tested for antibody activity, HRP followed by the substrate O-phenylene diamine. Several stable hybrid hybridoma clones were obtained and one clone was transplanted in mice for the production of ascitic fluid.

The ascitic fluid was fractionated by hydroxylapatite column chromatography [8] which resulted in five peaks in contrast to three peaks when the ascitic fluids of the parental lines were fractionated (Table 1). Peak 4 from the ascitic fluid of the hybrid hybridoma contained the bispecific antibodies. SDS-polyacrylamide gel electrophoresis showed that this fraction contained the heavy chains of both anti-AFP and anti-HRP antibodies [4].

The bispecific anti-AFP/anti-HRP antibodies could be used to build up an enzyme

Table 1. Antibody activity in ascitic fluid from hybrid hybridomas after hydroxylapatite column chromatography

Fractions	Antibody activity		
	Anti-HRP[a]	(Anti-AFP/ anti HRP)	Anti-AFP[a]
1	−	−	−
2	−	−	−
3	+ + +	(+)	(+)
4	+ +	+ + +	+ +
5	(+)	(+)	+ + +

[a] Tested by a solid-phase immunoassay with the incubation sequence: purified goat anti-mouse immunoglobulin, monoclonal antibody, HRP followed by the substrate or ^{125}J-labeled AFP.

immunoassay for the demonstration of AFP with the incubation sequence: monoclonal anti-AFP antibody with different epitope specificity at the solid phase, solution containing AFP, bispecific antibody, and HRP followed by the substrate.

C. Conclusion

These experiments demonstrate that hybrid hybridomas secreting bispecific monoclonal antibodies can be produced by fusing hybridoma cell lines and selecting hybrid hybridomas by using a FACS. For this purpose the parental cell lines are labeled by two different fluorescence markers. It is not necessary to convert the parental lines into selection medium-sensitive mutants and hybrid hybridomas can, therefore, be obtained in a relatively short time compared with the methods used so far [2, 3]. The technique presented here is a simple and effective method for the production of bispecific antibodies and can be applied to different systems. The bispecific monoclonal antibodies produced should be useful reagents to build up sensitive immunoassays and other immunological tests.

References

1. Nisonoff A, Rivers MM (1961) Arch Biochem Biophys 93:460
2. Milstein C, Cuello AC (1983) Nature 305:537
3. Martinis J, David GS, Bartholomew RM, Wang R (1983) In: Hollaender A, Jaskin AI, Roges P (eds) Basic biology of new developments in biotechnology. Plenum, New York, p 129
4. Karawajew L, Micheel B, Behrsing O, Gaestel M J Immunol Meth (to be published)
5. Micheel B, Fiebach H, Karsten U, Goussev AJ, Jazova AR, Kopp J (1983) Eur J Cancer Clin Oncol 19:1239
6. Ternynck T, Gregoire J, Avrameas S (1983) J Immunol Meth 58:109
7. Köhler G, Milstein C (1975) Nature 256:495
8. Stanker LH, Vanderlaan M, Juarez-Salinas H (1985) J Immunol Meth 76:157

Virology

Haematology and Blood Transfusion Vol. 31
Modern Trends in Human Leukemia VII
Edited by Neth, Gallo, Greaves, and Kabisch
© Springer-Verlag Berlin Heidelberg 1987

Henry Kaplan Award for J. C. Neil

K. Bister [1]

Poster Award, Virology Section

From the many excellent posters covering virological aspects of carcinogenesis, the contribution by James C. Neil and his colleagues was selected for this award by the poster awards selection committee.

In their contribution, Neil and coworkers describe the transduction of a T-cell antigen receptor β-chain gene by feline leukemia virus (FeLV). Although it is not yet known whether retroviruses carrying such a receptor gene in their genomes have any oncogenic properties, these viruses may be useful tools in studying both FeLV-induced leukemia and T-cell antigen receptor function.

[1] Otto-Warburg-Laboratorium, Max-Planck-Institut für Molekulare Genetik, Ihnestr. 73, 1000 Berlin 33, FRG

Haematology and Blood Transfusion   Vol. 31
Modern Trends in Human Leukemia VII
Edited by Neth, Gallo, Greaves, and Kabisch
© Springer-Verlag Berlin Heidelberg 1987

Viral Transduction of Host Genes in Naturally Occurring Feline T-Cell Leukaemias: Transduction of *myc* and a T-Cell Antigen Receptor β-Chain Gene

J. C. Neil[1], R. Fulton[1], T. Tzavaras[1], D. Forrest[1], R. McFarlane[1], and D. Onions[2]

A. Introduction

Feline leukaemia virus has been a particularly useful tool in cancer research since many of the naturally occurring tumours associated with this virus group have yielded recombinant retroviruses containing host-derived oncogenic information. The prevalence of transduction as an oncogenic mechanism was seen first in multicentric fibrosarcoma, a relatively rare tumour in FeLV-infected cats (Hardy et al. 1982; Besmer 1984). In a significant percentage of cases of this disease, oncogene-containing feline sarcoma viruses have been identified. More recently, we and others have found that in the more common FeLV-associated neoplasm, thymic lymphosarcoma, viral capture of the c-*myc* gene can occur (Neil et al. 1984; Levy et al. 1984; Mullins et al. 1984). Since the oncogenes carried by feline sarcoma viruses do not include *myc,* these reports provided the first evidence that *myc* may be a target for oncogenic activation by FeLV.

Further study of feline tumours revealed that c-*myc* could be affected either by viral transduction or by proviral insertion into the cellular gene locus (Neil et al. 1984, 1987; Forrest et al. 1987) although the majority of field-case tumours showed neither of these features. To gain more information on the cellular origin of the feline lymphoid tumours and to search for some distinguishing feature of those with activated *myc* genes, we

undertook an analysis of the state of rearrangement and expression of the genes encoding α and β chains of the T-cell antigen receptor. In the course of this analysis we discovered a novel FeLV provirus in which a full-length β-chain gene had been incorporated into the viral genome (Fulton et al. 1987). The present report describes this novel provirus and considers its possible significance in leukaemogenesis.

B. T-Cell Antigen Receptor Gene Rearrangements and Expression in Feline Leukaemias

Analysis of feline T-cell receptor genes was performed with cDNA probes derived from the human α (pJα6) and β (pB400) genes (Collins et al. 1985 b); these were kindly provided by Michael Owen (ICRF Tumour Immunology Labs, London). We found these probes to be strongly cross-reactive with the feline genes and their transcripts, although hybridisation was stronger with the β-chain than with the α-chain probe. For this reason, only the β-chain probe has been used to assess gene rearrangement.

The overall gene arrangement and transcript sizes appear similar for feline and human genes. Thus, as in the human and the murine Cβ loci (Gascoigne et al. 1984; Malissen et al. 1984; Sims et al. 1984) the feline Cβ coding sequence appears to be tandemly duplicated in germ-line DNA. Also, some of the feline tumours examined displayed rearrangement of both Cβ alleles with two distinct transcript sizes of 1.2 and 1.4 kb, which by analogy with human genes (Collins et al.

[1] Beatson Institute for Cancer Research, Bearsden, Glasgow
[2] University of Glasgow Department of Veterinary Pathology, Glasgow

Table 1. Rearrangements of T-cell antigen receptor β-chain gene in feline leukaemias

1. Thymic and multicentric lymphosarcomas

(a) *myc* gene involved		(b) No detected *myc* rearrangement	
FeLV v-*myc*	T3 +[a]	FeLV +ve	84904 −[c]
	F 422 +[a]		89407 +
	T17 +[b]		86800 +
	84793 +		T14 +
	T11 +		Q109 −
c-*myc*	T8 +	FeLV-ve	86503 −
Rearranged	T7 +		89960 +
	T5 +		T16 −
			T20 −

2. Other tumours

Spleen lymphosarcoma (FeLV-ve)			T9 +[d]
Alimentary	FeLV-ve	87416 −	
Lymphosarcomas[e]	FeLV +ve	87655 −	
		75800 −	
		83029 −	

Rearrangements of β-chain genes of T-cell antigen receptor were assessed by Southern blot hybridisation analysis. The Cβ probe hybridises to a 18 kb *Eco*RI fragment in germ-line DNA of most cats. Where possible, digests of DNA from tumour and uninvolved tissues (usually kidney) were run side by side. In some cases both germ-line bands were rearranged. In most cases the pattern of rearrangement was consistent with a monoclonal tumour outgrowth. However, tumour 86416 showed evidence of a bi-clonal nature. For all cases examined so far Northern blot analyses show that both α- and β-chain transcripts are expressed in cases with rearranged β-chain genes.
[a] All tumours induced experimentally by inoculation of GT3 and F422 viruses were also positive for gene rearrangement.
[b] Amplified due to FeLV transduction.
[c] *pim*-1 gene rearranged.
[d] c-*myc* amplified (Neil et al. 1984).
[e] Assumed to be of B-cell origin.

1985 a) correspond to abortive (D-J-C) and successful (V-D-J-C) joining events, respectively. The results of a survey of β-chain rearrangement are given in Table 1. The conclusions both from these data and from those of Northern blot analyses for the expression of α- and β-chain transcripts are that feline thymic tumours are heterogeneous with respect to maturity as assessed by T-cell receptor gene rearrangement and expression. However, the tumours involving c-*myc* activation, either by transduction or by proviral insertion, represent a homogeneous subset with mature characteristics (expressing both α- and β-chain transcripts).

C. A FeLV Provirus Containing a β-Chain T-cell Antigen Receptor Gene

Tumour T17 showed an anomalous pattern of β-chain mRNA both in size (>6 kb) and in abundance. Furthermore, DNA blots showed gross amplification of sequences hybridising to the human Cβ probe. Further Southern blot hybridisation analysis of tumour T17 showed that the amplified sequences could be resolved into a single, intensely hybridising fragment if digestion was performed with any of the enzymes which characterise the FeLV LTR (*Kpn*I, *Sma*I, *Pst*I and *Hinc*II) (Fig. 1). These data provide indirect but persuasive evidence that the amplification of β-chain sequences in tumour T17 was due to their presence *within* multiple FeLV proviruses.

Cloning was undertaken to isolate the novel proviral structures from tumour T17. From a library of size selected (15–23 kb), *Eco*RI-digested tumour DNA in lambda EMBL 4 we selected recombinants with various probes, including the human Cβ cDNA clone, FeLV v-*myc*, FeLV *env* and FeLV LTR. The clones we have isolated correspond to the proviruses containing Cβ sequences, proviruses containing v-*myc*, FeLV helper-type proviruses and the normal cellular loci of c-*myc* and Cβ.

Our initial efforts have focussed upon characterising the FeLV proviruses containing the Cβ-hybridising sequences. A 1.9-kb fragment containing the entire hybridising sequence was sequenced and found to contain a 1.2-kb host-derived sequence insert including the intact coding sequence of a β-chain T-cell receptor gene (Fulton et al. 1987; see Fig. 1). The β-chain gene appears to have undergone productive rearrangement since sequences clearly identifiable as those of Vβ, Dβ, Jβ and Cβ origin are seen. Intron sequences are missing, however, as might be expected if the sequence has been transmitted as part of a retroviral replication

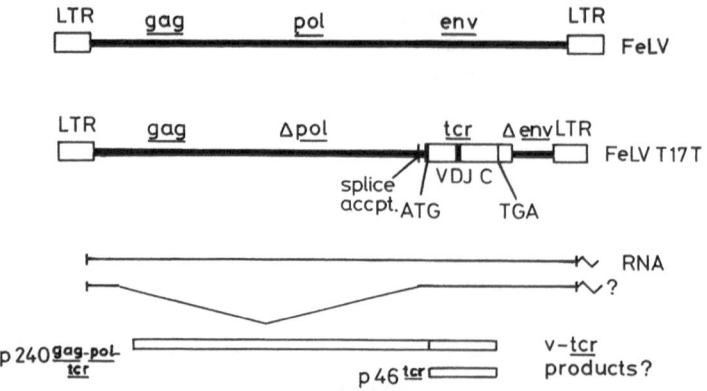

Fig. 1. Structure of the FeLV provirus (FeLV T17T) containing a T cell antigen receptor β-chain gene. Within the T17T provirus, the v-*tcr* gene replaces the 3′ end of *pol* and much of the *env* gene. The host-derived insert contains the complete coding sequence for a β-chain gene product including N-terminal signal peptide and variable, diversity, joining and constant region-derived sequences. The 3′ end of the insert appears to be coincident with the β-chain gene AATAAA sequence at the end of the 3′ untranslated region. As shown underneath, two modes of expression appear to be possible for the as yet uncharacterised v-*tcr* product. From genomic RNA read-through from *gag* and *pol* into *tcr* appears possible since the reading-frames are coincident. Alternatively, the splice acceptor site usually employed to generate *env* mRNA may serve to produce an RNA encoding a full-length β-chain product which is not fused to any viral protein

unit. The host-derived sequence replaces the 3′ end of *pol* and much of the FeLV *env* gene. The recombination junction is 7 base pairs upstream of the ATG, marking the beginning of the β-chain open reading frame which begins with the characteristic signal peptide for membrane insertion. The 3′ end of the host insert appears to be coincident with the polyadenylation signal (AATAAA). In this context the host-derived sequence (which we have designated v-*tcr*) could be expressed as a protein in two different ways. Firstly, since the *pol* reading frame is coincident with that of v-*tcr*, the gene may be expressed as a large fusion protein including *gag*, *pol*, and *tcr* sequences. Alternatively, the proximity of the splice acceptor site for the *env* mRNA means that a spliced subgenomic RNA could direct the synthesis of a v-*tcr* product which is neither truncated nor fused to viral sequences (Fig. 1). We are at present investigating these possibilities.

D. The *myc*-Containing Provirus in Tumour T17

Rather less information is available at present regarding the *myc*-containing provirus from tumour T17. Although EMBL 4 phage clones were readily obtained, full-length sub-clones have proved impossible to obtain thus far. Possible "poison" sequences have not yet been located in the provirus or its flanking sequences, but cloning in segments into plasmid vectors has allowed us to isolate possibly all the proviral structure. Since T17 represents the first recorded example of a "double transduction" event in which both host genes are present on separate proviruses, we wish to discover whether these recombinants arose independently or whether one recombinant provirus may have arisen from the other. Initial mapping suggests that the *myc* gene replaces *env*, as in the v-*tcr*-containing virus, however we do not yet know the precise 5′ and 3′ junctions.

E. Discussion

Although FeLV *myc* recombinant viruses appear to be potent initiators of tumour development, several features led us to consider that the FeLV v-*myc* genes may be insufficient for full neoplastic development. The first factor we considered is the latent period for FeLV *myc* virus-induced tumour development, which is shorter than that for helper FeLV but longer than that for many other v-*onc*-containing retroviruses. Also, analysis of integrated proviruses by Southern blot hybridisation with FeLV or v-*myc* probes indicated that even the short latency FeLV *myc* tumours represent monoclonal or oligoclonal outgrowths of virus-infected cells. Furthermore, these tumour cells could be established readily in culture in the absence of exogenous sources of interleukin 2 (IL-2), although such transformed cell lines could not be obtained in vitro even after a series of attempts to infect isolated T cells or bone marrow cell cultures (Onions et al. 1987).

While these phenomena may also be explained in other ways, we consider that the sum of the evidence points to secondary oncogenic events in vivo which we cannot so far reproduce in vitro. The finding here of a novel provirus containing a T-cell antigen receptor gene in the same tumour as a v-*myc* gene suggests a possible secondary oncogenic factor for this one case. In the majority of cases which do not show such proviruses we must seek other explanations. However, the observation that all of the tumours involving direct *myc* activation are of mature T-cell phenotype may provide a useful clue.

The oncogenic properties of v-*tcr* have not yet been tested by in vivo experiments. The primary tumour from T17 is no longer available and was in any case a very poor virus producer. We have therefore had to resort to transfection experiments to reconstruct virus complexes for inoculation into cats; these experiments are in progress. Predictably perhaps, initial experiments have shown no transforming potential of v-*tcr* for fibroblastic cells. Transfections into mature human T cells have been undertaken to discover whether the v-*tcr* gene product(s) can interact with human α chain and other T-cell receptor components and lead to membrane transport of the complex. At the same time, we will monitor any disturbance in growth or responsiveness to external stimuli (e.g. lectins, phorbol esters) which may give clues to the mode of action of v-*tcr*.

Our initial hypothesis was that v-*tcr* might cause constitutive activation of the antigen receptor in the absence of external antigen (Fulton et al. 1987). The rationale for this model was that the transmembrane region of v-*tcr* has a nonconservative change (met → lys) relative to the human and mouse *Cβ* sequences. Thus, in a manner akin to the proposed mechanism of activation of the *neu* gene (Bargmann et al. 1986), altered conformation might mimic the presence of extracellular ligand. This model now appears less likely for v-*tcr* in view of our finding that the cellular *Cβ* locus cloned from tumour T17 has the same transmembrane sequence as the viral gene (J.N. and R.F., unpublished results). The difference which we recorded (Fulton et al. 1987) may therefore be a species-specific change.

These results leave both the oncogenic significance and the possible modes of action of v-*tcr* as open questions. We will have to await the outcome of in vivo experiments for the answer to the first question. We may then have to address the possibility that the immunological specificity carried by v-*tcr* is the key to its oncogenic function. Recognition of a host or viral antigen seems possible, although the associated α chain might then be expected to play a contributory role. If self-reactivity is involved, we may speculate further that the v-*tcr* specificity would normally have been suppressed during thymic education of lymphocytes where specificity for host-MHC plus foreign antigen is learned (Bevan 1981). This self-reactivity may have been augmented in T17 by the retroviral capture of the important part of the immune effector involved in recognition. We might also propose that the role of v-*myc* in this case is to rescue (immortalise) a cell clone with autologous reactivity and "self-driven" proliferative capacity. Whatever the explanation, it is our hope that v-*tcr* may contribute in a wider sense to our understanding of normal and neoplastic T-cell growth.

Acknowledgements. We gratefully acknowledge the support of the Cancer Research Campaign for our research. Douglas Forrest and Theodore Tzavaras were supported by the Leukaemia Research Fund, while Ruth Fulton received a fellowship from the Scottish Home and Health Department.

375

References

1. Bargmann CI, Hung M-C, Weinberg RA (1986) Multiple independent activations of the *neu* oncogene by a point mutation altering the transmembrane domain of p185. Cell 45:649–657
2. Bevan MJ (1981) Thymic education. Immunol Today 2:216–219
3. Besmer P (1984) Acute transforming feline retroviruses. In: Vogt PK, Koprowski H (eds) Retroviruses 2. Springer, Berlin Heidelberg New York (Current topics in microbiology and immunology, vol 107)
4. Collins MKL, Kissonerghis A-M, Dunne MJ, Watson C, Rigby PWJ, Owen MJ (1985a) Transcripts from an aberrantly rearranged human T-cell receptor β-chain gene. EMBO J 4:1211–1215
5. Collins MKL, Tanigawa G, Kissonerghis AM, Ritter M, Price KM, Tonegawa S, Owen MJ (1985b) Regulation of T-cell receptor expression in human T-cell development. Proc Natl Acad Sci USA 82:4503–4507
6. Forrest D, Onions D, Lees G, Neil JC (1987) Altered structure and expression of c-*myc* in feline T-cell tumours. Virology 158:194–205
7. Fulton R, Forrest D, McFarlane R, Onions D, Neil JC (1987) Retroviral transduction of T-cell antigen receptor β-chain and *myc* genes. Nature 326:190–194
8. Gascoigne NRJ, Chien Y, Becker DM, Kavaler J, Davis MM (1984) Genomic organisation and sequence of T-cell antigen receptor β-chain constant and joining regions. Nature 310:387–391
9. Hardy WD Jr, Zuckerman E, Markovitch R, Besmer P, Snyder HW Jr (1982) Isolation of feline sarcoma viruses from pet cats with multicentric fibrosarcomas. In: Yohn D, Blakeslee J (eds) Elsevier/North-Holland, New York
10. Levy LS, Gardner MB, Casey JW (1984) Isolation of a feline leukaemia provirus containing the oncogene *myc* from a feline lymphosarcoma. Nature 308:853–856
11. Malissen M, Minard K, Mjolsness S, Kronenberg M, Goverman J, Hunkapiller T, Prystowsky MB, Yoshikai Y, Fitch F, Mak T, Hood L (1984) Mouse T-cell antigen receptor: structure and organisation of constant and joining gene segments encoding the β polypeptide. Cell 37:1101–1110
12. Mullins JI, Brody DS, Binari RC Jr, Cotter SM (1984) Viral transduction of the c-*myc* gene in naturally-occurring feline leukaemia. Nature 308:856–858
13. Neil JC, Hughes D, McFarlane R, Wilkie NM, Onions DE, Lees G, Jarrett O (1984) Transduction and rearrangement of the *myc* gene by feline leukaemia virus in naturally-occurring T-cell leukaemias. Nature 308:814–820
14. Neil JC, Forrest D, Doggett DL, Mullins JI (1987) The role of feline leukaemia virus in naturally-occurring leukaemias. Cancer Surv (in press)
15. Onions D, Lees G, Forrest D, Neil JC (1987) Recombinant feline leukaemia viruses carrying the *myc* gene rapidly produce clonal tumours expressing T-cell antigen receptor gene transcripts. Int J Cancer 40:40–45
16. Sims JE, Tunnacliffe A, Smith WJ, Rabbitts TH (1984) Complexity of human T-cell antigen receptor β-chain constant and variable region genes. Nature 312:541–545

Haematology and Blood Transfusion   Vol. 31
Modern Trends in Human Leukemia VII
Edited by Neth, Gallo, Greaves, and Kabisch
© Springer-Verlag Berlin Heidelberg 1987

Analysis of the Biological Role of Human Papilloma Virus (HPV)-Encoded Transcripts in Cervical Carcinoma Cells by Antisense RNA

M. von Knebel Doeberitz and L. Gissmann

A. Introduction

In cervical carcinomas and cell lines derived from them, human papilloma virus type 16 or 18 DNA has been found integrated into the host cell genome [6]. The chromosomal localization differs in different cell lines, as has been shown by in situ hybridization techniques (Mincheva et al., submitted for publication). The circular viral DNA is always disrupted in the E1/E2 open reading frame (ORF) by the integration event, and parts of the late viral genes can be deleted [6]. In contrast, the noncoding region containing promoter and enhancer sequences and the ORFs E6 and E7 are preserved. Northern blot analysis revealed that in all cell lines tested so far these ORF E6 and E7 are consistently transcribed into mRNA. Sequence analysis of cDNA clones derived from the three HPV 18-positive cell lines HeLa, SW 756, and C4-I revealed that the mRNAs consist of a 5′ viral sequence and a 3′ cellular sequence encoded by the flanking host cell DNA. Only the viral sequences give rise to major ORFs which may code for three putative proteins: E6, E7, and a spliced form of E6 (E6*) [5]. Therefore, it was speculated that these proteins are required for the characteristic growth pattern of these cervical carcinoma cells.

To analyze the biological role of the putative proteins within the cells we tried to specifically inhibit the translation by antisense RNA. The E6 and E7 ORFs were cloned in inverse orientation into a eukaryotic ex-

Institut für Virusforschung, Deutsches Krebsforschungszentrum, Heidelberg, FRG

pression vector and transferred into HPV 18-positive C4-I cervical carcinoma cells. Preliminary data suggest that expression of HPV 18 E6 and E7 antisense RNA may lead to inhibition of cell growth.

B. Results

The antisense RNA technique proved to be an intriguing approach to study the function of certain genes. Introduction of complementary RNA by expression vectors led to specific inhibition of gene expression and phenotypic conversion to "minus mutants" in several eukaryotic cells [2]. It was shown that complementary RNA strands hybridize within the cells, thereby inhibiting a normal nucleocytoplasmic transport and formation of an intact translation initiation complex [3, 4]. The excess of antisense RNA appears to be critical in such experiments.

To determine the influence of specific inhibition of HPV 18-encoded early mRNAs in HPV 18-positive cervical carcinoma cell lines, C4-1 cells were used as the test system; these cells contain only one viral genome copy per cell and express HPV 18 transcripts at a low level compared with other cell lines [6].

Expression vectors were constructed as shown in Fig. 1. The strong cytomegalovirus (CMV) immediate early promoter and enhancer element [1] (Pawlita, personal communication), was chosen to direct transcription of HPV 18 E6 and E7 sense or antisense mRNA. The HPV sequences were derived from a cDNA clone of the HPV 18-positive

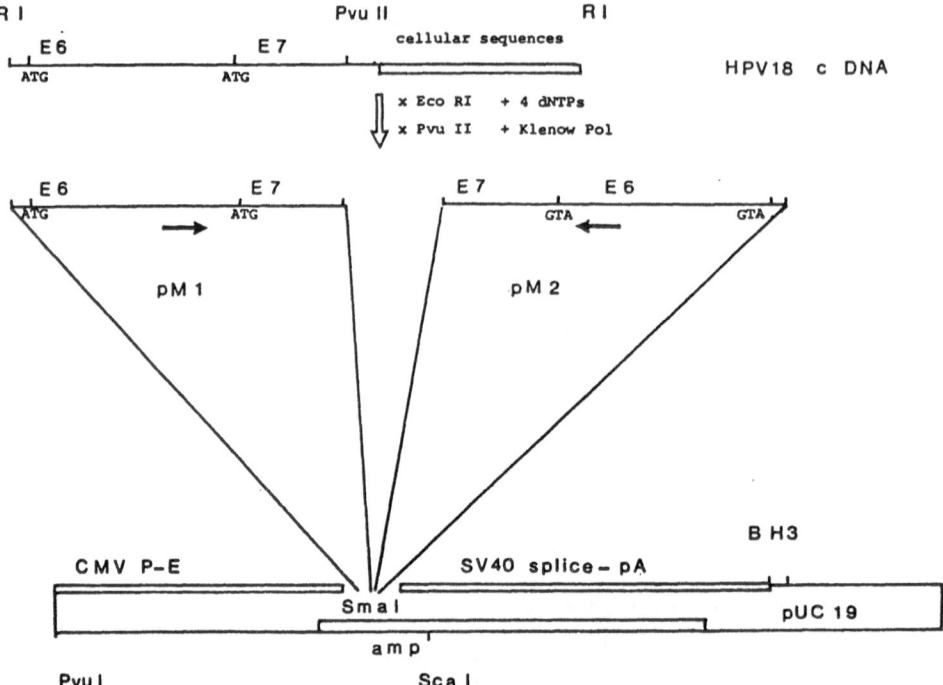

Fig. 1. Construction of expression vectors. Into the *Bam*HI site of a pUC19-derived plasmid containing the HCMV promoter (*P*) and enhancer (*E*) element (kindly provided by M. Pawlita) the *Bgl*II-*Bam*HI fragment derived from the pSV2 *β*-globin vector containing the SV40 early RNA-processing signals was cloned. The HPV 18 fragment derived from the cDNA clone (see text) was inserted into the *Sma*I site by blunt – end ligation. Clones with the HPV 18 E6 and E7 ORFs in both orientations were received and referred to as pM1 (sense) vector or pM2 (antisense) vector

cell line SW 756 [5]. This clone was used because it contains all HPV 18 E6 and E7 sequences in an unspliced form and covers 40 base pairs of the nontranslated 5′ sequence upstream from the E6 ATG start codon. At the nontranslated 5′ region the initiation complex is formed. Hybrid formation of the mRNA with a complementary RNA strand in this particular area was shown to be very important in other systems where antisense RNA was used to suppress gene expression [4]. To avoid interactions with other cellular transcripts, the cellular flanking sequence at the 3′ end of the E7 ORF was removed at the *Pvu*II site (see Fig. 1). The remaining HPV 18 sequences were cloned in both orientations downstream from the promoter and enhancer element. RNA processing signals were derived from the SV40 early region. Before transfection, performed by the calcium

phosphate technique, the DNA was linearized at the *Sca*I site which is distant to the transcription unit. It was either used as a monomer or ligated to oligomeres before introduction into the cells. To select transfected cell clones, a dominant marker plasmid (pSV2neo) was co-transfected in a ratio of 1 : 20, and culture dishes were screened for G418-resistant colonies.

When 20 µg pM2 antisense vector DNA (cut and ligated to oligomeres) were co-transfected with 1 µg pSV2neo DNA into 2.5×10^6 C4-1 cells and incubated in DMEM medium containing 10% FCS and 800 µg/ml G418, no surviving cells were found after 4 weeks (Table 1). After transfection of unligated pM2 antisense vector DNA one G418-resistant cell clone could be raised. When the sense mRNA expressing construct pM1 was transfected into C4-1

Table 1. Numbers of G418 – resistant cell clones in the different transfection experiments. Culture dishes were screened for colonies 4 weeks after transfection

C4-I carcinoma cells	pM1	pM2
DNA cleaved with *Sca*I	15	1
DNA cleaved with *Sca*I and ligated to oligomeres	40	0

C127 mouse fibroblasts	pM1	pM2
DNA cleaved with *Sca*I	5	7
DNA cleaved with *Sca*I and ligated to oligomeres	5	11

cells following the same protocol, 40 and 15 G418-resistant colonies formed respectively. Six of each group were raised to cell lines.

In control experiments HPV 18-negative C127 mouse fibroblasts were treated by the same protocol. As shown in Table 1, the same number of G418-resistant colonies formed when these cells were transfected with either ligated or unligated sense pM1 or antisense pM2 DNA.

Southern blot analysis of the one C4-I clone transfected with the pM2 antisense vector showed that the antisense RNA transcription unit is integrated in a rearranged pattern, while in C4-I clones transfected with the pM1 sense construct the transcription unit was not found to be rearranged. The C127 fibroblasts contained unrearranged transcription units after transfection of the sense or antisense plasmid. These data may suggest that expression of antisense RNA to HPV 18 transcripts in C4-I cells led to diminished cell viability.

To test whether this effect was due to the expression of antisense RNA in these cells we exchanged the CMV promoter and enhancer element with the inducible mouse mammary tumor virus long-terminal repeat. Equal numbers of G418-resistant cell clones grew out after transfection of the inducible

sense or antisense RNA-expressing vectors. We are presently analyzing the DNA and RNA of these clones, as well as possible effects of dexamethasone induction of the expression vectors on the growth characteristics of these cervical carcinoma cells.

C. Conclusions

The transfection experiments indicate that expression of antisense RNA to HPV 18 early transcripts in HPV 18-positive cervical carcinoma cells may lead to decreased growth properties of the cells. HPV 18-negative cells are not influenced by expression of sequences complementary to HPV 18 mRNA.

Because an apparently nonviable phenotype was rendered in this first set of experiments, it was not possible to correlate expression of antisense RNA to decreased growth rates of the C4-I cells directly. This could be achieved if expression of antisense RNA is directed by an inducible promoter element. It will be interesting to analyze whether gene expression of HPV 18 early ORFs E6 and E7 acts in a dose-dependent manner on the growth characteristics of cervical carcinoma cells.

References

1. Boshart M, Weber F, Jahn G, Dorsch-Häseler K, Fleckenstein B, Schaffner W (1985) Cell 41:521–530
2. Izant JG, Weintraub H (1985) Science 229:345–352
3. Kim SK, Wold BJ (1985) Cell 42:129–138
4. Melton DA (1985) Proc Natl Acad Sci USA 82:144–148
5. Schneider-Gädicke A, Schwarz E (1986) EMBO J 5:2285–2292
6. Schwarz E, Freese UK, Gissmann L, Mayer W, Roggenbuck B, Stremlau A, zur Hausen H (1985) Nature 314:111–114

Haematology and Blood Transfusion Vol. 31
Modern Trends in Human Leukemia VII
Edited by Neth, Gallo, Greaves, and Kabisch
© Springer-Verlag Berlin Heidelberg 1987

Transcription of Human Papillomavirus Type-18 DNA in Human Cervical Carcinoma Cell Lines *

A. Schneider-Gädicke and E. Schwarz

A. Introduction

DNA of human papillomavirus (HPV) type 16 or 18 has been identified in about 70% of all human cervical carcinomas analyzed so far [1] and in cell lines established from cervical carcinomas [2, 3]. In the malignant tumors and all cell lines, DNA of HPV 16 or 18 is integrated into the host cell genome. Integration consistently results in disruption of the viral genome within the open reading frame (ORF) E1, E2 region. With regard to the host cell genome, however, HPV 16/18 DNA integration seems to occur at different sites in different tumors and cell lines. Since tissue culture systems susceptible to transformation by HPVs were not available, we used the three HPV 18-positive cervical carcinoma cell lines HeLa, C4-1, and SW756 for a comparative analysis of HPV 18 transcription.

B. Results

HPV 18 transcription was studied by cDNA cloning and sequence analysis of HPV 18-positive cDNA clones isolated from the HeLa, C4-1, and SW756 cDNA library.

The HPV 18-positive cDNA clones of all three cell lines are derived from virus-cell fusion transcripts. They are composed of 3'-terminal host cell sequences spliced to 5'-proximal viral sequences. Splicing involves a

* The study was supported by the *Deutsche Forschungsgemeinschaft*
Institut für Virusforschung, Deutsches Krebsforschungszentrum, 6900 Heidelberg, FRG

viral splice donor site located a few nucleotides downstream from the start codon of HPV 18 ORF E1 (Fig. 1). The 3'-terminal cellular sequences are different in cDNA clones from the three cell lines and also differ – due to variable use of cellular splice acceptor sites – within the same cell line. They do not harbor long ORFs. Furthermore, no viral-cellular fusion ORFs of considerable protein-encoding capacity have been detected in the cDNA sequences. These data indicate that the chimeric viral-cellular transcripts do not contain the information for specific cellular proteins.

The 5' viral sequences are derived from the 5' part of the early region of HPV 18. Three types of cDNA clones can be distinguished due to the splicing patterns observed in the 5' HPV 18 sequences (Fig. 1). As potential protein-coding regions they contain ORFs E6 or E6*, followed in 3' by E7 and E1 (only in HeLa). Northern blot hybridizations with E6/E6* exon- and E1 exon-specific oligonucleotides revealed that mRNAs types 1 and 2 are present in C4-1 and SW756 cells, whereas types 2 and 3 (and type 1 in very small amounts) are present in HeLa cells. Primer extension experiments were performed to determine the 5' ends of the mRNAs. Several transcriptional initiation sites were identified, which are located directly at the A residue of the E6/E6* start codon or up to eight nucleotides upstream from it. These data indicate that a TATA box sequence located 35 nucleotides upstream from the E6/E6* ATG initiates transcription in all three cell lines. The very close proximity of the 5' ends of the mRNAs to the E6/E6* start codon may play a role in

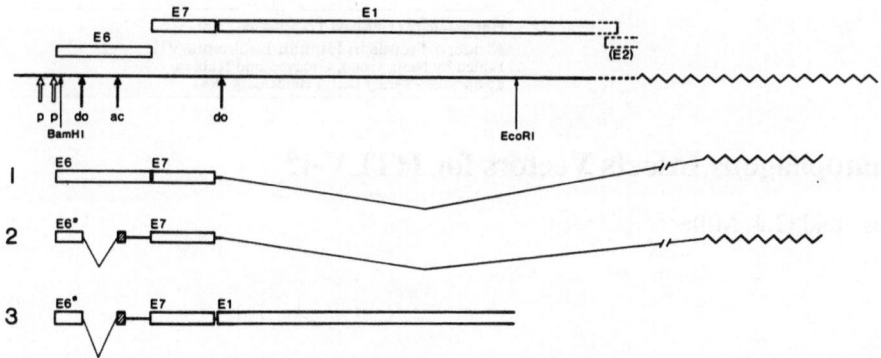

Fig. 1. Splicing patterns of HPV 18-positive cDNA clones from HeLa, C4-1, and SW756 cells. *Upper part:* The E6-E7-E1 region of the integrated HPV 18 DNA is shown together with the 3' flanking cellular sequences (indicated by *zig-zag lines*). ORFs are indicated by *open boxes*, the viral-cellular junctions by *dotted lines*. The positions of TATA box sequences (*p*), and splice donor (*do*) and splice acceptor (*ac*) sites are indicated. *Lower part:* Three types of cDNA clones can be distinguished according to the splice patterns of the 5'-terminal HPV 18 sequences. As possible protein-coding regions they contain ORFs E6 or E6*, followed in 3' by ORF E7 and E1 (type 3 is present only in HeLa cells). Intron sequences excised by splicing are represented as *thin, slanted lines*

regulating the synthesis of the E6/E6* and E7 proteins by shifting translation from the 5'-proximal cistron (E6 or E6*) to the second cistron (E7).

ORF E6* is generated by splicing (see Fig. 1) and encodes a putative protein of only 57 amino acids (aa) that shares the N-terminal 43 aa residues with the ORF E6 gene product. Generation of an E6* ORF due to splicing in E6 was not described for other papillomaviruses. Nucleotide sequence comparisons with other genital HPV DNAs revealed that only HPV 16, 18, and 33 contain possible splice sites at the corresponding positions, but HPV 6 and 11 do not, due to single nucleotide exchanges. Thus, it is tempting to speculate that mRNAs with an E6* splice pattern possibly encoding a E6* protein are specific for HPV types associated with genital carcinomas. Sequence comparisons revealed a certain homology between the putative E6* gene product and epidermal growth factors.

The similar transcription patterns of HPV 18 DNA in the three human cervical carcinoma cell lines indicate that expression of specific HPV 18 early genes (E6, E6*, E7) may have a functional role in the maintenance of the malignant phenotype of these cells.

References

1. Gissmann L (1984) Papillomaviruses and their association with cancer in animals and man. Cancer Surv 3:161–181
2. Boshart M, Gissmann L, Ikenberg H, Kleinheinz A, Scheurlen W, Hausen H zur (1984) A new type of papillomavirus DNA, its presence in genital cancer biopsies and in cell lines derived from cervical cancer. EMBO J 3:1151–1157
3. Schwarz E, Freese UK, Gissmann L, Mayer U, Roggenbuck B, Stremlau A, Hausen H zur (1985) Structure and transcription of human papillomavirus sequences in cervical carcinoma cells. Nature 314:111–114
4. Schneider-Gädicke A, Schwarz E (1986) Different human cervical carcinoma cell lines show similar transcription patterns of human papillomavirus type 18 early genes. EMBO J 5:2285–2292

Haematology and Blood Transfusion Vol. 31
Modern Trends in Human Leukemia VII
Edited by Neth, Gallo, Greaves, and Kabisch
© Springer-Verlag Berlin Heidelberg 1987

Are Haematophagous Insects Vectors for HTLV-I?

M. F. Greaves[1] and G. J. Miller[2]

A. Introduction

Human T-lymphotropic virus I (HTLV-I) and its associated malignancy, adult T-cell leukaemia [19, 30, 31, 37] are endemic in southern Japan [18, 26], the Caribbean Basin and neighbouring mainland America [1, 6, 10, 14, 23], and sub-Saharan Africa [5, 20, 38].

The natural history and mode of transmission of HTLV-I infection is largely unknown. Worldwide, the infection as indicated by the presence of antibodies is confined mostly to tropical areas of high humidity in Japan [36], the Caribbean and tropical South America [7, 23], and Central Africa [4, 5, 20, 38]. Sero-positivity for HTLV-I and the associated risk of adult T-cell leukaemia/lymphoma has been reported among immigrants to temperate regions from the Caribbean [10, 15]. More recently, southern Italy [22] and the Arctic regions [32] have been identified as possibly additional endemic regions. In the Caribbean, sero-positivity has been found almost entirely in people of African or part-African descent, although there are recent reports of HTLV-I-positive adults among Amerindians in Cayenne [11] and Venezuela [23] and Campuchian immigrants to Cayenne [11].

Earlier studies, especially in Japan, have suggested that HTLV-I might be transmitted by sexual contact [36], from mother to child via transplacental passage [21] or breast feeding [28], by blood transfusion [16], or by insect vectors [35]. Sexual transmission has been emphasised as a possible major route, but it cannot easily explain the demographic distribution of sero-positivity or the relatively high incidence of HTLV-I antibodies in children whose parents are sero-positive [17]. Neither does it adequately explain why the highest rates of sero-positivity should be observed in 70-year-old Japanese women.

B. A Role for Haematophagous Insects?

The possibility has been raised that Africans represent the natural host of HTLV-I, and that the virus was introduced in this way to the West Indies and perhaps also to Japan [13, 20]. In Britain, HTLV-I sero-positivity is found in first generation but very rarely in second generation West Indian people of African descent (Table 1) [15] (M.F. Greaves, T.A. Lister, S. Pegram and L. Chan, unpublished observations). Thus, the circumstances required for transmission may be largely confined to tropical and subtropical areas of high humidity, and – strikingly – to some Arctic regions [32]. Within endemic areas strong associations exist between sero-positivity to HTLV-I and evidence of exposure to arthropod-transmitted diseases such as filariasis [35], malaria [3] and equine encephalitis [23]. These relations might imply human transmission of HTLV-I by mosquitoes, shared environmental factors which promote the transmission of HTLV-I and arthropod-borne disease, or

[1] Leukaemia Research Fund Centre, The Institute of Cancer Research, London SW3 6JB, England
[2] Dept. of Epidemiology and Social Medicine, Albert Einstein College of Medicine, New York, NY, USA

Table 1. HTLV-I antibodies in United Kingdom residents of Caribbean origin

---

1. Relatives of HTLV-I [+] adult T-cell leukaemia patients:

   23 Relatives of 6 patients
   Sero-positive: 0/12 UK born (of Afro-
   Caribbean parentage)
   4/11 Caribbean born

2. Non-leukaemic serum donors (unrelated to ATL patients):

   Series 1: Hospital out-patients

   Sero-positive: 6/70 – all positives were born
   in Caribbean [15]

   Series 2: Hospital out-patients + normals
   Sero-positive: 0/70 UK born (of Afro-
   Caribbean parentage)
   6/130 Caribbean born

---

potentiation of the response to one infection by previous exposure to the other [3].

Involvement of mosquitoes or other haematophagous insects in the transmission of HTLV-I would go some way towards explaining the endemicity of this virus in Arctic regions where such insects are exceedingly common. Recent collaborative studies we have conducted on the Caribbean island of Trinidad provide, we believe, further support for the idea that insects might be vectors for HTLV-1 [25]. Between 1977 and 1981, blood samples were obtained for a cardiovascular survey of all adults aged 35–69 years and resident within a geographically defined area of Port-of-Spain, Trinidad [24]. In most respondents, sufficient serum had been stored for screening of the community for evidence of HTLV-I infection. As far as we are aware, this is the first systematic study of the distribution of HTLV-I sero-positivity in a total community.

The population of Trinidad is of African, Indian, European, Chinese, Lebanese and Syrian descent. The forbears of those of African origin arrived after 1776, coming either directly from West Africa or by way of neighbouring islands such as Grenada. People of Indian descent came from 1845 onwards, mostly from northern India. Smaller numbers of Chinese entered Trinidad after 1852.

Port-of-Spain lies on the coast of N.W. Trinidad and has a humid tropical climate. The survey was conducted in a defined area encompassing contiguous sectors of two suburbs of the city which we refer to as sectors A and B. Although in general the A-sector community is of lower socio-economic standing than sector B, there is no appreciable difference between Africans and Indians in living standards within the A sector.

Sera were screened for HTLV-I with an enzyme-linked immunosorbent assay (ELISA) [33]. Samples positive with this test were examined with an ELISA modification of a previously described competitive assay [40]. Only subjects whose sera were positive to both assays were considered sero-positive for HTLV-I.

Details of this study are published elsewhere [25]. Several important facts emerged: 1. Individuals of Asian (Indian) descent were infected at a lower rate (1.4%) than Afro-Caribbean blacks (7.0%). 2. As in Japan, sero-positivity rates were age and sex associated, the highest rates (12.3%) being observed in females over 65 years of age. 3. Black males living in the less-prosperous sector A were infected at a higher rate (5.4%) than those living in sector B (2.6%). 4. Sero-positivity was significantly ($P < 0.001$) associated with poor-quality housing. 5. Sero-positivity was significantly ($P < 0.025$) associated with living distances of less than 30 m from open water courses.

We have suggested [25] that, when taken together, the household clustering of HTLV-I infection (documented in Japan), the increased risk to adult females, the association with poor-quality housing and proximity to insect breeding sites (i.e. open, stagnant water) implicate an insect vector of intensively domestic habit. One candidate would be the mosquito species *Aedes aegypti*, which is known to have limited dispersal from its breeding grounds [27], but other domestic insects including mites and ticks would also be candidates. Women might be more likely to be infected than their husbands by virtue of their spending more time in the house and therefore incurring a greater risk of exposure. In the Caribbean region, non-black ethnic groups might be infected only by co-habitation with people of African descent who probably provide the host reservoir for the virus, and this would need to be prolonged if infectivity were very low. This might then explain why Indians, though infected with HTLV-I, have a much lower sero-positivity rate in Trinidad than do inhabitants of African origin.

The increasing sero-positivity with age still requires an explanation. One possibility is that it reflects the requirement for continuous exposure to potential sources of virus coupled with inefficient transmission. Another possibility is that the age association is merely a mirror of historical events, with young people now being infected at a much lower rate due, for example, to improving living conditions. We have assumed that if blood-sucking insects are capable of transmitting HTLV-I this will be via the purely mechanical transfer of infected lymphocytes. At this stage, however, it remains possible, though perhaps less likely, that insects serve as a biological vector supporting viral replication, as happens, for example, with the Japanese encephalitis arbovirus [34]. This is currently being investigated.

Finally, it is important in this context to re-emphasise the similarity between HTLV-I and bovine leukaemia virus (BLV) with respect to viral structure and disease similarities [8, 39]. Although BLV in developed countries may commonly be transmitted iatrogenically, there may well be a role for haematophagous insects as mechanical vectors, especially in tropical regions. Experimental evidence for this has been produced [2, 9, 12]. BLV does not, however, spread readily within a herd of cows, and physical contact is almost certainly required [29]. This might again implicate an insect vector other than common mosquitoes.

It is of interest that BLV can be experimentally transferred by injecting a sero-negative cow with 100 µl of blood or around 1000–2000 lymphocytes from an infected cow, but that this value drops by 3 orders of magnitude if the donor cow has a BLV-associated lymphocytosis (A. Burny, this volume). The latter corresponds to the transfer of less than 0.1% of the volume of a mosquito blood feed which could easily be carried on the mouthparts. Perhaps HTLV-I is effectively transmitted only by blood-sucking insects that have had an interrupted meal on a sero-positive individual with some degree of lymphocytosis. This might then explain the apparent need for close familial contact over a prolonged period.

It is clear that HTLV-I has been transmitted by blood transfusion in Japan [16], and we do not contest that infection can be spread via breast feeding or sexual contact. Although several modes of transmission may be possible, we hypothesise that insect vectors play a more significant role than has hitherto been appreciated.

Acknowledgements. The work reported here was supported by the Leukaemia Research Fund of Great Britain and will be reported in detail elsewhere. Our collaborators in this work include Dr. N. Byam and Dr. G. Beckles (Port of Spain, Trinidad), Dr. R. Kirkwood, Dr. D. C. Carson, Dr. L. Chan, Dr. L. Kinlen, Dr. T. A. Lister, Ms. S. M. Pegram and Ms. S. Claydon. We thank Ms. G. Parkins and Mrs. J. Needham for typing the manuscript.

References

1. Bartholomew C, Charles W, Saxinger C, Blattner W, Robert-Guroff M, Raju C, Ratan P, Ince W, Quamina D, Basdeo-Maharaj K, Gallo RC (1985) Racial and other characteristics of human T-cell leukaemia/lymphoma (HTLV-I) and AIDS (HTLV-III) in Trinidad. Br Med J 290:1243–1246
2. Bech-Nielsen S, Piper CE, Ferrer JF (1978) Natural mode of transmission of the bovine leukemia virus: role of blood-sucking insects. Am J Vet Res 39:1089–1092
3. Biggar RJ, Gigase PL, Melbye M, Kestens L, Sarin PS, Bodner AJ, Demedts P, Stevens WJ, Paluku L, Delacollette C, Blattner WA (1985) Elisa HTLV retrovirus antibody reactivity associated with malaria and immune complexes in healthy Africans. Lancet II:520–523
4. Biggar RJ, Johnson BK, Oster C, Sarin PS, Ocheng D, Tukei P, Nsanze H, Alexander S, Bodner AJ, Siongo TA, Gallo RC, Blattner WA (1985) Regional variation in prevalence of antibody against human T-lymphotropic virus types I and III in Kenya, East Africa. Int J Cancer 35:763–767
5. Biggar RJ, Saxinger C, Gardiner C, Collins WE, Levine PH, Clark JW, Nkrumah FK, Blattner WA (1984) Type-I HTLV antibody in urban and rural Ghana. Int J Cancer 34:214–219
6. Blattner WA, Gibbs WN, Saxinger C, Robert-Guroff M, Clark J, Lofters W, Han-

chard B, Campbell M, Gallo RC (1983) Human T-cell leukaemia/lymphoma virus-associated lympho-reticular neoplasia in Jamaica. Lancet II:61–64

7. Blattner WA, Kalyanaraman VS, Robert-Guroff M, Lister TA, Galton DAG, Sarin PS, Crawford MH, Catovsky D, Greaves M, Gallo RC (1982) The human type-C retrovirus, HTLV, in Blacks from the Caribbean region, and relationship to adult T-cell leukaemia/lymphoma. Int J Cancer 30:257–264

8. Burny A, Bruck C, Couez D, Deschamps J, Ghysdael J, Kettmann R, Mammerick M, Marbaix G, Portetelle D (1984) Enzootic bovine leukemia: its relevance as a model system for humen T-cell leukemia. In: Gallo RC, Essex ME, Gross L (eds) Human T-cell leukemia/lymphoma virus. Cold Spring Harbor Laboratory, New York, pp 17–24

9. Buxton BA, Schultz RD, Collins WE (1982) . Role of insects in the transmission of bovine leukosis virus. Potential for transmission by mosquitoes. Am J Vet Res 43:1458–1459

10. Catovsky D, Greaves MF, Rose M, Galton DAG, Goolden AWG, McCluskey DR, White JM, Lampert I, Bourikas G, Ireland R, Brownell AI, Bridges JM, Blattner WA, Gallo RC (1982) Adult T-cell lymphoma-leukaemia in Blacks from the West Indies. Lancet I:639–643

11. De The G, Gessain A, Gazzolo L, Robert-Guroff M, Najberg G, Calender A, M'Pnagi P, Brubaker G, Benslimane A, Fabry J, Strobel M, Robin Y, Fortune R (1986) Comparative seroepidemiology of HTLV-I and HTLV-III in French West Indies and some African countries. Cancer Res (in press)

12. Fischer RG, Leucke DH, Rehacek J (1973) Friend leukaemia virus (FLV) activity in certain arthropods. III. Transmission studies. Neoplasma 20:255–260

13. Gallo RC, Sliski A, Wong-Staal F (1983) Origin of human T-cell leukaemia-lymphoma virus. Lancet II:962–963

14. Gessain A, Jouannelle A, Escarmant P, Calender A, Schaffar-Deshayes L, The G de (1984) HTLV antibodies in patients with non-Hodgkin lymphomas in Martinique. Lancet I:1183

15. Greaves MF, Verbi W, Tilley R, Lister TA, Habeshaw J, Guo H-G, Trainor CD, Robert-Guroff M, Blattner W, Reitz M, Gallo RC (1984) Human T-cell leukaemia virus (HTLV) in the United Kingdom. Int J Cancer 33:795–806

16. Hino S, Kawamichi T, Funakoshi M, Kanamura M, Kitamura T, Miyamoto T (1984) Transfusion-mediated spread of the human T-cell leukaemia virus in chronic hemodialy-sis patients in a heavily endemic area, Nagasaki. Gann 75:1070–1075

17. Hino S, Yamaguchi K, Katamine S, Sugiyama H, Amagasaki T, Kinoshita K, Yoshida Y, Doi H, Tsuji Y, Miyamoto T (1985) Mother-to-child transmission of human T-cell leukemia virus type I. Gann 76:474–480

18. Hinuma T, Komoda H, Chosa T, Kondo T, Kohakura M, Takenaka T, Kikuchi M, Ichimaru M, Yunoki K, Sato I, Matsuo R, Takiuchi Y, Uchino H, Hanaoka M (1982) Antibodies to adult T-cell leukaemia-virus-associated antigen (ATLA) in sera from patients with ATL and controls in Japan: a nationwide sero-epidemiological study. Int J Cancer 29:631–635

19. Hinuma Y, Nagata K, Nakai M, Matsumoto T, Kinoshita K, Shirakawa S, Miyoshi I (1981) Adult T-cell leukemia: antigen in an ATL cell line and detection of antibodies to the antigen in human sera. Proc Natl Acad Sci USA 78:6476–6480

20. Hunsmann G, Schneider J, Schmitt J, Yamamoto N (1983) Detection of serum antibodies to adult T-cell leukaemia virus in non-human primates and in people from Africa. Int J Cancer 32:329–332

21. Komuro A, Hayami M, Fujii H, Miyahara S, Hirayama M (1983) Vertical transmission of adult T-cell leukaemia virus. Lancet I:240

22. Manzari V, Gradilone A, Barillari G, Zani M, Collalti E, Pandolfi F, de Rossi G, Liso V, Babbo P, Robert-Guroff M, Frati L (1985) HTLV-I is endemic in southern Italy: detection of the first infection cluster in a white population. Int J Cancer 36:557–559

23. Merino F, Robert-Guroff M, Clark J, Biondo-Bracho M, Blattner WA, Gallo RC (1984) Natural antibodies to human T-cell leukaemia/lymphoma virus in healthy Venezuelan populations. Int J Cancer 34:501–506

24. Miller GJ, Beckles GLA, Byam NTA, Price SGL, Carson DC, Kirkwood BR, Baker IA, Bainton D (1984) Serum lipoprotein concentrations in relation to ethnic composition and urbanization in men and women of Trinidad, West Indies. Int J Epidemiol 13:413–421

25. Miller GJ, Pegram SM, Kirkwood BR, Beckles GLA, Byam NTA, Clayden SA, Kinlen LJ, Chan LC, Carson DC, Greaves MF (1986) Ethnic composition, age, sex, and the location and standard of housing as determinants of HTLV-I infection in an urban Trinidadian community. Int J Cancer 38:801–808

26. Minwor M, Sugano H, Sugimura T, Weiss RA (eds) (1985) Retroviruses in human lymphoma/leukaemia. Japan Scientific Soc. Press, Tokyo

27. Morlan HB, Hayes RO (1958) Urban dispersal and activity of *Aedes aegypti*. Mosquito News 18:137–144
28. Nakano S, Ando Y, Ichijo M, Moriyama I, Saito S, Sugamura K, Hinuma Y (1984) Search for possible routes of vertical and horizontal transmission of adult T-cell leukaemia virus. Gann 75:1044–1045
29. Piper CE, Abt DA, Ferrer JF, Marshak RR (1975) Seroepidemiological evidence of the horizontal transmission of the bovine C-type virus. Cancer Res 35:2714
30. Poiesz BJ, Ruscetti FW, Gazdar AF, Bunn A, Minna JD, Gallo RC (1980) Detection and isolation of type-C retrovirus particles from fresh and cultured lymphocytes of a patient with cutaneous T cell lymphoma. Proc Natl Acad Sci USA 77:7415–7419
31. Reitz MS, Poiesz BJ, Ruscetti FW, Gallo RC (1981) Characterization and distribution of nucleic acid sequences of a novel type-C retrovirus isolated from neoplastic human T-lymphocytes. Proc Natl Acad Sci USA 78:1887–1891
32. Robert-Guroff M, Clark J, Lanier AP, Beckman G, Melbye M, Ebbesen P, Blattner WA, Gallo RC (1985) Prevalence of HTLV-I in arctic regions. Int J Cancer 36:651–655
33. Saxinger C, Gallo RC (1983) Application of an indirect ELISA microtest to the detection and surveillance of human T-cell leukemia/lymphoma virus (HTLV). Lab Invest 49:371–377
34. Shiraki H (1970) Japanese encephalitis. In: Debre R, Celers J (eds) Clinical virology. The

evaluation and management of human viral infections, chap 11. W.B. Saunders, Philadelphia, pp 155–175
35. Tajima K, Fujita K, Tsukidate S, Oda T, Tominaga S, Suchi T, Hinuma Y (1983) Seroepidemiological studies on the effects of filarial parasites in infestation of adult T-cell leukaemia virus in the Goto Islands, Japan. Gann 74:188–191
36. Tajima K, Tominaga S, Suchi T, Kawagoe T, Komoda H, Hinuma Y, Oda T, Fujita K (1982) Epidemiological analysis of the distribution of antibody to adult T-cell leukaemia-virus-associated antigen: possible horizontal transmission of adult T-cell leukaemia virus. Gann 73:893–901
37. Watanabe T, Seiki M, Yoshida M (1984) HTLV type I (US isolate) and ATLV (Japanese isolate) are the same species of human retrovirus. Virology 133:238–241
38. Williams CK, Saxinger WC, Alabi GO, Junaid TA, Blayney DW, Greaves MF, Gallo RC, Blattner WA (1984) HTLV-associated lymphoproliferative disease: report of 2 cases in Nigeria. Br Med J 288:1495–1496
39. Wong-Staal F, Gallo RC (1985) Human T-lymphotropic retroviruses. Nature 317:395–403
40. Tedder RD, Shanson DC, Jeffries DJ, Cheingsong-Popov R, Clapham P, Dalgleish A, Nagy K, Weiss RA (1984) Low prevalence in the UK of HTLV-I and HTLV-II infection in subjects with AIDS, with extended lymphadenopathy, and at risk of AIDS. Lancet II:125–128

Haematology and Blood Transfusion Vol. 31
Modern Trends in Human Leukemia VII
Edited by Neth, Gallo, Greaves, and Kabisch
© Springer-Verlag Berlin Heidelberg 1987

Neutralization and Receptor Recognition of Human T-Lymphotropic Retroviruses

R. A. Weiss, P. R. Clapham, A. G. Dalgleish, and J. N. Weber

A. Introduction

Like other enveloped viruses, the outer membrane antigens of retroviruses present target antigens for neutralizing antibodies, and also play a key role in interacting with cell-surface receptors for initial stages of infection. We have investigated these attributes of the envelopes of human T-lymphotropic retroviruses (Weiss 1985; Wong-Staal and Gallo 1985) and our studies are briefly summarized here.

The viruses investigated are human T-cell leukemia virus type-1 (HTLV-1), the etiologic agent of adult T-cell leukemia-lymphoma (ATL), HTLV-2, first isolated from the leukemic cells of a patient with T-cell hairy leukemia (Kalyanaraman et al. 1982) and present in a proportion of intravenous drug abusers (Tedder et al. 1984), and human immunodeficiency virus (HIV-1, HTLV-3/LAV) the causative agent of AIDS.

B. Neutralizing Sera for HTLV-1 and HTLV-2

HTLV-1 and HTLV-2 are not readily amenable to quantitative titration of infectivity because the virions are largely cell-associated. We have therefore employed a viral pseudotype technique for detecting neutralizing antibodies and for probing receptors. The pseudotypes are virions of vesicu-

Institute of Cancer Research, Chester Beatty Laboratories, Fulham Road, London SW3 6JB, England

lar stomatitis virus enveloped by the glycoproteins of HTLV-1 or HTLV-2 (Clapham et al. 1984), a system originally devised for avian retroviruses by Zavada (1972). Pseudotypes possess the neutralization and host range properties of the retrovirus, while replicating as VSV to produce cytopathic plaques in cell monolayers that can be assayed in a simple, quantitative way.

Using stocks of VSV(HTLV-1), we found that sera of infected subjects, whether healthy or suffering ATL, possessed neutralizing titers ranging from 1:50 to 1:50000 (Clapham et al. 1984). In collaboration with H. Hoshino, we showed that VSV(HTLV-1) pseudotypes prepared with Japanese or American HTLV-1 isolates did not distinguish by neutralization titer between sera from Japanese and British West Jamaican subjects (Hoshino et al. 1985).

For HTLV-2 neutralization, we have used a single isolate from an American patient (Kalyanaraman et al. 1982) for pseudotype preparation, and observed high neutralization titers in the sera of 4% of British intravenous drug abusers (Tedder et al. 1984). There is a slight degree of cross-neutralization between HTLV-1 and HTLV-2, but the heterologous titers are 100- to 1000-fold lower than the homologous titers (Clapham et al. 1984).

C. Common and Variable Antigens for HIV-1 Neutralization

We have also detected neutralizing activity in sera of subjects infected with HIV-1 (Weiss et al. 1985a, 1986). In a longitudinal

Table 1. Common and strain-specific neutralizing activities of human and rabbit sera to HIV-1[a]

Serum	Neutralizing titer for VSV (HIV-1)						
Strain origin (% env divergence)	RF Haiti 15	IIIB USA 0	MN USA 10	ARV-2 USA 15	MA-2 UK 10	Rut Tanzania >20	Z129 Zaire >20
Human							
British control							
1	10	10	250	6250	50	250	50
2	50	10	250	1250	50	250	50
3	10	–	250	250	10	250	50
4	50	10	250	1250	50	50	250
5	50	10	10	1250	10	50	250
6	250	–	10	1250	10	250	250
Ugandan control							
1	50	10	50	1250	50	10	250
2	250	10	–	1250	10	250	–
3	50	10	10	6250	250	250	50
4	50	10	10	1250	250	250	–
Rabbit							
Preimmune	–	–	–	–	–	–	–
Anti-gp130	–	50	10	–	10	–	–

[a] Data from Weiss et al. (1986).

study of initially asymptomatic male homosexuals known to be infected with HIV-1 for at least 3 years (Weber et al. 1987), the continued presence and a slightly rising titer of neutralizing anti-HIV-1 appears to correlate with a relatively good prognosis. However, a stronger correlation was found with low or no anti-gag serum activity (measured by radioimmunoprecipitation) and progression to AIDS or AIDS-related complex (ARC). We do not, at present, know whether some of the neutralizing activity may be directed to gag antigens, though this appears unlikely for VSV(HIV-1) pseudotypes, which are thought to assemble only membrane glycoproteins of the retrovirus.

Using VSV(HIV-1) pseudotypes prepared with seven different isolates of HIV-1 from USA, Haiti, Europe and Africa, we examined the specificity and variability of neutralizing epitopes (Weiss et al. 1986). Sera from Ugandan and British subjects selected for capacity to neutralize the RF (Haitian) isolate, showed significant neutralizing activity for almost all HIV-1 strains (Table 1). Interestingly, the ARV-2 pseudotype stock appeared to be most sensitive to neutraliza-

tion, whatever the origin of the anti-HIV human serum. By contrast to the cross-neutralization observed with human sera, we found in collaboration with L. Lasky and P. Berman that a rabbit serum raised by Lasky et al. (1986) against a recombinant gp130 molecule specific to the outer envelope glycoprotein of HIV-1, neutralized the strain from which the recombinant was made (HTLV-IIIB), but only two of the other six strains. Even the ARV-2 isolate that was so sensitive to human sera was not significantly neutralized by the anti-gp130 rabbit serum. Tests with further rabbit and guinea-pig sera raised against gp130 confirmed the strain-specificity of this antigen (Weiss et al. 1986).

The antigen targets for neutralization of HIV-1 thus appear to include epitopes common to widely divergent HIV-1 strains as well as variable antigens specific to individual strains and more closely related isolates. The presence of common neutralization antigens between HIV-1 strains differing by 20% or more in the envelope gene (Alizon et al. 1986; Starcich et al. 1986) is a promising finding for the development of vaccines.

D. Receptors for HTLV and HIV

HTLVs and HIV share a common property of tropism for T4$^+$ lymphocytes in vivo (Weiss 1985; Wong-Staal and Gallo 1985). ATL is a T4$^+$ neoplasm, while the salient feature of AIDS is the depletion of T4$^+$ T-helper cells. However, other cell types can be infected in vitro by HTLV-1 (Clapham et al. 1983) and by HIV-1 (Levy et al. 1985; Gartner et al. 1986). We investigated to what extent the cellular tropisms of HTLV and HIV are determined by the cell surface receptors for initiating infection, and identified the T4 (CD4) antigen itself as an important component of the HIV-1 receptor (Dalgleish et al. 1984).

Using VSV pseudotypes with envelopes of HTLV or HIV, we found that HTLV-1 and HTLV-2 recognise receptors on diverse types of human cells and mammalian cells of many species. Productive infection of cells by HTLV-1 not only blocks receptor availability to VSV(HTLV-1) but also to VSV(HTLV-2), indicating that these two viruses use a common receptor (Weiss et al. 1985 b). The recognition of a common cell surface receptor for HTLV-1 and HTLV-2 accords with the slight cross-neutralization of these viruses already noted, as there may be a common epitope of the external glycoprotein that binds to the receptor. We do not at present know the biochemical nature of the HTLV receptor.

Pseudotypes of HIV-1 plate only on cells expressing T4 antigen (Dalgleish et al. 1984). These may be T-helper lymphocytes or monocytes, such as the U937 cell line. Using monoclonal antibodies (mAbs) to T4 antigen, we found that pseudotype infection, and also induction of multinucleated syncytia by HIV-1, could be blocked in T4$^+$ T cells (Dalgleish et al. 1984) and U937 cells (Clapham et al. 1987). Infection by HIV-1 (Dalgleish et al. 1984) and treatment by TPA (Clapham et al. 1987) caused concomitant disappearance of T4 antigen and HIV-1 receptor from the cell surface without affecting the HTLV receptor. Other groups have also observed that mAbs specifically blocked infection by HIV-1 (Klatzmann et al. 1984) and binding of labelled HIV-1 virions (McDougal et al. 1986). Preliminary studies also indicate that HIV-2 (LAV-2;

Clavel et al. 1986) reception is also blocked by certain anti-T4 mAbs. Thus, the T4 antigen acts as a specific receptor on lymphocytes and monocytes for binding HIV.

The precise epitopes on the T4 antigen recognized by HIV-1 remain to be determined. In collaboration with Q. Sattentau and P. C. L. Beverley, we have analyzed a series of 25 different mAbs raised against T4 for ability to block each other and HIV-1 syncytium induction (Sattentau et al. 1986). The mAbs that interfere with HIV-1 reception fall into three noncompeting groups. Two block HIV-1 completely and the third only weakly. Some mAbs, e.g., OKT4 and OKT4c, fail to compete with the HIV-1 receptor at all. These epitopes are thought to be located near to the transmembrane domain of the T4 molecule. Although there is some degree of variation in T4 epitope expression on T lymphocytes from different African and Caucasian individuals, this was not correlated with susceptibility to HIV-1 infection in vitro and did not affect those epitopes most important for T4 binding (Sattentau et al. 1986).

We next examined whether the T4 antigen would act as a functional receptor for HIV-1 if expressed ectopically on the surface of unusual cell types. In collaboration with P. Maddon, R. Axel, and J. S. McDougal, the cDNA for the human *T4* gene was introduced into various human and mouse cell types via a retrovirus vector carrying a neomycin resistance gene as a dominant selectable marker (Maddon et al. 1986). Our findings, summarized in Table 2, show that human cells such as the immature T-cell line HSB2, the Burkitt's lymphoma line, Raji, and the cervical carcinoma line, HeLa, become susceptible to HIV-1 infection and replication upon expression of T4. On the other hand, transfection and expression of the human *T4* gene to mouse cells, including L3T4$^+$ mouse cells (the murine equivalent of human T4$^+$ lymphocytes), does not result in infection of HIV-1 or of the VSV(HIV-1) pseudotype. HIV-1 virions did, however, bind specifically to the surface of T4 transfected mouse cells and not to control mouse cells. Therefore, we conclude that T4 antigen is sufficient for HIV-1 attachment to the surface of mouse cells, but that some other human component, present in HeLa and Raji

389

Table 2. Interaction of HIV-1 with cells transfected with the human T4 gene[a]

Cell type[b]		HIV-1 virion binding	Syncytium induction	VSV (HIV-1) infection	HIV-1 replication[c]
Human					
HSB2	T cell	+	+	+	+
Raji	B cell	+	+	+	+
HeLa	Carcinoma	+	+	+	+
Murine					
3DT	T cell	+	−	−	−
L	Fibroblast	+	−	−	−
NIH-3T3	Fibroblast	+	−	−	−

[a] Data from Maddon et al. (1986).
[b] All control cells (transfected with neo vector alone or neo + human T8 gene) were universally negative for all HIV-1 interactions listed in the table.
[c] HIV-1 replication was assayed by production of reverse transcriptase, immunofluorescence for viral antigens, and induction of syncytia in indicator T cells.

cells, is necessary for functional penetration following attachment. It appears that the binding of virions alone is insufficient to trigger endocytosis of the ligand-receptor complex on mouse cells.

E. Conclusions

Our studies of virus neutralization serve to distinguish different strains of human retroviral pathogens and may eventually provide prognostic tools and aid the development of vaccines. Our receptor studies serve to distinguish the cellular tropisms of HTLVs and HIVs, and have identified certain epitopes of the T4 surface antigen as the binding receptor for HIV. Infection of T4[+] lymphocytes and monocytes by HIV-1 largely explains the immunodeficiency underlying the opportunistic infections and neoplasms evident in AIDS. The binding of free envelope glycoprotein to uninfected T4[+] cells when shed by infected cells may further exacerbate the immunodeficiency, as T4 antigen plays a functional role in cell interactions in the immune system (Dalgleish 1986).

References

1. Alizon M, Wain-Hobson S, Montagnier L, Sonigo P (1986) Genetic variability of the AIDS virus: nucleotide sequence analysis of two isolates from African patients. Cell 46:63–74
2. Clapham PR, Weiss RA, Dalgleish AG, Exley M, Whitby D, Hogg N (1987) Human immunodeficiency virus infection of monocytic and T-lymphocytic cells: receptor modulation and differentiation induced by phorbol ester. Virology 158:44–51
3. Clapham P, Nagy K, Weiss RA (1984) Pseudotypes of human T-cell leukaemia types 1 and 2: neutralization by patients' sera. Proc Natl Acad Sci USA 81:2886–2889
4. Clavel F, Guetard D, Brun-Vezinet F, Chamaret S, Rey M-A, Santos-Ferreira MO, Laurent AG, Dauguet C, Katlama C, Rouzioux C, Klatzmann D, Champalimaud JL, Montagnier L (1986) Isolation of a new human retrovirus for West African patients with AIDS. Science 233:343–346
5. Dalgleish AG (1986) The T4 molecule: function and structure. Immunology Today 7:142–144
6. Dalgleish AG, Beverley PCL, Clapham PR, Crawford DH, Greaves MF, Weiss RA (1984) The CD4 (T4) antigen is an essential component of the receptor for the AIDS retrovirus. Nature 312:763–767
7. Gartner S, Markovits P, Markovits DM, Kaplan MH, Gallo RC, Popovic M (1986) The role of mononuclear phagocytes in HTLV-III/LAV infection. Science 233:215–219
8. Hoshino HH, Clapham PR, Weiss RA, Miyoshi I, Yoshida M, Miwa M (1985) Human T-cell leukemia virus type I: pseudotype neutralization of Japanese and American isolates with human and rabbit sera. Int J Cancer 36:671–675

9. Kalyanaraman VS, Sarngadharan MG, Robert-Guroff M, Miyoshi I, Blayney D, Golde D, Gallo RA (1982) A new subtype of human T-cell leukemia virus (HTLV-II) associated with a T-cell variant of hairy cell leukemia. Science 218:571

10. Klatzman D, Champagne E, Chamaret S, Gruest J, Guetard D, Hercent T, Gluckman J-C, Montagnier L (1984) T-lymphocyte T4 molecule behaves as the receptor for human retrovirus LAV. Nature 312:767–768

11. Lasky LA, Groopman JE, Fennie CW, Benz PM, Capon DJ, Dowbenko DJ, Nakamura GR, Nunes WM, Renz ME, Berman PW (1986) Neutralization of the AIDS retrovirus by antibodies to a recombinant envelope glycoprotein. Science 233:209–212

12. Levy JA, Shimabukuro J, McHugh T, Casavant C, Stites D, Oshino L (1985) AIDS-associated retroviruses (ARV) can productively infect other cells besides human T helper cells. Virology 147:441–448

13. Maddon PJ, Dalgleish AG, McDougal JS, Clapham PR, Weiss RA, Axel R (1986) The *T4* gene encodes the AIDS virus receptor and is expressed in the immune system and the brain. Cell 47:333–348

14. McDougal JS, Kennedy MS, Sligh JM, Cort SP, Mawle A, Nicholson JKA (1986) Binding of HTLV-III/LAV to T4$^+$ T cells by a complex of the 110K viral protein and the T4 molecule. Science 231:382–385

15. Sattentau QJ, Dalgleish AG, Weiss RA, Beverley PCR (1986) Epitopes of the CD4 antigen and HIV infection. Science 234:1120–1123

16. Starcich BR, Hahn BH, Shaw GH, McNeely PD, Modrow S, Wolf H, Parks ES, Parks WP, Josephs SF, Gallo RC, Wong-Staal F (1986) Identification and characterisation of conserved and variable regions in the envelope gene of HTLV-III/LAV, the retrovirus of AIDS. Cell 45:637–648

17. Tedder RS, Shanson D, Jeffries D, Cheingsong-Popov R, Clapham P, Dalgleish A, Nagy K, Weiss RA (1984) Low prevalence in the UK of HTLV-1 and HTLV-II infection in subjects with AIDS, with extended lymphadenopathy, and at risk of AIDS. Lancet II:125–128

18. Weber JN, Clapham PR, Weiss RA, Parker D, Roberts C, Duncan J, Weller I, Carne C, Tedder RS, Pinching AJ, Cheingsong-Popov R (1987) Human immunodeficiency virus infection in two cohorts of homosexual men: Neutralising sera and association of anti-gag antibody with prognosis. Lancet I:119–122

19. Weiss RA (1985) Human T-cell viruses. In: Weiss RA, Teich NM, Varmus HE, Coffin J (eds) RNA tumor viruses, vol 2. Cold Spring Harbor Laboratory, New York, pp 404–485

20. Weiss RA, Clapham PR, Weber JN, Dalgleish AG, Berman PW, Lasky LA (1986) Variable and conserved neutralization antigens of human immunodeficiency virus (HIV-1). Nature 324:572–575

21. Weiss RA, Clapham PR, Cheingsong-Popov R, Dalgleish AG, Carne CA, Weller IVD, Tedder RS (1985a) Neutralization of human T-lymphotropic virus type III sera of AIDS and AIDS-risk patients. Nature 316:69–71

22. Weiss RA, Clapham PR, Nagy K, Hoshino H (1985b) Envelope properties of human T-cell leukemia viruses. Current topics in microbiol. Immunol 115:235–246

23. Wong-Staal F, Gallo RA (1985) Human T-lymphotropic retroviruses. Nature 317:395–403

24. Zavada J (1972) Pseudotypes of vesicular somatitis virus with the coat of murine leukemia and of avian myeloblastosis viruses. J Gen Virol 15:183–191

Haematology and Blood Transfusion Vol. 31
Modern Trends in Human Leukemia VII
Edited by Neth, Gallo, Greaves, and Kabisch
© Springer-Verlag Berlin Heidelberg 1987

Markers of HTLV-I-Related Virus in Hamadryas Baboon Lymphoma

A. F. Voevodin[1], B. A. Lapin[1], A. G. Tatosyan[2], and I. Hirsch[3]

A. Introduction

Our previous studies have shown that hamadryas baboons of the Sukhumi "high lymphoma" stock are infected with human T-lymphotrophic virus (HTLV)-I-related virus to a significantly higher degree than baboons of different lymphoma-free populations. Levels of anti-HTLV-I-related antibodies in prelymphomatous baboon sera were also significantly higher than those in matched controls [1, 2]. These studies posed the question of whether HTLV-I-like virus is etiologically related to baboon malignant lymphoma. The most informative indirect approach to the study of this possibility is the search for integrated provirus in baboon lymphoma DNA. Thus, we tested by Southern blotting PstI, BamHI, and EcoRI digests of high molecular weight baboon lymphoma DNA, using as a probe genome-length HTLV-I cloned in SstI site of pSP-65 vector (this molecular clone was kindly provided by Dr. R. Gallo). Ten PstI-digested lymphoma DNA samples (lymphomatous lymph nodes) were found positive (Table 1). The band pattern was similar to, but clearly different from, that characteristic for HTLV-I (cf. Figs. 1, 2, 4). At least three fragments (1.7 kb, 1.5 kb, and 1.1 kb) were observed in all samples (Table 1; Fig. 1). They were

thought to be internal fragments [3]. In each positive sample "individual" bands were also found that suggest monoclonal (or oligoclonal) integration of HTLV-I provirus into different sites in baboon lymphoma DNA (Fig. 1). This suggestion was proved correct by Southern analysis of BamHI and

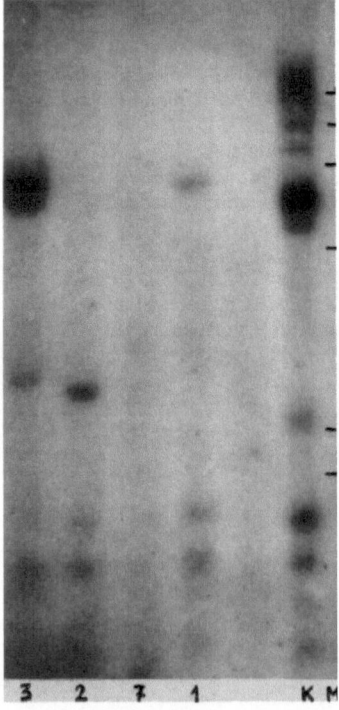

Fig. 1. Southern analysis of PstI digests of baboon lymphoma DNA. 1–10, sample numbers the same as in Table 1; K, baboon cell line (594S-F9) producing HTLV-I-like virus; M, Molecular size markers: 23.4, 9.4, 6.5, 4.4, 2.3, and 2.0 kb

[1] Institute of Experimental Pathology and Therapy, USSR Academy of Medical Sciences, Sukhumi, USSR
[2] All-Union Oncological Research Center, Moscow, USSR
[3] Institute of Sera and Vaccines, 10103 Prague, Czechoslovakia

Table 1. HTLV-I-related sequences in DNA of lymphomatous lymph nodes of hamadryas baboons

No.	Tumor no.	PstI digests		BamHI digests		EcoRI digests	
		+/−	internal fragments (in kb)	+/−	fragments (in kb)	+/−	fragments (in kb)
1.	PHL-1	++	1.7; 1.5; 1.1ᵃ	++	25; 15	++	20
2.	PHL-2	++	1.7; 1.5; 1.1ᵃ	++	24; 22	++	23.5
3.	PHL-3	++	1.7; 1.5; 1.1ᵃ	+++	14; 8; 4.1	+++	24; 5
4.	PHL-4	++	1.7; 1.5; 1.1ᵃ	+++	9	+++	23.4; 4.5
5.	PHL-5	++	1.7; 1.5; 1.1ᵃ	+	12; 7.5	NT	
6.	PHL-6	+	1.7; 1.5; 1.1ᵃ	+	13; 10; 7.6	+	23.5; 15
7.	PHL-7	+	1.7; 1.5; 1.1ᵃ		8.4; 5.8	−?	
8.	PHL-8	++	1.7; 1.5; 1.1ᵃ	++	8	+++	11.5; 9.4; 7
9.	PHL-9	+	1.7; 1.5; 1.1ᵃ	NT		++	24
10.	PHL-10	++	1.7; 1.5; 1.1ᵃ	NT		++	20; 12

+, weakly positive; ++, positive; +++, highly positive. NT, not tested.
ᵃ Junction fragments of different sizes were individual for each sample in Pst digests.

Ten μg of high molecular weight DNA was digested with the enzymes PstI, BamHI, and EcoRI under optimal conditions (5u/μg, 37° C overnight), electrophoresed through 1.2% (PstI) or 0.8% (BamHI, EcoRI) agarose, blotted to nitrocellulose filter in 20 × SSC according to Southern blotting. Hybridization was carried out with ^{32}P-labeled DNA of pMT-2 plasmid (pSP 65 vector containing genome-length insert of HTLV-I which represented approximately 70% of pMT-2) at 42° C for 40 h in the following solution −4 × SSC, 2 × Denhardt's solution, 0.5% Sodium dodecyl sulfate, 0.02M EDTA, 100 mg/ml sonicated denatured salmon sperm DNA, 50 mg/ml yeast RNA, 50% formamide 5×10^7 cpm probe DNA. Before this, filters were prehybridized in the same solution, but without probe DNA, for 16 h. Washing was carried out twice for 10 min at room temperature in 2 × SSC, five times for 15 min at 55° C in 2 × SSC + 0.1% SDS, and finally five times for 15 min at 55° C in 0.1 × SSC + 0.1% SDS. Filters were exposed to X-ray film with intensifying screens at −70° C for 5–10 days.

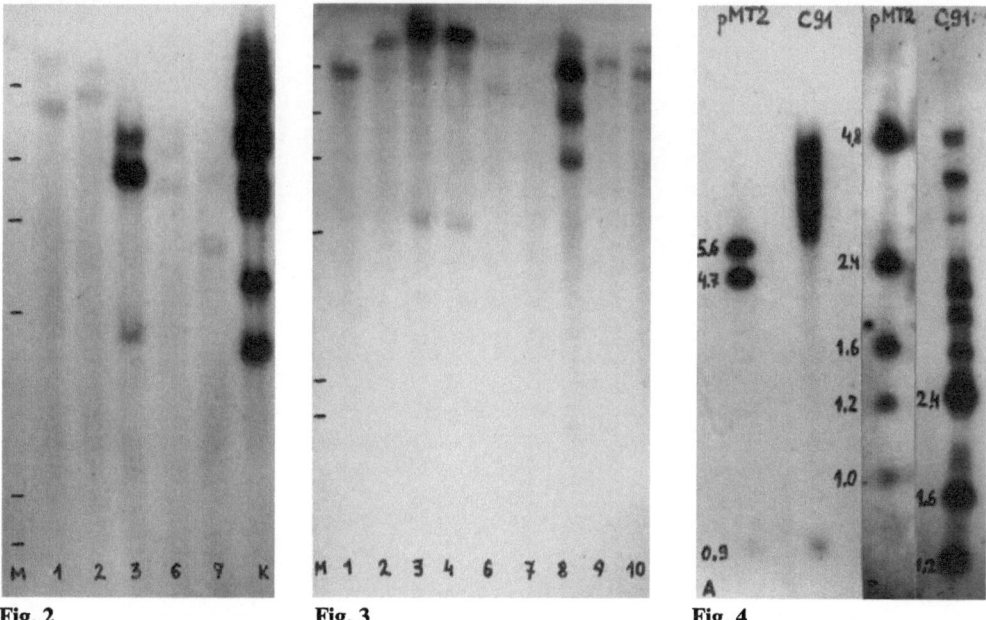

Fig. 2   Fig. 3   Fig. 4

Fig. 2. Southern analysis of BamH1 digests of baboon lymphoma DNA
Fig. 3. Southern analysis of EcoR1 digests of baboon lymphoma DNA
Fig. 4. Southern analysis of PstI (B) and BamHI (a) digests of positive-control cellular and plasmid DNA. C91, human cell line (C91-PL) producing HTLV-I

*Eco*RI digests of the same lymphoma DNA (Table 1; Fig. 2, Fig. 3). One to three large fragments were observed in each sample, all with individual size. In some cases, fragments were found which were smaller than the expected HTLV-I-like provirus size. These data suggested multiple integration of HTLV-like provirus(es) in some baboon lymphomas or the oligoclonal origin of these tumors, as well as integration of defective provirus(es) in several cases. HTLV-I-related sequences were not found in one sample of baboon normal lymph node DNA and three samples of muscle DNA isolated from lymphomatous animals.

B. Conclusions

1. HTLV-I-like provirus is integrated into DNA of baboon malignant lymphomas.

2. Baboon HTLV-I-like provirus is closely related to, but distinct from, HTLV-I.

3. In most cases the integration of HTLV-I-like provirus is multiple monoclonal, or the origin of these tumors is oligoclonal.

4. Defective HTLV-I-like proviruses are integrated into DNA of some baboon malignant lymphomas.

References

1. Lapin BA, Voevodin AF, Indzhiia LV et al. (1983) Bull Exp Biol Med v. XCV, 14–16 (in Russ)
2. Voevodin AF, Lapin BA, Yakovleva LA et al. (1985) Int J Cancer 36:579–584
3. Guo H, Wong-Staal F, Gallo R (1984) Science 223:1195–1196

Haematology and Blood Transfusion Vol. 31
Modern Trends in Human Leukemia VII
Edited by Neth, Gallo, Greaves, and Kabisch
© Springer-Verlag Berlin Heidelberg 1987

Replication and Pathogenesis of the Human T-Cell Leukemia/Lymphotropic Retroviruses

W. Haseltine *, J. Sodroski, and C. Rosen

A. Introduction

Human retroviruses represent an emerging class of complex pathogens involved in a wide variety of maladies, including leukemias and lymphomas, diseases of the central nervous system, and immune function impairment. These have recently been reviewed by Wong-Staal and Gallo. Four different types of human retroviruses have been isolated to date: the etiological agents of a malignant T cell leukemia/lymphoma, the virus HTLV-I which causes the disease ATLL, two viruses associated with more benign forms of T-cell leukemia (HTLV-II), and the etiological agent of the acquired immune deficiency syndrome and related disorders (HIV). Additionally, retroviruses of genomic organization similar to that of HIV but differing markedly in DNA sequence have recently been isolated among persons in West Africa (Kanki et al. 1985; Clavel et al. 1986).

As far as they have been characterized to date, the human retroviruses display interesting features of growth regulation not previously observed for the well characterized murine and avian retroviruses. The following presents a brief overview of the some of the unusual features of human leukemia viruses with some discussion of similar features in the bovine leukemia virus and simian T-cell leukemia virus, which have

genomic organization similar to that of the human T-cell leukemia viruses.

B. Pathogenesis

The T-cell leukemia and lymphoma induced by HTLV-I and -II all appear only after a very long incubation period, measured in decades (Catovsky et al. 1982). Infection is marked by seroconversion, but there is some evidence that seroconversion may occur only after very prolonged periods, ranging from 10 to 15 years from the time of infection at birth to the time of seroconversion in the teens. There is an absence of viremia in the patients and a notable lack of virus expression even in fresh tumor cell populations (Franchini et al. 1984). Stimulation of infected patient T cells with mitogens results in the expression of high levels of viral RNA and protein and the budding of virus particles (Poiesz et al. 1980).

T cells from infected patients can be made to transform normal peripheral blood T cells from uninfected people (Chen et al. 1983; Popovic et al. 1983; Miyoshi et al. 1981; Yamamoto et al. 1982). Such transformation is generally accomplished by co-cultivation and is very difficult to accomplish with cell-free virus. The transformed cells have the appearance of tumor cells, characterized both by a distinctive set of surface markers including the T4 antigen and by large lobulated nuclei similar to those of the tumor cells. The fresh tumors cells and cell lines immortalized by HTLV-I express abnormally high levels of the interleukin 2 (IL-2) surface receptor.

* Laboratory of Biochemical Pharmacology, Dana-Farber Cancer Institute, Department of Pathology, Harvard Medical School, Department of Cancer Biology Harvard School of Public Health

The absence of viremia in infected persons and the difficulty of free infection may help to explain the epidemiology of infection transmission. For most populations, including those in the Pacific rim, particularly Japan and Taiwan, and in the Caribbean, Africa, and the United States, transmission is limited to family contexts (Blattner et al. 1983). Transmission from mother to child and from infected male to female partner is documented, whereas transmission from infected female to male sex partners is thought to be rare. The virus is also transmitted by needle, either by blood transfusion or by hypodermic syringe. The latter route appears to be a significant factor in current transmission patterns of the virus, as large proportions of certain populations – for instance, intravenous drug abusers – have been found to be infected with either HTLV-I, HTLV-II, or HTLV-IV, depending upon the geographical region.

C. Genomic Organization

How might one explain the limited replication and the pathogenesis of these viruses in molecular terms?

The genomic structure of the human leukemia viruses differs from that of other retroviruses characterized to date except for the two very close relatives of these viruses, the simian T-cell leukemia virus type I (STLV-I) and, more distantly, the bovine leukemia virus (BLV). The latter, like HTLV-I, -II, and -V, is poorly infectious, and it is transmitted most commonly by the veterinarian needle. The unusual features of the organization of these viruses is pictured in Fig. 1. As with all other retroviruses the human leukemia retroviruses contain genes that encode the virion internal capsid proteins (*gag* gene proteins), genes that encode replication functions (reverse transcriptase, integrase, and protease), and genes that specify the exterior proteins which are embedded in the lipid layer that surrounds virion. The envelope protein is comprised of an exterior glycoprotein and an integral transmembrane protein. The organization of the virion structural genes and replicative genes is similar to that of the simplest avian, murine, and feline viruses.

The genome of HTLV-I, HTLV-II, and BLV viruses differs from that of other retroviruses by the presence of approximately 1500 nucleotides located between the 3' end of the envelope glycoprotein and the 3' LTR (long terminal repeat) (Seiki et al. 1983; Haseltine et al. 1984; Shimotohno et al. 1984). This region, called pX, has the capacity to encode multiple polypeptides of the size of 100 amino acids or greater. For an analysis of the coding capacity of the pX region of HTLV-I, see the review by Haseltine et al. (1984). Similar analyses indicate that the corresponding regions of HTLV-II and of BLV have the capacity to encode numerous polypeptides.

It has been demonstrated that the pX region of HTLV-I specifies at least three polypeptides which are made in infected, activated T cells (Kiyokawa et al. 1985). The largest of these proteins – of sizes 42 kD, 38 kD, and 36 kD for HTLV-I, II, and BLV, respectively – encode a protein that is located primarily in the nucleus (Goh et al. 1985; Slamon et al. 1985). Initially we have called this protein the *X-lor* protein for the product of the long open reading frame within the X region; however, we now refer to it as the *tat* gene product for *trans*-activator (see below) (Sodroski et al. 1985b). A subscript, tat_I, tat_{II}, or tat_{BLV} or tat_{STLV}, denotes the virus of origin. Approximately half the people infected with HTLV-I, whether symptomatic or not, produce antibodies to this protein. The *tat* protein is also called X or pX40 by others who have confirmed the existence of this gene product in HTLV-I and -II infected cells (Felber et al. 1986; Seiki et al. 1986).

The *tat* product is synthesized from a doubly spliced messenger RNA species

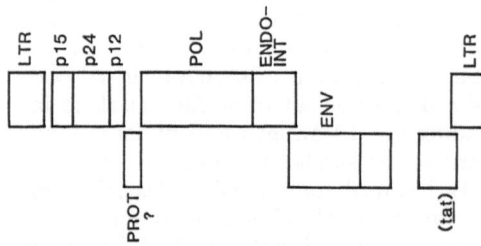

Fig. 1. Provirus structure of HTLV-I

which includes transcripts of portions of the 5' LTR, a small sequence located immediately 5' to the envelope gene, and the distal two-thirds of the pX region through the end of the 3' LTR (Sodroski et al. 1985b; Seiki et al. 1985; Wachsman et al. 1985; Aldovini et al. 1986).

It has recently been reported for HTLV-I that this same messenger RNA species encodes two other polypeptides from an overlapping reading frame (Fig. 1) (Kiyokawa et al. 1985; Nagashima et al. 1986). The initiating codons for the larger of these two polypeptides is located 5' to the site of initiation of the *tat* gene product. The same splice donor-acceptor combinations as is used for production of the *tat* gene product places the alternative open reading frame in the correct register with a second open reading frame which overlaps that used to produce the *tat* gene product. The product of this second initiation event is a 27 kD protein. The protein is phosphorylated and located predominantly in the nucleus (Kiyokawa et al. 1985). The protein is called pp27, denoting both its size and the observation that it is phosphorylated. A second polypeptide is also synthesized from the same reading frame as is the pp27 protein. This third product of the pX region is thought to be initiated at an AUG codon within the second coding exon of the messenger RNA. This protein is also phosphorylated and has an apparent molecular weight of 21 kD; it is located primarily in the cytoplasm.

It is notable that the genomes of HTLV-II (Shimotohno et al. 1985), STLV-I (Watanabe et al. 1985), and BLV (Sagata et al. 1985a, b) all possess the capacity to encode similar alternative reading frame polypeptides. Indeed, there is evidence that BLV, as does HTLV-I, in fact also encodes such proteins (Yoshinaka and Oroszlan 1985). It is a curosity that these proteins do not raise antibodies in infected people. No reactivity to these smaller proteins is observed in cattle or sheep infected with BLV. The complete coding capacity of these virus has not yet been fully explored. It is conceivable that other virally encoded proteins which are of low antigenicity in infected people are present in virus-infected cells.

D. Trans-Activation: The *tat* Protein

The phenomenon of *trans*-activating retroviral gene products was first reported for HTLV-I and -II (Sodroski et al. 1985b). It was observed that the LTRs of HTLV-I and -II function much more efficiently as promoter elements in infected than in uninfected cells (Fig. 2) (Sodroski et al. 1985b). A positive *trans*-activating genetic regulatory system requires at least two elements, the *trans*-activator product and a *cis*-acting responsive element.

The *trans*-activator product of HTLV-II was initially identified as the product of the HTLV-II pX open reading frame (Sodroski et al. 1985a). It has since been reported that the pX open reading frame of HTLV-I and of BLV also encodes a *trans*-activator (Rosen et al. 1986). Isogenic cell lines which differ only in their ability to express the long open reading frame product are capable of *trans*-activation. Gene expression directed by a plasmid which carries the *trans*-activator gene has been shown to stimulate the homologous LTR of HTLV-I, -II, and BLV (Sodroski et al. 1985a; Pashkalis et al. 1986; Rosen et al. 1986; Fujisawa et al. 1986). Plasmids constructed so as to eliminate the possibility of producing the pp27 and pp21 gene products are also capable of *trans*-activation as measured in transient cotransfec-

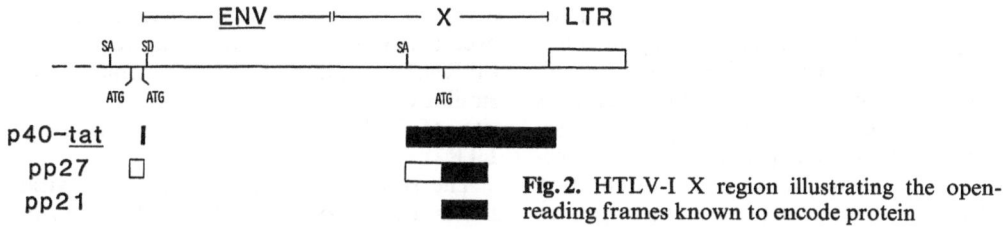

Fig. 2. HTLV-I X region illustrating the open-reading frames known to encode protein

tion assays (Kiyokawa et al. 1985). The LTR of HTLV-I can also be activated by the *tat* gene product of either HTLV-I or -II but not by the *tat* BLV product (Sodroski et al. 1985 a; Rosen et al. 1986).

The increase in LTR-directed gene expression induced by the *tat* genes is accompanied by an increase in the steady-state level of corresponding messenger RNA species (Sodroski et al. 1985 b; Felber et al. 1985). The increase in messenger RNA levels of heterologous genes directed by the LTR corresponds very roughly to the level of increase observed for protein expression. However, precise correspondence is difficult to document and post-transcriptional alterations in the efficiency of mRNA utilization cannot be ruled out entirely. A cautionary note is in order. At present *trans*-activation of viral genes is only inferred from the ability of the *trans*-activator proteins to increase the expression of heterologous genes directed by the HTLV LTRs. Direct induction of viral genes by the *trans*-activators has not yet been reported. Therefore the ability of the *tat* gene alone to stimulate the expression of viral genes is not established.

The *cis*-acting regulatory sequences, called TAR (*trans*-acting responsive region), were initially found to be located in the U3 region of the viral LTR, entirely 5′ to the site of initiation of viral RNA synthesis (Rosen et al. 1985). It was noted above that the U3 element of the HTLV-I and -II LTRs contained 21 nucleotide sequences repeated several times and that the sequences of these repeat units were preserved between HTLV-I and -II (Sodroski et al. 1984). It was also observed that except for these repeated sequences and for a short region near the site of RNA initiation, the sequences of the HTLV-I and -II LTRs are notably different as compared to the extent of conservation of other parts of the genomic sequences. Recently synthetic oligonucleotides which correspond to these 21-nucleotide long sequences have been demonstrated to convey a response to the *trans*-activator upon heterologous promoters (Shimotohno et al. 1986). The response to the *trans*-activator is observed when the 21-nucleotide repeat sequences are located proximal to the promoter and is irrespective of the orientation of the 21-nucleotide sequence with respect to

the promoter. In some experiments a single repeat unit suffices to convey the *trans*-activation response (Rosen et al., to be published) whereas others report that two or more 21-nucleotide long sequences, tandemly repeated, are required for the *trans*-activation effect. These repeat units are called TAR-21 sequences to denote the observation that they convey a responsive phenotype (Rosen et al., to be published).

Another cautionary note is appropriate. Although the TAR-21 sequences do permit increased expression of both homologous and heterologous promoters in the presence of the *trans*-activators, the response is weak and the level of expression of heterologous genes is one or two orders of magnitude below that observed for promoters and their natural configuration – even for promoters which contain 5′ deletions that preserve only the TAR-21 sequence located proximal to the promoter (Rosen et al. 1985). This observation suggests that promoter strength and inducibility depend upon the sequences adjacent to TAR-21.

Two other curious features of the viral promoters are notable. The promoter strength of HTLV-I is dependent upon sequences located 3′ to the site of RNA initiation, within the R and U5 regions of the LTR (Derse and Casey 1986; Rosen et al., to be published). A set of nested deletions originating in the U5 region of the HTLV-I LTR and extending to the site of RNA initiation results in a progressive weakening of promoter activity. Gene expression directed by such altered LTRs is inducible by the *trans*-activator genes, although the ultimate level of LTR-directed gene expression is progressively diminished both in the induced and uninduced states by these deletions. Evidently the R and U3 region of the viral LTR encodes sequences important for high-level LTR-directed gene expression. Location of these sequences 3′ to the site of RNA initiation raises the possibility that they may be involved in post-transcriptional regulatory events as well as in contributing to the rate of RNA initiation. Sequences which have similar effects are reported to exist 3′ to the site of RNA initiation within the BLV LTR.

The second notable feature of the viral LTRs lies in asymmetry in the function of the HTLV-I and -II sequences. The LTR of HTLV-I functions well as a promoter of heterologous genes in a wide variety of cell types, unrestricted as regards species or tissue of origin (Rosen et al. 1985). The activity of the HTLV-II LTR is markedly limited (Sodroski et al. 1985). It functions well in very few cell types. It is remarkable that the HTLV-II LTR does not function as a promoter in most human lymphoid cell lines, whether they be T or B cells. In fact, no promoter activity was observed in two human lymphoid cell lines that expressed a functional tat_{II} product (Sodroski et al. 1985a). The tat_{II} product in these cell lines was found to be capable of stimulating the HTLV-I LTR, while in the same cell lines no HTLV-II promoter activity was observed. It can be concluded that the HTLV-II promoter is either extremely fastidious as regards the requirement for cell-specified expression factors or that viral gene products of the *trans*-activator are required for activity of the HTLV-II LTR. Such other gene products cannot be supplied by the alternative reading frame product, pp27, as the HTLV-II LTR is inactive in the cell line that is reported to express both the HTLV-I *trans*-activator and pp27 proteins. The BLV LTR also displays a narrow cell line activity and is a very poor promoter in most uninfected cell types.

E. Transactivation: The pp27 and pp21 Proteins

A recent report by Inoue et al. (1986) indicates that the pp27 protein may play an important role in virus replication via a *trans*-acting mechanism. An integrated provirus deleted for the amino terminal portion of the *env* gene was found to be defective for RNA synthesis and for *gag* gene production. The deletion was such as to eliminate the 5′ coding exons of the *tat* and pp27 proteins. Transfection of a cell line containing this defective provirus with plasmids capable of expression of the *tat* and/or pp27 proteins revealed that *gag* gene synthesis was dependent upon both *tat* and pp27 gene expression from the transfected plasmids. Moreover, no *gag* gene RNA was detected upon transfection with the *tat* expressing plasmid alone.

This observation indicates that both the *tat* and pp27 proteins are needed for the expression of viral genes. Heterologous gene synthesis directed by the HTLV-I LTR, however, is not dependent on pp27, nor does the expression of pp27 markedly affect the rate of expression of such constructs (Rosen, Sodroski, Dokhelar, and Haseltine, unpublished observations).

The function of the pp27 gene resembles in a formal sense that of the *art* gene of HIV (Table 1). Neither pp27 nor *art* are required

Table 1

	None	tat_I	pp27	$(tat_I + pp27)$
LTR_I-heterologous gene	+	+ + + +	+	+ + + +
LTR_I-gag_I	−	−	−	+ + + +
LTR_I-tat_I	+	+	+	+
LTR_I-env_I		(unknown)		
LTR_{III}-heterologous gene	+	+	+	+

	None	tat_{III}	art	$(tat_{III} + art)$
LTR_{III}-heterologous gene	+	+ + +	+	+ + + +
LTR_{III}-gag_{III}	−	−	−	+ + + +
LTR_{II}-env_{III}	−	−	−	+ + + +
LTR_{III}-tat_{III}	+	+	+	+

LTR_I is the LTR of the HTLV-I virus.
LTR_{III} is the LTR of the HIV virus.
gag_I is the *gag* gene of the HTLV-I virus.
gag_{III} and env_{III} are the *gag* and *env* genes of HIV, respectively.
tat_I and tat_{II} are the *trans*-activators of the HTLV-I and HIV viruses, respectively.

for expression of heterologous genes under the control of the LTR. However, in the absence of a second gene product the *trans*-activator genes (*tat* genes) of these viruses are insufficient to permit expression of viral *gag* proteins. We nevertheless note that the *trans*-activator genes of both viruses can be synthesized in the absence of auxiliary proteins (Rosen, Sodroski, Dokhelar, and Haseltine, unpublished observations). For both viruses the regulatory genes are controlled independently from the structural genes.

Although the *art* and pp27 genes display a formal analogy in functional terms, such similarity does not necessarily imply that the mechanism of action is the same. The *trans*-activator gene of HTLV-I acts primarily as a transcriptional *trans*-activator of the viral LTR whereas the *trans*-activator of HIV is primarily a post-transcriptional activator. It remains to be tested whether the pp27 protein possesses an antirepression function as does *art*, although the preliminary genetics suggest that this is likely. Table 1 also shows that the *tat* genes of HTLV-I and of HIV do not reciprocally *trans*-activate the heterologous virus LTRs.

F. The Mechanism of Transformation

The process of in vitro formation of tumors by HTLV-I, -II, and BLV has not been fully characterized. Infection of T cells by the virus does not result in immediate tumor formation. Rather, tumors arise rarely (1 in 100–300 infected people over a lifetime). The role of viral genes in the transformation process is strongly inferred by epidemiological studies which link seropositivity to disease as well as the observation that T-cell tumors in infected people invariably contain at least one integrated copy of the provirus (Seiki et al. 1984). It is sometimes observed that tumors contain only the 3' portion of the genome. However, most of the tumors found in patients contain, as a minimum, the 5' LTR and the pX region.

T-cell tumors in patients are clonal with respect to the site of integration of the provirus (Seiki et al. 1983; Hahn et al. 1983). The long latent period and the clonal nature

of the tumors indicate that events in addition to infection of T cells with the virus are required for the appearance of malignant tumors. Such events may represent either secondary changes occurring within the infected cell, such as somatic mutations, or changes in the immunological status of the host.

Two additional observations indicate that the viral genes play an important role in the initiation and maintenance of tumors. Tumorigenesis by the avian, murine, and feline retroviruses which contain only those genes required for virion formation and virus replication depend upon activation of cellular growth regulatory genes. This conclusion is reached from the observation that independent, virally induced tumors contain proviruses that are found integrated near the same cellular genes. Such is not the case for tumors induced by HTLV-I or BLV, for which no repeated chromosomal sites of integration have been observed in naturally occurring tumors (Seiki et al. 1983; Hahn et al. 1983). It is therefore inferred that viral genes themselves play a key role in the initiation and maintenance of the tumor phenotype.

The role of the viral genes in the transformation process is also inferred from in vitro transformation studies. Primary T cells can be immortalized by co-cultivation with infected cells treated with mitomycin C. In contrast to role cultures, recipient cell cultures continue to proliferate without continued antigen stimulation in the presence of the T-cell growth factor, IL-2. Eventually immortalized cells emerge from such cultures (Chen et al. 1983; Popovic et al. 1983; Miyoshi et al. 1981; Yamamoto et al. 1982). The expanding population of T cells is initially polyclonal with respect to the site of provirus integration. Cell lines that are monoclonal with respect to the sites of viral integration eventually emerge from the population and dominate the culture. Such cell lines may remain dependent upon IL-2 for growth or may become capable of IL-2 independent growth, depending on cell culture conditions. Such immortalized primary cells are typically T4$^+$ cells as are most HTLV-I induced tumors. T8$^+$ cell lines can be derived by co-cultivation of mitomycin-treated infected cells with primary populations of lymphocytes enriched for cells which bear the T8 antigen (DeRossi et al. 1985).

It is possible that cell lines established from patient cells are not derived from tumors themselves but represent immortalization of the normal patient T cells by a mechanism analogous to that described for immortalization of T cells via co-cultivation. In this regard Waldmann and colleagues have found the T-cell receptor beta gene rearrangement in patient and tumor cells to differ (T. Waldmann, personal communication).

Events that occur between the initiation of infection and establishment of IL-2 dependent or independent T-cell lines have not been well characterized. Selection of specific fast growing clones may occur both in infected patients as well as in vitro. It is possible that secondary changes occur within the infected cell which permit rapid growth. Alternatively, the clonality of the tumor cells may represent selection of a cell population which expresses high levels of viral proteins that promote cellular growth.

G. Induction of the IL-2 Receptor by the *Trans*-activator Gene

The promoter of the IL-2 receptor and the IL-2 genes have been cloned. Cotransfection of the promoters placed 5' to reported genes, such as the chloramphenicol acetylase transferase gene, with the *trans*-activator gene of HTLV-I has been shown to increase the level of expression of the IL-2 gene promoter (W. Greene, personal communication and our unpublished observations). The level of expression of the genes under the control of the IL-2 promoter was found be increased slightly in similar experiments. The *trans*-activator gene of HTLV-II has also been shown to increase the level of expression of the IL-2 receptor gene, albeit more weakly than that observed for the tat_I gene, at least in the particular experimental configuration used.

These observations suggest that the *trans*-activator gene of HTLV-II can contribute to the growth properties of the T cell by deregulation of genes which normally control T-cell proliferation in response to antigen stimulation. Such a model for T-cell transformation must include the additional consideration that the expression of the viral genes is dependent upon T-cell activation. Thus, an infected resting T cell should not be transformed as the viral genes are not expressed.

Although simple, this explanation for transformation does not suffice to account for the clinical observations with ATLL patients. If *tat* genes were sufficient to induce both IL-2 and IL-2 receptors, infection should lead to transformation. However, malignant growth of T cells in infected patients is a rare event. It is also possible that the pp27 and pp21 proteins play a role in the activation of cellular genes.

H. Summary

The broad outlines of mechanisms of tumorigenesis by the HTLV-I family of viruses are beginning to emerge. The viruses encode at least three genes in addition to the genes (*gag, pol,* and *env*) required for virus replication. These additional genes encoded for by the X region are likely to affect in a specific fashion the growth of lymphocytes. The *tat* gene appears to mimick at least part of the response of mature lymphocytes to recognition of the cognate antigen. That is, in T-lymphocytes the tat_I gene seems to induce the IL-2 and IL-2 receptor genes (W. Greene et al. 1986). The alternative reading-frame proteins, pp21 and pp27, have some similarity of cellular proteins that are associated with G_0 to G_1 transitions and may contribute to the transformed phenotype in cooperation with the *tat* gene.

The expression of viral genes in infected lymphocytes, the *tat* gene and pp21 and pp27 proteins, and possibly other viral genes (since the coding capacity of the X region is not exhausted by the *tat* and pp21 and pp27 proteins) may be sufficient to account for the transformation of T cells in culture. A secondary change in the infected cells in culture is not required to explain the outgrowth of cells which are clonal with respect to the site of viral genomic integration, as selection of the most rapidly growing infected cell could account for this observation.

The case of infected patients is more complex. Infection of T cells with the HTLV-I or

-II virus is not sufficient to produce malignant disease. Failure of the virus to induce malignancy in all infected T cells may be attributed to diverse causes. It is possible that viral gene expression is suppressed in most infected T cells. Certainly no viral RNA is detected in peripheral lymphocytes of infected patients which include the tumor cells themselves. Transcriptional repression of viral genes in infected cells is a sufficient explanation for the failure of the virus to transform most T cells in patients.

It is also possible that T cells which do express viral antigens are eliminated by the immune system. The observation that many tumor cell lines derived from patients contain deletions of virus structural proteins is consistent with this notion. Patients infected with HTLV-I and -II do show good immune responses to virion structural proteins.

An additional explanation may lie in homeostatic regulatory mechanisms of the immune response itself. Lymphocytes are thought to possess regulatory mechanisms that limit their proliferation response to antigen recognition. The early proliferative response of T cells in response to the presence of the cognate antigen is followed by reestablishment of a resting phase. Stabilization of the stimulated population of T cells was thought to involve activation of an internal cellular program of a repressive nature. Interaction of the activated T cells with other components of the immune system may also contribute to reestablishment of the resting state. It is conceivable that the homeostatic mechanisms regulating T-cell proliferation also regulate HTLV-I and -II gene expression and thereby limit the growth of infected cells in patients. In this view, malignant transformation by HTLV-I and -II requires bypass of the normal homeostatic mechanisms of growth control of lymphocytes. Such bypass may occur either by a secondary intracellular change that occurs in the infected cells or it may be due to a systemic failure of normal immunoregulatory mechanisms. Either process could give rise to a tumor cell population, the first by outgrowth of a cell which contains a secondary genetic lesion, and the second by overgrowth of the infected cell population by fast growing infected cells as is observed in cell culture.

The molecular biology and in vivo replication of the virus also provide some insight into the mechanisms of transmission into the virus. This family of viruses seems to be either poorly infectious or altogether noninfectious for uninfected cells. For establishment of infection it is likely that viral gene products transferred from an infected cell by cell fusion are required. The infectious unit may well be an infected cell rather than a cell previrion. In this context the X genes of this family of viruses are required for replication and may be viewed as replicative genes. Tumorigenesis may be a byproduct of the natural replicative cycle of this family of viruses.

References

1. Aldovini A, De Rossi A, Feinberg MB, Wong-Staal F, Franchini G (1986) Molecular analysis of a deletion mutant provirus of type I human T-cell lymphotropic virus: evidence for a doubly spliced x-lor mRNA. Proc Natl Acad Sci USA 83:38–42
2. Blattner WA et al. (1983) J Infect Dis 147:406–412
3. Clavel F et al. (1986) Science 233:343–346
4. Catovsky D et al. (1982) Lancet I:639–643
5. Chen IS et al. (1983) Proc Natl Acad Sci USA 80:7006–7009
6. De Rossi A et al. (1985) Virology 163:640–645
7. Derse D, Casey JW (1986) Science 231:1437–4411
8. Felber BK, Paskalis H, Kleinman-Ewing C, Wong-Staal F, Pavlakis GN (1985) Science 229:675–679
9. Franchini G et al. (1984) Proc Natl Acad Sci USA 81:6207–6211
10. Greene W et al. (1986) Science 232:877
11. Hahn B et al. (1983) Nature 305:340–341
12. Haralabos P, Felber BK, Pavlakis GN (1986) Cis-acting sequences responsible for the transcriptional activation of human T-cell leukemia virus type I constitute a conditional enhancer. Proc Natl Acad Sci USA 83:6558–6562
13. Haseltine WA et al. (1984) Science 225:419–421
14. Inoue JI, Seiki M, Yoshida N (1986) Febs Lett 209:187–190
15. Josephs SF, Wong-Staal F, Manzari V, Gallo RC, Sodroski JG, Trus MD, Perkins D, Patarca R, Haseltine WA (1984) Long terminal repeat structure of an American isolate of type I human T-cell leukemis virus. Virology 139:340–345

16. Kanki PJ et al. (1986) Science 232:238–243
17. Kiyokama T, Seiki M, Iwashita S, Imagawa K, Shimiza F, Yoshida M (1985) p27^{x-III} and p21^{x-III}, proteins encoded by the pX sequence of human T-cell leukemia virus type I. Proc Natl Acad Sci USA 82:8359–8363
18. Kunitada S, Masako T, Tsoshiyuki T, Masanao M (1986) Requirement of multiple copies of a 21-nucleotide sequence in the U3 regions of human T-cell leukemia virus type I and type II long terminal repeats for *trans*-acting activation of transcription. Proc Natl Acad Sci USA 83:8112–8116
19. Miyoshi I (1981) Nature 294:770–774
20. Nagashima K, Yoshida M, Seiki M (1986) A single species of pX mRNA of human T-cell leukemia virus type I encodes *trans*-activator p40^x and two other phosphoproteins. J Virol 60:394–399
21. Poiesz B et al. (1981) Proc Natl Acad Sci USA 77:7415–7419
22. Popovic M et al. (1983) Proc Natl Acad Sci USA 80:5402–5406
23. Rice NR, Stephens RM, Couez D, Deschamps J, Kettmann R, Burny A, Gilden RV (1984) Virology 138:82–93
24. Rosen CA, Sodroski JG, Haseltine WA (1985) Proc Natl Acad Sci 82:6502–6506
25. Rosen CA, Sodroski JG, Willems L, Kettmann R, Campbell K, Zaya R, Burny A, Haseltine WA (1986) The 3' region of bovine leukemia virus genome encodes a *trans*-activator protein. EMBO 5(10):2585–2589
26. Sagata N, Yasunaga T, Tsuzuku-Kawamura J, Ohishi K, Ogawa Y, Ikawa Y (1985a) Complete nucleotide sequence of the genome of bovine leukemia virus: its evolutionary relationship to other retrovirus. Proc Natl Acad Sci USA 82:677–681
27. Sagata N, Yasunaga T, Igawa Y (1985b) Two distinct polypeptides may be translated from a single splice mRNA of the X genes of human T cell leukemia and bovine leukemia virus. FEBS Lett 192:37–42
28. Seiki M et al. (1983a) Proc Natl Acad Sci USA 80:3618–3622
29. Seiki M et al. (1983b) Nature 309:640–642
30. Seiki M, Hikikoshi A, Taniguchi T, Yoshida M (1985) Science 228:1532–1534
31. Seiki M, Inoue J, Takeda T, Yoshida M (1986) Direct evidence that p40^x of human T-cell leukemia virus type I is a *trans*-acting transcriptional activator. EMBO 5(3):561–565
32. Shimotohno et al. (1984) Proc Natl Acad Sci USA 81:6657–6661
33. Shimotohno K, Takahashi Y, Shimizyi N, Golde DW, Chen ISY, Miwa M, Sugimara T (1985) Complete nucleotide sequence of an infectious clone of human T-cell leukemia virus type II: an open reading frame for the protease. Proc Natl Acad Sci USA 82:3101–3105
34. Slamon DJ, Shimotohno K, Cline MJ, Golde DW, Chen ISY (1984) Science 226:61–65
35. Slamon DJ, Press MF, Souza LM, Murdock DC, Cline MJ, Golde DW, Gasson JC, Chen ISY (1985) Science 228:1427–1430
36. Sodroski J, Rosen C, Wong-Staal F, Salahuddin SZ, Popovic M, Arya S, Gallo RC, Haseltine WA (1985a) Science 227:171–173
37. Sodroski J, Rosen C, Goh WC, Haseltine W (1985b) Science 228:1430–1434
38. Wachsman W, Golde DW, Temple PA, Orr EC, Clark SC, Chen ISY (1985) Science 228:1534–1537
39. Watanabe T, Seiki M, Tsujimoto H, Miyoshi I, Hayami M, Yoshida M (1985) Sequence homology of the simian retrovirus genome with human T-cell leukemia virus type I. Virology 114:59–65
40. Yamamoto M et al. (1982) Science 217:737–740
41. Yoshinaka Y, Oroszlan S (1985) Bovine leukemia virus post-envelope gene coded protein: evidence for expression in natural infection. Biochem Biophys Res Com 131:347–354

Haematology and Blood Transfusion   Vol. 31
Modern Trends in Human Leukemia VII
Edited by Neth, Gallo, Greaves, and Kabisch
© Springer-Verlag Berlin Heidelberg 1987

Complete Nucleotide Sequences of Functional Clones of the Virus Associated with the Acquired Immunodeficiency Syndrome, HTLV-III/LAV

L. Ratner [1], A. Fisher [2], L. L. Jagodzinski [3], R.-S. Liou [3], H. Mitsuya [4], R. C. Gallo [2], and F. Wong-Staal [2]

There is considerable evidence that the human T-lymphotropic virus type III/lymphadenopathy-associated virus (HTLV-III/ LAV) is the etiological agent in the acquired immunodeficiency syndrome (AIDS) and AIDS-related syndromes [1]. The most convincing line of evidence is the recapitulation with in vitro infection of the major manifestation of the disease, depletion of T4 cells [2]. Definition of the viral determinants of this lymphocytopathic activity is critical to understanding the pathogenesis of AIDS. With this goal in mind we have established an in vitro model which will facilitate this analysis. In this system, plasmid clones with the full HTLV-III/LAV proviral sequence are transfected into normal human umbilical cord blood mononuclear cell cultures. This results in production of virus particles with a morphology typical of HTLV-III/LAV and in death of the cell culture (Fig. 1).

To provide the basic information for utilization of this assay system, we have determined the complete nucleotide sequence of the biologically active proviral clone HXB2 [3]. Eighty nucleotide substitutions are noted, compared to the previously reported HTLV-III/LAV sequence for clone BH10 [4]. Insertions of two and three nucleotides in HXB2 compared to BH10 were recog-

nized in noncoding regions, as well as a deletion of one copy of a 36-nucleotide, tandemly repeated sequence in the overlap of *gag* and *pol*. Most notable is the lack of alterations in the size and location of each of the seven previously identified viral genes [3].

Polymorphism is also noted in the predicted amino acid sequences of the viral protein products of HXB2 compared to the other sequenced HTLV-III/LAV viruses. *Gag, pol,* and *sor* are relatively well conserved, with 0.6%–3.6%, 1.0%–4.0%, and 0.5%–10.9% amino acid substitutions respectively. *Tat, trs, env,* and *3'orf* are more polymorphic, with 0.0%–11.6%, 5.2%–16.3%, 1.7%–17.5%, and 2.9%–16.0% amino acid substitutions respectively. A number of amino acid insertions and deletions are also noted. The relationships of these sequence variations to alterations in neutralizing epitopes, receptor binding domains, and other biological characteristics of the virus remain to be determined. The use of molecularly cloned viruses generated from this in vitro system will provide reagents for approaching these problems.

The biological activity of several other HTLV-III/LAV clones was also tested in umbilical cord blood mononuclear cells and the T4+ cell line, ATH8 [3]. To test the functional capabilities of clone BH10, the missing portions of the provirus were complemented with long-terminal repeat sequences from HXB2. The resultant clone gave rise to a lymphocytopathic virus. Clone HXB3 has been partially sequenced and appears to be closely related to HXB2, differing at only 63 of 3890 positions in the 3' por-

---

[1] Division of Hematology/Oncology, Washington University, St. Louis, MO
[2] Laboratory of Tumor Cell Biology, National Cancer Institute, Bethesda, MD
[3] Biotech Research Laboratories, Inc., Rockville, MD
[4] The Clinical Oncology Program, National Cancer Institute, Bethesda

ANALYSIS OF HTLV-Ⅲ/LAV TRANSFECTED CELLS

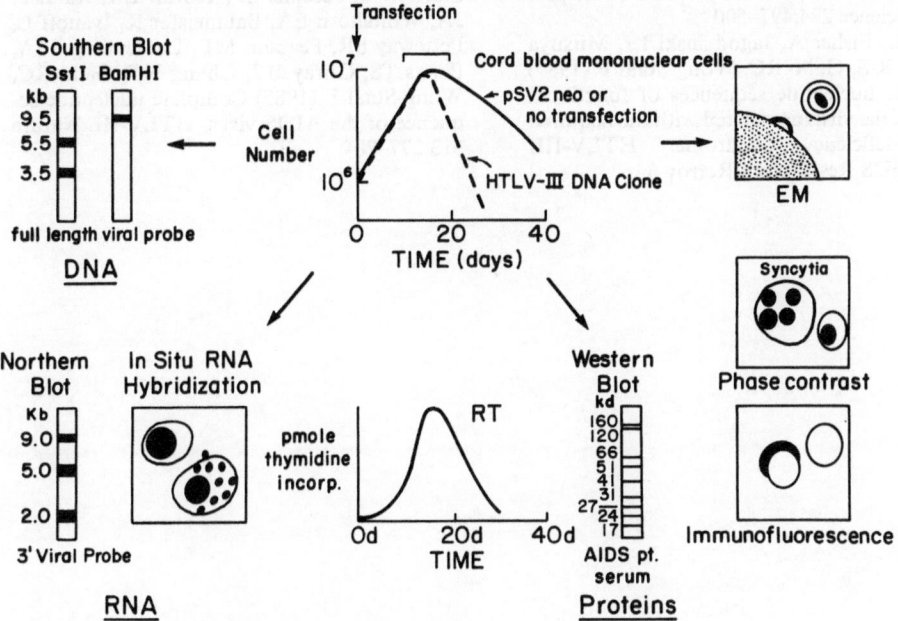

Fig. 1. An in vitro model system for AIDS. The schematic drawing depicts the major characteristics of the transfection system for analysis of the biological activity of HTLV-III/LAV DNA clones. The *top-center* drawing shows the growth curve of umbilical cord blood mononuclear cells after transfection with a plasmid lacking HTLV-III/LAV DNA sequences (pSV2neo) or a plasmid with the full HTLV-III/LAV provirus. Parameters measured 7–25 days after transfection include analysis of viral DNA by Southern blot, of viral RNA by Northern blot or in situ hybridization, of viral proteins by reverse transcriptase assays, Western blot, immunofluorescence for *gag* or *env* products, or phase-contrast microscopy for syncytia formation, and of the expression of particles with a morphology characteristic of HTLV-III/LAV

tion of the genome. A notable difference between HXB2 and HXB3, however, is the presence of a termination codon in *3'orf* of HXB2 and the lack of this sequence in HXB3. Viruses generated from HXB2 and HXB3 have similar replicative and cytopathic abilities. This finding, together with additional data on clones with deletions in *3'orf* (see Fisher et al., this volume), suggests that *3'orf* plays no essential role in the ability of HTLV-III/LAV either to replicate or to kill T4-lymphocytes.

Thus, these data provide the basic information essential for utilization of this system to construct clones of HTLV-III/LAV with alterations in the viral genome and for their assay in human lymphoid cells. Appli-

cation of this system has yielded a variant with markedly attenuated cytopathic activities but normal replication (see Fisher et al., this volume). Further applications should provide information essential to understanding the pathogenesis of cell killing in AIDS and lead to approaches to the treatment and prevention of this disease.

References

1. Gallo RC, Wong-Staal F (1985) A human T-lymphotropic retrovirus (HTLV-III) as the cause of the acquired immunodeficiency syndrome. Ann Int Med 103:679–689
2. Popovic M, Sarngadharan MG, Read E, Gallo RC (1984) Detection, isolation, and continu-

ous production of cytopathic retroviruses (HTLV-III) from patients with AIDS and pre-AIDS. Science 224:497–500

3. Ratner L, Fisher A, Jagodzinski LJ, Mitsuya H, Liou R-S, Gallo RC, Wong-Staal F (1987) Complete nucleotide sequences of functional clones of the virus associated with the acquired immunodeficiency syndrome, HTLV-III/ LAV. AIDS Res & Hum Retrov 3

4. Ratner L, Haseltine W, Patarca R, Livak KJ, Starcich B, Josephs SF, Doran ER, Rafalski JA, Whitehorn EA, Baumeister K, Ivanoff L, Petteway SR, Pearson ML, Lautenberger JA, Papas TS, Ghrayeb J, Chang NT, Gallo RC, Wong-Staal F (1985) Complete nucleotide sequence of the AIDS virus, HTLV-III. Nature 313:277–284

Haematology and Blood Transfusion   Vol. 31
Modern Trends in Human Leukemia VII
Edited by Neth, Gallo, Greaves, and Kabisch
© Springer-Verlag Berlin Heidelberg 1987

LAV/HTLV-III: Fine-structure Analysis, Localization of Structural Proteins, and Detection of Envelope Antigens by Patient Sera

G. Pauli [1], E. Hausmann [2], R. Weiss [3], P. Clapham [3], J. Schneider [4], G. Hunsmann [4], R. C. Gallo [5], M. D. Daniel [6], M. A. Koch [2], and H. Gelderblom [2]

LAV/HTLV-III was investigated by thin-section and immunoelectron microscopy. Formation of the virion takes place at the cell membrane. The inner components are assembled concomitant with budding, as is characteristic of type-C oncovirinae. Different from type-C viruses and typical for the subgroup of lentivirinae, these components in immature particles form an 18-nm broad, electron-dense spherical shell apposed to the viral membrane. After budding the structural components are rearranged ("maturation"). The electron-dense nucleoid formed is surrounded by a prismatic electron-opaque core shell 4–5 nm thick [1]. From immunocryoultramicrotomy, using monoclonal as well as monospecific antibodies, we concluded that the core shell is built up by p24. The inner leaflet of the envelope is covered by a 5–7-nm electron-dense layer with p18 antigenicity.

Adjacent to this layer we observed electron-dense "lateral bodies" with unknown composition and function. Knobs on the viral envelope can be demonstrated with tannic acid-treated samples. While on budding or immature particles a uniform fringe of equidistantly spaced spikes is visible, which can be labelled with anti-gp120 and/or anti-gp41 antibodies, mature virions lack these projections partially or completely. The spontaneous loss of knobs seems to be rapid. This became particularly evident when parallel cultures harvested at different times were investigated. Five- to 7-day-old cultures only rarely contained spiked particles. The knobs, about 70–80 per virion, have a height of 9 nm above the unit membrane and a diameter of 15 nm. They are connected to the virion via stalks 7–8 nm thick [2].

When patient sera were investigated by IEM it could be shown that LAV/HTLV-III-infected individuals carry antibodies directed against different viral proteins. IEM revealed a qualitative correlation of labelling intensity of viral envelope components and neutralizing capacity. The presence of antibodies in patients and the assumption that envelope proteins are also shed in vivo have important implications. First, protecting antibodies might be captured by shed proteins and are therefore not available for neutralization. Second, circulating immune complexes (CIC) can be involved in the pathogenicity of LAV/HTLV-III. CIC of unknown composition have been frequently observed in ARC and AIDS patients. An improvement of clinical symptoms after plasmapheresis of CIC has been reported [3]. The question whether LAV/HTLV-III antigens are involved in the formation of CIC can be answered by the characterization of such complexes.

[1] Institut für Virologie der FU Berlin
[2] Robert-Koch-Institut des Bundesgesundheitsamtes
[3] Institute of Cancer Research, Chester Beatty Laboratories, London
[4] Deutsches Primatenzentrum, Göttingen
[5] National Cancer Institute, Bethesda, MD
[6] New England Regional Primate Res. Center, Southborough

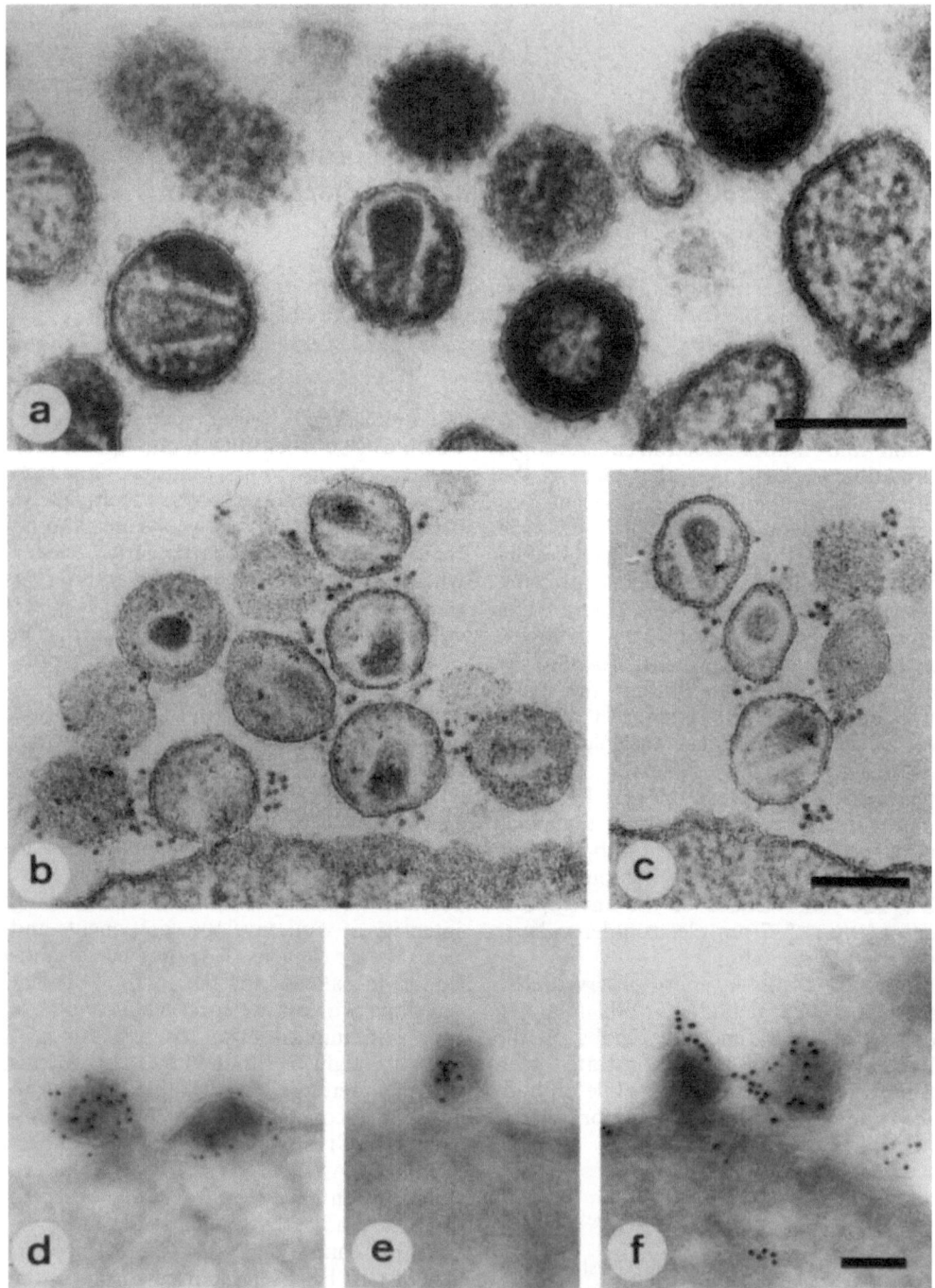

Fig. 1. a Ultrathin sections of LAV/HTLV III particles after treatment with tannic acid and Epon embedding. "Immature" particles just after budding are densely studded with knobs. The viral RNP is closely apposed to the viral membrane as a concentric shell. "Mature" particles lack the fringe of projections and show an elongated tubular core and ill-defined "lateral bodies". **b, c** Pre-embedding IEM of LAV/HTLV III using anti-gp120 (**b**) or anti-gp41 (**c**) peptide antisera. **d, e** Immuno-gold labelling of ultrathin cryosections after incubation with a p24-specific monoclonal antibody (**d**) and a monospecific anti-p24 antibody (**e**). **f** Labelling after incubation with anti-p18 hyperimmune serum leads to a shell-like distribution of the marker

References

1. Gelderblom H, Özel M, Pauli G (1985) T-Zell-spezifische Retroviren des Menschen: Vergleichende morphologische Klassifizierung und mögliche funktionelle Aspekte. Bundesgesundhbl. 28:161–171
2. Gelderblom HR, Hausmann EHS, Özel M, Pauli G, Koch MA (1987) Fine structure of human immunodeficiency virus (HIV) and immunolocalization of structural proteins. Virology 156:171–176
3. Kiprov DD, Lippert R, Sandstrom E, Jones FR, Cohen RJ, Abrams D, Busch DF (1985) Acquired immunodeficiency syndrom (AIDS)-apheris and operative risk. J Clin Apheresis 2:427–440

Haematology and Blood Transfusion   Vol. 31
Modern Trends in Human Leukemia VII
Edited by Neth, Gallo, Greaves, and Kabisch
© Springer-Verlag Berlin Heidelberg 1987

Transfusion-Acquired HIV Infection Among Immunocompromised Hosts

R. Marlink, K. Anderson, M. Essex, and J. Groopman

Introduction

Since the surveillance definition of acquired immunodeficiency syndrome (AIDS) excludes patients who have other etiologies of immunodeficiency, transfusion – associated HIV disease in immunocompromised hosts has not been described. We have studied the transmission of HIV to 25 immunocompromised cancer patients through the transfusion of blood components harvested from a single asymptomatic seropositive donor prior to the initiation of blood bank serologic screening. Recipients and their intimate contacts/family members were traced, and serologic, virologic, immunologic, and medical evaluations were performed.

Results

In this study, we documented nearly uniform transmission of HIV via blood products from a single donor to immunocompromised patients with cancer. The asymptomatic index blood component donor, nine of ten living recipients of his blood products, and cryopreserved sera available from two decreased recipients demonstrate HIV seropositivity by all available serologic techniques at a median of approximately 1 year after transfusion. The recovery of HIV from cultures of peripheral blood mononuclear cells (PBMC) of seven of nine seropositive

recipients, coupled with significant decreases in the T4:T8 ratio in seven of eight seropositive recipients, further confirms that these patients are infected with this retrovirus (Table 1).

The *only* recipient tested who remains seronegative at >2 years after transfusion received only one unit of fresh frozen plasma from the seropositive donor. Since fresh frozen plasma contains few leukocytes and is frozen then thawed prior to use, this patient may not have received a significant inoculum of infectious virus. Overall, HIV transmitted by transfusion to immunocompromised hosts appears to have an extremely high attack rate (Table 2).

Although many of the 25 recipients have died from their underlying cancer, HIV – related clinical sequelae have been noted in eight recipients (seven seropositive and one unable to be tested). To date, these sequelae have included hematologic abnormalities and opportunistic infections, together with lymphadenopathy and wasting (Table 3). The median time to development of these sequelae has been less than 1 year. This latent period in our adult immunocompromised patients resembles that of the pediatric HIV-infected population.

The HIV serologic profiles of the immunocompromised patients analyzed by native and recombinant gp41 Western blot (WB) and by radioimmunoprecipitation (RIP) were similar to serologic profiles of previously healthy high-risk seropositive individuals. Furthermore, as shown by RIP, the envelope proteins gp160 and gp120 appear to be the most immunogenic in this population.

Dept. of Cancer Biology, 665 Huntingdon Avenue, Boston, Massachusetts 02115, USA

Table 1. HIV serologic and virologic studies

Recipient patient	Interval from transfusion to ELISA seropositivity for HIV antibodies (days)	Interval from transfusion to HIV culture positivity (days)	Interval from transfusion to death (days)	T4:T8[a] at time of ELISA seropositivity for HIV antibodies
1	686	714[b]	–	0.20
2	384	659[b]	–	0.21
3	423	(647) (culture-negative)	–	1.26
4	553	643[b]	–	0.57[d]
5	380	322[c]	–	qns[a]
6	331	387[b]	–	0.21
7	323	343[b]	–	qns
8	402	615[b]	–	0.30
9	237	(267 and 322) (culture-negative)	–	0.31
10[e]	(807) (seronegative)	(807) (culture-negative)	–	1.21
13	26	NT	43	NT
21	12	NT	55	0.02

NT, not tested.

[a] Anti-T4 and anti-T8 monoclonal antibodies were used to enumerate helper-inducer and cytotoxic-suppressor cells within recipient's PBMC. Normal T4:T8 ratio is 1.5–2.5.

[b] HIV culture positivity was not documented at the same time as ELISA evidence of HIV antibody was obtained, owing either to the time of testing or to the need for repeated cultures; but this does not imply a temporal sequence for viral culture positivity and seropositivity for HIV in recipient patients.

[c] Patient 5 underwent autologous bone marrow transplantation at 256 days after transfusion as treatment for neuroblastoma and was HIV culture-positive but ELISA-seronegative at 66 days after transplant (322 days after transfusion). ELISA seroconversion was documented 58 days after cultures were positive, at 380 days after transfusion.

[d] The quantity of PBMC available was not sufficient to permit accurate phenotypic analysis.

[e] Patient 10 is the only living recipient to have received fresh frozen plasma and remains HIV seronegative and culture-negative, as well as in good health, 807 days after transfusion.

The commercial enzyme-linked immunosorbent assays (ELISA) were false-negative in three cases (patients 5, 8, and 21) on the basis of concomitant positive native WB, recombinant gp41 WB, and/or RIP with banding indicative of HIV antibodies. This false-negative ELISA "window" was during seroconversion and may be prolonged in immunocompromised hosts.

A correlation was noted between the clinical status of the patients and the presence of serum-neutralizing antibodies. The two transfusion recipients who manifested neutralizing activity (patients 1 and 3) remain asymptomatic, one after prolonged thrombocytopenia which has resolved.

The one sexual partner of a recipient who has tested positive for seroconversion is also asymptomatic and has high neutralizing titers. The seropositive blood donor is also asymptomatic, repeatedly culture-negative for HIV, and has high titers of serum-neutralizing activity. In contrast, seven of nine seropositive recipients who lack neutralizing activity have manifested severe clinical complications indicative of HIV infection. These observations strongly support the view that an in vitro assay for neutralizing antibody, utilizing a stringent cut-off of $\geq 90\%$ inhibition of HIV infection, may have clinical and prognostic significance.

Table 2. Characterization of HIV antibodies

Recipient patient	Day after transfusion	ELISA[a]	WB		RIP[d]	Neutralizing antibody[e]
			Native[b]	Recombi-nant gp41[c]		
1	714	+	+	+	+	+
2	384	+	+	+	+	−
	659	+	+	+	+	
3	423	+	+	NT	+	+
	647	+	+	+	+	
4	553	+	+	+	+	−
5	322	−	+	+	+	−
	380	+	+	+	+	
6	387	+	+	+	+	−
7	323	+	+	+	+[f]	−
	343	+	+	+	+	
8	267	−	−[g]	−	+	−
	296	−	NT	NT	+	
	337	−	NT	NT	+	
	402	+	NT	NT	+	
	443	+	+	+	+	
9	269	+	+	+	+[f]	−
10	807	−	−	−	−	−
13	43	+	+	+	+	−
21	2 days before transfusion	−	+	+	+[f]	−
	12	+	+	+	+	−
Intimate contact of recipient						
1	686	+	+	+	+	+
6	331	−	−	−	−	−
7	323	−	NT	NT	NT	NT
13	476	−	NT	NT	NT	NT
21	620	−	−	−	−	−
23	629	−	NT	NT	NT	NT
25	370	−	NT	NT	NT	NT

NT, not tested.

[a] Positive (+) or negative (−) by repeated ELISA.

[b] Presence of bands at p24 or gp41 and of at least one other band characteristic of HIV infection (gp 120, p64/53, p34, or p17) is positive on native WB.

[c] Presence of band at gp41 on recombinant gp41 WB is positive (+).

[d] Presence of definite bands in the envelope region gp 160–120 is positive (+). Other characteristic bands (p55, p27, p24, and p17) are usually also seen on RIP.

[e] Neutralizing activity of a patient's or family members sera against HIV is determined using a modification of the assay described by Robert-Guroff et al. Neutralization is arbitrarily defined using a stringent cut-off of $\geq 90\%$ inhibition of HIV infection compared to control cultures with known HIV seronegative sera.

[f] Presence of band on RIP at gp 160/120 only.

[g] Presence of band on native WB at p24 only.

Table 3. HIV clinical sequelae[a]

Recipient patient	Status (day after transfusion)	Day after transfusion when HIV seropositive seropositive by ELISA	Manifestation of HIV infection (day after transfusion)
2	Alive (745)	384	*Pneumocystis carinii* pneumonia (745)
3	Alive (718)	423	Immune thrombocytopenic purpura, resolved (233)
5[b]	Deceased (411)	380	Persistent thrombocytopenia (286) *Pneumocystis carinii* pneumonia (411)
6	Alive (459)	331	Persistent thrombocytopenia (56)
7	Deceased (365)	323	*Pneumocystis carinii* pneumonia (365)
8	Alive (718)	402	Recurrent cryptococcal meningitis (266) Lymphadenopathy, wasting and lymphopenia (456)
14	Deceased (194)	NT	Lymphopenia and Candida esophagitis (169) Undefined pneumonia (194)
21[c]	Deceased (54)	12	Cytomegalovirus pneumonia (54)

NT, not tested

[a] HIV clinical sequelae observed by 1 March 1986.

[b] Patient 5 underwent autologous bone marrow transplantation at 256 days after transfusion as treatment for neuroblastoma and was HIV viral-culture-positive but ELISA seronegative at 66 days after transplant (322 days after transfusion). ELISA seroconversion was documented 58 days after cultures were positive, at 380 days after transfusion.

[c] Patient 21 underwent autologous bone marrow transplantation 18 days before the transfusion of platelets from the seropositive donor. At 30 days after transplant (12 days after transfusion) she was seropositive, and at 66 days after transplant (54 days after transfusion) she died of cytomegalovirus pneumonia.

Summary

This survey suggests that HIV infection in immunocompromised hosts is characterized by a high attack rate, short incubation time to clinical sequelae, and WB and RIP seropositivity which may precede evidence of antibodies by ELISA by weeks or months. The functional properties of patients' serum antibodies, such as neutralizing activity against HIV in vitro, may correlate with clinical course.

References

1. Allan JS, Coligan JE, Barin F et al. (1985) Sience 228:1091–1094 – Centers for Disease Control (1985) MMWR 34:373–375
2. Cabradilla CD, Groopman JE, Lanigan J (1986) Biotechnology 4:128–133
3. Church JA, Isaacs H (1984) J Petdiatr 105:731–737
4. Robert-Guroff M, Brown M, Gallo RC (1985) Nature 316:72–74
5. Scott GB, Buck BE, Leterman JG, Bloom FL, Parks WP (1984) N Engl J Med 310:76–81

Haematology and Blood Transfusion   Vol. 31
Modern Trends in Human Leukemia VII
Edited by Neth, Gallo, Greaves, and Kabisch
© Springer-Verlag Berlin Heidelberg 1987

Restricted Neutralization of Divergent HTLV-III/LAV Isolates by Antibodies to the Major Envelope Glycoprotein

Th. J. Matthews[1], A. J. Langlois[1], W. G. Robey[2], N. T. Chang[3], R. C. Gallo[4], P. J. Fischinger[2], and D. P. Bolognesi[1]

A. Summary

By analogy to other retroviruses, the major envelope glycoprotein – gp120 – of HTLV-III/LAV is a probable target for neutralizing antibody. This antigen has been purified from H9 cells chronically infected with the HTLV-III$_B$ prototype strain. Several goats immunized with the gp120 produced antibodies that neutralized infection of H9 by the homologous virus isolate. These same sera failed to neutralize the divergent HTLV-III$_{RF}$ isolate. Individuals infected with HTLV-III/LAV commonly develop antibodies to gp120 which could be isolated using the gp120 antigen coupled to an immunoadsorbent resin. The antibody fraction that bound tightly to such a resin was found to neutralize the III$_B$ but not the RF isolate in a fashion similar to that of the goat anti-gp120 sera. However, the nonbinding fraction (effluent) from the resin also contained neutralizing activity which was able to block infection by both virus isolates with similar efficacy. Human antibodies to the other virus envelope gene product, the transmembrane gp41, were also affinity-purified utilizing the recombinant peptide 121, but they failed to influence infection by either virus isolate.

B. Introduction

Human T-cell lymphotropic virus type III (HTLV-III) is a pathogenic human retrovirus that is structurally and genetically related to the subfamily Lentivirinae [1]. Epidemiological studies combined with virus isolation and antibody detection in acquired immunodeficiency syndrome (AIDS) or AIDS-related complex (ARC) cases, especially in blood donors and recipients, have defined the association of HTLV-III infection with AIDS [2–5]. The virus contains an RNA genome capable of coding for at least six gene products [6–9]. The envelope (env) gene products and the internal structural gene (*gag*) products are the most antigenic in man because antibodies to them are readily detectable in patients by a variety of tests [4, 10–12]. We [15] and others [10, 12] have recently reported some of the characteristics of the HTLV-III envelope gene products. The primary gene product of this gene is a 160000 dalton glycosylated protein (gp160) that is processed by proteolysis into a gp120 external glycoprotein and a gp41 transmembrane protein [10, 12, 15].

Purification of HTLV-III gp120 to homogeneity was possible through the use of infected cells or cell culture fluids as the source of the glycoprotein [16]. The purified material is immunogenic in goats, horses, and rhesus monkeys in that antibody to gp120

[1] Department of Surgery, Duke University Medical School, Durham, North Carolina 27710, USA
[2] Office of Director, National Cancer Institute-Frederick Cancer Research Facility (NCI-FCRF), Frederick, Maryland 21701, USA
[3] Center for Biotechnology, Baylor College of Medicine, Houston, Texas 77025, USA
[4] Laboratory of Tumor Cell Biology, National Cancer Institute, National Institutes of Health, Bethesda, Maryland 20892, USA

both precipitated gp120 and neutralized the infectivity of HTLV-III in cell culture. These results suggest that the establishment of protective humoral immunity to HTLV-III may be theoretically possible in man [16].

Neutralization of HTLV-III/LAV by naturally occurring human antibodies has been observed by several investigators with varying degrees of efficiency depending on the type of assay utilized [13, 14, 17]. However, two major issues concerning the specificity of virus neutralization require resolution. First, it has not been demonstrated that the antibodies in HTLV-III/LAV-infected individuals neutralize virus through reactivity with a virus-encoded gene product. Second, it is not known to what extent the neutralizing activity relates to the genetic diversity of the various isolates which is found in large part in the envelope gene of the virus [18, 19]. The exterior-envelope-encoded product of HTLV-III/LAV has been identified as gp120 [10, 11, 15, 20] and, by analogy to other retrovirus systems, is likely to represent the major target of neutralizing antibodies [21]. Interspersed within this gene are both hypervariable and conserved regions [19], both of which may contribute to formation of epitopes involved in virus neutralization. Retroviruses can also incorporate cellular antigens into their envelope structure, and it is known that antibodies to leukocyte alloantigens can neutralize virus infectivity [22]. Recent studies suggest that HLA-DR molecules can be found in association with HTLV-III/LAV and that some AIDS-related sera contain antibodies to these determinants [23].

In this study it was our aim to examine the role of the HTLV-III envelope gene product, gp120, as a target for neutralizing antibody and to assess the impact of gp120 polymorphism on such antibodies. We have compared the ability of heterologous antisera raised against purified gp120 and gp120 affinity-purified human antibodies to block infection by the homologous virus isolate, HTLV-III$_B$, as well as by the widely divergent Haitian HTLV-III$_{RF}$ isolate [18]. The nucleotide sequences of these two isolates predict a 21% difference in amino acid residues in the corresponding gp120 polypeptides [19]. Both isolates readily infect the H9 cell line [18, 24], and it was thus possible to compare directly the activity of the various antibodies on these two dissimilar genotypes under the same assay conditions.

C. Materials and Methods

I. Cells

Uninfected H9 cells, H9 cells chronically infected with HTLV-III$_B$, and H9 chronically infected with the Haitian isolate HTLV-III$_{RF}$ have been described [18, 24]. Cells were maintained in RPMI 1640 (GIBCO, Grand Island, New York) supplemented with 20% fetal calf serum, penicillin (100 units/ml), and streptomycin (100 µg/ml).

II. Virus

Virus stocks were prepared from 100 ml cultures of chronically infected H9 cells that had been passed into fresh medium 24 h before harvesting. Cells were removed by centrifugation, and the supernatants were filtered through a 0.45 µm Millipore filter and frozen at −70 °C in 1 ml aliquots. The infectious titer of the virus stocks was measured in the following manner. Tenfold dilutions were made in growth medium, and 0.1 ml of each dilution was added to six well plates (Falco Labware) containing 1×10^5 H9 cells in 0.2 ml growth medium. The medium volume was doubled daily for 6 days. On the 7th day, cell clumps were disrupted and the culture volume was reduced to 0.5 ml. Fresh medium was added as before for 2 more days, after which growth of virus in the cultures was monitored on the basis of sedimentable reverse transcriptase (RT) activity (see below). The infectious titer of the virus stocks was taken as the highest dilution that yielded RT activity at least 20-fold that of background activity. Both the HTLV-III$_B$ and RF isolates yielded virus stocks ranging in titer from 10^4 to 10^5 infectious units/ml.

III. Neutralization Assay

The virus stocks were diluted with growth medium to give 1000 infectious units per 0.1 ml, and that volume was added to individual wells of the six Falcon well plates. Fourfold dilutions of test sera were made in growth medium, filtered (0.45 μm Millipore), and 100 μl of each dilution was added in duplicate to the virus-containing wells. The plates were incubated at 37 °C for 30 min, after which 1×10^5 H9 cells were added to each well in a volume of 0.1 ml. Fresh medium was added each day as described above, and the cultures were tested for virus release 10 days later. For that purpose, cells were removed by centrifugation and the supernatants assayed for RT activity. Briefly, virus was concentrated from 3 ml of culture fluid by precipitation with polyethylene glycol (PEG) and resuspended in 0.12 ml of Triton X-100 containing lysis buffer as described [25]. Duplicate 10 μl samples were tested for RT activity using poly (rA) p(dT) 12–18 as template primer [24, 25]. The results are expressed as average counts per minute per 10 μl sample assayed. The neutralizing titer of individual sera was defined as the reciprocal of the serum dilution required to inhibit RT activity by 50% in relation to no serum controls.

IV. Antigens

The purification and characterization of gp120 from H9 cells chronically infected with HTLV-III$_B$ is described elsewhere [26]. Briefly, the antigen was isolated by affinity chromatography from cell lysates. The sequence of the N-terminal 18 amino acid residues matched that predicted by the corresponding env gene nucleotide sequence of the BH10 clone of HTLV-III$_B$ [7]. A similar procedure was used to isolate gp120 from HTLV-III$_{RF}$. The recombinant peptide 121 is encoded by sequences in the transmembrane gp41 env gene and is specifically reactive with most, if not all, HTLV-III antibody-positive human sera [27].

V. Affinity Chromatography

Immunoadsorbent resins were prepared by coupling the purified gp120 (about 0.5 mg) or the peptide 121 (about 5 mg) to cyanogen-bromide-activated Sepharose 4B (Pharmacia) [28]. Two ml of test serum was incubated with these resins for about 2 h at room temperature. Nonbinding protein was washed from the resins with phosphate-buffered solution (PBS) until no further A280 absorbing material was detected. This flow through fraction was collected as effluent (usually 20–30 ml). The resins were further washed with 10 bed volumes of PBS (discarded). The bound fraction was eluted with 4 M magnesium chloride and dialyzed against PBS. The effluent was concentrated to about 2 ml and rechromatographed over the resins as before. This process was repeated so that each serum was passed over the indicated resins a total of three times. The eluate fractions were pooled together, and both the final effluent fraction and the eluate pool were concentrated to 2 ml through an Amicon PM10 filter.

D. Results

I. Neutralization
by Unfractionated Human Serum

We have examined the ability of human serum to block infection of H9 cells in an assay system similar to that described by Robert-Guroff et al. [14], except that the end-point measurements for virus infection were based on development of sedimentable RT or levels of viral p24 antigen in the supernatant of challenged cells. A comparison of these tests using a human AIDS serum is shown in Table 1. Over 100 HTLV-III antibody-positive sera have been tested, about 90% of which were found to prevent infection completely at low-serum dilutions (1 : 8). This effect was titratable such that it was possible to assign to individual sera a specific neutralization end point based on the reciprocal of the serum dilution required to block RT activity by 50%. The most active of the sera tested yielded neutralization titers of about 500–1000 when assayed in this manner. Patient sera positive for antiviral antibodies with no neutralizing activity in these experiments were from individuals who either had recently seroconverted (2–6 months) or were in late stage of disease. At a serum dilution of 1–8 or higher, none of 55 antibody-negative sera showed any inhibi-

Table 1. Neutralization of HTLV-III as measured by RT and viral p24 antigen

Serum dilution[a] (Reciprocal)	RT[b] (cpm)	p24[c] (ng/ml)
8	2 500	< 1
32	1 700	< 1
128	70 000	100
2048	82 000	140
No serum	68 000	130

[a] Serum from an AIDS patient was tested for neutralization of HTLV-III$_B$, as described in Sect. B.
[b] Ten days after infection, virus was concentrated from a 3 ml portion of cell-free supernatant for measurement of RT.
[c] A second portion of cell-free supernatant at 10 days was made in 0.5% Triton X-100 and tested for viral p24 antigen, using a competition radio-immunoassay developed by E.I. DuPont de Nemours and Company, Wilmington, Delaware. The lower limit of detection with this assay is about 1 ng/ml of culture supernatant.

tory activity. A compendium of these results will be reported elsewhere and in general are in agreement with those of Robert-Guroff et al. [14].

An example of a titration of a strongly neutralizing serum taken from an individual with PGL (persistent generalized lymphadenopathy) is shown in Fig. 1. Each dilution of serum was tested on 1000 infectious units of

both the HTLV-III$_B$ and HTLV-III$_{RF}$ isolates. Both viruses were effectively neutralized with 50% neutralization titers of 700 for the III$_B$ and 600 for the RF isolates – not a significant difference in this assay. To date, we have titrated 15 antibody-positive human sera against these two virus prototypes. Of the sera tested, seven failed to neutralize either virus, while the remaining sera blocked infection by both viruses with no more than a twofold difference in titer.

II. Neutralization by Goat Anti-HTLV-III$_B$ gp120 Sera

As described elsewhere [26], purified gp120 from HTLV-III$_B$ was used to obtain heterologous sera from two goats. One of these animals (NATIVE) received antigen exposed only to 4 M magnesium chloride and 0.1% Triton X-100. The other animal (PAGE) received the gp120 following sodium dodecyl sulfate (SDS) denaturation and electrophoresis as a final purification step. The antigens (50 µg per immunization) were administered intradermally in Freund's complete adjuvant twice over a 5-week period, after which the sera utilized for these studies were taken. We have reported elsewhere [26] that both of these animals developed antibodies that were capable of neutralizing the homologous HTLV-III$_B$ virus isolate. Thus, the

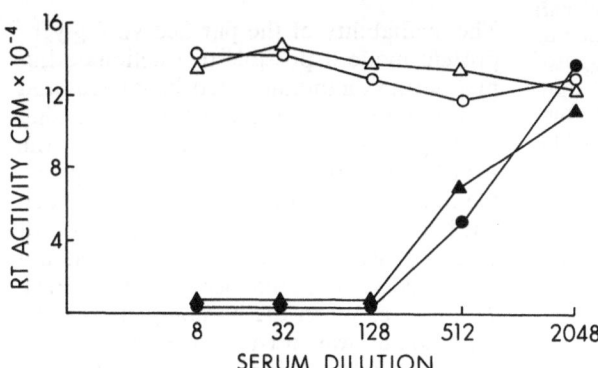

Fig. 1. Titration of human serum for neutralization of HTLV-III$_B$ and HTLV-III$_{RF}$. Sera were obtained from a seronegative laboratory worker (*open*) and a seropositive bisexual with persistent generalized lymphadenopathy (*closed*). Serial fourfold dilutions of each sera were incubated for 30 min with 1000 infectious units of each HTLV-III$_B$ (*circles*) and HTLV-III$_{RF}$ (*triangles*). The virus-sera mixtures were added to H9 cells, and virus propagation was monitored 10 days later on the basis of sedimentable RT activity in the supernatant of the cultured cells

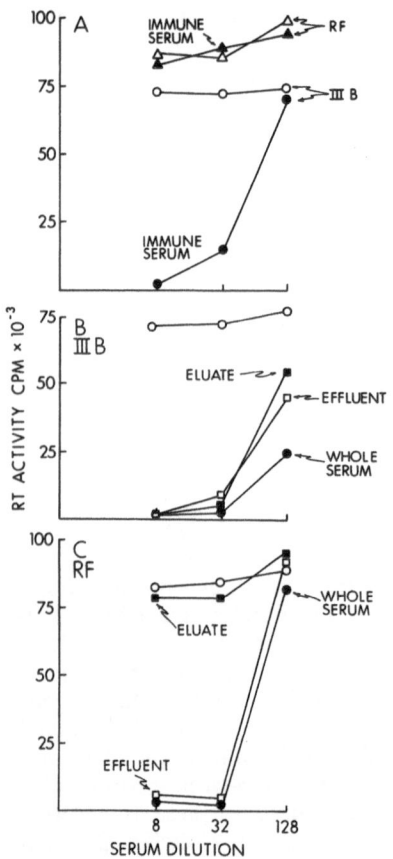

Fig. 2a–c. Titration of goat anti-HTLV-III$_B$ gp120 serum (**a**) and human serum fractions (**b** and **c**) for neutralization of HTLV-III$_B$ and HTLV-III$_{RF}$. In **a**, dilutions of preimmune goat serum (*open*) and immune goat serum (*closed*) were tested for their ability to block infection of the HTLV-III$_B$ isolate and the HTLV-III$_{RF}$ isolate. Panels **b** and **c** a 2 ml sample of serum from a seropositive homosexual with PGL was fractionated on an immunoadsorbent resin containing HTLV-III$_B$ gp120. Untreated serum, flow-through or effluent fraction, and eluate fraction were titrated for neutralizing activity against the III$_B$ isolate (**b**) and the RF isolate (**c**). Virus production in the presence of normal human serum is indicated by the *open circles* in **b** and **c**

SDS treatment did not irreversibly destroy epitopes that can induce neutralizing antibodies. The relative activity of the PAGE serum on the divergent HTLV-III$_{RF}$ isolate in comparison to the homologous HTLV-III$_B$ is shown in Fig. 2a. Again, this serum

completely blocked infection by HTLV-III$_B$ at a dilution of 1–8 and yielded a titer of about 50. In contrast, there was no effect on the RF isolate, and the immune and preimmune bleeds from this animal were essentially identical. Each serum has been tested on both isolates three times, and the results of each experiment were the same as shown in Fig. 2.

Binding studies indicate that the inability to neutralize the RF isolate is not related to an overall lack of recognition by these goat sera. For example, in the solid-phase binding experiment shown in Table 2, the PAGE goat serum gave essentially equivalent levels of binding to the gp120 of HTLV-III$_B$ and HTLV-III$_{RF}$. It failed to react with recombinant peptide 121, and this is consistent with the apparent specificity of that serum for the gp120 portion of the envelope gene. Other radioimmunoprecipitation (RIP) and Western blot experiments (not shown) confirmed the results set out in Table 2. We conclude from these studies (a) that the neutralizing epitopes on the glycoprotein are only a subset of a larger number of potentially immunogenic sites on the molecule, and (b) that the neutralizing epitopes recognized by the goat sera are not conserved on the two divergent isolates studied here.

III. Neutralization by Human Antibodies Directed to gp120

The availability of the purified viral glycoprotein made it possible to fractionate human serum on immunoadsorbent resins and to estimate the proportion of neutralizing activity which can be attributed to the HTLV-III$_B$ gp120. Moreover, it was possible to analyze further the specificity of such antibodies with respect to neutralization of divergent isolates. An example of a serum fractionated in this manner is shown in Figs. 2b and 2c. When the homologous HTLV-III$_B$ isolate was used as the target virus (panel B), neutralizing activity could be detected in both the antibody-binding (eluate) and nonbinding (effluent) fractions. Even after repeated passes over the gp120 resin, we were unable to remove all of the neutralizing activity from the effluent. When serum fractions were tested in Western blot

Table 2. Antibody binding to gp120 of divergent isolates

Serum[b]	HTLV-III$_B$ gp120 cpm	HTLV-III$_{RF}$ gp120 cpm	Recombinant p121 cpm
Preimmune goat (1/100)	2600 ± 100	2800 ± 200	3800 ± 200
Goat anti-gp120 (1/100)	35700 ± 700	33900 ± 800	4400 ± 200
Normal human (1/10)	1800 ± 200	1600 ± 200	2900 ± 300
Human PGL (1/10)	15200 ± 400	17500 ± 600	31000 ± 600

[a] Solid-phase immunoassay was performed as described [17], except that binding antibody was monitored with ^{125}I-SpA (200000 cpm) per well. About 200 ng of each antigen was added per well of Immulon 1 microtiter strips (Dynatech Lab. Inc., Alexandria, Virginia), and sera were tested in triplicate.

[b] Sera were tested at the dilutions indicated in a final volume of 200 µl. The goat sera containing wells were incubated with 100 µl of rabbit anti-goat IgG (Cappel) at a 1–300 dilution before addition of ^{125}I-SpA.

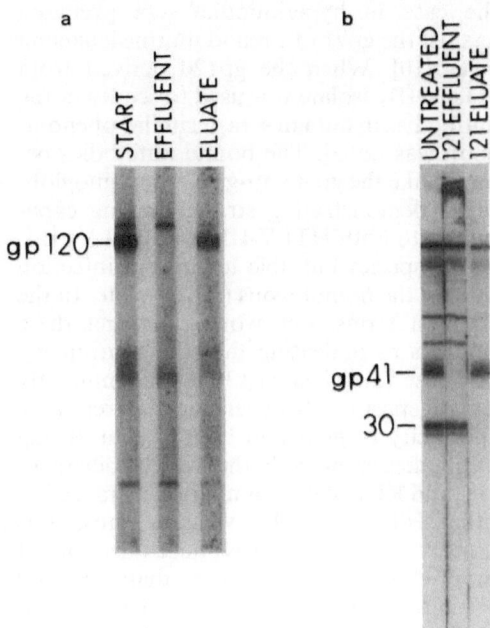

Fig. 3 a, b. Western blot analysis of human sera fractionated on affinity resins bearing gp120 (**a**) and p121 (**b**). In **a**, the serum fractions from the gp120 resin as shown in Figs. 2b and 2c were tested for binding to partially purified HTLV-III$_B$ gp120 by the Western blot technique, using ^{125}I-SpA to localize antibody. In **b**, serum from an AIDS patient was fractionated on the p121 affinity resin and tested for binding to disrupted HTLV-III$_B$ virus proteins by the Western blot procedure. Serum and serum fractions were incubated with appropriate nitrocellulose strips at a dilution of 1–100

(Fig. 3 a) and plate-binding assays, we found no evidence of anti-gp120 antibodies remaining in the effluent fraction, and essentially all of the reactivity in whole serum (Table 2) was found in the tightly binding antibody fraction which was subsequently eluted from the resin. However, when measured by immunoprecipitation of radioiodinated gp120, considerable activity was also noted in the effluent fraction (not shown). This confirms earlier conclusions that RIP analyses are the most sensitive and accurate measure of antibodies to the gp120 [29] (see Discussion for further elaboration of this point).

The results when HTLV-III$_{RF}$ was used as a target for neutralization were qualitatively different (Fig. 2 c). Of note is the fact that the activity against RF in the effluent fraction is essentially indistinguishable from that in untreated serum. In contrast, the material in the eluate had no detectable activity against the divergent RF strain. Although the absolute titers differed, three other human sera fractionated in this manner gave the same qualitative results shown in Figs. 2 b and 2 c. In all cases, the eluate fractions neutralized the III$_B$ but not the RF isolate, while the effluent fractions blocked infection by both viruses. Thus, we conclude that human serum commonly contains anti-gp120 antibodies that neutralize infection by HTLV-III in a fashion that is restricted with respect to divergent isolates. The identity of the more broadly neutralizing antibodies represented in the effluent is uncertain at this time. It is possible that these antibodies are also directed against the gp120 but bind with insufficient avidity, to be totally removed by antigen isolated from a single virus genotype. Alternatively, other viral or cellular antigens may be involved as suggested earlier.

IV. Human Serum Fractionated by Recombinant Peptide 121

All known retroviruses contain a second *env*-gene-encoded product, a transmembrane polypeptide, that under certain conditions can also serve as a target antigen for neutralizing antibody [30]. The analogous polypeptide in the case of HTLV-III has been identified as gp41 [12]. Since almost all antibody-positive human sera react with gp41, as with gp120, it was therefore a good candidate for an additional target for neutralizing antibodies. We thus performed similar analysis, as shown in Figs. 2b and 2c, using an affinity column containing the recombinant peptide 121 [27]. This molecule contains only about one-half the gp41 sequences, but a major portion of the immunodominant epitopes of gp41 [27]. In three of the six sera tested, it was possible to remove all gp41 reactivity by Western blot analysis with the p121 resin, as shown in Fig. 3b. Sensitive plate-binding assays using the 121 recombinant peptide also failed to detect antibodies in the effluent fraction. Both these measures are more effective than RIP assays for measuring antibodies to gp41, unlike the situation with gp120 [10].

Analysis in the neutralization assay revealed that the bound fractions failed to neutralize either the III_B or RF isolates, while the effluent fractions showed only a modest reduction in titer, probably resulting from manipulative losses rather than from any specific effects. Rabbit serum raised against p121 also failed to neutralize the virus, even though it reacted strongly with gp41 (not shown). These results do not rule out the possibility that neutralization targets exist on gp41 which are not contained in the recombinant peptide 121. Nevertheless, on the basis of those sera from which we were able to remove all detectable gp41 reactivity,

we feel this antigen does not play a major role in neutralization under the conditions used.

E. Discussion

The experiments described here focus attention on the polymorphism in the gp120 envelope region of HTLV-III/LAV. On the one hand, polyclonal sera raised in goats (and in other animal species; unpublished results) bound with similar efficacy to widely divergent gp120 species, but their ability to neutralize the infectivity of the respective viruses was much more restricted. It is possible that further immunization may overcome the apparent type specificity, as has proven to be the case in hyperimmune sera prepared against the gp71 of Freund murine leukemia virus [10]. When the gp120 derived from $HTLV-III_B$ isolate was used to sequester the antibodies in human sera, a similar phenomenon was noted. The bound antibodies behaved like the goat anti-gp120 immunoglobulins, demonstrating strong binding capabilities to both $HTLV-III_B$ and $HTLV-III_{RF}$ gp120 species but able to prevent infection of only the homologous (III_B) isolate. In the simplest terms, one would interpret these findings as indicating that the neutralizing response to a given gp120 is predominantly isolate-specific. However, the apparent type specificity of goat and human neutralizing antibodies seen with the widely divergent III_B and RF isolates cannot be generalized to other HTLV-III/LAV viruses. Thus, it is quite possible that cross-neutralization of more closely related viruses than III_B and RF does occur through antibodies directed against the gp120 of a single isolate.

Analysis of the antibody fraction that did not bind to the $HTLV-III_B$ gp120 resin raises a number of additional questions. First, antibodies are present in this fraction which, in spite of their lack of binding activity to the immobilized gp120, neutralize not only the $HTLV-III_B$ but also the highly divergent $HTLV-III_{RF}$ isolate. It is possible that these antibodies represent low-affinity immunoglobulins with significant neutralizing potential. An argument in favor of this is the fact that in RIP assays, one can readily detect anti-$HTLV-III_B$ gp120 antibodies in the effluent fraction. It is not clear why these antibodies do not bind the immobilized antigen well, but it is possible that there is a better opportunity for multivalent binding and resultant stabilization of the complex when the antigen is in solution.

Other possibilities exist, however, which could explain the presence of neutralizing activities in human sera which are not related to gp120. Potential targets for neutralization include other viral antigens such as the gp41 transmembrane envelope component, which is highly immunogenic in man and known to represent a target for neutralization in animal retroviruses, albeit in the presence of complement [30]. Our studies demonstrate that at least in the absence of complement, anti-gp41 antibodies do not play a detectable role in virus neutralization and do not account for the neutralizing activity in the gp120 unbound fractions. In addition, antibodies directed against leukocyte alloantigens which can associate with the budding virion may also be targets for neutralization, as demonstrated with feline leukemia virus [22]. The presence of antibodies to HLA in HTLV-III/LAV-infected individuals has also been documented, as has the association of HLA chains with HTLV-III$_B$ [23]. Therefore, it is conceivable that at least some portion of the unbound fraction may contain such antibodies, and studies are in progress to determine this and the antibodies' potential role in virus neutralization.

Our studies represent a first step in defining the epitopes of the HTLV-III/LAV gp120 that are associated with biologically important functions and the degree to which these epitopes are immunogenic in man. The present results clearly demonstrate that this viral antigen can serve as a target for neutralizing antibodies. It is not yet known what portions of the gp120 are involved, but our results demonstrate that there is at least one such epitope that is polymorphic, i.e. not conserved in the HTLV-III$_B$ and HTLV-III$_{RF}$ isolates. If conserved sequences that can also serve as neutralizing epitopes are present, the goats immunized with gp120 have yet to recognize these regions. Likewise, it was not possible to isolate broadly reactive human neutralizing antibodies by immunoaffinity chromatography, using gp120 obtained from a single isolate. The latter result, however, could be due to other limitations of the technique, including avidity and/or steric accessibility to the epitopes in question. Because of these considerations, we cannot conclusively eliminate the possibility that conserved sites serve as targets for neutralizing antibody. The broad reactivity commonly observed with antibody-positive human sera might be due to such conserved sites or, alternatively, these might reflect a response by the individuals exposed to multiple virus genotypes. A more definitive answer to this question must await studies similar to those described here, ones utilizing purified gp120 from other prototypic strains (e.g., RF) as well as field isolates. Our results, however, raise the possibility that multiple gp120 immunogens might be required to generate antibodies that would neutralize the full spectrum of divergent viruses which exist in the population. Even if this were achievable, either naturally or through vaccination, much more needs to be learned about the role of virus neutralization in protection against HTLV-III/LAV infection.

Acknowledgements. This research was supported by NIH Program Project CA5862-06. We wish to thank Natalie Cates, Carl Stone, and Charlene McDanal for their expert technical assistance.

References

1. Gonda MA, Wong-Staal F, Gallo RC, Clements JT, Narayan O, Gilden RV (1985) Science 227:173–177
2. Gallo RC, Salahuddin SZ, Popovic M, Shearer GM, Kaplan M, Haynes BF, Palker TJ et al. (1984) Science 224:500–503
3. Shaw GM, Hahn B, Arya SK, Groopman JE, Gallo RC, Wong-Staal F (1984) Science 226:1165–1171
4. Sarngadharan MG, Popovic M, Bruch L, Schupbach J, Gallo RC (1984) Science 224:506–508
5. Safai B, Groopman JE, Popovic M, Schupbach J, Sarngadharan MG, Arnett K, Sliski NA, Gallo RC (1984) Lancet I:1438–1440
6. Wain-Hobson S, Sonigo P, Danos O, Coles S, Alizon M (1985) Cell 40:9–17
7. Ratner L, Haseltine W, Patarca R, Livak KJ, Starcich B, Josephs SF, Doran ER et al. (1985) Nature 313:277–284

8. Muesing MA, Smith DH, Cabradilla CD, Benton CV, Lasky LA, Capon DJ (1985) Nature 313:450–458
9. Sodroski J, Patarca R, Rosen CA, Wong-Staal F, Haseltine WA (1985) Science 229:74–77
10. Allan JS, Coligan JE, Barin F, McLane MF, Sodroski JG, Rosen CA, Haseltine WA, Lee TH, Essex M (1985) Science 228:1091–1093
11. Barin F, McLane MF, Allan JS, Lee TH, Groopman JE, Essex M (1985) Science 228:1094–1096
12. Veronese FD, DeVico AL, Copeland TD, Oroszlan S, Gallo RC, Sarngadharan MG (1985) Science 229:1402–1405
13. Weiss RA, Clapham PR, Cheingsong-Popov R, Dalgleish AG, Carne CA, Weller IVD, Tedder RS (1985) Nature 316:69–72
14. Robert-Guroff M, Brown M, Gallo RC (1985) Nature 316:72–74
15. Robey WG, Safai B, Oroszlan S, Arthur LO, Gonda MA, Gallo RC, Fischinger PJ (1985) Science 228:593–595
16. Matthews TJ, Langlois AJ, Robey WG, Chang NT, Gallo RC, Fischinger PJ, Bolognesi DP (in press) Proc Natl Acad Sci USA
17. Ho DD, Rota TR, Hirsch MS (1985) N Engl J Med 312:649–650
18. Wong-Staal F, Shaw GM, Hahn BH, Salahuddin SZ, Popovic M, Markham P, Redfield R, Gallo RC (1985) Science 229:759–762
19. Starcich BR, Hahn BH, Shaw GM, McNeely PD, Modrow S, Wolf H, Parks ES et al. (in press) Science
20. Montagnier L, Clarel F, Krust B, Chamaret S, Rey F, Barre-Sinoussi F, Chermann JC (1985) Virology 144:283–289
21. Schafer W, Bolognesi DP (1977) Contemp Top Immunobiol 6:127–167
22. Lee TH, Essex M, de Noronha F, Azocar J (1982) Cancer Res 42:3995–3999
23. Arthur L et al. (in press) J Immunol
24. Popovic M, Sarngadharan MG, Read E, Gallo RC (1984) Science 224:497–500
25. Poiesz BJ, Ruscetti FW, Gazdar AF, Bunn PA, Minna JD, Gallo RC (1980) Proc Natl Acad Sci USA 77:7415–7419
26. Robey WG, Arthur LO, Matthews TJ, Langlois A, Copeland TD, Oroszlan S, Bolognesi DP, Gilden RV, Fischinger PJ (in press) Proc Natl Acad Sci USA
27. Chang TW, Kato I, McKinney S, Chanda P, Barone AD, Wong-Staal F, Gallo RC, Chang NT (1985) Biotechnology 3:905–909
28. Porath J, Kristiansen T (1975) In: Neurath H, Hill RL (eds) The proteins, vol 1. Academic, New York, p 95
29. Essex M, Allan J, Kanki P, McLane MF, Malone G, Kitchen L, Lee TH (1985) Ann Intern Med 103:700–703
30. Fischinger PJ, Schafer W, Bolognesi DP (1976) Virology 71:169–184

Haematology and Blood Transfusion   Vol. 31
Modern Trends in Human Leukemia VII
Edited by Neth, Gallo, Greaves, and Kabisch
© Springer-Verlag Berlin Heidelberg 1987

Interaction of Viral and Cellular Factors with the HTLV-III * LTR Target Sequences In Vitro

V. Heisig. T. Benter, S. F. Josephs, M. R. Sadaie, T. Okamoto, R. C. Gallo, and F. Wong-Staal

A. Summary

The location of *cis*-acting regulatory sequences within the long terminal repeat (LTR) of the human T-cell lymphotropic virus type III was determined by eukaryotic cell transfection and chloramphenicol acetyltransferase (CAT) assay or in vitro cell-free transcription. A 160 base pair (bp) region of the LTR at position −104 to 56 is required for *trans*-activation (cap site 1). A 24 bp enhancer element (EHE) capable of increasing the rate of transcription, irrespective of orientation, is located between nucleotides −105 to −80. It contains two 10 bp repeats. Three Sp1 binding sites (Sp1 III-I) are located between −78 and −45. A deletion of Sp1 III allowed for limited TATIII response while the presence of a functional enhancer restored the activity in HTLV-III infected cells. Complete loss of transcriptional activity and CAT gene expression could be attributed to the absence of EHE and Sp1 III-I at position −48. However, reinsertion of the enhancer restored accurate initiation but at a decreased level suggesting that the presence of a Sp1 binding site is not a prerequisite for the accurate initiation of transcription but is required for transcriptional activation independent of a promoter. The presence of a negative regulatory element (NRE) has been demonstrated by removal of the 5′ part of U3 to position −117.

Nucleotide sequences around the cap site and poly (A) site contain a *trans*-activator response element (TRE) and could be arranged into a unique secondary structure. A deletion of four nucleotides TCTGAGCCTGGG*AGCT*C causes a loss of three dimer linkage sequence binding. The CAT gene enzyme expression is completely abolished but transcriptional activity remains at reduced level.

B. Introduction

Human T-lymphotropic virus type III (HTLV-III, LAV-1, HIV), the virus causing the acquired immunodeficiency syndrome (AIDS), can infect OKT 4+ human T-cell lines in culture [13]. A high level of virus expression is observed after 1 week. This high gene expression results, at least in part, from transcriptional [7] and post-transcriptional activation [2, 9]. In both mechanisms the virus encoded *trans*-activator protein TATIII is involved. The target site of this protein (*trans*-acting responsive element, TAR) is part of the LTR downstream of the RNA initiation site [10]. Other regulatory elements within the LTR have been detected: a negative regulatory element (NRE), an EHE [10], and three binding sites for the Sp1 protein[4].

In this study various deletion mutants of the LTR have been tested to locate *cis*-acting regulatory regions responsive to the virus associated *trans*-acting regulatory factors at transcriptional and post-transcriptional levels.

---

* HTLV-III/LAV = HIV

Laboratory of Tumor Cell Biology, Developmental Therapeutics Program, National Cancer Institute, Bethesda, Maryland 20892, USA

C. Material and Methods

I. Cell Lines

H9 and HTLV-III infected human H9 T-lymphocytes (H9/III) were maintained in RPMI-1640 medium supplemented with 10% fetal bovine serum (FBS). Hela cells, S3, were grown in MEM with 10% FBS.

II. Plasmid Constructions

Plasmids pSVOCAT, pSV2CAT, and pRSVCAT have been previously described [11]. pC15CAT (Fig. 1) was constructed by blunt ending the *Pst*I cDNA insert of C15 [1], ligation of *Hin*dIIIlinkers, and and subsequent ligation of the resulting fragment into the *Hin*dIII site of pSVOCAT. The 5′ deletion mutants were derived from pC15CAT, which contains a portion of 3′ orf, U3 and the majority of the R region, by cleavage at the *Kpn*I site, digestion with *Bal*31 exonuclease, blunt-ending and the addition of a unique *Xba*I site. These 5′ mutants include pCD12CAT (no deletion within the LTR, ca. 50 bp, *Knp*I site), pCD7CAT (deletion to −278), pCD16CAT (−176), pCD23CAT (−117), pCD52CAT (−65), and pCD54CAT (−48). Nucleotide 1 was assigned as determined by nuclease S1 mapping [12]. Synthetic oligonucleotides of HTLV-III sequences (EHE) from −105 to

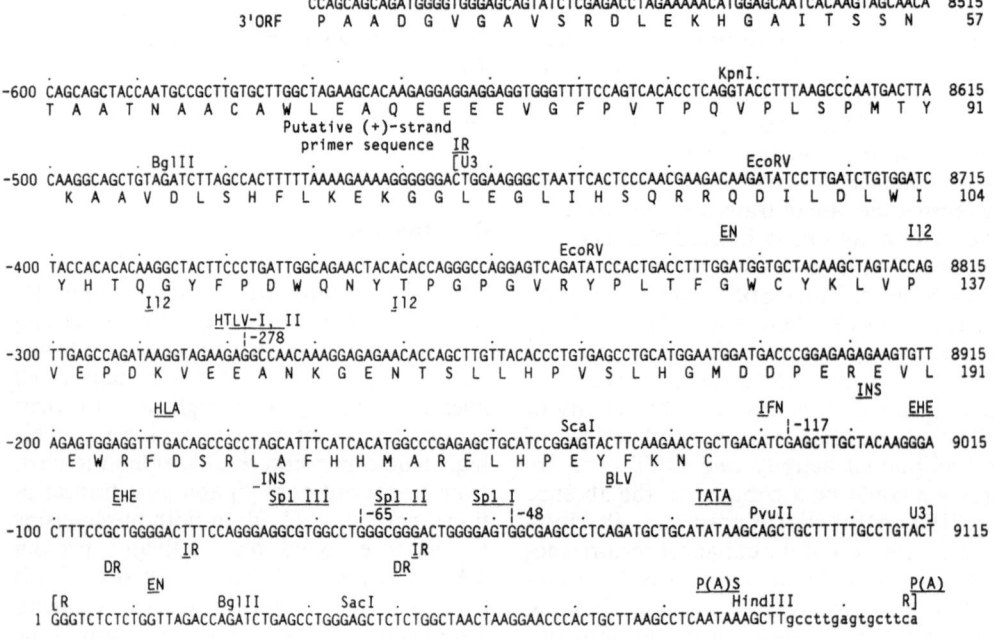

Fig. 1. Sequence of pC15CAT. Numbers on the right of each line are according to Ratner et al. [8]. The 5′ deletion clones schematized in Fig. 2a and b are indicated by vertical lines followed by the distance of each from the transcriptional start site at 1 (position 9116). Shown are the portion of the coding region for 3′ orf which terminates at position −125 (8991). The LTR sequences begin at −454 bp (8662) from the CAP site. The promoter signal (TATA) is at −27 and the polyadenylation signal [P(A)S] at position 74. Bases written in lower case letters from 84 to the polyadeny-

lation site [P(A)] at 98 were deleted from the C15 insert during the construction of C15CAT and replaced by the bacterial chloramphenicol transferase gene. Sequences homologous to other genes as previously reported and EN are underlined. *IL-2*, interleukin 2; *HTLV-I, -II*, human T-lymphotropic viruses type I and II; *IF*, gamma interferon; *INS*, insulin gene; *EHE*, enhancer; *Sp1 III-I*, Sp1 binding sites (−77 to −46); *EN*, core enhancer consensus sequences; and *DR* or *IR*, direct or inverted repeats

−80 were placed in front of pCD52CAT (−65) and pCD54CAT (−48) in sense orientation which results in pCD52ECAT and pCD54ECAT (*GGGACTTTCCGCTG GGGACTTTCC*ATCTAGA −65 or −48), or antisense orientation which results in pCD52EWCAT and pCD54EWCAT (*GGAAAGTCCCC*AGCG*GAAAGTCCC*TCTAGA −65 or −48). pVHHCAT (5′–3′) and pVHHWCAT (3′–5′) were constructed by cloning the 3′ HindIII fragment of pHXB2gpt [3] into pSVOCAT. DNA templates for in vitro transcription were prepared by cleavage with NcoI. For the deletion mutants within the TRE, pCD23CAT was digested with SacI (pCD23ΔSCAT), BglII and SacI (pCD23ΔBSCAT), BglII and HindIII (pCD23ΔBHCAT), or SacI and HindIII (pCD23ΔSHCAT) and self ligated. pCD23ΔSHaCAT is a replacement of the SacI and HindIII fragment (38 to 80) by a oligonucleotide sequence from 39 to 56. The extent of each deletion was confirmed by DNA sequencing analysis [6] and revealed that the resulting mutants pCD23ΔSCAT and pCD23ΔSHaCT lacked, after ligation, the HindIII fragment containing tailing sequences.

III. Eukaryotic Cell Transfections and CAT Assays

In general, 10 μg of plasmid DNA was transfected into approximately 10^7 lymphocytes using the DEAE-dextran method. Cell extracts were prepared by three freeze and thaw cycles 48 h post-transfection. CAT assays were performed as described previously [11].

IV. In Vitro Transcription

Nuclear extracts were prepared from H9 HTLV-III infected cells (H9/IIIE) [7] and whole cell extracts from Hela cells (Hela CE) [5]. Standard in vitro transcription mixtures (25 μl) contained 12 m*M* HEPES (pH 7.9), 60 m*M* KCL, 7 m*M* MgCl, 0.2 m*M* EDTA, 1.3 m*M* DTT, 10% glycerol, 50 μM each of ATP, CTP, and UTP, 5 μ*M* GTP plus 10 μCi of [$^{-32}$P] GTP, 4 m*M* creatine phosphate, 0.4 μg of poly [d(I-C)]: poly [d(I-C)]

as a carrier, 10 μl of Hela whole cell extract (Hela CE), and 0.4 μg (16 μg/ml) of template DNA. Extraction of RNA products, denaturation with glyoxal, and agarose (1.8%) gel electrophoresis followed. To quantitate the in vitro transcripts, gel slices were cut and the radioactivity was counted.

D. Results

To identify transcriptional regulatory elements, recombinant plasmids containing the bacterial chloramphenicol acetyltransferase (CAT) gene with various deletions from the 5′ end of the HTLV-III LTR, detailed in Fig. 1, were investigated in an in vitro cellfree system or transfected into H9 or infected H9 cells for CAT enzyme level determination.

In a second series of deletions, we examined nucleotide sequences surrounding a possible hairpin structure in the terminal redundancy (R). Table 1 summarizes the results of these experiments.

I. Identification of Negative Regulatory Regions

The activity of the individual 5′ LTR deletion mutants was tested by co-transfection experiments with pHXB2gpt, transfection into H9 or H9/III, or by in vitro transcription. A small deletion of ca. 50 nucleotides (pCD12CAT) into the 3′orf sequences of pC15CAT significantly increased the level of CAT gene expression in co-transfection (twofold) and transfection (fourfold) experiments. Additional deletions from −278 (pCD7CAT) to −117 (pCD23CAT) showed no further increase. However, we also examined a plasmid, pVHHCAT which contains the 3′ end of envelope, 3′orf, U3, and R sequences derived from an infectious provirus. In contrast to pC15CAT, the level of CAT gene expression was increased and values are comparable to pCD12CAT (Table 1, Experiment 2). To determine if the level of CAT enzyme activity reflects their in vitro transcriptional activities, we tested pCD12CAT, pCD7CAT, pCD16CAT, and pCD23CAT in an in vitro cell-free system with or without preincubation of nuclear ex-

Tabelle 1. CAT activity and in vitro transcription activity of LTR recombinants and controls

Plasmid	Description	Co-transfection with pHXB2gpt(a)	Absolute CAT activity				In vitro transcription activity (c)	
			Exp 1 (b)		Exp 2 (b)		Hela CE	
		H9	H9	H9III	H9	H9III / H9	H9	H9/IIIE
		(16 h) (30 min)	(30 min)	(15 h)	(20 min)	(20 min)		
pVHHCAT	pHXB2gpt(5'-3')	NT	NT	NT	2.4±0.34	92.7± 1.3	NT	NT
pC15CAT	C15	24.1 (0.0)	0.3	5.1±0.5	0.1±0.0	20.8	NT	NT
pCD12CAT	Del KpnI	44.9	2.0	39.4±5.9	0.7±1	88.8±10.9	2	8
pCD7CAT	-278	46.4	2.6±0.3	58.0±9.8	NT	NT	2	9
pCD16CAT	-176	58.4	2.1±0.3	60.5±12.3	NT	NT	3	9
pCD23CAT	-117	21.4	1.1±0.1	55.9±3.2	0.4	97.5	4	10
pCD52CAT	-65	2.1	0.0	1.6±0.5	0.1±0.0	32.1±0.0	1	2
pCD52ECAT	EHE(5'-3')-65	NT	NT	NT	0.4±1.0	99.0±0.0	NT	7
pCD52EWCAT	EHE(3'-5')-65	NT	NT	NT	0.9±0.3	99.2±0.1	NT	NT
pCD54CAT	-48	0.0	0.0	0.0	0.0±0.0	0.0±0.0	0	1
pCD54ECAT	EHE(5'-3')-48	NT	NT	NT	0.2±0.0	26.7±0.0	NT	4
pCD54EWCAT	EHE(3'-5')-48	NT	NT	NT	0.2±0.0	30.8±1.0	NT	NT
pCD23ΔSHaCAT	-117 to 56	NT	1.0	40	NT	NT	1	7
pCD23ΔSHCAT	-117 SacI-HindIII	NT	1.0	0.0	16.7	1.2±0.3	NT	NT
pCD23ΔBHCAT	-117 BglII-HindIII	NT	NT	NT	0.1	0.0	0	3
pCD23ΔSCAT	-117 SacI	NT	1.0	NT	0.2	0.0	1	4
pCD23ΔBSCAT	BglII-SacI	NT	1.0	0.0	0.2	0.1	0	2
pVHHWCAT	pHXB2gpt(3'-5')	NT	NT	NT	0.1±0.0	0.0	NT	NT
pSVOCAT	CAT	NT	NT	NT	0.0±0.0	0.0±0.0	NT	NT
pSV2CAT	SV 40	NT	NT	NT	6.7±1.5	2.6±0.0	NT	NT
pRSVCAT	RSV	(2.9)	61.0	0.5±0.1	48.4±3.4	18.8± 4.8	NT	NT

[a] Co-transfection using HTLV-III LTR CAT plasmids and pHXB2gpt in H9 cells. Absolute activies are average valuese for two independent experiments 48 h post-transfection. pC15CAT and pRSVCAT values in parentesis are transfections without pHXB2gpt.

[b] Plasmids were transfected into the indicated cells and CAT assays were performed on extracts after 48 h. The values show percent conversion per time of chloramphenicol to acetylated metabolites. Transfections were done in triplicate.

[c] Ratio of CAT enzyme activities of H9 (16 or 15 h) and H9/III (30 or 20 min).

[d] Run-off RNAs were obtained from in vitro transcription of indicated plasmids after digestion with NcoI. Values indicate relative radioactivity between 0 and 10.

NT, not tested; Exp, Experiment; Del, deletion.

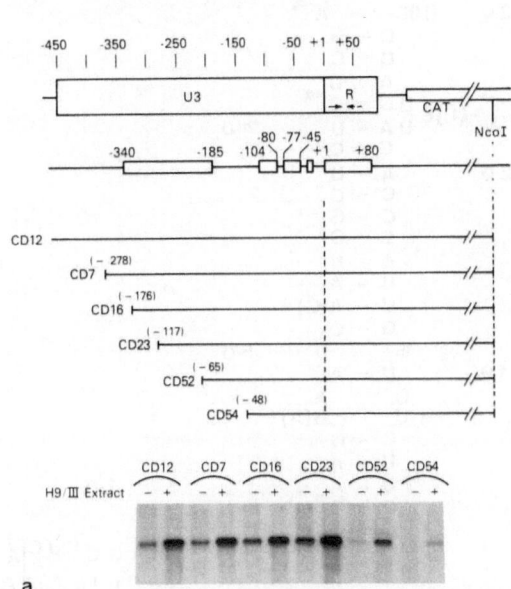

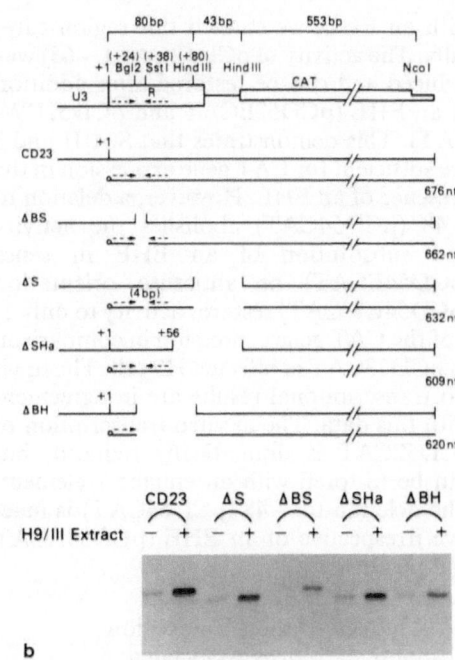

Fig. 2a, b. 5′ (a) and 3′ (b) deletion plasmids of pC15CAT. Deletions were made as described in the material and methods section. pCD12CAT (CD12) contained a small deletion at the *Kpn*I site. Each plasmid is numbered corresponding to the distance in nucleotides from the transcriptional start site 1. The 3′ deletion is constructed from plasmid pCD23CAT (CD23) and indicated as △BS, △S, △SHa, and △BH. Sizes of the transcripts are labeled in nucleotides (*nt*). Autoradiogramms of the in vitro transcription experiments are shown with (+) or without (−) H9/III extract

tract prepared from HTLV-III infected H9 cells (H9/IIIE). Deletions to position −117 showed gradual enhancement of transcription after incubation with H9/IIIE (Fig. 2, Table 1). Experiments at the post-transcriptional and transcriptional level indicate the presence of an negative regulatory element around the *Kpn*I site and 5′ part of U3.

II. Location of an HTLV-III Enhancer Element

The level of CAT gene expression was substantially decreased with plasmids containing deletions extending to −117 (pCD23CAT). We concluded that the reduced activity might reflect the removal of an EHE, a direct repeated sequence of 10 nucleotides from −104 to −80. If this is the case, substitution would restore functional gene enzyme activity. The data in Table 1 demonstrate indeed that the gene expression was activated after insertion of an EHE independent of orientation in pCD52ECAT or pCD52EWCAT and comparable to pCD12CAT.

III. Importance of Sp1 Binding Sites

Binding of the nuclear transcriptional factor Sp1 has been shown to be specific for GC rich regions [4]. Experiments in which regions of DNA were protected from reagents by specifically bound proteins indicated that the region −77 to −46 contains three tandem, closely spaced Sp1 binding sites of variable affinity (Fig. 1).

To determine if Sp1 binding sites influence the gene expression at transcriptional or post-transcriptional level in combination with an EHE, we studied this region carefully. The activity of pCD52CAT (-65) was reduced and can be restored after addition of an EHE (pCD52ECAT and pCD52EWCAT). This demonstrates that Sp1 II and I are sufficient for CAT gene expression in the presence of an EHE. However, a deletion to -48 (pCD54CAT) abolishes the activity and substitution of an EHE in sense (pCD54ECAT) or antisense orientation (pCD54EWCAT) restores activity to only 1/3 of the CAT gene expression in comparison to pCD23CAT in infected H9 cell. The in vitro transcriptional results are in agreement with this data. The in vitro transcription of pCD52CAT is dramatically reduced, but can be restored with an enhancer element. The deletion to -48 (pCD54CAT) is inactive irrespective of an EHE (pCD54ECAT and pCD54EWCAT).

IV. Characterization of a Region Responsive to Virus-Associated Trans-Acting Regulatory Factors

Previous studies have shown that heterologous promoter and enhancer sequences could be placed in front of a region from -17 to 80 of the HTLV-III LTR [10]. Specific elements in this region are recognized by factors present in response to virus infection. To determine the location of these elements responsive to *trans*-acting regulatory factors we deleted sequences around a possible hairpin structure (Fig. 3). For these experiments pCD23CAT, a plasmid with high CAT gene activity, was used for all deletions in the R region. A deletion of 54 bp (pCD23ΔBHCAT) inactivates CAT gene activity completely and decreases in vitro transcription (Fig. 2 b). pCD23ΔSHCAT, a deletion of 40 bp, shows high promoter activity of Exp2 (Table 1), but CAT expression in infected cells are low in Exp1 and 2. The in vitro transcription is comparable to pCD23ΔSHCAT. Two deletions of 14 bp and 4 bp around the hairpin structure, pCD23ΔBSCAT and pCD23ΔSCAT, are inactive in the CAT gene expression system. The in vitro transcription of pCD23ΔSCAT shows transcripts at decreased level. A deletion of 18 bp between 56 and 84 (pCD23ΔSHaCAT) gave values comparable to pCD23CAT.

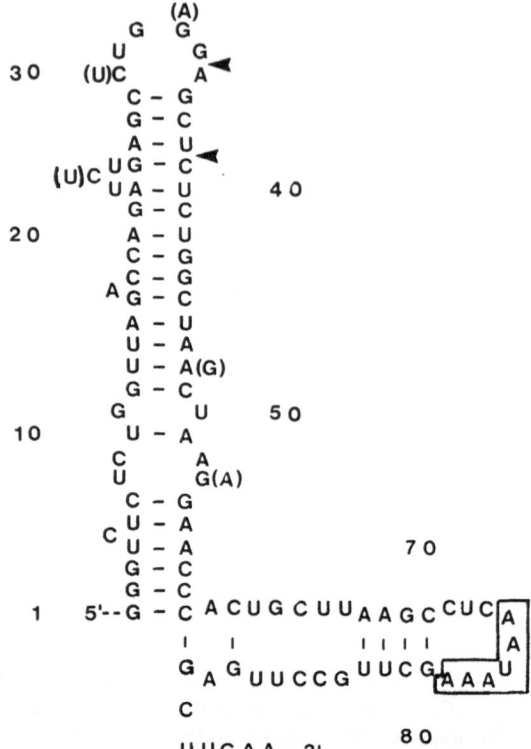

Fig. 3. Possible secondary structure of the nucleotide sequences around the cap site and poly(A) site of C15. In *parentheses* are variation of other virus isolates [8], *arrow* indicates the deletion of four nucleotides (pCD23ΔSCAT). The polyadenylation signal is *boxed*

E. Discussion

The *cis*-acting regulatory elements located within a 160 bp region of the HTLV-III LTR have been described in an in vitro transcription system or CAT gene enzyme expression assay. The presence of the NRE has been demonstrated on the transcriptional and post-transcriptional level by removal of the 5′ part of the 3′ orf and U3 to -117 of pC15CAT. In addition we found differences in CAT gene enzyme response between pC15CAT and pVHHCAT. A explanation for the low activity of pC15 (ca. $^1/_4$ of pCD12CAT) might be a negative regulation of sequences between the *Xho*I and *Kpn*I site. A dramatic loss of transcriptional and CAT enzyme activity upon deletion of sequences between -117 to -65 suggested the presence of a strong positive-regulatory element. A substitution of the EHE (-104 to -81) restored CAT gene activity and in vitro transcription. However, we can not conclude from this experiment that all of these 24 inserted base pairs are needed for enhancement; one of the 10 bp repeat might be sufficient for *trans*-activation.

Three Sp1 binding sites have been identified from -78 to -45 [4]. Complete loss of transcriptional activity could be attributed to the absence of Sp1 III-I. However, reinsertion of the EHE at -54 (pCD54ECAT and pCD54EWCAT) restored the accurate initiation at the transcriptional level, suggesting that the presence of Sp1 binding sites are not a prerequisite for the accurate initiation of transcription. This findings implicate also that one important component of the virus transcriptional unit interacts with the cellular transcription factor, Sp1, and that this factor must function in conjunction with transcriptional elements located downstream of the RNA initiation site to mediate the response of the LTR to viral *trans*-activation.

Sequences surrounding the site of genomic RNA initiation respond to viral-associated *trans*-acting regulatory factors in the presence of the enhancer. This TRE, including Sp1 II and I, that we have mapped to the region -65 to 56, overlaps the promoter, suggesting *trans*-activation may occur via an increased rate of transcriptional initiation. A deletion to 56 (pCD23ΔSHaCAT) showed transcriptional and CAT gene enzyme activity comparable to pCD23CAT. However, a small deletion of four nucleotides (pCD23ΔSCAT) resulted in an complete loss of CAT gene enzyme expression and remaining in vitro transcriptional activity at decreased level. This observation sug-

gested the possibility that at least part of the increase of the HTLV-III LTR directed gene expression in infected cells might be due to post-transcriptional events, including mRNA stability and transport or initiation of protein synthesis. We can arrange the sequences of TRE into a secondary structure (Fig. 3). If for example pCD23ΔSCAT is configured as proposed, a loss of three dimer linkage binding sites may result in an inactivation of CAT gene expression due to post-transcriptional events, but the activity at the transcription level could be decreased.

References

1. Arya SK, Guo C, Josephs SF, Wong-Staal F (1985) Science 229:69–73
2. Feinberg MB, Jarrett RF, Aldovini A, Gallo RC, Wong-Staal F (1986) Cell 46:807–817
3. Fisher AG et al. (1986) Nature 320:367–371
4. Jones KA, Kadonaga JT, Luciw PA, Tjian R (1986) Science 232:755–759
5. Manley JL, Fire A, Samuels M, Sharp PA (1983) Meth Enzyme 101:568–582
6. Maxam AM, Gilbert W (1977) Proc Natl Acad Sci USA 74:560–564
7. Okamoto T, Wong-Staal F (1986) Cell 47:29–35
8. Ratner L, Chang NT, Gallo RC, Wong-Staal F (1985) Nature 313:277–284
9. Rosen CA, Sodrowski JG, Goh WC, Dayton AI, Lippke J, Haseltine WA (1986) Nature 319:555–559
10. Rosen CA, Sodrowski JG, Haseltine WA (1985) Cell 41:813–823
11. Seigel LJ, Ratner L, Josephs SF, Derse D, Feinberg MB, Reyes GR, O'Brien SJ, Wong-Staal F (1986) Virology 148:226–231
12. Starcich B, Ratner L, Josephs SF, Okamoto T et al. (1985) Science 227:538–540
13. Wong-Staal F, Gallo RC (1985) Nature 317:395–403

Haematology and Blood Transfusion   Vol. 31
Modern Trends in Human Leukemia VII
Edited by Neth, Gallo, Greaves, and Kabisch
© Springer-Verlag Berlin Heidelberg 1987

Improvement of HIV Serodiagnosis

I. Wendler [1], J. Schneider [1], F. Guillot [1], A. F. Fleming [2], and G. Hunsmann [1]

Summary

Experience is described with four different assays to detect antibodies against the HIV. ELISA tests using HTLV-III from two different cell lines or the bacterially synthesized envelope peptide ENV(80)-DHFR were compared with the confirmatory immunoprecipitation assay. A total of 831 sera – 678 from Germany and 155 from Zambia – were examined. The specificity of the ENV(80) ELISA was found to be superior to the two virus ELISAs and equivalent to the immunoprecipitation. The diagnostic value of the ENV(80) ELISA test was confirmed with European and African sera.

Serological assays for the detection of antibodies to the human immunodeficiency virus (HIV), earlier named LAV, human T-lymphotrophic virus (HTLV)-III, or ARV, are important for identifying individuals infected with such a virus and for epidemiological research on the acquired immunodeficiency syndrome (AIDS) and related diseases. Four different methods are widely used to determine HIV antibodies.

In the enzyme-linked immunosorbent assay (ELISA), antigen adsorbed to beads or wells of microtitre plates is incubated with sera to be tested. Bound immunoglobulins are detected by a second enzyme-linked anti-antibody. The amount of first antibodies bound is quantitated by the colour-producing enzyme reaction. Numerous commercial ELISAs are available.

For Western blotting, viral proteins are separated electrophoretically in the presence of sodium dodecyl sulfate (polycrylamide gel electrophoresis) (PAGE) and transferred to a nitrocellulose membrane. Antibodies binding to viral proteins on the membrane are visualized with an anti-antibody linked to an enzyme catalysing a colour reaction.

In the immunofluorescence assay, virus-producing or non-infected cells as negative controls are fixed onto slides and then incubated with patients' sera. Subsequently, antibodies recognizing viral proteins are visualized under a fluorescence microscope with a second fluorescein-labelled anti-antibody.

For immunoprecipitation (IP), lysates of virus-producing cells labeled with radioactive amino acids are incubated with patients' sera. The immunocomplexes are collected by adsorption to protein A sepharose and subsequently separated by PAGE. Precipitated radiolabelled proteins are identified by autoradiography. IP is an expensive and sophisticated assay. On the other hand, it is highly specific because native viral polypeptides are selected out of a large excess of cellular proteins and characterized by PAGE according to their molecular weight (Fig. 1).

The ELISA is most suitable for screening large numbers of sera for HIV antibodies. However, our own experience and interlaboratory tests regularly performed among German blood banks have shown that the ELISA gives a substantial number of false positive results which have to be sorted out by time-consuming confirmatory assays [1]. More seriously, up to 5% of positives may

---
[1] Deutsches Primatenzentrum Göttingen, Kellnerweg 4, D-3400 Göttingen, FRG
[2] Tropical Diseases Research Centre, 9, Ndola, Zambia

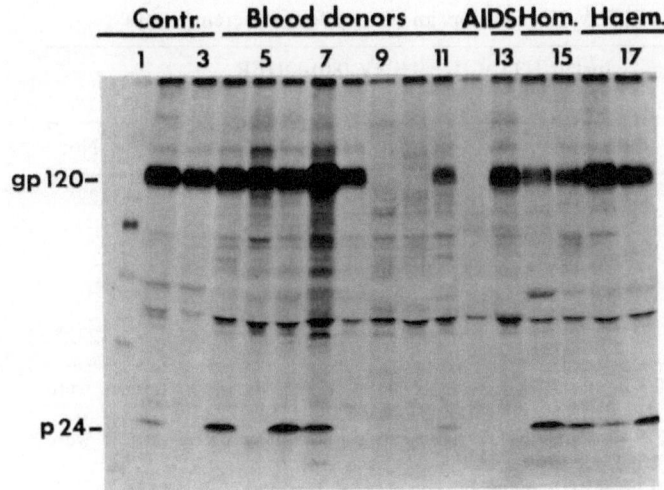

gp 120—

p 24—

Contr. | Blood donors | AIDS Hom. Haem.
1 3 5 7 9 11 13 15 17

Fig. 1. Immunoprecipitations of HIV polypeptides confirm results of the ELISA. Cell extracts of H9/HTLV-III cells labelled for 4 h with ^{35}S-cysteine were reacted with ELISA-positive sera from blood donors (4–12), AIDS patients (13), homosexuals (14, 15) and haemophiliacs (16, 17). Gp120 and p24 were detected as the predominant immunoreactive polypeptides in HTLV-III infected cells

be missed in the primary ELISA screening [2]. False-positive results occur when antibodies bind to cellular antigens, e.g., histocompatibility antigens [3], or proteins derived from medium contaminating the antigen preparation. False-negative results are probably due to the low concentration of the viral membrane protein gp120 in the virus preparation. Gp120 is mainly detected by serum antibodies in the IP assay [4]. However, it is lost considerably during virus preparation and density gradient purification [5]. Therefore, sera with low titres or sera which recognize only gp120 may be missed in the screening ELISA.

To obtain a highly specific and sensitive ELISA, the essential antigenic determinants have to be presented in high concentrations free of non-viral proteins. The antigen for the ELISA and other HIV tests is most commonly derived from the H9/HTLV-IIIB cell line [6]. In our experience, virus harvested from these cultures by two sedimentation steps contains a great excess of contaminating proteins from cells and medium. We have established a cell line permanently producing HTLV-IIIB by infecting the human Jurkat mature T-cell line [7]. Jurkat/HTLV-III cells release 10–15 times more virus than the H9/HTLV-III line. Moreover, such virus preparations are less contaminated with non-viral proteins, as shown by PAGE analyses and determination of specific RT activity. To normalize ELISAs performed with

different antigen stocks, the relative optical density (OD) of each serum was calculated by dividing its OD through the OD of a positive control serum run on the same plate.

A comparison of sera tested in the ELISA with antigen derived from H9/HTLV-III or Jurkat/HTLV-III has shown that the relatively pure virus from Jurkat cells allows a clearer differentiation between positive and negative sera (Table 1). ELISA results of all sera were compared with those obtained by IP. In our experience, IP is the most specific and sensitive HTLV-III antibody assay (Fig. 1). IP positive and negative sera overlap in their relative OD in the ELISA. This range extended from 0.1 to 0.25 with antigen from Jurkat/HTLV-III cells, but from 0.1 to 0.6 when H9/HTLV-III cultures were used as antigen source. Sera attaining OD values within the range of uncertainty were classified as $+/-$.

A pronounced enhancement of specificity and sensitivity is expected from second generation ELISA tests, which use bacterially produced antigens. In these tests, the essential antigenic determinants can be offered in great quantity and purity.

In our laboratory, the diagnostic potential of a bacterially produced peptide of the HIV *env* gene was tested. A synthetic DNA fragment of 240 base pairs coding for a peptide homologous to a conserved region of the gp41 transmembrane glycoprotein of HIV was expressed in *E. coli* as a N-terminal fu-

431

Table 1. Detection of antibodies against HTLV-III in European sera by four different assays

IP[a]		H9/HTLV-III ELISA[a]		Jurkat/HTLV-III ELISA[a]		ENV (80)-DHFR ELISA[b]		IP[b]	
Score[c]	No.	Score[d]	%[e]	Score[f]	%	Score[g]	%	Score	No.
+	111	+	57	+	77	+	95	+	225
		+/−	42	+/−	23	+/−	2		
		−	1	−	0	−	3		
		+	3	+	0	+	3		
		+/−	40	+/−	3	+/−	1		
−	68[h]	−	57	−	97	−	96	−	272[h]

[a] The same 179 sera derived from AIDS patients, AIDS risk groups or healthy blood donors were tested comparatively by IP, H9/HTLV-III ELISA and Jurkat/HTLV-III ELISA.
[b] The same 497 seca derived from AIDS patients, AIDS risk groups or healthy blood donors were tested comparatively by IP and ENV (80)-DHFR ELISA.
[c] Sera precipitating gp120 or additional viral proteins were recorded as positive.
[d] Sera with a relative OD below 0.1 were scored as negative. Positivity was recorded when a serum gave a relative OD of at least 0.6 (see text).
[e] Percent of IP + or − sera.
[f] Sera with a relative OD below 0.1 were scored as negative. Positivity was recorded when a serum gave a relative OD of at least 0.25 (see text).
[g] Sera with OD below 0.15 were scored as negative. Positivity was recorded when a serum gave an OD of at least 0.25.
[h] Including sera which were not tested by IP, since they gave clear negative results in other different screening assays.

Table 2. Detection of antibodies against HTLV-III in African sera by three different assays

IP		Jurkat/HTLV-III ELISA			ENV (80)-DHFR ELISA		
Score[c]	No.	Score[f]	No.	%[g]	Score[g]	No.	%
+	27	+	27	100	+	26	96
		+/−	0	0	+/−	0	0
		−	0	0	−	1	4
−	128[h]	+	2	2	+	0	0
		+/−	44	34	+/−	3	2
		−	82	64	−	125	98

For footnotes see Table 1.

sion protein to dihydrofolate reductase [8]. The resulting ENV(80)-DHFR peptide was enriched to high purity by affinity chromatography and used as antigen in an ELISA [9]. A total of 497 sera from German individuals with AIDS, from AIDS risk groups and from healthy blood donors were evaluated by IP and ELISA, using the ENV(80)-DHFR peptide as antigen. The results show that the ENV(80) ELISA is a valuable screening assay for HTLV-III antibodies (Table 1). The results of the ENV(80) ELISA and IP agreed in 95% of the sera. However, the Jurkat/HTLV-III ELISA agreed with IP in only 77%. No clear statement was possible for 2% of the sera tested with the ENV(80) ELISA. Accordingly, the latter was ten times more accurate than the Jurkat/HTLV-III ELISA. Even more uncertain and false-positive results were obtained in the H9/HTLV-III ELISA. The specificity of the ENV(80) ELISA is comparable to that of the IP. Three per cent of the sera scoring as positive in either test were missed in the other assay. This discrepancy between ENV(80) ELISA and IP may be explained by the genomic heterogenicity found in LAV/HTLV-III variants [10–13].

The high specificity of the ENV(80) ELISA compared to the HTLV-III ELISA was also confirmed in a study comprising 155 sera from tropical Africa (Table 2). In conventional ELISAs, reactions of African sera are often difficult to interpret. The presence of high titres of antimalarial and other antibodies and immunocomplexes in these sera leads to a high frequency of false-positive and uncertain results [14, 15]. As summarized in Table 2, the ENV(80) ELISA is 96%–98% specific when applied to African sera. However, early seroconversion was obviously not detected in one patient, who had antibodies in the IP against gp120 but not gp41. HIV antibody tests which work reliably in Africa are urgently needed to assess the prevalence of viral infection and the spread of the AIDS epidemic through this continent.

Further improvement of the ENV(80) ELISA should be possible when the antigen is supplemented with peptides corresponding to other conserved regions of the viral envelope and/or core protein.

Acknowledgements. We thank H. Buss, R. Jung, A. Jurdzinski, S. Mader, D. Schreiner and S. Sievert for expert technical assistance, and C. Schalt for typing the manuscript. The gift of the ENV(80) peptide from Hoffmann-La Roche is gratefully acknowledged.

References

1. Hunsmann G, Wendler J, Schneider J (1986) The LAV/HTLV-III antibody test: methods, scoring and implications. AIFO 1:22–25
2. Schneider J, Wendler I, Bayer H, Hunsmann G (1987) Zur Bedeutung der Serumantikörperbestimmung gegen humane lymphotrope Retroviren. Ärztliches Laboratorium 33:45–47
3. Kühnl P, Seidl S, Holzberger G (1985) HLA DR4 antibodies cause positive HTLV-III antibody ELISA results. Lancet 1:122–1223
4. Schneider J, Bayer H, Bienzle U, Hunsmann G (1985) A glycopolypeptide (gp100) the main antigen detected by HTLV-III antisera. Med Microbiol Immunol 134:39–42
5. Montagnier L, Clavel F, Krust B, Chamaret S, Rey F, Barre-Sinoussi F, Chermann JC (1985) Identification and antigenicity of the major envelope glycoprotein of lymphadenopathy-associated virus. Virology 144:283–289
6. Popovic M, Sarngadharan MG, Read E, Gallo RC (1984) Detection, isolation and continous production of cytopathic retroviruses (HTLV-III) from patient with AIDS and pre AIDS. Science 224:497–500
7. Wendler I, Jentsch KD, Schneider J, Hunsmann G (1987) Efficient replication of HTLV-III and STLV-III mac in human Jurkat T-cell cultures. Med Microbiol Immunol 176:273–280
8. Certa U, Bannwarth W, Stüber D et al. (1986) Subregions of a conserved part of the HIV gp41 transmembrane protein are differentially recognized by antibodies of infected individuals EMBO J 5:3051–3056
9. Schneider J, Wendler I, Guillot F, Hunsmann G, Galatti H, Schoenfeld H-J, Stüber D, Mous J (1987) A new ELISA test for HTLV-III antibodies using a bacterially produced viral env gene product. Med Microbiol Immunol 176:47–51
10. Wain-Hobson S, Sonigo P, Danos O, Cole S, Alizon M (1985) Nucleotide sequence of the AIDS virus. Cell 40:9–17
11. Ratner L, Haseltine W, Patarca R et al. (1985) Complete nucleotide sequence of the AIDS virus, HTLV-III. Nature 131:277–284
12. Sanchez-Pescador R, Power MD, Barr PJ, Steimer KS, Stempien MM, Brown-Shimer SL, Gee WW, Renard A, Randolph A, Levy JA, Dina D, Luciw PA (1985) Nucleotide sequence and expression of an AIDS-associated retrovirus (ARV-2). Science 227:484–492
13. Muesing MA, Smith DH, Cabradilla CD, Benton CV, Lasky DJ, Capon DJ (1985) Nucleic acid structure and expression of the human AIDS/lymphadenopathy retrovirus. Nature 313:450–485
14. Hunsmann G, Schneider J, Wendler I, Fleming AF (1985) HTLV positivity in Africans. Lancet 26:952–953
15. Wendler I, Schneider J, Gras B, Fleming AF, Hunsmann G (1986) Seroepidemiology of human immuno deficiency virus in Africa. British Med J 293:782–785

Haematology and Blood Transfusion   Vol. 31
Modern Trends in Human Leukemia VII
Edited by Neth, Gallo, Greaves, and Kabisch
© Springer-Verlag Berlin Heidelberg 1987

Incidence of LAV/HTLV-III-Positive Blood Donors

R. Laufs

In January 1985 we started to screen all blood donors of the blood bank of the University clinics in Hamburg Eppendorf (UKE) for LAV/HTLV-III antibodies [1, 2]. Of the 7624 donors examined up until July 1985, 10 were positive in the enzyme-linked immunosorbent assay (ELISA), the IFT, and the Western blot analysis. All of the LAV/HTLV-III-positive donors were male; the mean age was 34 years; nine out of the ten LAV/HTLV-III positives were homosexual and one out of the ten had had multiple contacts with prostitutes.

Each of the stock donors who were LAV/HTLV-III-positive at the first examination had donated blood 8–95 times prior to detection of the infection. Fourteen out of 16 recipients followed back until 1981 are LAV/HTLV-III-positive. From two of the donors and the two recipients of their blood we isolated LAV/HTLV-III using two procedures: the detection of reverse transcriptase after in vitro cocultivation of their lymphocytes with normal lymphocytes, and the demonstration of the viral antigens in the Western blot analysis, using the supernatants of those cultures. The *env* and core proteins of LAV/HTLV-III were demonstrated in the supernatants of the isolates.

Among the recipients of LAV/HTLV-III-positive blood there is a higher rate of AIDS in infants than in adults, and the mean incubation period is 4.5 years. In the United States, up to June 1986, 384 cases of AIDS attributed to blood transfusion had been reported, and we have to expect an increasing number in the years ahead.

From May to September 1985 about 0.02% of donors in West Germany proved to be LAV/HTLV-III-positive. In the large cities, where AIDS occurs more frequently, the frequency of positive donors was much higher: in Berlin it was 0.14% and in Hamburg 0.10%. In the second half of 1985 the prevalence of LAV/HTLV-III-positive donors dropped sharply in Hamburg from 0.1%–0.003%.

Although 35% of the donors tested were female and 65% were male, more than 90% of ELISA- and Western-blot-positive donors were men. The female donors, however, were overrepresented in the false ELISA-reactive blood samples; 44% of the latter were of female origin. About 20%–30% of the ELISA-reactive sera could be confirmed as positive in the Western blot analysis. This may be partly due to the fact that the H9 cell line used for the growth of LAV/HTLV-III contains the HLA DR-4 antigen; 10 out of 27 commercial DR-4 antisera were positive in the ELISA for LAV/HTLV-III antibodies.

No cases of LAV/HTLV-III infection have been attributed to the use of immunoglobulins, commercial hepatitis B antisera, or the licensed hepatitis B vaccines.

The remaining problems for the screening of blood donors are the seronegative LAV/HTLV-III carriers and the blood donations of freshly infected persons who carry the

Institute for Medical Microbiology and Immunology, University of Hamburg, FRG virus but are still seronegative. These problems could be diminished by the introduction of an antigen test. The fact that the risk of acquiring LAV/HTLV-III in Hamburg by blood transfusion has already significantly decreased demonstrates the great progress made in the screening of blood donors for LAV/HTLV-III antibodies.

References

1. Kühne P, Seidl S, Holzverger G (1985) HLA-DR 4 antibodies cause positive HTLV-III Elisa results. Lancet I:1222
2. Laufs R, Sibrowski W, Karch H, Busch H, von Eisenhart-Rothe B, Roos D (1985) AIDS-Virusinfektionen bei Blutspendern. Dtsch Ärzteblatt 48:3593–3598

Haematology and Blood Transfusion   Vol. 31
Modern Trends in Human Leukemia VII
Edited by Neth, Gallo, Greaves, and Kabisch
© Springer-Verlag Berlin Heidelberg 1987

Growth of the HTLV-III Strain of Human Immunodeficiency Virus in Different Cell Types

E. M. Fenyö and B. Åsjö

The major immunological abnormality in the acquired immunodeficiency syndrome (AIDS) appears to be a quantitative defect in the T4 antigen-positive helper/inducer T-

Department of Virology, Karolinska Institutet, Stockholm, Sweden

cell subset. AIDS is etiologically linked to a retrovirus, designated human immunodeficiency virus (HIV), that has been shown to selectively infect T4 antigen-positive lymphoid cells in vitro [1]. Since virus replication in vitro is associated with a pronounced cytopathic effect, it has been suggested that

Table 1. Growth of the HTLV-IIIB isolate in different cell types

Cell type[a]	T4[b] antigen positive cells (%)	Virus[c] dose (cpm × 10^3/ 10^6 cells)	No. of experiments	Weeks after infection					
				1			2		
				RT	IF[d] (%+)	CPE[e]	RT	IF (%+)	CPE
PBMC		32	15	26		+	72		+
Monocytes		180	3	68.4		−	31		−
		180	1	31		−	9.7		−
T-cell lines									
H9		75	10	8	10	+	35	64	+
		2.5	2	−		−	−		−
HUT-78		60	1	5.8		+	143		++
		12	1	2.8		+	65		++
Karpas45		70	2	4.8	7	+	293	83	+++
Molt-3		50	2	−	−	−	−	−	−
Monocytoid cell line and derived clones									
U937 parental	<10	150	1	−		−	−		−
U937 clone 4	<10	1800	1	6.5		−	3		−
U937 clone 1	50–60	350	1	1.3		−	1.7		+
U937 clone 16	>95	100	15	80	95	+++			
		25	2	15		++			+++
		2.5	2	0.4		−	5.8		++
Malignant glioma cell lines									
138	0	100	2	−	−	−	−	2	−
373	0	100	2	−	−	−	−	−	−
489	0	100	2	−	−	−	−	−	−

Footnote see p. 438.

immunodeficiency in vivo is a result of the virus killing the T4 cells. To gain further insight into the virus-cell interactions we studied the replication of the HTLV-IIIB strain of HIV in different cell types.

Peripheral blood mononuclear cells (PBMC) from blood donors were separated by Ficoll-Isopaque and treated with 2.5 mg/ml phytohemagglutinin (PHA-P, Difco) for 3 days prior to infection [2]. Monocytes were obtained by harvesting the surface-adherent cells 24 h after separation of PBMC and either exposing them to OKT3 antibodies and C' (negative selection) or submitting them to FACS selection of M3 antigen-positive cells (positive selection). Both PBMC and monocyte cultures could readily be infected with HTLV-IIIB and yielded reverse transcriptase-positive culture fluids 1 week after infection (Table 1). PBMC cultures showed slight cytopathic changes. Virus production descreased by the 3rd week, probably due to depletion of virus-sensitive T4-positive cells. Monocyte cultures showed no cytopathic changes during the first 2 weeks after infection. From the 3rd week on, cell loss occurred due to gradual cell death.

All four T-cell leukemia lines could be infected by the HTLV-IIIB isolate. H9, HUT-78, and Karpas45 cultures produced small amounts of virus the first week after infection. Large amounts of virus were produced during the second week when the majority of cells became infected, as shown by immunofluorescence with monoclonal antibodies to viral core proteins p24 and p15. The particular Molt-3 line used began virus production with a 4-week delay. Virus spread was also slower in these cultures, since only 50% of cells were virus antigen positive 6 weeks after infection. Cultures of all T-cell lines showed cytopathic changes simultaneously with virus production. In the case of H9, HUT-78, and Molt-3 cells, cell death could be

3			4			9			Continuously producing line established	Virus detected by co-cultivation with U937–16
RT	IF (%+)	CPE	RT	IF (%+)	CPE	RT	IF (%+)	CPE		
2.5	—		0.5	—						
Gradual cell death										
3.0	—		Gradual cell death							
64	70	+	110	80	++				yes	
—	—	—	64		++					
135		+	161		—				yes	
134		+	49		—				yes	
104		+++							no	
—	—	—	72	5	+				yes	
—	—	—	—			79	90	—	yes	
12	—		19		—	170		—	yes	
35		++	65	70	—				yes	
									no	
		+++								
—	—	—	—	20	—	—	—	—	no	+
—	—	—	—	—	—	—	—	—	no	—
—	—	—	—	—	—	—	—	—	no	—

437

compensated by the addition of uninfected cells, and eventually a continuously virus-producing line, no longer showing cytopathic changes, could be established. In Karpas45 cultures, however, the cytopathic changes led to extensive cell death, and no producer line could be established.

The U937 monocytoid cell line was originally derived from a histiocytic lymphoma [3]. It has retained a basic phenotype corresponding to that of an immature monocyte [4]. The cell line is inducible by various agents to phenotypic alterations similar to those of normal monoblasts undergoing differentiation. It has recently been cloned, and several clonal lines with different properties have been derived. Susceptibility to infection with HTLV-IIIB and sensitivity to cytopathic changes following infection correlated with the expression of T4 antigen on the cell surface [5]. The parental U937 line and one of its subclones, clone 4, had less than 10% T4-positive cells; hence, productive infection could be established only after a long latency (parental line) or with a high virus inoculum (clone-4 line). These lines showed no or only marginal cytopathic effects.

The clone-1 line contained 50%–60% T4-positive cells and showed moderate susceptibility to infection. Cytopathic changes, even if pronounced, could be overcome in the infected cultures by the addition of uninfected cells, and in each case a producer line could be established. Similarly, the U937 parental and clone-4 lines, once infected, gave rise to continuously virus-producing lines. The clone-16 line contained more than 95% T4-positive cells and was the line most sensitive to infection and to cytopathic changes. Cell death was so extensive following infection that no continuously virus-producing line could be established. The clone-16 line thus resembled monocytes in its prompt virus production but was similar to the Karpas45 T-cell line in its sensitivity to cytopathic changes. The results suggest that the T4 molecule may also play a role in the effector mechanisms leading to cytopathic changes as recorded by cell death.

None of the malignant glioma cell lines used [6, 7] in these experiments appeared to be T4 antigen positive. In spite of this, one of the lines, MG138, could be infected with the HTLV-IIIB isolate [8]. Infection appears to be latent rather than productive, since only a minority of cells in the MG138 culture show transient expression of viral antigens. No virus production could be detected in these cultures. However, the presence of virus could be demonstrated through cocultivation with sensitive target cells, U937 clone 16 in the present experiments. Through contact with the monocytoid cells the virus present in the glioma cells can be transmitted and can give rise to a fully productive infection. The fact that the T4 antigen-negative glioma cells do not show any cytopathic effect provides further support for the notion that the T4 antigen is necessary for the cytopathic effect after virus infection.

In conclusion, T-lymphoid, monocytoid, and glioma cell lines can be infected with HIV. Whereas infection is productive in T-lymphoid and monocytoid cells, glioma cells appear to be latently infected. Cells with low expression or apparent lack of T4 antigen do not show cytopathic changes after virus infection. This suggests that the T4 antigen is necessary for the cytopathic effect after virus infection.

Footnote of Table 1, p. 436:

[a] Peripheral blood mononuclear cells were grown in RPMI medium supplemented with 10% fetal calf serum (FCS), 10% T-cell growth factor (Cellular Products), 45 IU of sheep anti-human α-interferon serum, and 2 µg/ml polybrene (PB). Monocytes, T-cell lines, and monocytoid cell lines were grown in RPMI medium with 10% FCS and 2 µg/ml PB. Malignant gliomas were grown in Eagles MEM with 10% FCS and PB.

[b] Indirect membrane immuniofluorescence with the *Fab* fragment of an anti-T4 monoclonal antibody (received from Dr. Ellis Reinherz) and fluorescein isothiocyanate (FITC)-labeled rabbit anti-mouse IgG (Dakopatts, Glostrup, Denmark).

[c] Estimated by reverse transcriptase activity (RT) [5].

[d] Immunofluorescence on methanol-fixed cells with monoclonal antibodies to HTLV-III p24 and p15.

[e] Cytopathic effect: syncytia formation and cell death; $+$, $< 5\%$ of cells, $+ +$, 5%–50%, $+ + +$, $> 50\%$ of cells show CPE.

Acknowledgements. We thank Dr. R.C. Gallo, NIH, Bethesda, for the H9 cell line and the HTLV-IIIB virus strain, Dr. A. Karpas, Cambridge, for the Karpas 45 cell line, Drs. M. Gidlund and F. Chiodi for their collaboration, and Mrs. B. Lind and A. von Gegerfelt for their expert technical assistance.

This work was supported by grants from the Swedish Cancer Society (1089-B87-10XB) and the Swedish Medical Research Council (K86-16H-7737-01A).

References

1. Klatzmann D, Champagne E, Chamaret S, Gruest J, Guetard D, Hercend T, Gluckmann JC, Montagnier L (1984) T-lymphocyte T4 molecule behaves as the receptor for human retrovirus LAV. Nature 312:767–768
2. Åsjö B, Morfeldt-Månson L, Albert J, Biberfeld G, Karlsson A, Lidman K, Fenyö EM (1986) Replicative capacity of human immunodeficiency virus from patients with varying severity of HIV infection. Lancet II:660–662
3. Sundström C, Nilsson K (1976) Establishment and characterization of a human histiocytic lymphoma cell line (U-937). Int J Cancer 17:565–577
4. Nilsson K, Ivhed I, Forsbeck K (1985) In: Andersson L-C, Gahmberg CG, Ekblom P (eds) Gene expression during normal and malignant differentiation. Academic Press, New York, pp 57–72
5. Åsjö B, Ivhed I, Gidlund M, Fuerstenberg S, Fenyö EM, Nilsson K, Wigzell H (1987) Susceptibility to infection by the human immunodeficiency virus (HIV) correlates with T4 expression in a parental monocytoid cell line and its subclones. Virology 157:359–365
6. Westermark B, Pontén J, Hugosson R (1973) Determinants for the establishment of permanent tissue culture lines from human gliomas. Acta Pathol Microbiol Scand [A]81:791–805
7. Pontén J, Macintyre EM (1968) Long-term culture of normal and neoplastic human glia. Acta Pathol Microbiol Scand 74:465–486
8. Chiodi F, Fuerstenberg S, Gidlund M, Åsjö B, Fenyö EM (1987) Infection of brain-derived cells with the human immunodeficiency virus. J Virol 61:1244–1247

Haematology and Blood Transfusion Vol. 31
Modern Trends in Human Leukemia VII
Edited by Neth, Gallo, Greaves, and Kabisch
© Springer-Verlag Berlin Heidelberg 1987

Nonhuman Primate Models of Human Hematological Malignancies

B. A. Lapin [1]

Tremendous progress has been achieved in cancer research in the past decade. It is widely accepted that the major breakthrough is in the field of oncogenes. However, this direction of cancer research has not yet contributed significantly to an understanding of the etiology of human leukemia. On the other hand, in the past few years we have witnessed a renaissance in the field which I would call "classical virology." It began with the isolation by Gallo and coworkers [1] of the first human retrovirus, HTLV-I, implicated in the etiology of adult T-cell leukemia/lymphoma [2, 3].

Here I will describe some aspects of a nonhuman primate model of human lymphoma which we and our collaborators in many countries have been working with for almost 20 years. This model was studied within the framework of the above-mentioned classical virological approach, and we have found many interesting and unique parallels with the human system.

The story began almost 20 years ago, when, with the aim of isolating a hypothetical human leukemia virus, we inoculated some baboons of our colony with pooled fresh blood of leukemia patients. We were too optimistic and expected that in a few months we would have a human leukemia virus in our hands. But after a year the inoculated animals did not show any symptoms of leukemia. Our optimism sharply decreased, and due to some difficulties in keeping these monkeys in strict isolation we

transferred them to open-air compounds where they had close contact with untreated animals.

To our surprise, approximately 2 years after the inoculation, some of the treated animals developed malignant lymphoma (Fig. 1), and, totally unexpectedly, some of their untreated neighbors developed the same disease. It should be noted that our monkey colony was established in 1927 and we now have the eleventh generation of baboons born in captivity. However, we had never seen lymphoma in this simian species before the introduction of human leukemic material.

Quite frankly, we still do not know what role this human leukemic material played in the development of malignant lymphoma in our baboons. Nevertheless, it appeared, and with these cases an outbreak of malignant lymphoma started; to date almost 270 baboons have died of this disease. The mortality of the disease fluctuates, being around 1.8%–2% per year in a susceptible age-group, which consists of animals over 3–4 years of age (see Table 1). There are now 1200 baboons in this age-group in our baboon stock, and this means that every year we register up to 20 animals as dead or killed because of malignant lymphoma [4, 5].

Our first impression was that the disease was monomorphic. But later on, after thorough morphological investigations, we came to the conclusion that there were many morphological variants of the baboon malignant lymphoma. In some cases we observed Hodgkin-type lymphomas; the rest of the cases were non-Hodgkin types including lymphoblastic, prolymphocytic, immu-

---

[1] Institute of Experimental Pathology and Therapy, USSR Academy of Medical Sciences, Sukhumi, USSR

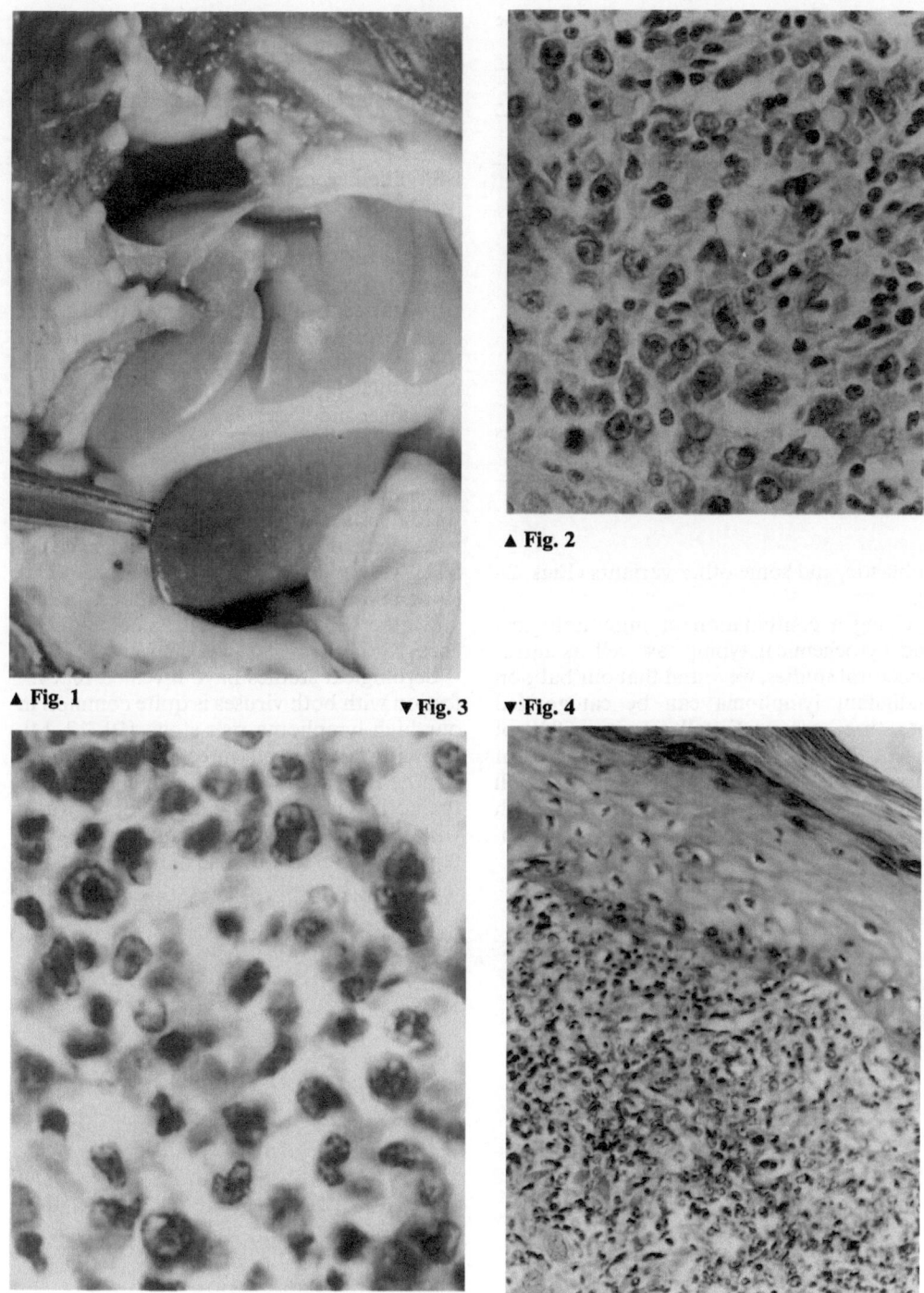

Fig. 1. Spleno- and hepatomegaly in baboon with malignant lymphoma
Fig. 2. B-cell immunoblastic non-Hodgkin's lymphoma
Fig. 3. T-cell immunoblastic non-Hodgkin's lymphoma
Fig. 4. Skin proliferation in baboon with T-cell non-Hodgkin's lymphoma

Table 1. Lymphoma mortality among the baboons of the Sukhumi monkey colony

Year	Number of adult baboons in the stock	Mortality	
		Number	%
1966	346	0	0
1967	365	1	0.27
1968–1980		179	1.85
1981	1126	16	1.42
1982	1041	18	1.73
1983	1254	13	1.04
1984	1140	14	1.22
1985	1248	18	1.44
1986 (September)	1281	17	1.33

Total number of baboons dead of hemoblastosis
−276

noblastic, and some other variants (Figs. 2–4).

Using a combination of immunological and cytochemical typing, as well as ultrastructural studies, we found that our baboon malignant lymphoma can be categorized into three groups: T-cell (around 50% of cases), B-cell lymphoma (around 40% of cases), and "null," or non-T-, non-B-cell lymphoma (around 10% of cases). Both helper and suppressor phenotypes were observed in the T-cell lymphoma group.

The disease could be transmitted with the cell-containing materials, and we started our attempts to isolate the viruses which might be responsible for the development of the disease. We isolated two types of oncogenic viruses. The first was a B-lymphotropic EBV-like herpesvirus which we called *Herpesvirus papio* (HVP) [5, 6]. This virus is very closely related to EBV [7]. It immortalizes primate B-lymphocytes in vitro and has antigens cross-reacting with corresponding EBV antigens [8]. The genome structure of both viruses is the same, and the overall homology of EBV and HVP DNAs approximates 40% [7].

The second virus is a C-type retrovirus which belongs to the HTLV-I family [9, 10]. It is closely related to HTLV-I but there are some differences [11, 12] (Fig. 5). Although we did not compare baboon HTLV-I-like virus with various simian isolates called STLV-I, we have many reasons to suspect a close relationship between baboon isolate and other STLV-I, as well as some differences.

Serological studies have revealed that infection with both viruses is quite common in our high-lymphoma-risk stock [10, 12–14]. The prevalence of infection with both viruses increases with age, which indicates the horizontal transmission of these viruses within the colony. HVP virus is more contagious than STLV-I. The data presented il-

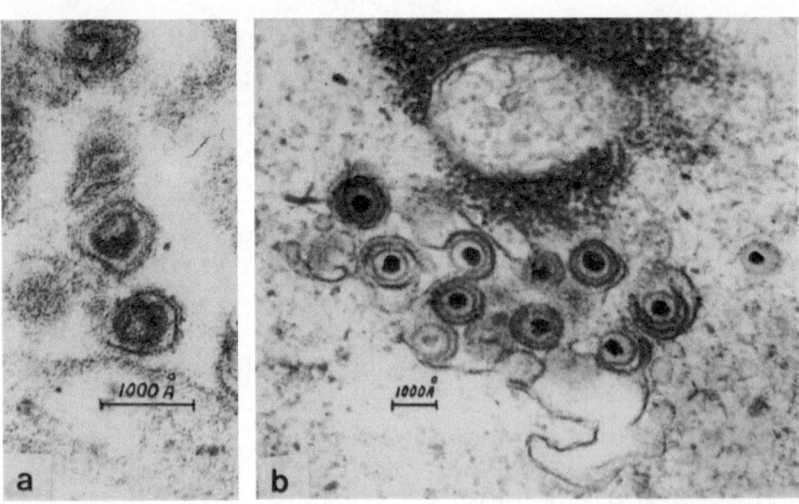

Fig. 5. a Type-C retrovirus; **b** herpesvirus

lustrate the dynamics of the infections in high-lymphoma-risk stock. It should be noted that similar studies of ours with wild animals have shown some of them also to be infected with both HVP and STLV-I. But in this case the prevalence of infection was much lower, especially in the case of STLV-I.

The level of antibodies against both viruses increases in the prelymphoma period and as a rule decreases after lymphoma development. HVP-specific DNA has been found in lymphomatous spleen tissues and some normal baboon tissues [15]. We have also demonstrated the presence of integrated STLV-I provirus in the DNA of malignant lymph nodes. The integration was monoclonal, and in some cases we found several integrated proviruses, including defective ones [12].

All these baboon lymphomas occurred in our main stock, which we called a high-lymphoma-risk stock. As controls we have another stock composed of animals imported directly from the wilderness, that have never had contact with the high-risk stock animals. This control stock numbers approximately 600 animals, a over a period of 15 years we have observed no cases of malignant lymphoma.

Thus, the material presented here shows great similarities between baboon lymphomas and those in human beings. The discovery of the two viruses HVP and STLV-I in baboon malignancy, with integration of STLV-I provirus into the DNA of lymphomatous tissue, and the characteristic dynamics of antibody titers with their elevation in the prelymphoma period make it possible to conclude that baboon malignant lymphoma is associated with DNA and RNA oncogenic viruses.

References

1. Poiesz BJ, Ruscetti FW, Mier SW, Woods AM, Gallo RC (1980) T-cell lines established from human T-lymphocytic neoplasias by direct response to T-cell growth factor. Proc Natl Acad Sci USA 77:6815–6821
2. Hinuma Y, Nagata K, Nanaoka M, Nakai M, Matsumoto T, Kinoshita K, Shirakava S, Miyoshi I (1981) Adult T-cell leukemia antigen in an ATL cell line and detection of antibodies to the antigen in human sera. Proc Natl Acad Sci USA 78:6476–6480
3. Yoshida M, Seiki M, Yamaguchi K, Takatsuki K (1984) Monoclonal integration of human T-cell leukemia provirus in all primary tumors of adult T-cell leukemia suggests causative role of human T-cell leukemia virus in the disease. Proc Natl Acad Sci USA 81:2534–2537
4. Lapin BA (1985) Hematopoietic diseases in non-human primates. In: Deinhardt F (ed) Proceedings XIIth Symposium for comparative research on leukemia and related diseases, Hamburg 7–11 July, p 277
5. Lapin BA (1985) EBV-related baboon virus. In: Mathé G, Reizenstein P (eds) Advances in the biosciences, vol 50. Pathophysiological aspects of cancer epidemiology. Pergamon, Oxford, p 163
6. Agrba VZ, Yakovleva LA, Lapin BA, Sangulija IA, Timanovskaya VV, Markaryan DS, Chuvirov GN, Salmanova EA (1975) The establishment of continuous lymphoblastoid suspension cultures from cells of haematopoietic organs of baboons (*Papio hamadryas*) with malignant lymphoma. Exp Pathol 10:318–332
7. Falk L, Deinhardt F, Nonoyama M, Wolfe LG, Bergolz C, Lapin BA, Yakovleva LA, Agrba V, Henle G, Henle W (1976) Properties of baboon lymphotropic herpes virus related to Epstein-Barr virus. Int J Cancer 18:798–807
8. Rabin H, Neubauer R, Hopkins R, Dzhikidze E, Shevtsova Z, Lapin BA (1977) Transforming activity and antigenicity of an Epstein-Barr-like virus from lymphoblastoid cell lines of baboons with lymphoid disease. Intervirology 8:240–249
9. Lapin BA, Voevodin AF, Indzhiia LV, Yakovleva LA, Gallo RC (1983) Some aspects on the etiology of leukemias in primates, including man (in Russian). Bull Exp Biol Med v. XCY; 14–16
10. Voevodin AF, Lapin BA, Yakovleva LA, Ponomaryeva TI, Oganyan TE, Razmadze EN (1985) Antibodies reacting with human T-lymphotropic retrovirus (HTLV-I) or related antigens in lymphomatous and healthy hamadryas baboons. Int J Cancer 36:579–584
11. Guo HG, Wong-Staal F, Gallo RC (1984) Novel viral sequences related to human T-cell leukemia virus in T cells of seropositive baboon. Science 223:1195–1197
12. Voevodin AF, Lapin BA, Tatosyan AG, Hirsch I (1985) Markers of HTLV-I-related virus in hamadryas baboon lymphoma. In this volume

13. Neubauer RH, Rabin H, Strnad BC, Lapin BA, Yakovleva LA, Indzhiia EV (1979) Antibody responses to herpes virus papio antigens in baboons with lymphoma. Int J Cancer 23:186–192

14. Voevodin AF, Yakovleva LA, Lapin BA, Ponomarjeva TI (1983) Increased antibody responses to herpes virus papio (HVP) antigens in pre-lymphomatous baboons (*Papio hamadryas*) of the Sukhumi high lymphoma stock. Int J Cancer 32:637–639

15. Djatchenko AG, Kokosha IV, Lapin BA, Yakovleva LA, Agrba VZ (1980) The revealing of the herpes virus DNA in the tissues of lymphomatous and healthy Sukhumi baboons (in Russian). J Exp Onkol 2:31–33

Haematology and Blood Transfusion   Vol. 31
Modern Trends in Human Leukemia VII
Edited by Neth, Gallo, Greaves, and Kabisch
© Springer-Verlag Berlin Heidelberg 1987

Modelling of Malignant Lymphoma in Rabbits, Using Oncogenic Viruses of Non-Human Primates

L. A. Yakovleva, V. V. Timanovskaya, A. F. Voevodin, L. V. Indzhiia, B. A. Lapin, M. T. Ivanov, and D. S. Markaryan

The discovery of lymphoid B-lymphotropic herpesvirus-producing cell lines from M. arctoides peripheral lymphocytes (MAL-1) producing their own lymphotropic virus HVMA was reported earlier [1]. Subsequently, two more M. arctoides virus-producing lymphoid cell lines (MAL-2, MAL-3) were discovered in our laboratory. The cells of some baboon lymphoid cultures, parallel with B-lymphotropic herpesvirus, produced C-type retrovirus antigenically similar to human T-lymphotropic virus (HTLV)-I. The cells of MAL-1, MAL-2 and MAL-3 cultures also produced B-lymphotropic herpes-

Institute of Experimental Pathology and Therapy, USSR Academy of Medical Sciences, Sukhumi, USSR

virus, and small amounts of retrovirus particles were revealed (Fig. 1). Furthermore, it was reported that a number of Old World monkeys, including M. arctoides, can be the carriers of simian T-lymphotropic virus (STLV) related to HTLV-I [3].

One of our research aims was to a achieve a simplified modelling of virus-associated malignant lymphoma, which we have been investigating in primates. Tests in some laboratory animals, including rabbits, on their sensitivity to B-lymphotropic herpesviruses of baboons (HVP) failed to give positive results. At the same time, some reports appeared on the transformation of rabbit lymphocytes in vitro caused by HTLV-I [2].

Six young grey rabbits bred in Sukhumi (each weighing 500–600 g) were inoculated

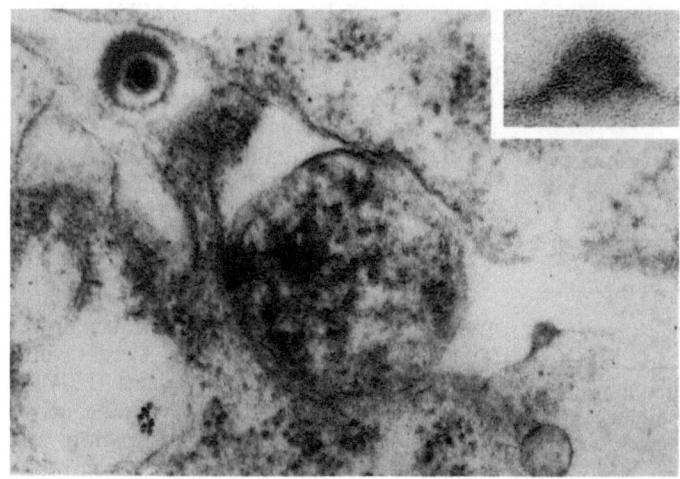

Fig. 1. Type-C and herpesvirus particles in tissue culture MAL-3 cells; × 60 000 and × 200 000

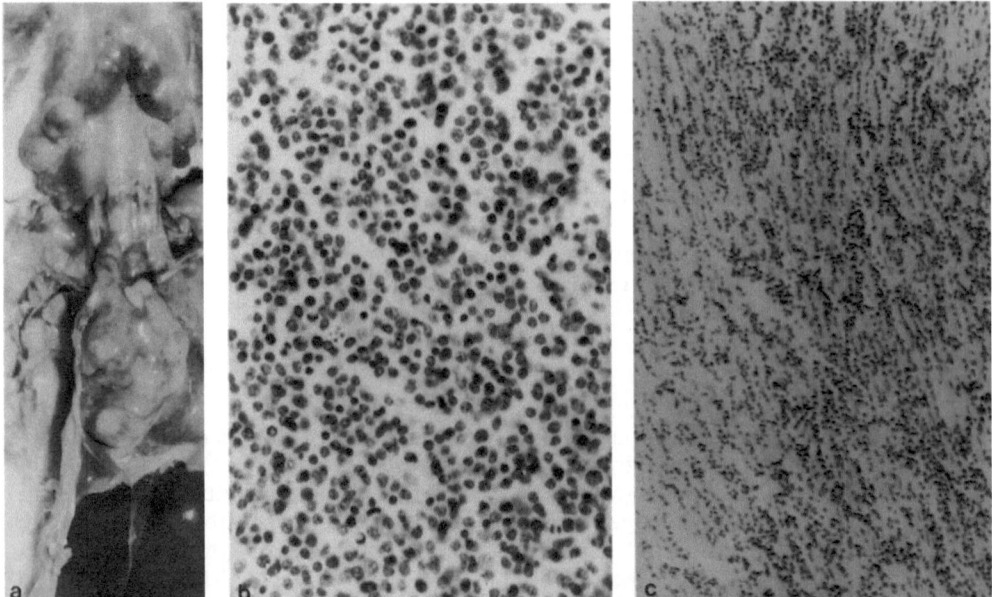

Fig. 2. a The neck lymph nodes, thymus and heart involvement in induced rabbit malignant lymphoma. Proliferation of malignant lymphoma cells in lymph node (**b**) and heart (**c**). Haematoxylin and eosin, × 500 (**b**) and × 160 (**c**)

intramuscularly with M. arctoides cell cultures (MAL-1, MAL-2, MAL-3). Inoculation led to the development of malignant lymphomas in all six rabbits. The first signs of the process were revealed 20–25 days after inoculation, and after 35–40 days the lymphoma acquired a generalized character. The sites mostly affected were popliteal lymph nodes, pelvic, mesenteric and neck lymph nodes as well as spleen, kidneys (rarely), liver, thymus, skin and bone marrow (Fig. 2). The injection of tumour materials from one animal into three others was successful in one case. We have also succeeded in causing generalized lymphoma by injection of cell-free filtrated supernatant of MAL-3 culture. Cultivation of the tumour cells of one of the rabbits led to the establishment of suspension lymphoid cell culture (RT-I), which now has 18 passages. Growing factor supplement was not needed. Culture cells had no B-lymphoid markers (Table 1) and have so far not revealed the presence of B- or T-lymphotropic viruses. Tumour cells, including those being cultivated, possess rabbit karyotype.

In six control animals, inoculated with materials of MAL-1, MAL-2 and MAL-3 cultures heated at 56 °C for 1 h, a 4-month observation has revealed no tumour occurrence.

The sera of a rabbit inoculated with homogenate of rabbit lymphoma (induced by a mixture of MAL-2 and MAL-3 cells) were tested against Epstein-Barr virus (EBV)-, HTLV-I and STLV-I positive and negative target cells before and after inoculation, using an indirect immunofluorescence test

Table 1. Testing of tumour and mononuclear peripheral blood cells of a rabbit inoculated with MAL-2 culture cells

Source of cells	SIg$^+$ cells (%)[a]
Tumour	14.0
Mononuclear from blood	28.8

[a] Cells were tested in a direct immunofluorescent test with the use of fluorescein isothiocyanate-conjugated swine anti-rabbit immunoglobulins (Dakopatts, Denmark).

446

Table 2. Reactivity of first passage rabbit sera against EBV/HVP and HTLV/STLV-I positive/negative cells in an indirect immunofluorescence test[a]

Target cells / Rabbit sera	Human B cells		Human T cells		Baboon B cells	Rabbit cells
	EBV-VCA/ EA− HTLV-I− (Raji)	EBV-VCA/ EA+ HTLV-I− (P3HR-I)	HTLV-I+ EBV− (C9I-PL)	HTLV-I− EBV− (H9)	HVP+ STLV-I+ BEV+ (594S-F9)	? ? (OK-I)
Before inoculation	−	−	−	−	−	−
After inoculation day 36	−	+[d]	++[c]	+[c]	+[b]	++[c]
After inoculation day 60	−	++[b]	+[c]	±[c]	++[b]	+[c]

[a] Rabbit was inoculated by homogenate of tumour induced by a mixture of MAL-2 and MAL-3 in another rabbit.
[b] Brilliant cytoplasmic fluorescence, low percentage of positive cells (5%–10%).
[c] Faint cytoplasmic fluorescence in practically all cells.
[d] Intensity of fluorescence

(Table 2). The preinoculation serum was negative against all types of target cells. The reactivity pattern of the postinoculation sera suggested the presence of antibodies against EBV/HVP antigens and against cell antigen(s) shared by human T cells and cultured rabbit tumour cells during lymphoma development.

The results of the present research show high oncogenicity for rabbits inoculated with M. arctoides lymphoid cell cultures. It is possible that the occurrence of tumours in rabbits after the injection of MAL-1, MAL-2 and MAL-3 cultures is associated with simultaneous expression of EBV-like B-lymphotropic herpesvirus and perhaps C-type retrovirus.

References

1. Lapin BA, Timanovskaya VV, Yakovleva LA (1985) Herpesvirus HVMA: a new representative in the group of the EBV-like B-lymphotropic herpesviruses of primates. In: Neth R et al. (eds) Modern trends in human leukemia VI. Springer, Berlin Heidelberg New York Tokyo, pp 312–313 (Haematology and blood transfusion, vol 29)
2. Miyoshi J, Yoshimoto S, Taguchi H, Kubonishi J, Fujishita M, Ohtsuki Y, Shiraishi Y, Akagi T (1983) Transformation of rabbit lymphocytes with T-cell leukemia virus. Gann 74, 1:1–4
3. Watanabe T, Seiki M, Hirayama Y, Yoshida M (1986) Human T-cell leukemia virus type-1 is a member of the African subtype of simian viruses (STLV). Virology 2:385–388

Haematology and Blood Transfusion   Vol. 31
Modern Trends in Human Leukemia VII
Edited by Neth, Gallo, Greaves, and Kabisch
© Springer-Verlag Berlin Heidelberg 1987

Retrovirus-Induced Malignant Histiocytosis in Mice: A Model for the Human Disease

J. Löhler [1], T. Franz [1], K. Klingler [1], W. Ostertag [1], and R. Padua [2]

Malignant histiocytosis, also known as histiocytic medullary reticulosis or malignant reticulosis, is a hematopoietic neoplastic disorder characterized by proliferation of abnormal histiocytes and of their precursors, with mostly a rapidly fatal course [1, 2]. Clinical findings are fever, jaundice, pancytopenia, and enlargement of liver, spleen, and lymph nodes. The etiology of the disease is unknown, although viral infections have been suggested as playing a role [3]. The study of its pathogenesis has been hampered by the lack of a suitable animal model. However, we have recently described a novel retrovirus inducing a systemic neoplastic disease in mice which is strikingly reminiscent of malignant histiocytosis in humans [4].

A new isolate of a murine retrovirus with spleen focus-forming activity – the AF-1 or, as it is now designated, malignant histiocytosis sarcoma virus (MHSV) – was derived from sarcomas that had been induced on passage of a cloned Friend helper virus in newborn BALB/c mice. Subsequently, the transforming defective subunit of the MHSV complex was cloned in NRK cells. Injection of the MHSV into mice revealed its unique capacity to transform macrophage precursor cells. MHSV-sensitive DDD mice (Fv-2^s and Fv-2^r) rapidly develop splenomegaly, hepatomegaly, and pancytopenia after intravenous infection and die within the first

25 days of the disease. Histological examination showed the proliferation of histiocytic tumor cells in bone marrow, spleen, lymph nodes, and liver, with a final infiltration of all major parenchymal organs (Fig. 1). Permanent cell lines established from MHSV-infected DDD or BALB/c mice, histiocytic tumor cells in situ, and cells of serially transplanted tumors all exhibited differentiation-specific antigens, intracellular enzyme patterns, and phagocytic ability characteristic of mononuclear phagocytes (Table 1). Mice

Table 1. Histochemical, immunohistochemical, and functional characterization of histiocytic tumor cells in MHSV-infected DDD mice, and permanent cell lines derived from tumor-bearing DDD mice

	Tumor cells in spleens of DDD mice	Permanent cell lines	
		HA15/A[a]	HA15/S[b]
Non specific esterase	+	+	+
Lysozyme	+	+	+
Alkaline phosphatase	–	–	–
F4/80 antigen	+	+	+
Pan-B-cell antigen	–	–	–
Thy-1	–	–	–
Phagocytosis	+	+	+

[a] Slow-growing adherent cells resembling macrophages.
[b] Predominantly suspended growing cells resembling monoblasts.

[1] Heinrich-Pette-Institut für Experimentelle Virologie und Immunologie an der Universität Hamburg, FRG
[2] Marie Curie Memorial Foundation, Research Institute, The Chart, Oxted, UK

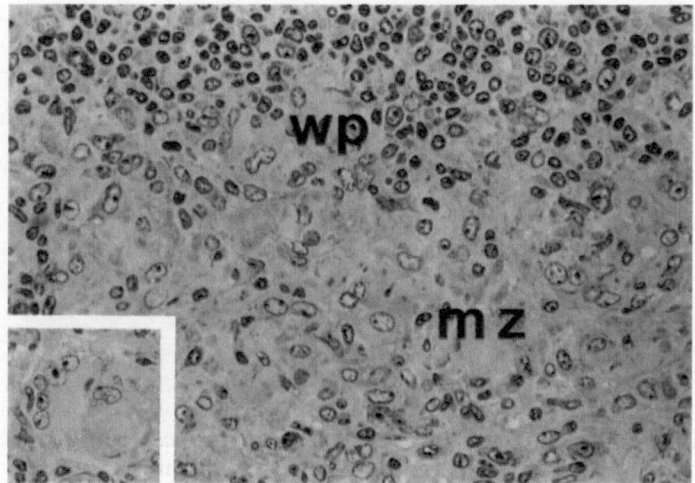

Fig. 1. Spleen of DDD mouse 8 days after infection with MHSV. Proliferation of histiocytic tumor cells in the marginal zone (*mz*) of the white pulp (*wp*). The *inset* shows a multinuclear giant cell. Toluidine blue; × 187

infected with MHSV show a large relative increase in myeloid precursor cells (CFU-C). Examination of these CFU-C in spleen and bone marrow of infected DDD mice showed that the normal distribution of CFU-C (CFU-G 25%, CFU-M 25%, CFU-GM 50%) was shifted toward a predominance of macrophage colonies: approximately 95% of the spleen CFU-C of infected DDD mice were CFU-M. Most of these CFU-C proliferated in the absence of growth factors, which are required for the growth of CFU-M of uninfected animals. Partial nucleotide sequence analysis of molecularly cloned MHSV shows that MHSV has a unique F-MuLV-related long terminal repeat with one large deletion and duplications within the direct repeat. MHSV contains, like Harvey and Kirsten sarcoma virus, rat VL30 sequences, and the *ras* oncogene of MHSV encodes a p21 protein (Padua et al., in preparation).

In conclusion, symptoms and pathological alterations of the histiocytic neoplastic disorder in mice caused by the MHSV share many features with the malignant histiocytosis of man. Irrespective of a possibly different etiology of the human and murine malignancies, we hope that studying this animal model will provide more insight into the mechanisms operating in the pathogenesis of the fatal human disease.

References

1. Rappaport H (1966) In: Atlas of tumor pathology, sect 3, fasc 8. Armed Forces Institute of Pathology, Washington, pp 49–63
2. Byrne GE Jr, Rappaport H (1973) Gann Monogr Cancer Res 15:145–162
3. Editorial (1983) Lancet I:455–456
4. Franz T, Löhler J, Fusco A, Pragnell I, Nobis P, Padua R, Ostertag W (1985) Nature 315:149–151

449

Haematology and Blood Transfusion   Vol. 31
Modern Trends in Human Leukemia VII
Edited by Neth, Gallo, Greaves, and Kabisch
© Springer-Verlag Berlin Heidelberg 1987

Oncogenes: Clinical Relevance

U. R. Rapp, S. M. Storm, and J. L. Cleveland

The last 10 years have seen something of a revolution in experimental carcinogenesis, sparked by the discovery of oncogenes [1–3]. The first such gene and most of the ones that followed [1] have been isolated as part of the genome of a tumor-inducing retrovirus. Mostly obtained from birds and mice, these viral oncogenes are nearly identical to genes present in normal cells and, because of their high degree of evolutionary conservation, could be used directly to isolate their human counterparts.

What implicated these genes in chemically induced and natural tumors? First indications came from oncogene transduction experiments with retroviruses and chemically transformed mouse and rat cells [4–6]. The transduction experiments led to the isolation of new oncogene-carrying viruses [5, 7, 8], but proof of the supposition that cellular oncogenes were involved in chemical carcinogenesis came from another quarter. Gene transfer methods using transfection of chromosomal DNA had become more efficient [9, 10], and their application to the search for transforming genes in chemically transformed mouse cells was successful [11]. The advent of molecular cloning greatly accelerated the identification of transfected, focus-inducing DNA, thus leading to the following central findings.

DNA from transformed cells was active, while DNA from untransformed cells had very little or no activity. The transforming DNA was related to one of several groups of

known viral oncogenes, the *ras* oncogenes. Similar transforming DNA could be isolated from human tumor cell lines and biopsies, whereas normal control tissue was negative. Comparison of *ras* oncogene DNA from tumor and normal tissue revealed point mutations at specific codons in transforming *ras* genes, which increased their focus-forming activity [for a review see reference 12]. Thus, it was established that at least some chemically transformed cells and cells in natural tumors differed from their normal progenitors in the biological activity and primary structure of a class of cellular oncogenes, the *ras* family. Curiously, first experiments testing DNA from a wide variety of tumors yielded only transforming *ras* genes, even though the cells were known to harbor a fair number of other oncogenes previously identified in retroviruses. While this was sometimes looked upon as a blessing, indicative of the fact that all tumors were the result of one basic malfunction, other lines of investigation suggested otherwise. Activation of human oncogenes by translocation was discovered (*myc, abl*) [for a review see reference 13], and amplification of cellular oncogenes (*myc* family, Ki-*ras*) was observed in certain tumors [2, 14]. More recently, DNA transfection also led to identification of other, non-*ras*-related oncogenes [15–19], and thus it was established that a variety of cellular oncogenes were involved in the development of human tumors.

Was oncogene activation cause or consequence of tumor development? In animal systems, it could clearly be shown to occur as an early, presumably initiation, event [20, 21]. In human tumors, some changes, such

Laboratory of Viral Carcinogenesis, Division of Cancer Etiology, National Cancer Institute, National Institutes of Health

as oncogene amplification [22, 23] and perhaps activation by translocation [24], as well as at least two documented cases of mutational activation of *ras* genes, appeared to be late events [25, 26]. This does not exclude the possibility that other oncogenes had become active early in the same tumors; in fact, the combined data from in vivo carcinogenesis, animal models, and human pathology make it likely that oncogenes are involved in initiation, maintenance, and progression of human tumors [2, 3]. But the process of carcinogenesis is definitely more complex.

A major disappointment with tumor-derived *ras* genes was the observation that, as a rule, they were not able to induce in one step a fully transformed phenotype in the presumed progenitor cells. Inspiration again came from the tumor virus sector, where cooperation between two or more genes for transformation had previously been observed [27–29], and high-efficiency transformation of primary cells in culture with specific combinations of viral and tumor-derived oncogenes was accomplished [30–33]. While the in vitro experiments could only suggest what might be going on *in vivo, owing* to the artificial nature of culture conditions and the limited variety of cell types of which they allowed study, support for the

concept of cooperating oncogenes in natural settings came from work with retroviruses carrying multiple cell-derived oncogenes or a single oncogene in the company of a supposed helper gene [33]. In fact, it was work with a dual oncogene-carrying retrovirus that established the phenomenon of synergistic transformation in vivo [32, 34] consistent with its behavior in vitro [32, 34, 35].

However, the mere fact that certain combinations of oncogenes accelerate tumor induction in birds and mice does not directly address the question of the role of oncogene synergism in human tumor development, and to date there is no example of the isolation of multiple active oncogenes from a primary human tumor. Moreover, the true assay for the transforming potential of a tumor-derived oncogene, i.e., incorporation into tumor progenitor cells by gene replacement or at least addition, and implantation of these cells at various doeses into their natural site, has yet to be performed. Nevertheless, it seems reasonable to expect that multiple, weakly transforming oncogenes, presumably activated successively, are involved in the development of perhaps the majority of human tumors.

What are cellular oncogenes and what is their normal role in cellular physiology? The

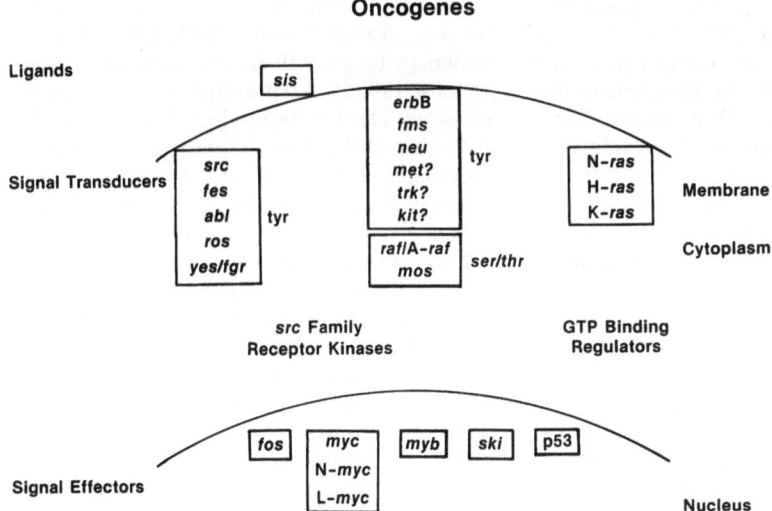

Fig. 1. Schematic representation of oncogenes grouped in the cell according to their amino acid sequence relatedness, cellular location, and position in the signal transduction pathway of growth factors

Table 1. Human oncogene map

Chromosome

1. N-*ras*, c-SK, NGF
2. *fos*, N-*myc*
3. *raf*-1
4. *raf*-2, IL-2
5. *fms*
6. *myb*, c-Ki-*ras*-1
7. ERV3, *erb*-B, A-*raf*-2 *met*
8. *myc*, *mos*
9. *abl*
10.
11. c-Ha-*ras*-1
12. c-Ki-*ras*-2, *int*-1
13. RB-1 (retinoblastoma)
14.
15. *fes* (*fps*), ERV2
16.
17. *erb*-A1, *erb*-A2
18. ERV1
19.
20. *src*
21.
22. *sis* (PDGF)
X. c-Ha-*ras*-2, A-*raf*-1

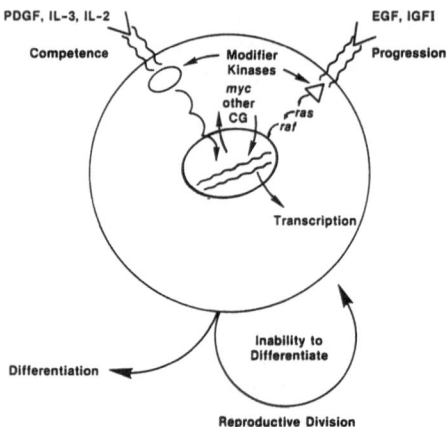

Fig. 2. Schematic representation of proto-onco-genes involved in the signal transduction path-ways of growth factors. *PDGF*, platelet-derived growth factor; *IL-3, IL-2*, interleukin 3 and 2; *EGF*, epidermal growth factor; *IGF-1*, insulin-like growth factor 1; *CG*, "competence" genes; ≋, re-ceptors

functions of several such genes have recently been identified [36–38] or approximated [34, 39–42]. Figure 1 shows a compilation of the best-studied oncogenes according to their location in the cell, sequence relatedness, en-zymatic activity, and known or presumed function in the signal transduction pathway of growth factors [34, 43]. Table 1 gives the chromosomal locations of oncogenes in hu-mans. Briefly, there are three major func-tional groups: ligands [*sis* = platelet-derived growth factor (PDGF) gene-derived], recep-tors, and cytoplasmic transmitters (two large families, *src* and *ras*) and genes for nu-clear proteins, at least one of which (*myc*) appears to function as a central relay for growth factor signal transduction [34, 39–41]. The largest superfamily of known onco-genes is the *src* family, which contains trans-membrane receptors [*erb*B, derived from the epidermal growth factor (EGF) receptor; *fms*, related to the colony-stimulating factor (CSF)-1 receptor; and *neu*, *met*, and *trk*, de-rived from receptors for unknown ligands], and both membrane-associated (*src*, a form of *abl*) and cytoplasmic protein kinases (c-*raf*, A-*raf*, and *mos*). In general, these kin-

ases have specificity for tyrosine, with the ex-ception of the *raf* family and *mos*, which have associated kinase activity specific for serine and threonine [44]. The second, grow-ing cytoplasmic/membrane-associated fam-ily is the *ras* family, which appears to have to do with cyclic nucleotide metabolism and guanosine triphosphate (GTP) binding [12].

The most prominent of the nuclear genes are *myc*, *fos*, and *myb*, which have all been shown to be growth-factor-regulated in ex-pression [39, 45–47] and might in turn medi-ate growth factor signals [40, 41]. Another il-lustration of the growth factor connection of oncogenes is to be found in Fig. 2, which places various genes in a scheme built on earlier observations made by others [48, 49] in the course of study of growth regulation of BALB 3T3 fibroblasts. Under certain conditions, these cells require sequentially two qualitatively distinct ligands – PDGF, which was called a competence factor, fol-lowed by EGF, a progression factor – before they enter S-phase. Treatment of cells with PDGF induces a set of "competence" or early G1 genes, [48] to which belong onco-genes such as *myc* and *fos* and R-*fos* [50], at least one of which can partially [40] or com-pletely [41], presumably depending on dose, replace the cell's need for the inducing fac-

Table 2. Human tumors frequently associated with a specific oncogene

Burkitt's lymphoma	c-*myc*
CML	*abl*
Neuroblastoma	N-*myc*
Lung carcinoma	c-*raf*-1
Stomach cancer	c-*raf*-1 (sporadic?)

tor. On the basis of experiments in growth factor abrogation [41], oncogene synergism [32, 34, 51], and the relationship of *ras* and *raf* oncogenes [43, 52, 53], the latter two were placed in the progression pathway of growth regulation, with *raf* located downstream of *ras*. One possibility for connecting the two pathways, consistent with the observed synergisms and the enzymatic activity of *raf* as well as with properties of *myc*, is the activation of *myc* by *raf* via phosphorylation [43, 54].

Thus, the conclusion from the above findings is that oncogenes are relevant to human oncology. Their deregulated function presumably causes the loss of growth control in malignant cells. Does this knowledge help us in diagnosis or treatment of clinical cancer? The answer is no, or not yet. Although there are a few types of human tumors in which a specific oncogene is consistently involved (presumably activated), such as chronic myelocytic leukemia (CML) [55, 56], Burkitt's lymphoma [13, 57–59], and perhaps lung and stomach cancer [18, 43, 60; Table 2], most tumors appear to be variably associated with a variety of oncogenes, if they yield activated oncogenes at all. There is some hope, however, that with the isolation of additional oncogenes and improved histological typing, a list of preferred oncogenes may be emerging which is typical for certain tumors. It is likely to be a list of genes rather than a single one because, as indicated in Fig. 2, oncogenes appear to belong in signal transmission pathways from cell surface to the nucleus, where presumably each pathway involves the agency of multiple oncogene products, any one of which may be able to deregulate the chain. In any case, there is some hope that different tumor types may be distinguishable on the basis of oncogene profiles, which would provide a set of functional rather than structural tumor markers.

What might be the consequence of identifying such markers? So far, there is no evidence that oncogene typing would be useful for early diagnosis or treatment of tumors, except for certain familial cases of retinoblastoma, where the DNA probe that is being used, however, is not an oncogene probe but a RFLP probe. Using such probes, the presence of a predisposing retinoblastoma chromosome 13 (Table 1) in one case was detected in amniocentesis material, and early surgery on the infant probably saved his life [61].

There are also familial cases of renal carcinoma which may involve *raf* and *myc* oncogenes [43, 62], and other rare familial tumors associated with distinct chromosomal abnormalities [24] for which a similar approach may become applicable in the future. Moreover chromosomal site changes or specific gene changes involved in hereditary cancer may also occur in sporadic tumors of the same type, and their identification may thus become important for establishing tumor-specific (onco)-gene profiles in individual patients. Another example of the clinical use of oncogene- or oncogene-related DNA probes is a breakpoint specific probe characterizing the translocation that activates the *abl* oncogene in CML. Current technology allows detection of translocation-positive CML cells in cell mixtures at the level of 1%, and this probe is therefore presently being evaluated in clinical trials to determine the effect of various treatment regimens at the level of the target cell.

Oncogene probes have also become clinically useful for diagnosis of unrelated genetic diseases. For example, the *raf*-2 pseudogene is currently the closest RFLP marker for Huntington's chorea [63], and the active *met* oncogene probe is used to help in the diagnosis of people with a predisposition to cystic fibrosis [64–66]. Thus, oncogene probes are today clinical tools important for diagnosis and treatment of certain human tumors as well as for diagnosis of two of the four most common noncancerous human hereditary diseases. Moreover, we are only beginning to explore what other consequences of specific oncogene expression in tumors might be exploited in the future. To list a few ongoing investigations: (a) Production of transforming growth factors by tu-

Table 3. *raf* oncogenes

---

2 active genes in man: c-*raf*-1 and A-*raf*-1
c-*raf*-1 on chromosome 3p25; site altered in several epithelial neoplasias
  Gene expressed in many tissues
A-*raf*-1 on chromosome Xp21
  Gene expressed in select tissues
Genes encode 74- and 69-kd cytosolic proteins with associated serine/threonine kinase activity
  Function in signal transduction downstream of *ras*
Oncogenic activation can be achieved by truncation
Both genes have pseudogenes: c-*raf*-2 and A-*raf*-2
  c-*raf*-2 marks Huntington's chorea

---

mors and excretion in urine are being studied and may become of diagnostic and/or prognostic value [67]. (b) We are determining the possibility of immunity induction to altered oncogenes in cancer patients. (c) There is some hope that expression of specific oncogene constellations in a cell will alter their physiology such that they now differ from their normal progenitors predictably in sensitivity to metabolic poisons or other cell regulators.

Since at least some growth factor receptors are cellular oncogenes and some tumor cells show autocrine secretion, efforts are under way to develop receptor-blocking agents in order to stop or slow down cancer cell growth. Unfortunately, cancer-specific receptors have yet to be identified, and we already know that tumor cells can become receptor-independent by switching to oncogenes capable of intracellular mitogen signal transmission [40, 41]. It is therefore especially worthwhile to focus on modes of inactivation of intracellular oncogenes, particularly those such as *raf* which are located at the effector end of the growth factor signal transduction chain. Indeed, there is preliminary evidence suggesting that *raf* protein kinase activity is regulated at the level of the protein, thus providing us with a target site to which to fit a downregulating agent.

Many of the techniques and approaches discussed above are being used in our laboratory to evaluate the role of *raf* oncogenes in lung carcinoma, the most common tumor of Western man.

The general properties of *raf* oncogenes are summarized in Table 3. c-*raf*-1 was first implicated in lung cancer because of its chromosomal map position at 3p25, a site that is

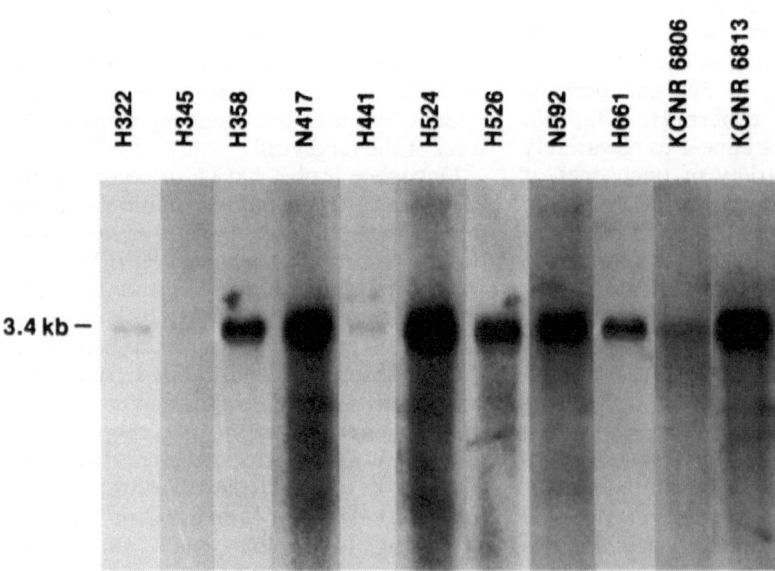

Fig. 3. Expression of c-*raf*-1 in human lung cancer cell lines. Poly(A)+mRNA from the indicated small-cell lung cancer cell lines was purified and analyzed using Northern blot procedures for c-*raf*-1 RNA. The size of the c-*raf* RNA is shown in kilobases (*kb*)

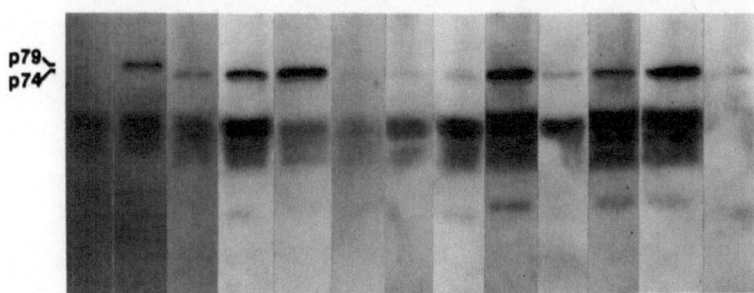

Fig. 4. Western analysis of c-*raf* proteins in human lung cancer cell lines. Unlabeled extracts of cells were affinity-purified using c-*raf* C-terminal specific anti-SP63 antibody. The extracts were electrophoresed, blotted, and reacted with anti-SP63 serum and ^{125}I protein A. As a negative control, c-*raf* immunoprecipitates from mouse 3T3 cells were reacted with anti-p15 *gag* serum and ^{125}I protein A. For comparison of levels of *raf,* 3T3 cells transformed by v-*raf* (3T3/3611) are shown. Sizes of proteins are indicated in kilodaltons (*kd*)

frequently altered in small-cell lung cancer [43, 60, 68]. Expression of c-*raf*-1 was therefore determined in lung cancer cell lines and biopsy material by Northern blotting (Fig. 3), Western blotting (Fig. 4), and immunohistochemistry with *raf*-specific antibodies, a highly sensitive technique applicable to biopsy material (data not shown). c-*raf*-1 RNA and protein of normal size are expressed in the majority of lung tumors of all histological types, whereas they are low or undetectable in normal lung (unpublished results). Thus, c-*raf*-1, sporadically amplified *myc* family genes [2], and occasionally occurring mutation-activated Ki-*ras* oncogenes [12, 69, 70] are candidate components of the machinery that drives the uncontrolled growth of these tumors. But how can we determine whether *raf* is an "activated" oncogene in these cells, given the fact that it is of normal size? Work with full-length, normal c-*raf*-1 cDNA has suggested that while amino terminal truncation of the molecule is a common structural change typical of several transforming versions of the gene, high-level expression of the normal gene may also facilitate transformation. The levels of c-*raf*-1 protein in lung tumor cells are well within the range observed in c-*raf*-1 cDNA transformed mouse cells (unpublished results). Nevertheless, because of the lack of telltale

signs of oncogenic activation, it remains to be determined whether *raf* oncogene and also *myc* gene functions play a role in the maintenance of the transformed phenotype of lung tumor cells.

Assuming that c-*raf*-1 is involved in lung carcinoma, is there evidence to suggest that *raf* transformed cells are more sensitive than control cells to potential negative growth regulators? We have examined the effects of a variety of substances in ongoing experiments and observed inhibitory actions of two reagents, the C-kinase activator TPA on *raf* transformed mouse cells and hydrocortisone for transformed rat, but not control cells (Fig. 5 a, b). These are preliminary data, and there may exist other agents, more suitable for clinical application, which are more effective, but these experiments serve to illustrate that there is a basis for the hope that tumor cells may have an altered or increased sensitivity to (negative) growth modulators.

To evaluate further the effects of potential negative growth regulators experimentally in vivo, we have developed an animal model system for the induction of lung carcinoma (Fig. 6). Transplacental treatment with ethylnitrosourea of NFS (female) mated with AKR (male) mice, followed by promotion with butylated hydroxytoluene (BHT), results in rapid tumor development, starting at

455

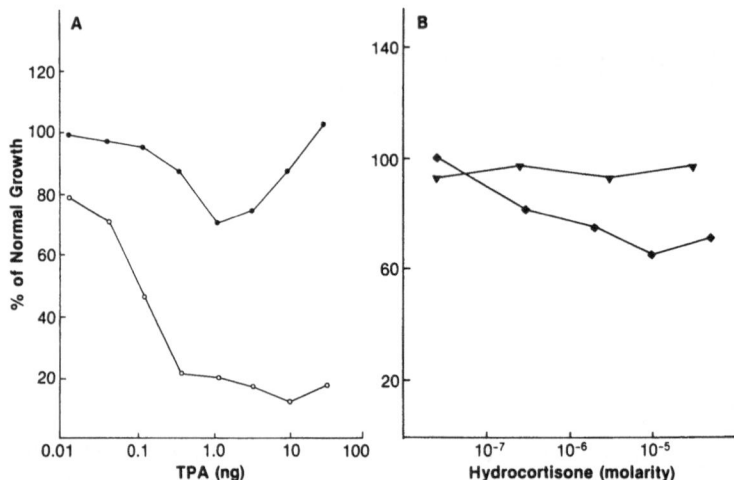

Fig. 5 a, b. Growth inhibition of mouse NIH/3T3 (**a**) and rat FRE3A (**b**) *raf*-transformed cells with TPA (**a**) and hydrocortisone (**b**), respectively; sub-confluent cultures of control (●, ▼) and v-*raf* transformed (○, ◆) cells were treated with the dose of TPA and hydrocortisone indicated, and after 4 days were pulsed with [^{125}I] IdUrd for the last 24 h to determine levels of DNA synthesis. In-

corporation of [^{125}I] IdUrd is expressed in terms of percent normal growth of untreated control cultures. A minor fraction of flat revertant cells present in the transformed parent culture is resistant to growth arrest by hydrocortisone. On microscopic inspection of LTR-*raf* transformed rat cells treated with 10^{-5} molar hydrocortisone only flat revertants were apparent (data not shown)

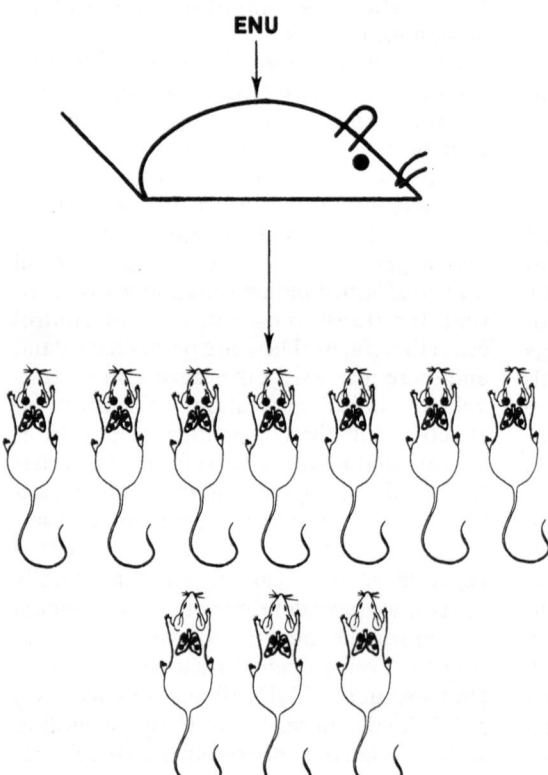

Fig. 6. Induction of lung adenocarcinoma and lymphoma in mice treated with ethylnitrosourea (*ENU*). Pregnant NFS females (mated with AKR males) were injected transplacentally with ENU, and weanling-age F1 mice were promoted with weekly injections of butylated hydroxytoluene (BHT). The incidence of tumor induction in F1 mice is shown diagrammatically; about 70% of animals develop a T-cell lymphoma and nearly 100% develop lung adenocarcinoma

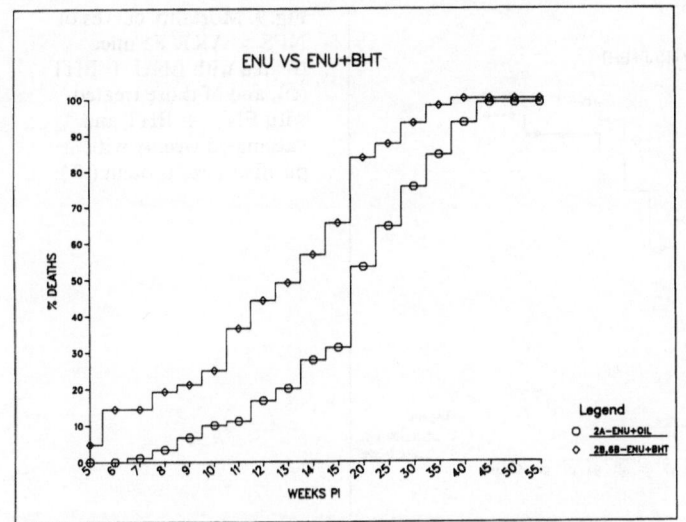

Fig. 7. Mortality curves for NFS × AKR F1 mice treated in utero with ENU (○) and mice treated with ENU followed by weekly promotion with BHT (◇). Fifty percent of mice treated with ENU + BHT died with a mean latency of 13 weeks, whereas those treated with ENU alone died with a mean latency of 20 weeks. Vaccinations with control proteins were ineffective

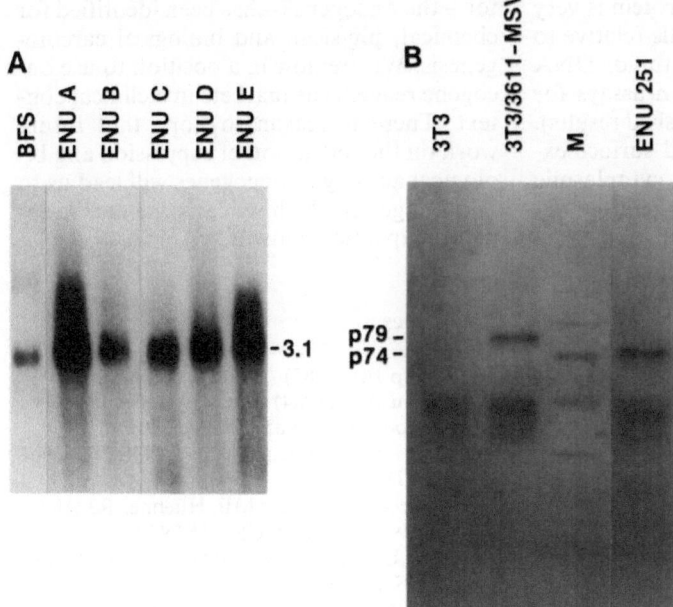

Fig. 8 a, b. Expression of c-*raf*-1 mRNA (**a**) and protein (**b**) in ENU-induced lung adenocarcinoma and lymphoma. **a** Levels of c-*raf*-1 poly(A)+ mRNA (5.0 μg) isolated from three T-lymphomas (ENU A–C) and two lung adenocarcinoma (ENU D and E) were compared to levels found in a murine T-cell line, BFS. **b** Western analysis of levels of c-*raf*-1 protein in an ENU-induced lymphoma (ENU 251) compared to those found in v-*raf* 3611-MSV transformed mouse fibroblast cells. p79 is the size (in kd) of the *gag*-v-*raf* fusion protein of 3611-MSV, whereas p74 is the size of c-*raf*. *M*, ^{14}C molecular weight standards. As a negative control, c-*raf* immunoprecipitates from mouse 3T3 cells were reacted with p15 *gag* antibody and [125I] protein A

457

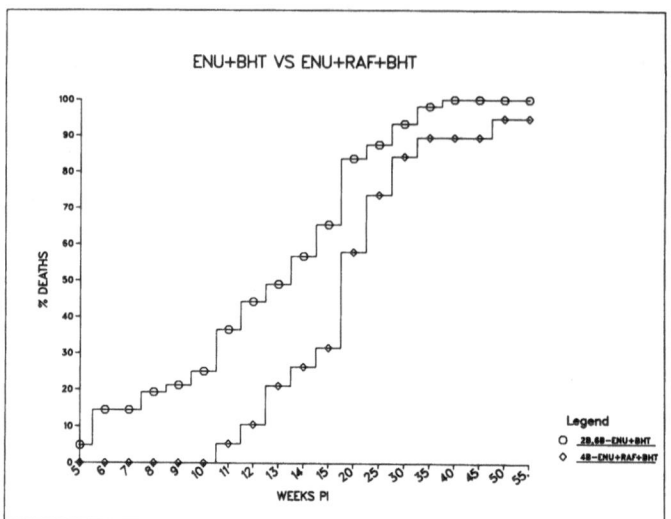

ENU+BHT VS ENU+RAF+BHT

Fig. 9. Mortality curves of NFS × AKR F1 mice treated with ENU + BHT (○), and of those treated with ENU + BHT and vaccinated weekly with purified v-*raf* protein (◇)

5 weeks of age (Fig. 7). Two types of tumors result – lung adenocarcinoma (80%–100%) and T-cell lymphomas (60%–70%). Expression of c-*raf*-1 RNA and protein is very high in both types of tumor cells relative to control tissue (Fig. 8 a, b), and tumor DNA is positive in DNA transfection assays for focus-forming activity (unpublished results). Live cell fluorescence suggested surface expression of the predominantly cytoplasmic *raf* protein in tumor cells. We therefore decided to test whether induction of an immune response to *raf* oncogene protein in these mice would affect tumor development, and observed significant effect of *raf* protein vaccination on the BHT-promoted early phase of tumor incidence, whereas no long-term protection was achieved (Fig. 9).

The *raf* oncogene may not be the best choice for study of the potentials of immune modulation of tumor growth, since it is predominantly located in the cytoplasm of cells [43]. Receptor-related oncogenes which become structurally altered in tumors may be more promising. However, the rules on how to induce a cellular immune response, which is presumably the critical element in host defense against tumor growth, are only becoming established. It may be that intracellular antigens are in fact more efficient in triggering a cytotoxic T-cell response [71]. In any case, the experiments with *raf* serve to illuminate some of the strategies for control of

tumor growth that may hold promise for the future.

In the last 10 years, a common denominator – the oncogenes – has been identified for chemical, physical, and biological carcinogenesis. We are now in a position to use oncogene reagents as markers in a clinical context. There is reason to hope that future work on the regulation of expression and biological activity of oncogenes will lead us to knowledge on which we can base new rational therapeutic regimens.

References

1. Bishop JM (1983) Ann Rev Biochem 52:301
2. Varmus HE (1984) Ann Rev Genet 18:553
3. Weinberg RA (1985) Science 230:770
4. Rapp UR, Todaro GJ (1978) Science 201:821
5. Rasheed S, Gardner MB, Huebner RJ (1978) Proc Natl Acad Sci USA 75:2972
6. Rapp UR, Todaro GJ (1980) Proc Natl Acad Sci USA 77:624
7. Rapp UR, Reynolds FH Jr, Stephenson JR (1983) J Virol 45:914
8. Rapp UR et al. (1983) Proc Natl Acad Sci USA 80:4218
9. Graham FL, van der Eb AJ (1973) Virology 52:456
10. Shih C et al. (1979) Proc Natl Acad Sci USA 76:5714
11. Parada LF, Weinberg RA (1983) Mol Cell Biol 3:2298

12. Barbacid M (1986) Human Oncogenes. In: Devita, Hellman, Rosenberg (eds) Important advances in oncology. Lippincott, Philadelphia, pp 3–22
13. Klein G (1983) Cell 32:311
14. Alitalo K et al. (1983) Proc Natl Acad Sci USA 80:1707
15. Cooper CS et al. (1984) Nature 311:29
16. Schechter AL et al. (1984) Nature 312:513
17. Fukui M et al. (1985) Proc Natl Acad Sci USA 81:5954
18. Shimizu K et al. (1985) Proc Natl Acad Sci USA 82:5641
19. Martin-Zanca D, Hughes SH, Barbacid M (1986) Nature 319:743
20. Sukumar S, Notario V, Martin-Zanca D, Barbacid M (1983) Nature 306:658
21. Balmain A, Ramsden M, Bowden GT, Smith J (1984) Nature 307:658
22. Kohl NE et al. (1983) Cell 35:359
23. Brodeur GM et al. (1984) Science 224:1121
24. Rowley JD (1980) Ann Rev Genet 14:17
25. Tainsky MA, Cooper CS, Giovanella BC, Vande Woude GF (1984) Science 225:643
26. Albino AP et al. (1984) Nature 308:69
27. Houweling A, van den Elsen PJ, van der Eb AJ (1980) Virology 105:537
28. Rassoulzadegan M et al. (1982) Nature 300:713
29. van den Elsen PJ et al. (1982) Gene 18:175
30. Land H, Parada LF, Weinberg RA (1983) Nature 304:596
31. Ruley HE (1983) Nature 304:602
32. Rapp UR et al. (1985) J Virol 55:23
33. Graf T et al. (1986) In: Genetics, cell differentiation and cancer, 7th Annual Bristol-Myers Symposium on Cancer Research
34. Rapp UR et al. (1985) In: Haveman K, Sorenson GD, Gropp C (eds) Peptide hormones in lung cancer. Springer, Berlin Heidelberg New York Tokyo, p 221 (Recent results in cancer research, vol 99)
35. Blasi E et al. (1985) Nature 318:667
36. Waterfield MD et al. (1983) Nature 304:35
37. Doolittle RF et al. (1983) Science 221:275
38. Downward J et al. (1984) Nature 307:521
39. Kelly K, Cochran BH, Stiles CD, Leder P (1983) Cell 35:603
40. Armelin HA et al. (1984) Nature 310:655
41. Rapp UR et al. (1985) Nature 317:434
42. Sherr CJ et al. (1985) Cell 41:665
43. Rapp UR, Cleveland JL, Bonner TI (1986) In: Curran, Reddy, Skalka (eds) The oncogene handbook
44. Moelling K et al. (1984) Nature 312:558
45. Greenberg ME, Ziff EB (1984) Nature 311:433
46. Muller R, Bravo R, Burckhardt J (1984) Nature 312:20
47. Kruijer W et al. (1984) Nature 312:711
48. Pledger WJ, Stiles CD, Antoniades HN, Scher CD (1977) Proc Natl Acad Sci USA 74:4481
49. Cochran BH, Reffel AC, Stiles CD (1983) Cell 33:939
50. Cochran BH, Zullo J, Verma IM, Stiles CD (1984) Science 226:1080
51. Cleveland JL et al. (1986) J Cell Biochem 30:195
52. Smith MR, DeGudicibus SJ, Stacey DW (1986) Nature 320:540
53. Huleihel M et al. (1986) Mol Cell Biol 6:2655
54. Rapp UR, Bonner TI, Cleveland JL (1985) In: Gallo, Stehelin, Varnier (eds) Retroviruses and human pathology. Humana, New Jersey, p 449
55. Heisterkamp N et al. (1983) Nature 306:239
56. Groffen J et al. (1984) Cell 36:93
57. Battey J et al. (1983) Cell 34:779
58. Adams JM et al. (1983) Proc Natl Acad Sci USA 80:1982
59. Dalla-Favera R et al. (1982) Proc Natl Acad Sci USA 79:7824
60. Bonner TI et al. (1984) Science 223:71
61. Cavenee WK et al. (1986) In: Cold Spring Harbor Symp Quant Biol Vol LI:829
62. Drabkin HA et al. (1985) Proc Natl Acad Sci USA 82:6980
63. Gusella JF et al. (1986) In: Cold Spring Harbor Symp Quant Biol
64. Knowlton RG et al. (1985) Nature 318:380
65. White R et al. (1985) Nature 318:382
66. Wainwright BJ et al. (1985) Nature 318:384
67. Sherwin SA et al. (1983) Cancer Res 43:403
68. Whang-Peng J et al. (1982) Science 215:181
69. Shimizu K et al. (1983) Nature 304:497
70. Capon DJ et al. (1983) Nature 304:507
71. Townsend ARM et al. (1986) Cell 44:959

Haematology and Blood Transfusion   Vol. 31
Modern Trends in Human Leukemia VII
Edited by Neth, Gallo, Greaves, and Kabisch
© Springer-Verlag Berlin Heidelberg 1987

Retroviruses with Two Oncogenes

D. Stehelin and P. Martin

A. Introduction

Less than a decade ago the first retroviral oncogene was discovered [1] and shown to derive from a normal cellular gene [2]. To date over 20 different retroviral oncogenes have been found, all derived from cellular counterparts. How a single oncogene can cause cancer is still not fully understood. Natural cancers are known to involve multistep molecular changes, raising a paradox, as compared to cancers induced by retroviral oncogenes. To turn a cellular gene into an active retroviral oncogene, an overexpression due to the very potent retroviral promoter may suffice in a few cases, whereas in most cases several modifications are probably required. These modifications might involve enhanced transcription, truncation of

Inserm U 186, Institut Pasteur, 15 Rue C. Guerin, 59019 Lille, France

the gene, specific mutations, deletions or insertions (Fig. 1) as well as the viral route of transmission.

In this respect a retroviral oncogene may then be regarded as a single gene having accumulated stepwise, through many replication cycles and selections by researchers (these viruses do not exist in nature) several modifications in order to become a potent cancer gene. Such a process represents a somewhat artificial situation difficult to be challenged for statistical reasons by a cellular oncogene during the lifetime of the host cells. Nevertheless, cellular oncogenes that were identified through retroviruses seem to be involved in some natural cancers, where they are for example deregulated through chromosomal translocation (c-myc) or mutations [13] (c-ras). Although they appear much "weaker" transforming genes than their viral counterparts, they legitimate the use of retrovirus as tools. It follows that nat-

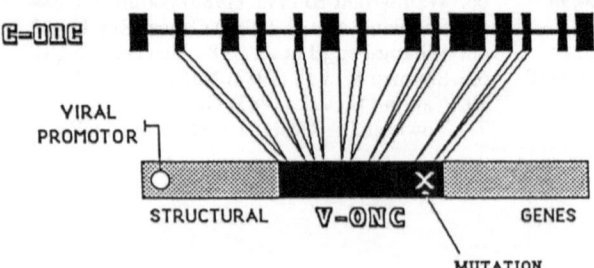

- Transduction of a truncated gene

- Linkage to structural viral genes

- Transcription under a strong viral promotor

- Possible mutations in the transduced gene

Fig. 1. Possible differences between v-*onc* and c-*onc*

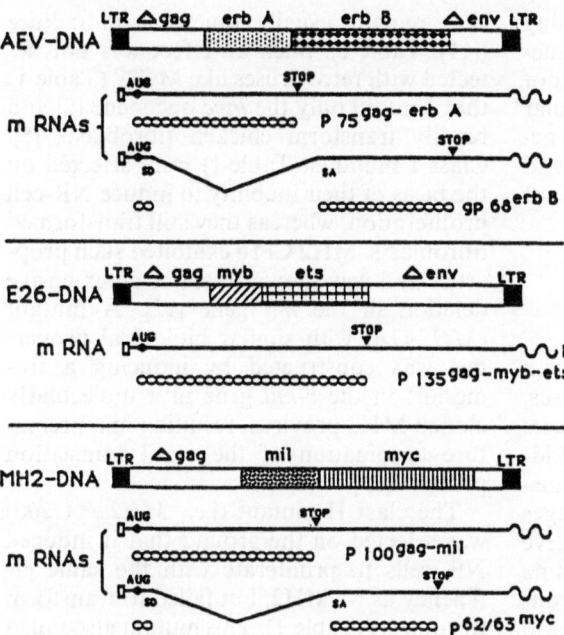

Fig. 2. Retroviruses with two onco-genes

ural cancers are likely to involve single alter-ations on several distinct genes that cooper-ate in the tumorigenic process. Recently, a first example of cooperation was demon-strated by in vitro studies showing that the activated *ras* and *myc* oncogenes could transform a rat embryo fibroblast in a way that neither gene could achieve alone [3] and some human tumor cell lines were found to contain the cellular *ras* and *myc* oncogenes both altered. How can we identify more such cooperative genes? Retroviruses may again represent useful tools. In 1979, studying acute avian leukemia retroviruses, we raised the possibility [4] that some retroviruses undergoing modifications could have, among those transduced, not one, but two distinct cellular genes that could cooperate in the viral transformation processes. There are now three examples of such retroviruses (Fig. 2) that we would like to review briefly.

B. Avian Erythroblastosis Virus

The genome of avian erythroblastosis virus (AEV) contains the two oncogenes *erbA* and *erbB* [5]. Deletion mutants in one or the other oncogene have shown that in adult bone marrow the erbB product transforms

erythroblasts which subsequently cannot mature properly anymore. The erbA prod-uct alone does not modify erythroid cells in a detectable way [6]. In contrast, wild type AEV tightly blocks erythroid cells at an im-mature stage (erythroid colony forming units or CFUe) [7]. Thus, erbA potentiates the transforming activity of the *erbB* gene product. The nucleotide sequencing of the *erbA* gene appears unrelated to any of the oncogenes characterized so far and related to carbonic anhydrases, enzymes known to play a major role in red blood cells, the pro-genitors of which are precisely the target cells for AEV. Other studies performed on embryonic tissue of the primitive streak indi-cate that AEV affects also target cells that appear to precede the BFUe stage.

C. Avian Erythroblastosis Virus E26

The genome of E26 virus contains the two oncogenes *myb* and *ets* [8], expressed in in-fected cells as a triple fusion protein P130$^{gag-myb-ets}$ [5]. E26 appears able to transform un-committed erythroid-myeloid hemopoietic cells as well as cells committed in the ery-throid and myeloid lineages (see Moscovici et al., this volume). How the two oncogenes *myb* and *ets* are involved in the transforming properties of E26 virus awaits the construction of mutants deleted in one or the other of the genes. We recently obtained a molecular clone of E26 provirus that is biologically active (D. Leprince et al., in preparation) and that should facilitate the construction of such mutants.

D. Mill-Hill-2 Retrovirus

The avian retrovirus Mill-Hill-2 (MH2) is a replication defective retrovirus that causes, like other avian *myc*-containing retroviruses (MC29, CMII, OK10), mainly liver and kidney carcinomas in the chicken, and transforms chicken fibroblasts and macrophages in culture [5]. MH2 appears more aggressive than the other *myc*-containing viruses in its tumorigenic potential and its genome contains a second oncogene, *mil* [9], yielding in infected cells the two onc proteins P100$^{gag-mil}$ and p62/63^{myc} [10]. In order to examine the respective roles of the two proteins in the transformation process, we attempted the isolation of spontaneous or constructed mutant expressing properly only the *mil* or only the *myc* oncogene product. Two classes of spontaneous mutants were isolated by Calothy's group (Institut du Radium, Orsay, France) using fibroblasts and neuroretinal (NR) cells prepared from 7-day-old chicken embryos. The choice of this latter cell system was bound to the observation that MH2 wild type virus was shown to stimulate the growth and to transform NR cells

Table 1. Characterization of *MH2* mutants

Virus	Fb1 T	NR		Apparent functional oncogene
		M	T	
MC29	+	−	−	*myc*
wt MH2	+	+	+	*myc* + *mil*
MH2 Cl 16	+	−	−	*myc* ⎫ (Class I)
MH2 OB	+	−	−	*myc* ⎭
MH2 PA 200	−	+	−	*mil* ⎫ (Class II)
MH2 LI 200	−	+	−	*mil* ⎭

Fb1, fibroblasts; NR, neuroretinal cells; T, transformed; M, mitogenized; wt, wild type

that remain usually quiescent in culture ([11]; Table 1). Such an effect was not detected with retroviruses like MC29 (Table 1) that contain only the *myc* oncogene [2] and readily transform chicken fibroblasts [5]. Class I mutants (Table 1) were selected on the basis of their inability to induce NR-cell proliferation, whereas they still transformed fibroblasts. MH2 Cl 16 exhibited such properties and was shown to suffer an extensive deletion in the *mil* gene [12]. A mutant (*MH2-OB*) with similar biological properties was constructed by inducing a frameshift in the *v-mil* gene in a molecularly cloned MH2 provirus, resulting in a premature termination of the v-mil translation product [13].

The class II mutant (i.e., *MH2 PA 200*) was selected on the ground that it induced NR cells to proliferate with the same efficiency as wt-MH2, but failed to transform fibroblasts (Table 1). This mutant also failed to morphologically transform NR cells and showed upon analysis that it was extensively deleted in the *myc* gene [14]. A mutant (*MH2 LI 200*) with similar biological properties (Table 1) was constructed by inducing a frameshift in the *v-myc* gene of molecularly cloned MH2 provirus that resulted in a premature termination of the v-myc translation product.

The results presented here [13] indicate that the ability to induce sustained proliferation and transformation of NR cells from 7-day-old chicken embryos is a remarkable property distinguishing MH2 among other *myc*-containing retroviruses, and requiring the coordinate expression of both *mil* and *myc* oncogenes. Class I mutants lacking a functional *mil* gene (*MH2 Cl 16, MH2 OB*) do not induce NR-cell proliferation nor transformation, although they still transform fibroblasts (and macrophages [15]). Conversely, mutants expressing only the *mil* oncogene (*MH2 PA 200, MH2 LI 200*) induce NR cell proliferation without morphological transformation.

So far, the viral *myc* oncogene (or the large T of polyomavirus) was shown to cooperate with the EJ bladder carcinoma activated *ras* oncogene (or middle T of polyomavirus) for rat embryo fibroblast transformation [3]. We show now that the *myc* oncogene can also cooperate with the *mil* oncogene (the latter being structurally related to the *src*-gene family [16]) for the transformation of NR cells. Thus, the *myc* oncogene may cooperate with two distinct types of oncogenes depending on the cell types considered. Whether *myc* plays a key role in two distinct pathways leading to transformation, or whether the three types of oncogenes (*myc*-, *ras*-, and *mil*-like) belong to a single pathway leading to cell-growth stimulation, where transformation can occur when some of them become deregulated, whereas others might be perhaps constitutively expressed at specific stages of cell maturation or in specific cell types, remains to be examined. Earlier work on polyoma might be recalled in this respect. Although the oncogenes of this virus were not shown to have cellular counterparts, the large *T* and middle *T* polyoma genes were shown to cooperate for fibroblast transformation, as do the activated *myc* and *ras* genes, respectively [17]. In addition, the middle T was shown [18] to bind specifically in the transformed fibroblast the cellular protein pp60^{src} that was shown activated in the complex.

In conclusion, research is slowly beginning to unwrap the cooperation of genes in normal and pathological cell-growth stimulation, and retroviruses with double oncogenes represent convenient tools in such investigations. They have allowed discovery of three new oncogenes (*erbA*, *ets*, and *mil*) that potentiate previously described oncogenes (*erbB*, *myb*, and *myc*, respectively) in their transforming activity or allow these viruses to transform new target cells. Whether the corresponding couples of cellular oncogenes participate in the formation of natural human cancers is under investigation.

References

1. Stéhelin D, Guntaka RV, Varmus HE, Bishop JM (1976) J Mol Biol 101:349–365
2. Stéhelin D, Varmus HE, Bishop JM, Vogt PK (1976) Nature 260:170–173
3. Land H, Parada LF, Weinberg RA (1983) Nature 304:596–602
4. Roussel M et al. (1979) Nature 281:452–455
5. Graf T, Stéhelin D (1982) Biophys Biochim Acta 651:245–271
6. Frykberg L et al. (1983) Cell 32:227–238
7. Samarut J, Gazzolo L (1982) Cell 28:921–929
8. Leprince D et al. (1983) Nature 306:395–397
9. Coll J et al. (1983) Embo J 2:2189–2194
10. Pachl C, Biegalke B, Linial M (1983) J Virol 45:133–139
11. Calothy G et al. (1979) Cold Spring Harbor Symp Quant Biol 44:983–990
12. Martin P et al. (1985) J Virol 57:1191–1194
13. Bechade et al. (1985) Nature 316:559–562
14. Martin P et al. (1986) Virology (in press)
15. Graf T et al. (1986) Cell 45:357–364
16. Galibert F et al. (1984) EMBO J 3:1333–1338
17. Cuzin F (1984) Biophys Biochim Acta 781:193–204
18. Courtneidge SA, Smith AE (1983) Nature 303:435–439

Haematology and Blood Transfusion   Vol. 31
Modern Trends in Human Leukemia VII
Edited by Neth, Gallo, Greaves, and Kabisch
© Springer-Verlag Berlin Heidelberg 1987

Activation of the *met* Proto-oncogene in a Human Cell Line *

M. Dean[1], M. Park[1], K. Kaul[1], D. Blair[2], and G. F. Vande Woude[1]

The *met* oncogene was identified in the MNNG-HOS cell line, derived by extensive treatment of a human osteosarcoma cell line (HOS) with *N*-methyl-*N*-*N'*-nitrosoguanidine (MNNG) [1]. DNA from MNNG-HOS cells was used to transform NIH/3T3

[1] BRI-Basic Research Program, NCI-Frederick Cancer Research Facility, Frederick, Maryland
[2] Laboratory of Molecular Oncology, National Cancer Institute, Frederick, Maryland, USA
* Research sponsored by the National Cancer Institute, DHHS, under Contract NO. NO1-CO-23909 with Bionetics Research, Inc. The contents of this publication do not necessarily reflect the views or policies of the Department of Health and Human Services, nor does mention of trade names, commercial products, or organizations imply endorsement by the U.S. Government.

mouse fibroblast cells, and the transforming gene (*met*) was isolated from one of these NIH/3T3 transformants [2] (Fig. 1 a).

The activated *met* allele in MNNG-HOS cells is rearranged with sequences from another gene (Fig. 1). This second gene appears to provide the promoter for the activated *met* oncogene and has been named *tpr* for "translocated promoter region" [3]. The *tpr* locus has been mapped by somatic cell hybridization analysis to human chromosome 1 [3], whereas *met* mapped to chromosome 7 [2, 4]. Therefore, the *met* oncogene has been activated by a DNA rearrangement involving portions of chromosomes 1 and 7.

We examined the expression of the *met* and *tpr* sequences in HOS, MNNG-HOS, and transformed NIH/3T3 cells. As shown

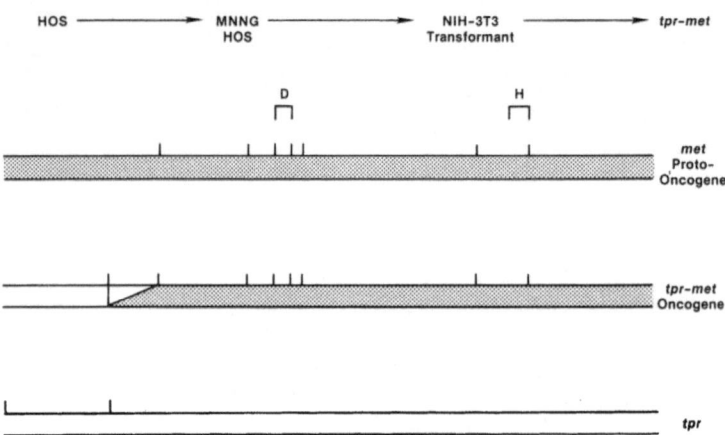

Fig. 1. Diagram of the *met* oncogene rearrangement. HOS cells treated with MNNG gave rise to MNNG-HOS cells. DNA from MNNG-HOS cells is capable of morphologically transforming mouse NIH/3T3 cells, and the *tpr-met* gene was isolated from a transformant

Table 1. *met* and *tpr* mRNA species

Probe	Size of mRNA species[a] (kb) in		
	HOS cells	MNNG-HOS cells	NIH/3T3 transformants
met	9.0, 7.0, 6.0	9.0, 7.0, 6.0	—
tpr-met	—	5.0	5.0
tpr	10.0	10.0	—

[a] mRNA species were determined by RNA blot hybridization, using *met* and *tpr* DNA as probes.

in Table 1, analysis with a *tpr* probe revealed an mRNA species of 10 kb in both HOS and MNNG-HOS cells. HOS and MNNG-HOS cells expressed *met* mRNAs of 9, 7 and 6 kb. However, analysis with probes from the 3′ end of the *met* gene and the 5′ end of *tpr* detected a hybrid 5.0-kb *tpr-met* transcript in MNNG-HOS cells [3] (Table 1), which is also found in NIH/3T3 cells transformed by MNNG-HOS DNA. We conclude that the gene rearrangement that activated the *met* locus results in the appearance of a hybrid mRNA transcript.

To determine the structure of the *met* gene product, we have begun to determine the nucleotide sequence of the coding regions. We have published the sequence of several *met* exons and demonstrated that *met* exhibits homology with the tyrosine kinase family of oncogenes and growth factor receptors [4]. We have recently isolated several *met* cDNA

clones from a library prepared from A431 human squamous cell carcinoma cells. The longest clone obtained was 1.6 kb, and when the nucleotide sequence was translated, the sequence was found to contain a single, long, open reading frame. Figure 2 shows the *met* sequence in one-letter amino acid code and compares it with several other tyrosine kinase genes.

The *met* gene is most extensively homologous to the human insulin receptor gene [5] and the v-*abl* oncogene from Abelson murine leukemia virus [6]. The homology is mostly confined to the kinase domain of the proteins and reaches 50%–60% at the amino acid level. However, the carboxy terminus of *met* is significantly different from that of the other members of the family. Therefore, although *met* is homologous to the tyrosine kinases, it is not identical to any other known member of that gene family.

Previous studies mapped the rearrangement of the *tpr-met* gene to a 3.4-kb *Eco*RI fragment [3]. To determine the nucleotide sequence of the breakpoint, we used *met* and *tpr* probes flanking the site of rearrangement to screen a λ phage library of human placental DNA. The rearrangement was mapped to small fragments present in the placental *met* and *tpr* phage clones. These fragments and a portion of *tpr-met* were cloned into M13 vectors and the nucleotide sequence was determined.

Figure 3 shows a portion of a sequencing gel of the *tpr* and *tpr-met* genes surrounding the chromosomal breakpoint. The se-

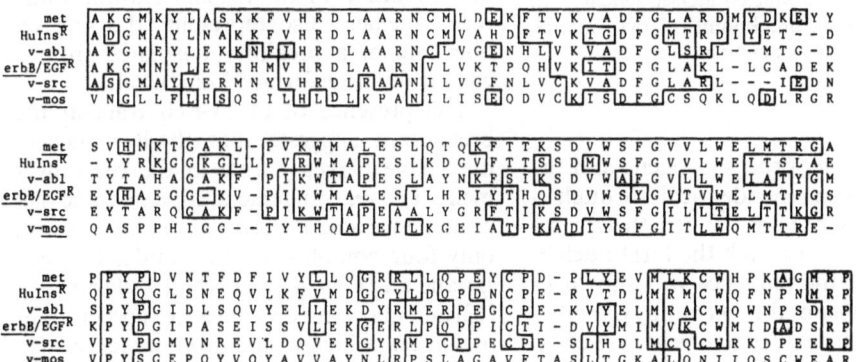

Fig. 2. Amino acid comparison of *met* with several protein kinases. The kinase domain of *met* is compared with the homologous region of the human insulin receptor (HuIns[R]), viral *abl* gene, *erb*B/epidermal growth factor receptor, viral *src* and *mos* genes

465

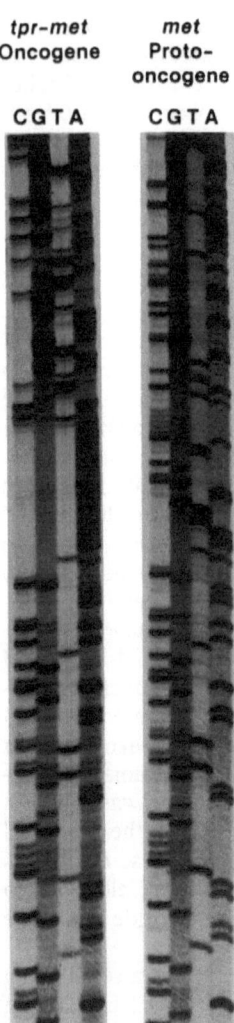

tpr–met
Oncogene

met
Proto-
oncogene

C G T A   C G T A

Fig. 3. Portion of a nucleotide-sequencing gel showing the *tpr–met* breakpoint. *C,* cytosine; *G,* guanine; *T* thymine; *A,* adenine

quences of the *met* proto-oncogene and the *tpr–met* oncogene are identical through a stretch of 21 A residues. When the *tpr* sequence was used to search the NIH nucleotide data base, the sequence was shown to contain a member of the *Alu* family of highly repetitive sequences. These repeats are often followed by poly A-rich stretches, and the one in *tpr* is localized just upstream from the 21 A residues at the breakpoint. Therefore, the DNA rearrangement leading to the ac-

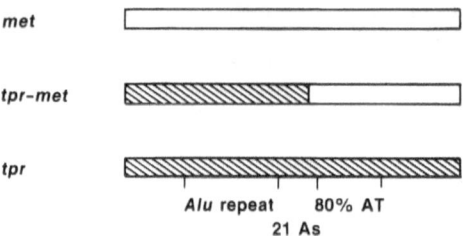

met

tpr–met

tpr

Alu repeat   80% AT
21 As

Fig. 4. Structure of the *tpr–met* breakpoint. Schematic of the rearrangement showing the position of the *Alu* repetitive element, 21 A residues, and the A-T-rich region flanking the breakpoint

tivation of *met* is located within this A-T rich region at the end of an *Alu* repeat.

Figure 4 is a schematic diagram of the *met* breakpoint region. The *met* and *tpr–met* genes are identical beyond the breakpoint for 600 residues, except for a single point mutation (not shown). Beyond the rearrangement site, on the *tpr* gene, is a stretch of 120 residues that are 80% A-T rich. Although chromosomal rearrangements have been observed in a wide variety of malignant cells [7], to our knowledge, this is the first time a chromosomal breakpoint has been sequenced in a nonhematopoietic cell. The nucleotide sequences of several other breakpoint sites have been determined and include rearranged c-*myc*, immunoglobulin heavy and light chain genes [8, 9], *bcll* [10], and T-cell receptor genes [11]; however, many of these rearrangements involve immunoglobulin switch-region sequences [8, 10] and are probably restricted to lymphoid cells. Our determination of the *tpr–met* chromosomal rearrangement also represents the first sequencing of a breakpoint isolated from a chemically transformed human cell.

The presence of an A-rich tract at the breakpoint suggests that these sequences may have played a role in the rearrangement. The rearrangement appears to be illegitimate because it occurred in a region with only four homologous nucleotides between *tpr* and *met* (Fig. 4a). MNNG is clastogenic [12] and may have created a free end in either *met* or *tpr*, which would promote rearrangement. Alternatively, the A-T-rich region of *tpr* may have contributed to the rearrangement. These regions may exist in a single-stranded structure and may be more susceptible to cleavage. Chromosomal regions with increased lability (fragile sites) have been described previously and have been proposed as playing a role in chromosomal rearrangement [13]. In fact, many fragile sites are induced by agents that interfere with thymidine metabolism [12]. It will be interesting to see whether *tpr* maps to any of the fragile sites located on chromosome 1.

The MNNG-HOS cell line used in our study arose after 7 days of MNNG treatment to HOS cells [1]. We cannot be sure that MNNG participated in the *tpr-met* rearrangement, but it is an interesting possibility. The principal action of MNNG on double-stranded DNA is the methylation of the N-7 position of guanine [14]. A pair of G residues is located in *tpr* just 3' to the breakpoint (not shown). MNNG is also capable of methylating adenine [14]; thus, MNNG-induced modification of residue(s) at the breakpoint may have contributed to the rearrangement. Besides the breakpoint, the only other change detected between *tpr-met* and placental DNA is a G-to-T transition. This alteration could be a polymorphic difference between individuals, could have arisen during transfection or cloning, or could have occurred as a consequence of MNNG treatment. At any rate, it is clear that massive mutation of the *tpr-met* gene did not occur in MNNG-HOS cells.

The expression of a truncated tyrosine kinase domain appears to be a common activation mechanism for this family of oncogenes. In addition to *tpr-met,* rearranged *bcr-abl* and *trk* genes have been isolated from human tumor DNA [15, 16]. Furthermore, retroviral insertion within the chicken epidermal growth factor receptor results in the expression of a truncated (*erb*B) kinase activity [17]. We are currently investigating the role, if any, of the *tpr* sequences in the transforming ability of the *tpr-met* oncogene.

The human *met* oncogene is located on a portion of chromosome 7 associated with nonrandom deletion in secondary acute nonlymphocytic leukemia patients [18]. Although we have not found any direct evidence of the fact that *met* plays a role in acute nonlymphocytic leukemia, an interesting outcome of that work is the discovery that *met* is very tightly linked to the gene for cystic fibrosis [19]. Cystic fibrosis is a recessive genetic disorder characterized by abnormal exocrine gland function. Cells from patients with cystic fibrosis show abnormal regulation of chloride ion transport and impaired secretion in response to β-adrenergic agents (inducers of adenylate cyclase). Although it may seem unlikely that *met* is involved in this pathway, several proto-oncogenes appear to be involved in signal transmission [20]. Recent evidence suggests that chloride channels can be phosphorylated by a tyrosine kinase [21] and that tyrosine kinases can cooperate with adenylate cyclase to modulate gene expression [22]. Clearly, the tyrosine gene family plays important roles in the cellular control of growth, differentiation, and metabolism.

References

1. Rhim JS, Park DK, Arnstein P, Heubner RJ, Weisburger EK (1975) Nature 256:751–753
2. Cooper CS, Park M, Blair DG, Tainsky MA, Huebner K, Croce CM, Vande Woude GF (1984) Nature 311:29–33
3. Park M, Dean M, Cooper CS, Schmidt M, O'Brien SJ, Blair DG, Vande Woude GF (1986) Cell 45:895–904
4. Dean M, Park M, LeBeau M, Robins T, Diaz M, Rowley J, Blair D, Vande Woude GF (1985) Nature 318:385–388
5. Ullrich A, Bell JR, Chen EY, Herrera R, Petruzzelli LM, Dull TJ, Gray A, Coussens L, Liao Y-C, Tsubokawa M, Mason A, Seeburg PH, Grunfeld C, Rosen OM, Ramachandran J (1985) Nature 313:756–761
6. Reddy EP, Smith MJ, Srinivasan A (1983) Proc Natl Acad Sci USA 3623–3627
7. Yunis JJ (1983) Science 221:227–236
8. Calame K, Kim S, Lalley P, Hill R, Davis M, Hood L (1982) Proc Natl Acad Sci USA 99:6994–6998
9. Neuberger MS, Calabi F (1983) Nature 305:240–243
10. Tsujimoto Y, Jaffe E, Cossman J, Gorham J, Nowell PC, Croce CM (1985) Nature 315:340–343
11. Denny CT, Yoshika Y, Mak TW, Smith SD, Hollis GF, Kirsch IR (1986) Nature 320:549–551
12. Perry P, Evans HJ (1975) Nature 258:121–125
13. LeBeau MM (1986) Blood 67:849–858
14. Lawley PD, Thatcher CJ (1970) Biochem J 116:693–707

15. Shtivelman E, Lifshitz B, Gale RP, Canaani E (1985) Nature 315:550–553
16. Martin-Zanca D, Hughes SH, Barbacid M (1986) Nature 319:743–748
17. Yamamoto T, Nishida T, Miyajima N, Kawai S, Ooi T, Toyoshima K (1983) Cell 35:71–78
18. Yunis J (1984) Cancer Genet Cytogenet 11:125–137
19. White R, Woodward S, Leppert M, O'Connell P, Hoff M, Herbst J, Lalouel J, Dean M, Vande Woude GF (1985) Nature 318:382–384
20. Bishop JM (1985) Cell 42:23–28
21. Mohamed AH, Stekk TL (1986) J Biol Chem 261:2804–2809
22. Ran W, Dean M, Campisi J (1986) Proc Natl Acad Sci USA 83:8216–8220

Haematology and Blood Transfusion Vol. 31
Modern Trends in Human Leukemia VII
Edited by Neth, Gallo, Greaves, and Kabisch
© Springer-Verlag Berlin Heidelberg 1987

Molecular-Genetic Analysis of *myc* and *c*-Ha-*ras* Proto-oncogene Alterations in Human Carcinoma

P. G. Knyazev, S. N. Fedorov, O. M. Serova, G. F. Pluzhnikova, L. B. Novikov, V. P. Kalinovsky, and J. F. Seitz

A. Introduction

The results of recent studies on the molecular biology of cancer suggest the abnormal expression of cellular proto-oncogenes in the process of carcinogenesis [1]. The activation of proto-oncogenes, i.e., their conversion into cellular oncogenes, is associated with gene structural alterations and mutations resulting in the unregulated production of oncoproteins, matched by deranged biological function of the latter. Recently, "mixed" variants of *ras*-family gene activation were established. They involve both amplification and point mutations in one of the "hot" codons [2, 3].

The present study deals with the analysis of alterations of *v*-*myc*-related sequences and *c*-Ha-*ras* proto-oncogenes occurring in primary tumors, metastases, homologous with cancer-intact tissues and peripheral blood leukocytes of cancer patients.

B. Materials and Methods

Genomic DNAs from tumors of the breast, ovary, lung, thyroid, colon, and stomach and homologous normal tissues were prepared as described [4], digested with restriction endonucleases, electrophoresed in 0.8% agarose gels, denatured, and transferred to nitrocellulose filters [5]. Filters were hybridized with ^{32}P-labeled (nick-translated) *v*-*myc* [6] or *hu*-*c*-Ha-*ras* [7] probes under stringent conditions, washed, dried, and exposed to ORWO film.

The N. N. Petrov Research Institute of Oncology, USSR Ministry of Health, Leningrad, USSR

C. Results and Discussion

Amplification of *myc*-specific sequences was observed in seven of 21 DNA samples obtained from human breast carcinomas (Table 1). Three DNAs (BrC2, BrC1, BrC23) contained additional *myc*-bands, besides a 12.0-kbp *Hind*III-*c*-*myc* germline, and were characterized by a high degree of amplification (20- and 100- to 150-fold) that may be regarded as *c*-*myc* gene rearrangement (Fig. 1) [8].

Analysis of DNAs from 11 thyroid carcinomas revealed 5- to 10- and 60- to 80-fold *c*-*myc* amplification in two samples (ThC3, ThC6). In the DNA with the higher degree of amplification we saw additional amplified *myc*-fragments of the same size as those in breast carcinomas (Fig. 1, Table 1).

Extra copies of the *c*-Ha-*ras* gene were registered in the samples of breast and thyroid with superamplification of *c*-*myc* (Fig. 2).

DNAs of 12 patients with ovarian cancer were analyzed, and there was *c*-*myc* amplification in primary bilateral and metastatic tumors of three of them (OvC7, OvC11, OvC16; Fig. 3, Table 1). *C*-*myc* alterations can be observed in poorly differentiated tumors characterized by an aggressive clinical course. An increase in the copy number of *myc*-related sequences has been also identified in the DNAs of peripheral blood leukocytes from two ovarian cancer patients (Fig. 3) [9].

The analysis of ten lung tumors showed *c*-*myc* amplification in two squamous carcinomas. In the only undifferentiated large-cell carcinoma tested amplification of maybe

Table 1. Amplification of *myc*-related sequences in human tumors of different localizations and histotypes

Tumor localization	Tumor histotype	Number of tested tumors/ Number of tumors with amplification	Copy number	Presence of rearrangements[a]
Breast	Ductal invasive carcinoma	17/6	5– 10 100–150	+
	Mucinous carcinoma	1/0		
	Medullar carcinoma	1/0		
	Tubular carcinoma	1/1	100–150	+
	Papillary carcinoma	1/0		
	Lobular fibroadenomatosis	1/0		
Total		22/7		
Ovary	Serous cystadenocarcinoma	13/4	5– 10	
	Serous cystadenocarcinoma metastasis	5/1	5– 10	
	Undifferentiated cystadenocarcinoma	6/2	10– 15	
	Undifferentiated cystadeno-carcinoma metastasis	4/1	5– 10	
	Mucinous borderline cystadenoma	1/0		
	Endometrioid adenomyoma	1/0		
	Dermoid tumor	1/0		
	Thecoma	1/0		
Total		32/8		
Lung	Keratinizing squamous cell carcinoma	6/1	10– 15	
	Non-keratinizing squamous cell carcinoma	3/1	10– 15	
	Undifferentiated large cell carcinoma	1/1	15– 20	+
Total		10/3		
Thyroid	Papillary carcinoma	9/2	5– 10 60– 80	+
	Follicular carcinoma	1/0		
	Undifferentiated spindle-cell carcinoma metastasis	1/0		
	Papillary carcinoma metastasis	1/0		
	Follicular adenoma	1/0		
Total		13/2		
Colon	Adenocarcinoma	11/1	40– 50	+
	Signet-cell carcinoma	1/0		
	Adenoma	6/0		
Total		18/1		
Stomach	Adenocarcinoma	9/0		
	Signet-cell carcinoma	1/0		
	Undifferentiated carcinoma	4/1	15– 25	+
Total		14/1		
Total		110/22		

[a] Presence of *myc*-related sequences containing restriction fragments different from the corresponding ones for *c-myc* locus

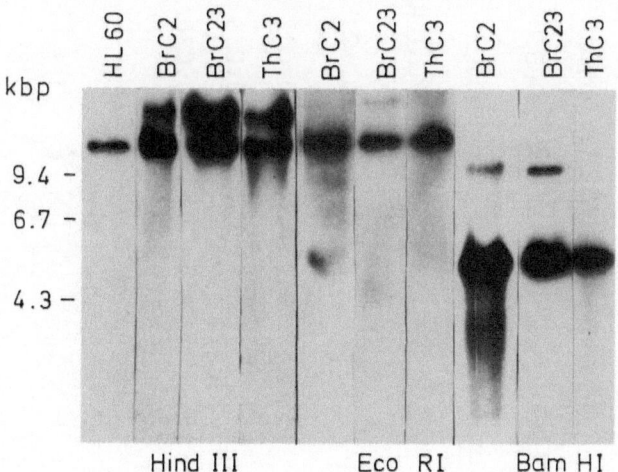

Fig. 1. Restriction analysis of *myc*-related sequences in breast (*BrC*) and thyroid (*ThC*) tumors

kbp

9.4 -
6.7 -

4.3 -

Hind III   Eco RI   Bam HI

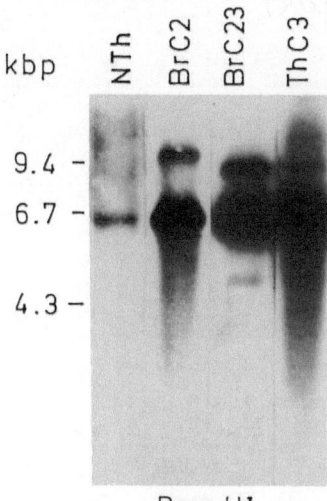

kbp

9.4 -
6.7 -

4.3 -

Bam HI

Fig. 2. Restriction analysis of *c-Ha-ras* proto-on-cogenes in breast (*BrC*) and thyroid (*ThC*) tumors as compared with normal thyroid tissue (*NTh*)

L-myc (6.6-kbp *Eco*RI-fragment) could be seen. All three tumors were highly metastatic and aggressive.

Myc-amplification is rather frequent in breast, ovarian, and lung tumors (seven of 21, eight of 28, three of ten respectively) and less so in thyroid (two of 12), stomach (one of 14), and colorectal (one of 12) malignancies (Fig. 4, Table 1).

We failed to detect amplification of *myc*-specific sequences in 13 DNA samples from benign tumors of the colon, ovary, thyroid, and breast (Table 1).

Forty-five samples of DNA obtained from normal lung tissue and gastric and colonic mucosa were examined for any alterations of *myc* proto-oncogenes developing in uninvolved tissues homologous with cancer tissues. Extra copies of *myc*-related sequences were identified in three of them. In two cases (lung and gastric tissues) the degree of amplification and length of amplified *myc*-fragments corresponded with those observed in tumors of the same patients. In one instance we were able to identify the amplification of *myc*-specific sequences in the DNA of colonic mucosa only, and there was none in the colon carcinoma of this patient (Fig. 5) [10].

The latter findings, as well as evidence of *myc* gene amplification in blood-circulating leukocytes, corroborate the concept of cancer as a general disease.

Summarizing the results obtained, we can conclude that the phenomenon of *myc*-gene family amplification appears to be common in human primary and metastatic tumors (22 of 98). Our observations are in line with those of J. Yokota and colleagues [11], who detected the above phenomenon in 11% of epithelial tumors tested. Perhaps the somewhat higher frequency of *myc*-gene amplification in our study can be explained by the application of a *v-myc*-specific probe for detecting a *c-myc* germline containing restriction fragments as well as bands characteristic for other genes of the *myc* family or rearranged *c-myc*.

471

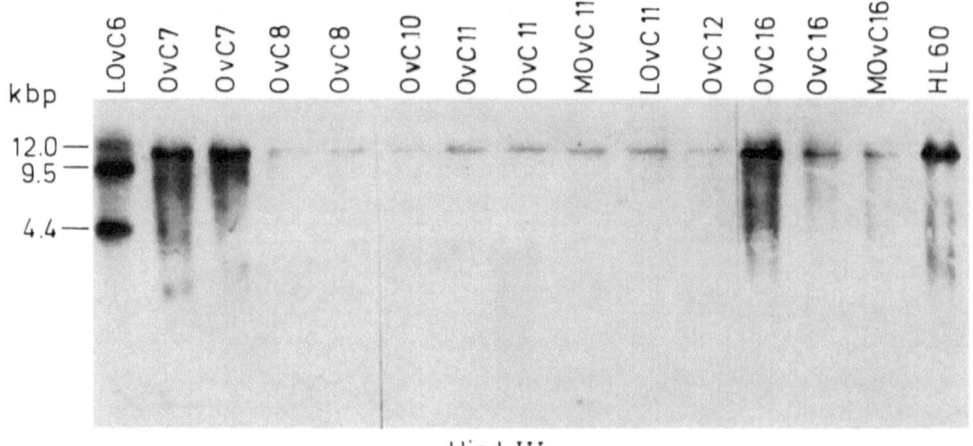

Hind III

Fig. 3. Restriction analysis of *myc*-related sequences in ovarian tumors (*OvC*), metastatic tumors of patients with ovarian cancer (*MOvC*), and blood-circulating leukocytes of ovarian cancer patients (*LOvC*)

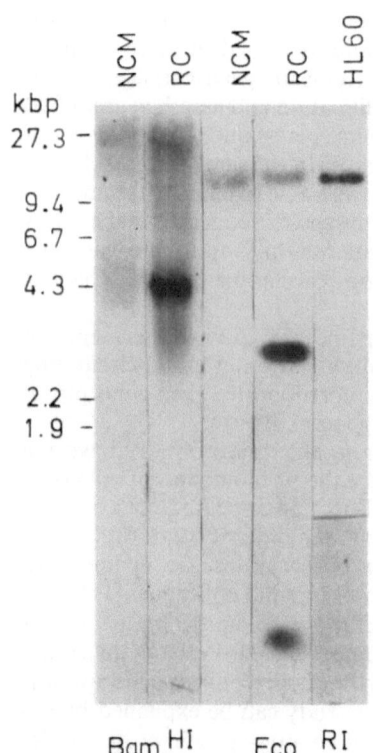

Bam HI   Eco RI

Fig. 4. Restriction analysis of *myc*-related sequences in rectal tumor (RC) and normal colonic mucosa (NCM) of same patient

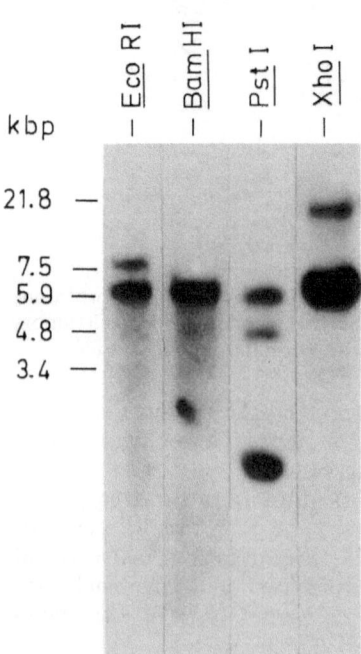

Fig. 5. Restriction analysis of *myc*-related sequences in colonic mucosa of a patient with colonic carcinoma

The finding of abnormal (amplified) *c-myc* and *c*-Ha-*ras* proto-oncogenes in a few breast and thyroid tumors confirms the hypothesis that these two genes somehow cooperate in the process of carcinogenesis.

In most cases *myc*-gene amplification was matched by poor cell differentiation and an aggressive clinical course of the tumor.

The study revealed that *myc* and *c*-Ha-*ras* proto-oncogene activation contributes to tumorigenesis through the mechanism of gene amplification and oncogene cooperation.

References

1. Cooper GM, Lane MA (1984) BBA 738:9–20
2. Taya Y, Hosogoi K, Hirohashi S (1984) EMBO J 3:2943–2946
3. Rio G, Barrous M, Tordjam J (1984) Annu Rep Fr Acad Sci 14:575
4. Maniatis T, Fritsch EF, Sambrook J (1982) Molecular cloning. Cold Spring Harbor, New York
5. Southern EM (1975) J Mol Biol 98:503–517
6. Vennström J, Moscovici C, Goodman HM, Bishop JM (1981) J Virol 39:625–631
7. Ellis RW, DeFeo D, Marya JM, Young HA, Shih TY, Chang EH, Lowy DR, Scolnick EM (1980) J Virol 36:408–420
8. Plushnikova GF, Serova OM, Knyazev PG, Fedorov SN, Novikov LB, Valdina EA, Moiseenko VM, Semiglazov VF, Vagner RI, Seitz JF (1987) Exp Oncol 9:15–17
9. Serova OM (1987) Exp Oncol 9:25–27
10. Seitz JF, Fedorov SN, Serova OM, Kalinovsky VP, Knyazev PG, Melnikov RA (1985) Vopr Onkol 31:52–56
11. Yokota J, Tsunetsugu-Yokota Y, Battifora H, Le Fevre C, Cline MJ (1986) Science 231:261–265

Haematology and Blood Transfusion   Vol. 31
Modern Trends in Human Leukemia VII
Edited by Neth, Gallo, Greaves, and Kabisch
© Springer-Verlag Berlin Heidelberg 1987

Interaction of Promoters and Oncogenes During Transfection

L. Z. Topol, A. G. Tatosyan, and F. L. Kisseljov

DNA transfection in recipient NIH3T3 mice cells is most widely used for identification of transforming genes in human tumor cells [1]. We showed earlier that c-Ha-*ras* proto-oncogene from a human malignant glioma cell line (U 251 Mg) was active in transfection experiments. In primary U 251 Mg cells, c-Ha-*ras* gene was present in a single copy but amplified in transfected NIH3T3 cells [2].

For the purpose of further analyzing this system, we studied the influence of exogenous promoters on molecular-genetic processes which occur during transfection of genetic material. As a source of promoter, we used pLTR 1.5 plasmid which was subcloned from pPR c11 plasmid containing Rous sarcoma virus (RSV) provirus [3]. The pLTR 1.5 clone contained the intact LTR of RSV and the 5′ leader sequence of the viral genome.

This plasmid was cotransfected in NIH3T3 cells with DNA containing amplified c-Ha-*ras* from nude mice tumors developed as a result of the injection of the cells transfected by DNA from a human malignant glioma cell line [2] or with DNA from the normal NIH3T3 cells. In both cases, 7 days after cultivation in vitro, the cells (2×10^6) were injected into nude mice. In the first case, tumors developed in a 2-week period, and in the second one a little later. DNA from these cells was analyzed for LTR sequences and the activation of cell proto-oncogenes by molecular hybridization tests

[4] using nick-tranlated LTR and oncogene probes [5]. Where cotransfection included pLTR 1.5 and DNA from NIH3T3 cells in the DNA of nude mice, the size of LTR-con-

Fig. 1. The analysis of pLTR 1.5 sequences in the genome of nude mice tumors induced by the injection of NIH3T3 cells transfected by various DNA preparations. *1* NLTR 1 (first round); *2* NLTR 2 (first round of the second experiment); *3* NLTR 1-1 (second round); *4* NLTR 1-2 (second round of the second experiment); *5* NIH3T3. Restriction with *Eco*RI. Washing conditions: 65 °C 0.1 × SSC, 0.1% SDS. Probe: ^{32}P-pLTR 1.5

Institute of Carcinogenesis, Cancer Research Center, Moscow, USSR

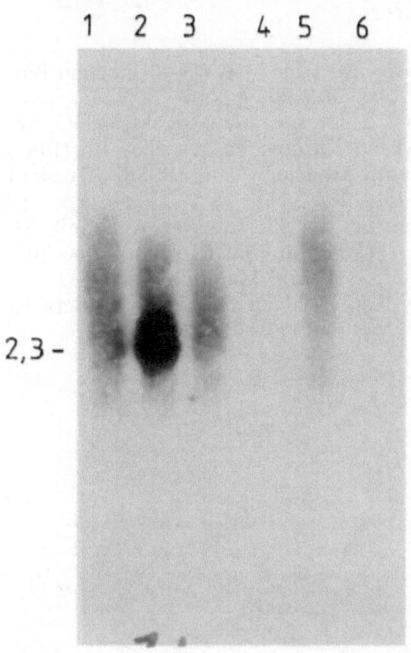

Fig. 2. Sequences specific for *fos* in RNA of nude mice tumors induced after the injection of NIH3T3 cells transfected by various DNAs. *1* NIH 3T3; *2* NLTR 1 (first round); *3* NLTR 1-1 (second round); *4* NMg 1-1 (second round); *5* NMg LTR 1 (first round); *6* NMg LTR 1-1 (second round). Probe: ^{32}P-*fos*

taining fragments was different in the first and the second rounds of transfection (Fig. 1).

On the basis of these data, we suppose that the integrated LTR can activate one of the cell proto-oncogenes. We tested several oncogenes (*fes, src, myc,* Ha-*ras, sis, abl, mos, fos*) and found that in this type of tumors c-*fos* oncogene transcription takes place. According to the results of Northern blotting, this RNA was represented by a 2.3-kb transcript (Fig. 2). The data obtained from blot hybridization with DNA of the tumors restricted with *Eco*RI and *Bam*HI indicate that no structural rearrangements in the c-*fos* gene were found.

Injection into nude mice of NIH3T3 cells cotransfected by pLTR 1.5 and DNA with amplified human c-Ha-*ras* gene also resulted in the development of tumors, which were designated as N MgLTR. The tumors also appeared in further rounds of transfection. In the genome of these tumors, the integration of LTR and pBr 322 plasmid sequences was shown (Fig. 3); the integrated site was localized in the plasmid region because after *Eco*RI restriction, an internal LTR RSV 0.3-kb fragment could also be detected. This is confirmed by Pst I digestion. Blot analysis showed that the integrated pLTR 1.5 se-

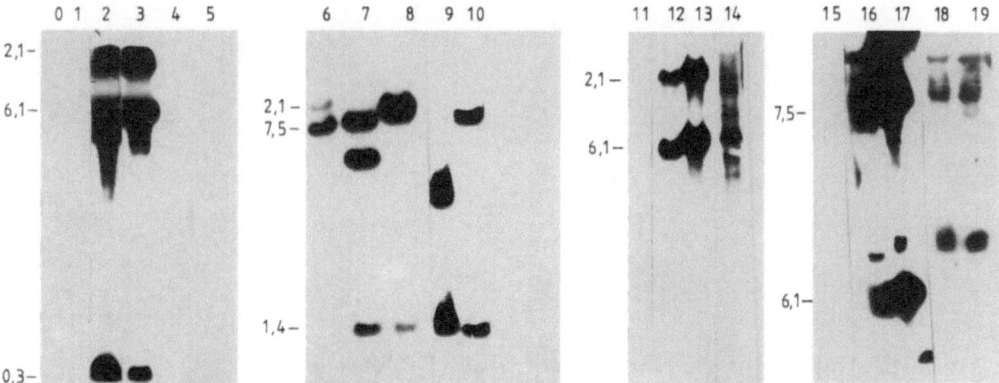

Fig. 3. Analysis of the genome of nude mice tumors – NMg LTR1 (first round) and NMg LTR 1-1 (second round). DNA preparations: *0* NLTR 1 (first round); *1, 11, 15* NIH3T3; *2, 6, 7, 8, 16* NMg LTR 1 (first round); *14* Np EJ-*ras* (nude mice tumor after transfection pEJ-*ras*-plasmid); *3,* *10, 13, 17* NMg LTR (second round); *4* NMg 1 (first round); *5, 18* NMg 1-1 (second round); *9* pLTR 1.5; *16* NMg 1-1-1 (third round). Restriction; *0–5, 11–14 Eco*RI; *6 Bam*HI; *7 Bam*H 1 + Pst 1; *8–10, 15–19* Pst1. Probes: *0–10* ^{32}P pLTR 1.5; *11–14* ^{32}P-pBr 322; *15–19* ^{32}P EJ-*ras*

quences in the genome of tumor cells were amplified (Fig. 3) in comparison to NLTR tumor DNA. The status of amplification is preserved for the human Ha-*ras* oncogene as well. We suppose that the integrated pLTR 1.5 and Ha-*ras* sequences are associated in one and the same locus of cell genome. Thus, LTR cotransfection with two different types of mouse DNA (tumor and normal) is accompanied by various molecular-genetic events, but the final result is the acquisition of oncogenic potential by NIH3T3 cells.

References

1. Cooper GM, Lane M-A (1984) Biochim Biophys Acta 738:9–20
2. Topol LZ, Tatosyan AG, Nalbaldyan NG, Revazova ES, Grofova M, Kisseljov FL (1985) Doklady Academii Nauk SSSR (Russian) 280:1261–1263
3. Ambartsumyan NS, Tatosyan AG, Enikolopov GN (1982) Mol Biol (Russian) 16:66–70
4. Southern E (1975) J Mol Biol 98:503–533
5. Rigby PW, Dichman H, Rhodes C, Berg PJ (1977) Mol Biol 113:237–251

Haematology and Blood Transfusion Vol. 31
Modern Trends in Human Leukemia VII
Edited by Neth, Gallo, Greaves, and Kabisch
© Springer-Verlag Berlin Heidelberg 1987

Conversion of *ras* Genes to Cancer Genes

K. Cichutek and P. H. Duesberg

The cellular precursor of Harvey and Balb sarcoma virus, termed proto-*ras*, from certain tumors registers most frequently as an apparent cancer gene in the gene transfer assay with NIH 3T3 cells [1–4]. The viral *ras* gene is a dominant transforming gene that elicits all features of oncogenic transformation in a single step upon transfer into established and primary human and animal fibroblast cells [5]. This encodes a single transforming protein of 21 kDA, p21 Ha-*ras*, which is presumed to be involved in the growth regulation of cells similar to G-proteins [6, 7]. However, the role of the cellular *ras* gene as a human cancer gene is debatable, as only 10% of the DNAs from certain cancer cells produce foci of transformed NIH 3T3 cells in the transfection assay. No consistent correlation between *ras* activation and any special type of human cancer is observed, thus 3T3-transforming proto-*ras* may not be necessary for malignancy [8, 9].

Activation of proto-*ras* in the 3T3 cell assay is due to point mutations in codons 12, 13, 59 or 61 [10–12]. The *ras* coding region in viruses also differs from the coding region of proto-*ras* in normal cells at codon 12 (Balb SV) [13] and codons 12 and 59 (HaSV) [14]. By analogy with the proto-*ras* genes, these point mutations are also thought to activate viral *ras* in sarcoma viruses [15]. To test this hypothesis, parts of viral *ras* including codons 12 (*Hind*III-*Pvu*II fragment; proviral DNA clones: pA12, pB12) or 12 and 59 (*Sac*II-*Fsp*I fragment: pA1259-1 or *Hind*III-*Fsp*I fragment: pA1259-2) were ex-

Department of Molecular Biology, University of California, Berkeley, CA, USA

changed in proviral DNA clones against the corresponding fragments of normal rat proto-*ras* 2. One proviral DNA clone derived from pA1259-2 included a *Sac*I-deletion of *ras* sequence directly 5′ of the p21 coding region (pA1259-2△Sc) (see Figs. 1, 2). Transfection of proviral DNA clones into NIH 3T3 cells (from S. Aaronson, NIH, Bethesda) clearly showed that viral *ras* containing normal codons 12 or 12 and 59 maintain a transforming function (Fig. 3). With clones pA12, pB12, pA1259-2 and pA1259-2△Sc only a minor reduction of transforming efficiency was observed, whereas pA1259-I showed tenfold less transforming efficiency (Table 1).

Finally, the complete coding region of normal rat p-*ras* 1 (including introns) was inserted into retro viruses to construct pApras1X and pBpras1. Both proviral clones showed efficient transforming function in NIH 3T3 cells (see Fig. 2 and Table 1). A slight delay of focus formation of 2–3 days already observed with pA1259-1 and pA1259-2 was most pronounced with pApras1X and pBpras1, probably due to the splicing out of introns during the first rounds of virus replication. Infection of primary Fischer rat embryo fibroblasts with virus derived from pApras1X DNA demonstrated transforming ability similar to wild type virus (Fig. 3). A few of these viruses will be reisolated and sequenced to verify the identity of the introduced codons of p21.

Inoculation of 10^4–10^5 ffu of each virus derived from the proviral clones described above into 1–5 day old Balb/c mice resulted in death of the animals within 2–8 weeks. Typical signs of malignancy, such as tumor

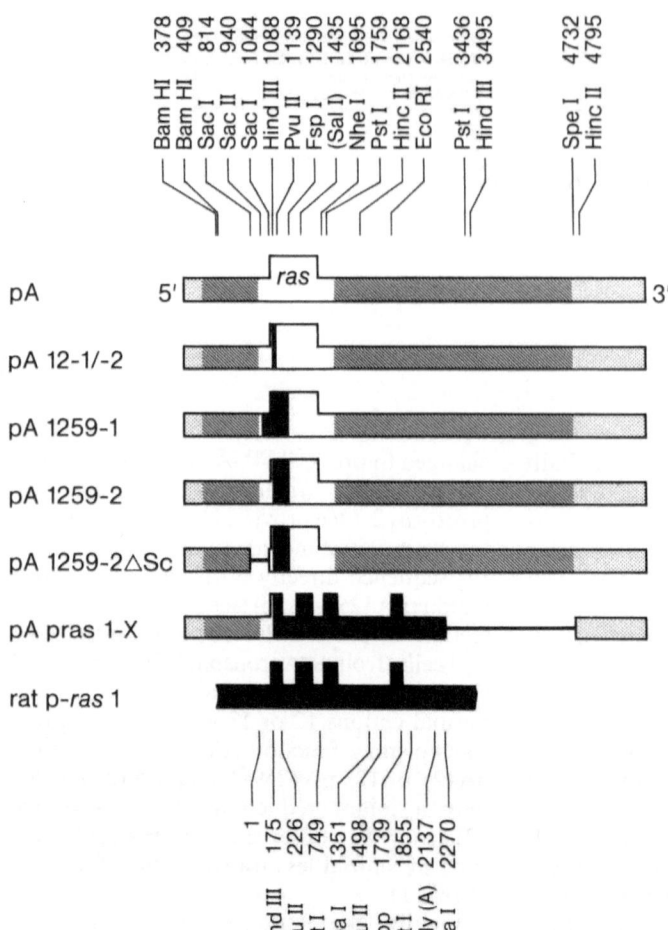

Fig. 1. Genetic structure of proviral DNA of Harvey sarcoma virus, rat proto-*ras* 1 and recombinant virus constructs

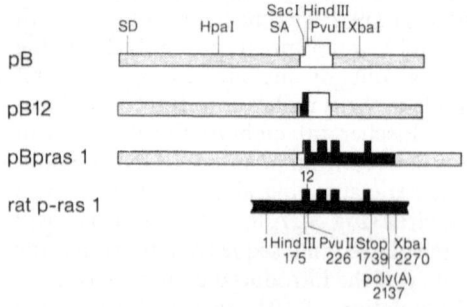

	ffu/µg	Latency period
pB	150–300	10 d
pB12	150–250	10 d
pBpras1	10	15 d

Fig. 2. Genetic structure of proviral DNA of Balb sarcoma virus, rat proto-*ras* 1 and recombinant constructs. The table shows the latent period in days for transforming activity after transfection into NIH 3T3 cells in the presence of Moloney MLV

478

Table 1. Transforming activity of proviral DNA of wild type and recombinant Harvey sarcoma virus after transfection into NIH 3T3 cells

Clone	Ras codon				Foci per µg DNA	Days first seen
	12	59	122	MLV		
pA	v	v	v	+	1000–2000	4
pA	v	v	v	−	40	14
pA12-1/-2	p	v	v	+	1000–2000	4
pA12-1/-2	p	v	v	−	4	14
pA1259-1	p	p	v	+	100– 200	6– 8
pA1259-2	p	p	v	+	300– 400	5– 6
pA1259-2△Sac	p	p	v	+	1000–1500	4
pApras2	p	p	p	+	0	–
pApras1-X	p	p	p	+	140– 160	10–14

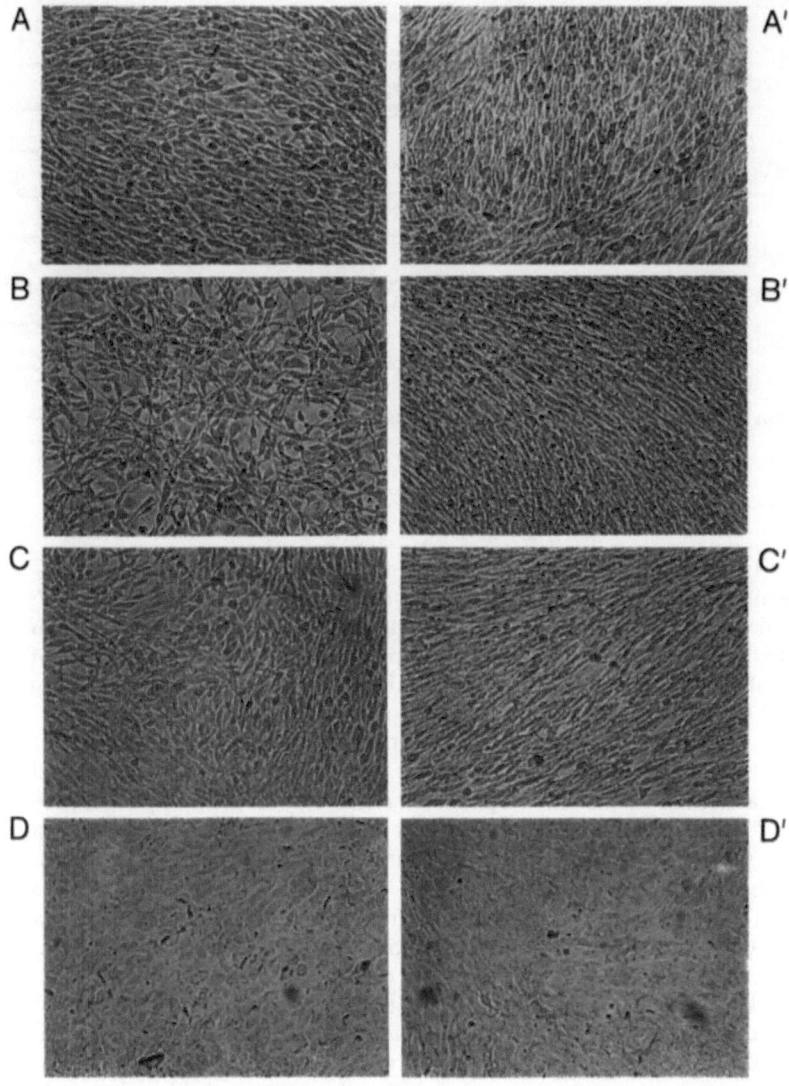

Fig. 3 A–D, A′–D′. Mouse NIH 3T3 cells (**A–D**) and primary Fischer rat cells (**A′–D′**) infected with wild type (**A** and **A′**) and recombinant Harvey sarcoma viruses pA12-2 (**B** and **B′**), pA1259-2 (**C** and **C′**), **D** and **D′** and helper virus (Moloney-MLV)

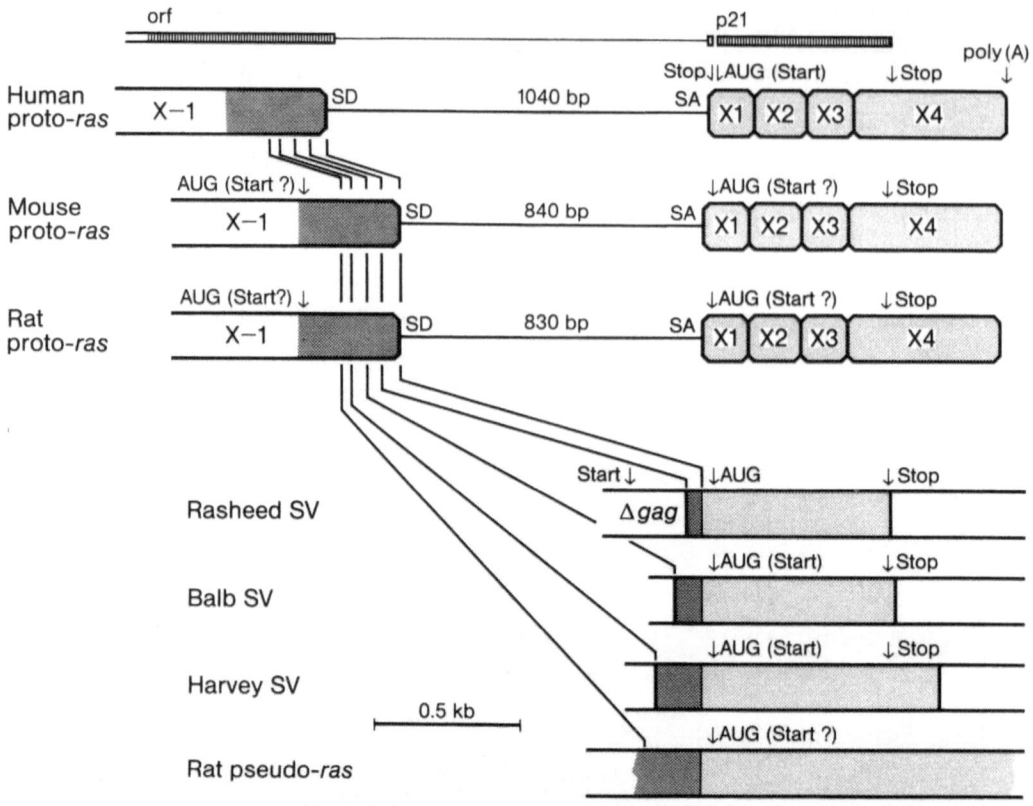

Fig. 4. Sequence comparison between *ras*-containing sarcoma viruses and human, mouse, and rat proto-*ras* genes

formation at the site of injection (sarcoma) or dark nodules in spleen and liver (erythroblastosis), were observed with wild-type and recombinant viruses. It is concluded that the transforming function of viral *ras* is independent of virus-specific point mutations in codons 12 or 59.

Sequence comparison between viral *ras* in HaSV, Balb SV and Rasheed SV, which expresses a p29 gag-*ras*[Ha] protein, and normal proto-*ras* 1 from rat (B. Rapoport, personal communication), mouse (J. Ihle, personal communication), and humans revealed a common border of homology at position 1037 of HaSV (Fig. 4). About 1 kb upstream the homology picks up again. At the homology junction perfect splice donor and splice acceptor sequences are present in the proto-*ras* genes. It is concluded that proto-*ras* 1 in humans, rats, and mice contains a previously undetected 5′ exon, termed exon-1, that is only partially present in HaSV, Balb SV, and Rasheed SV. Truncation of exon-1 of p-*ras* 1 and therefore truncation of the normal proto-*onc* gene occurred during transduction into the retroviruses [16].

Therefore we propose that substitution of the native promoter and as yet undefined upstream regulatory regions by the promoter of a retrovirus convert proto-*ras* to a transforming gene. Morphological transformation of 3T3 cells by intact proto-*ras* genes with point mutations may reflect a biochemical effect that enhances tumorigenicity, but does not initiate malignant transformation like viral *ras* genes. It is consistent with this view that 3T3 cells transform spontaneously at high frequency and that untreated 3T3 cells are aneuploid and already tumorigenic [17].

References

1. Taparowski E, Suard Y, Fasano O, Shimizu K, Goldfarb M, Wigler M (1982) Nature 300:762–765

2. Reddy EP, Reynolds RK, Santos E, Barbacid M (1982) Nature 300:149–152

3. Kraus MH, Yuasa Y, Aaronson SA (1984) Proc Natl Acad Sci USA 81:5384–5388

4. Tabin CJ, Bradley SM, Bargmann CI, Weinberg RA, Papageorge AG, Scolnick EM, Dhar R, Lowy DR, Chang EH (1982) Nature 300:143–149

5. Bishop JM, Varmus H (1985) In: Weiss R, Teich N, Varmus H, Coffin J (eds) RNA tumor viruses. 2nd Ed., pp 249–357

6. Lochrie MA, Hurley JB, Simon MI (1985) Science 228:96–99

7. Hurley JB, Simon MI, Teplow DB, Robishaw JD, Gilman AG (1984) Science 226:860–862

8. Feinberg AP, Vogelstein B, Droller MJ, Baylin SB, Nelkin BD (1983) Science 220:1175–1177

9. Eva A, Tronick SR, Gol RA, Pierce JH, Aaronson SA (1983) Proc Natl Acad Sci USA 80:4926–4930

10. Bishop JM (1983) Annu Rev Biochem 52:301

11. Varmus HE (1984) Annu Rev Genet 18:553

12. Duesberg PH (1985) Science 228:669–677

13. Reddy EP, Lipman D, Andersen PR, Tronick SR, Aaronson SA (1985) J Virol 53:984–987

14. Dhar R, Ellis RW, Shih TY, Oroszlan S, Shapiro B, Maizel J, Lowy D, Scolnick E (1982) Science 217:934–937

15. Tabin CJ, Weinberg RA (1985) J Virol 53:260–265

16. Cichutek K, Duesberg PH (1986) Proc Natl Acad Sci USA 83:2340–2344

17. Greig RG, Koestler TP, Trayner TP, Corwin SP, Miles L, Kline T, Sweet R, Yokoyama S, Poste G (1985) Proc Natl Acad Sci USA 82:3698–3701

Haematology and Blood Transfusion   Vol. 31
Modern Trends in Human Leukemia VII
Edited by Neth, Gallo, Greaves, and Kabisch
© Springer-Verlag Berlin Heidelberg 1987

Identification of the Bovine Leukemia Virus Transactivating Protein (p34^x)

L. Willems, R. Kettmann, D. Portetelle, and A. Burny

A. Introduction

Enzootic bovine leukosis (EBL) has been recognized as a neoplasm of infectious origin for half a century. The agent, bovine leukemia virus (BLV), is a retrovirus discovered in 1969 in short-term cultures of peripheral lymphocytes from animals with persistent lymphocytosis, a benign response to BLV infection. A virus distantly related to BLV was more recently identified as the etiological agent in the vast majority of cases of adult T cell leukemia and named for that reason human T-lymphotropic virus I (HTLV-I) [20]. The pathologies of BLV- and HTLV-I-induced diseases are notably similar, namely absence of chronic viremia, a long latency period, and lack of preferred integration sites in tumors. A second human virus, called HTLV-II, was identified in the Mo T cell line, derived in 1976 from the spleen of a patient with T cell-variant hairy cell leukemia [2, 10]. Other isolates of HTLV-I and -II have since been obtained around the world. Both viruses not only transform normal T-lymphocytes but might also very well be involved in a number of degenerative diseases of the nervous system.

The genomes of HTLV-I and -II show a nucleic acid sequence homology of about 60%. Relatedness between HTLV-I and BLV varies from 30% to more than 50%,

according to the genes under consideration [22, 23, 27]. Sequence similarities between the virion proteins of BLV, HTLV-I, and HTLV-II have also been reported [3, 18]. Moreover, the three viruses have in common the fact that they contain several overlapping open reading frames located between the *env* gene and the 3′ long terminal repeat (LTR). In these three cases, proteins coded by that region of the genome have been shown to transactivate the LTR of the provirus, hence their generic name of *tat* proteins (for transactivation of transcription) [13, 31, 34].

As a 34- to 38-kD protein predominantly located in the nucleus of the infected cell [28], the putative *tat* BLV product p34^x [26] is highly similar to the 42- and 38-kD products encoded by HTLV-I and HTLV-II [6, 32]. That transactivating proteins play key roles in tumor induction and maintenance is strongly suggested by the observation that the 5′LTR and 3′ region of the provirus are always conserved in BLV-induced tumors, even in cases where extended proviral deletions have occurred [12]. The lack of – or the very limited – expression of the *tat* gene product in BLV-induced tumors, even those propagated in vitro, argues in favor of BLV acting as an inducer of the neoplastic process and not as a maintenance determinant.

In this study we identified the protein product of the long open reading frame (LOR) gene, transcribed it in the SP6 system, and produced p34^x protein in reticulocyte lysates. The expressed native protein was used as an antigen to raise rabbit polyclonal antibodies. We further showed that most tumorous cattle and infected sheep

Faculty of Agronomy, 5800 Gembloux, Belgium, Department of Molecular Biology, University of Brussels, 1640 Rhode-Saint-Genèse, Belgium
L. Willems is *Aspirant* and R. Kettmann *Maître de Recherche* of the National Fund for Scientific Research.

harbor antibodies to p34[x]. Combined with the transactivation effect observed by Rosen et al. [26] with the same gene construct, our data strongly suggest that p34[x] is the *tat* gene product.

B. Results

Fetal lamb kidney (FLK)-BLV polyA[+] RNA was used as a template for cDNA synthesis. The double-stranded cDNA, annealed with *Eco*RI linkers, was cloned in λgt10. The library was screened with probes 1, 2, 3, and 4, as illustrated in Fig. 1. According to the known sequence of BLV provirus [22, 23, 27, 29], and in comparison with the HTLV-I and HTLV-II systems, it was inferred that the subgenomic mRNA coding for p34[x] should contain sequences hybridizing to probes 1 and 2 but that it should be devoid of sequences complementary to probe 4. Probe 1 partly corresponds to the LOR encompassing the information for 308 amino acids. Probe 2 expands over the 3' end of the *pol* gene, the *env*, and the 5' part of the X region. Among the clones satisfying the above requirements, one (BL-1) was selected, subcloned in pBR322, amplified, and sequenced by the dideoxynucleotide

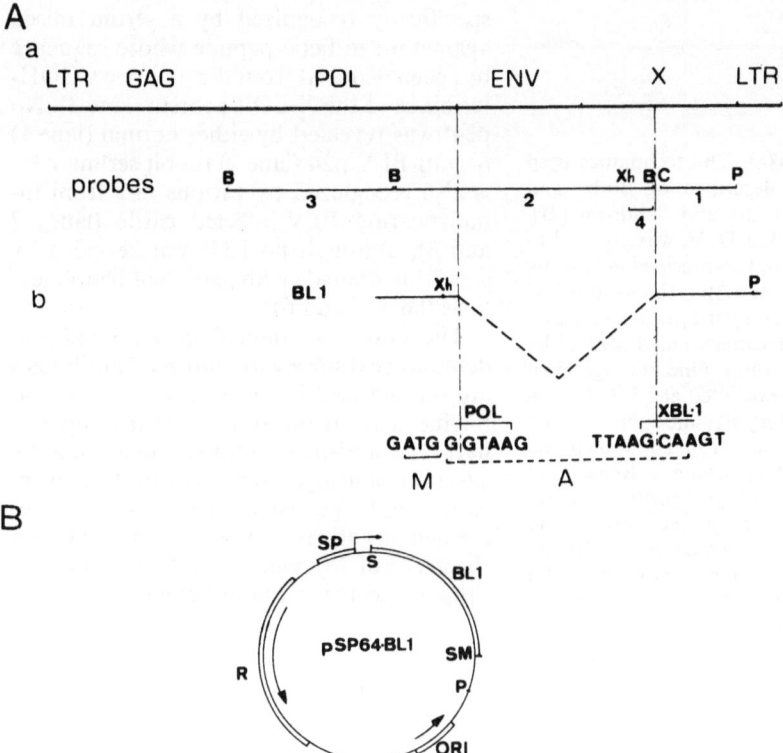

Fig. 1 A, B. Characterization of the BL1-cDNA and construction of the expression plasmid pSP64-BL1.
A *a:* Localization of the BLV probes on the BLV provirus. *B, Bam*HI; *C, Cla* I; *P, Pvu*II; *Xh, Xho*I. These probes were identified by DNA sequencing (not shown) and have been used previously [14]. *b:* Schematic representation of the BL1-cDNA clone. The splicing site between the methionine (*M*) initiation codon (at positions 4868–4870) [28, 29] and the entire BL-1 LOR (beginning at position 7246) generates an alanine (*A*) codon [30]. The two restriction endonucleases *Xho*I (*Xh*) and *Pvu*II (*P*) were used to subclone the coding region of BL-1 into the pSP64 plasmid.
B Construction of plasmid pSP64-BL-1. The *Xho*I-*Pvu*II fragment of BL-1 was subcloned into the *Sal*I (*S*)–*Sma*I (*SM*) sites of the pSP64 plasmid [17], according to Maniatis et al. [15]. *SP*, SP6 promoter; *ORI*, replication origin; *R*, ampicillin resistance gene; *P, Pvu*II

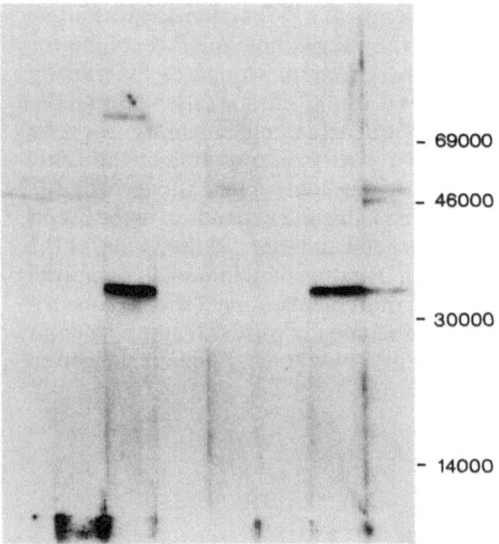

1 2 3 4 5 6 7 8 9

- 69000
- 46000
- 30000
- 14000

Fig. 2. Expression of p34^x. The techniques used were essentially those described by Butler and Chamberlin [1] and Renart and Sandoval [21]. Briefly, 5 μg of pSP64-BL1 DNA was digested to completion with PvuII and transcribed in vitro by the SP6 RNA polymerase (Amersham) at 37 °C for 2 h. RNA was capped by means of a cap analogue (m^7 G ppp G, Pharmacia) as described by the Amersham manufacturer. One microgram of the capped RNA was translated at 37 °C for 1 h in 20 μl of rabbit reticulocyte lysate supplemented with unlabeled amino acids [19]. The translation products were analyzed according to Renart and Sandoval [21]. The blotted p34^x protein was revealed by 50 μl of sera to be tested and 5×10^4 cpm of ^{125}I-labeled protein A (specific activity: 3×10^7 cpm/μg). *Lane 1*, normal rabbit serum; *lane 2*, rabbit anti-p24 polyclonal serum; *lane 3*, rabbit serum raised [7] against synthetic peptide RFPRDTSEPPLS of the p34^x protein [23]; *lane 4*, normal bovine serum; *lanes 5 and 6*, persistent lymphocytosis sera of cows 285 and 928 respectively; *lanes 7 and 8*, bovine tumor cases 15 and 82; *lane 9*, molecular weight markers

method. It was shown to contain 2353 base pairs consisting of 993 bp from the 3′ end of the pol gene ending at the splice-donor sequence GATGG/GTAAG and of 1360 bp from the X region including 924 bp representing the LOR (or putative tat gene) and, starting at CAAGT, a fragment immediately following the splice-acceptor sequence

TCTTTTAAG (Fig. 1). The BL-1 clone thus derived from a spliced mRNA whose AUG is very close to the end of the pol message, 44 nucleotides downstream from the putative AUG of env mRNA.

The BLV restriction fragment (XhoI-PvuII) containing the coding region of BL-1 was subcloned into the pSP64 plasmid. The recombinant plasmid was used to transform the HB101 strain of *Escherichia coli*. RNA from this clone was synthesized in vitro by the SP6 RNA polymerase and translated into a 34 000-dalton protein (p34^x) in rabbit reticulocyte lysates.

Figure 2 illustrates Western blot experiments performed with reticulocyte lysates expressing p34^x. A 34 000-dalton product is specifically recognized by a serum raised against a synthetic peptide whose sequence has been deduced from the putative COOH-terminus of the X LOR protein (lane 3). No p34^x was revealed by either normal (lane 1) or anti-BLV p24 (lane 2) rabbit serum. p34^x is also recognized by various sera from tumor-bearing BLV-infected cattle (lanes 7 and 8), although no p34^x was revealed by sera from animals with persistent lymphocytosis (lanes 5 and 6).

The data encountered in a limited epidemiological survey for anti-p34^x antibodies are summarized in Table 1. Most (22 of 24) bovine sera from tumor-bearing animals harbored anti-p34^x antibody, detectable by Western blotting. Many sera (6 of 8) from cattle with persistent lymphocytosis remained negative. Almost all BLV-infected sheep (23 of 25), whether in tumor phase or simply infected, without hematological dis-

Table 1. Response of BLV-infected animals to p34^x

Species	Stage of the disease	Western blot analysis	
		−	+
Cattle	Persistent lymphocytosis	6	2
	Tumorous case	2	22
Sheep	Antibody carrier to BLV gp51	0	6
	Tumorous case	2	17

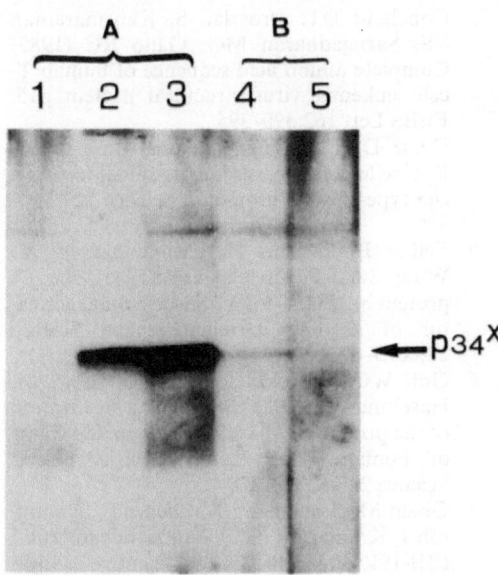

A   B

1   2   3   4   5

←—p34^x

Fig. 3. Comparison of in vivo and in vitro synthesized p34^x. p34^x was expressed as described in the legend to Fig. 2. Subcellular localization of p34^x has been described previously [6]. *A,* In vitro synthesized p34^x. *Lane 1,* normal rabbit serum; *lane 2,* rabbit serum raised against synthetic peptide RFPRDTSEPPLS of the p34^x; *lane 3,* rabbit serum raised against p34^x made in reticulocyte lysates. *B,* FLK nuclei lsyate. *Lane 4,* rabbit serum raised against synthetic peptide RFPRDTSEPPLS of the p34^x; *lane 5,* rabbit serum raised against p34^x

orders, reacted positively with p34^x. The latter result possibly reflects the high susceptibility of sheep to BLV infection and the high level of BLV replication in lymphoid and epithelioid sheep cells. Bovine cells are less susceptible to BLV replication, a fact reflected by the persistent, rather low antibody titer found in BLV-infected cattle. In general, anti-BLV antibody titers increase to high values (10^5) only in the tumor stage of the disease. We are thus inclined to think that detection of anti-p34^x antibody in BLV-infected non-tumorous cattle might require even more sensitive techniques.

Reticulocyte lysates programmed by BL-1 RNA were injected (three successive injections of 40 μl lysates at 2-week intervals) into a rabbit and elicited an excellent anti-p34^x response. This rabbit polyclonal antibody (Fig. 3, lane 3) and the antisynthetic peptide rabbit serum (Fig. 3, lane 2) revealed

the presence of p34^x in SP64-BL-1 RNA-programmed reticulocyte lysates. The same antisera also recognized a p34^x product in a nuclear extract of BLV-infected FLK cells (FLK-BLV) (Fig. 3, lanes 4 and 5). The straightforward interpretation of these data is that the proteins made in vitro or in vivo are very similar, thus ruling out significant posttranslational modifications.

A plasmid expressing the BL-1 information was used in co-transfection experiments with a plasmid containing the chloramphenicol acetyl transferase (CAT) gene under the control of the BLV LTR. The spectacular increase of CAT expression demonstrates that p34^x is a powerful transactivator of BLV LTR in the cell system used [26].

It is an established fact that the level of transactivation and, hence, viral gene expression depend upon the cell line examined, thus suggesting that cell proteins are mandatory and play a role in proviral transcription [4, 5, 24–26, 31–34]. Through such interactions, it is commonly inferred that infection by HTLV-I, -II, or BLV leads not only to activation of viral genes but also to modification of expression of normal cellular genes, and this can be a first step toward malignant transformation. In the HTLV-I and -II systems, genes such as IL-2, the IL-2 receptor, and genes for class-II proteins of the major histocompatibility complex are target candidates for *tat* 1 [8] and *tat* 2. The functional similarity between the BLV and HTLV transactivator products suggests that expression of the tat_{BLV} product (p34^x) may induce expression of cellular genes involved in target cell proliferation. Overexpression of a few genes, however, does not explain the entire transformation process, because of the long latency period and monoclonality of the tumor. We are thus led to speculate that BLV-induced leukemogenesis is a multistep mechanism initiated by *tat*.

We propose two explanations for the fact that p34^x expression is the first event in a cascade leading to cell transformation and leukemia or lymphosarcoma. Moreover, the very limited expression of p34^x in cultured tumor cells indicates that maintenance of transformation is independent of p34^x expression [11].

Explanation 1: Expression of p34^x leads with low frequency to expression of a cell protein critical for cell proliferation, modulating positively its own expression and acting as a repressor of p34^x expression. A model of this kind of interaction is the λ phage system in the interplay between genes C_{II} and C_I for establishment of lysogeny.

Explanation 2: Expression of p34^x induces with low frequency chromosomal abnormalities that definitely stabilize the transformed state. There are numerous examples of chromosomal rearrangements in neoplasia, such as the translocation of the Philadelphia chromosome in CML [9], the various translocations affecting the *myc* oncogene in Burkitt's lymphomas [35], and the chromosome breaks *bcl* 1 and *bcl* 2 in B cell lymphomas [36, 37]. Taking as an example a situation recently described in yeast [16], we imagine that p34^x expression leads with low frequency to an imbalance of histone-class proteins, which in turn induces chromosome abnormalities.

Cultured BLV-induced tumor cells systematically show karyotypic aberrations (Yu G, in preparation). It remains to be seen whether they are present in vivo or induced during establishment of the culture.

Finally, it can also be hypothesized that explanations 1 and 2 can be combined, chromosomal abnormality being a facultative consequence of p34^x expression.

Leukemogenesis by BLV is a complicated network of interactions, among which p34^x plays the initial role. It contributes to bringing the target cell into the transformed state; from then on, the cell proliferates and expands as the tumor clone.

Acknowledgements. This work was financially supported by the *Fonds Cancérologique de la Caisse Générale d'Epargne et de Retraite* and the Ministry of Agriculture.

References

1. Butler E, Chamberlin M (1982) Bacteriophage SP6 – specific RNA polymerase. J Biol Chem 257:5772–5778
2. Chen I, McLaughlin J, Gasson JC, Clark SC, Golde DW (1983) Molecular characterization of genome of a novel human T-cell leukaemia virus. Nature 305:502–505
3. Copeland DT, Oroszlan S, Kalyanaraman VS, Sarngadharan MG, Gallo RC (1983) Complete amino acid sequence of human T-cell leukemia virus structural protein p15. FEBS Lett 162:390–395
4. Derse D, Caradonna SJ, Casey JW (1985) Bovine leukemia virus long terminal repeat: a cell type-specific promoter. Science 227:317–320
5. Felber B, Paskalis H, Kleinman-Ening C, Wong-Staal F, Pavlakis GN (1985) The pX protein of HTLV-I is a transcriptional activator of its long terminal repeat. Science 229:675–677
6. Goh WC, Sodroski J, Rosen C, Essex M, Haseltine WA (1985) Subcellular localization of the product of the long open reading frame of human T-cell leukemia virus type 1. Science 227:1227–1228
7. Green M, Brackmann K, Lucher L, Symington J, Kramer T (1983) Human adenovirus 2 EIB-19K and EIB-53K tumor antigens; anti-peptide antibodies targeted to the NH$_2$ and COOH termini. J Virol 48:604–615
8. Greene WC, Leonard WJ, Wano Y, Svetlik PB, Peffer NJ, Sodroski JG, Rosen CA, Goh WC, Haseltine WA (1986) Trans-activator gene of HTLV-II induces IL-2 receptor and IL-2 cellular gene expression. Science 232:877–880
9. Heisterkamp N, Stephenson JR, Groffen J, Hansen PF, de Klein A, Bartram CR, Grosveld G (1983) Localization of the c-abl oncogene adjacent to a translocation breakpoint in chronic myelocytic leukaemia. Nature 306:239–242
10. Kalyanaraman VS, Sarngadharan MG, Robert-Guroff M, Miyoshi I, Blayney D, Golde D, Gallo RC (1982) A new subtype of human T-cell leukemia virus (HTLV-II) associated with a T-cell variant of hairy cell leukemia. Science 218:571–573
11. Kettmann R, Cleuter Y, Grégoire D, Burny A (1985) Role of the 3' long open reading frame region of bovine leukemia virus in the maintenance of cell transformation. J Virol 54:899–901
12. Kettmann R, Deschamps J, Cleuter Y, Couez D, Burny A, Marbaix G (1982) Leukemogenesis by bovine leukemia virus: proviral DNA integration and lack of RNA expression of viral long terminal repeat and 3' proximate cellular sequences. Proc Natl Acad Sci USA 79:2465–2469
13. Lee TH, Coligan JE, Sodroski JG, Haseltine WA, Salahuddin JZ, Wong-Staal F, Gallo RC, Essex M (1984) Antigens encoded by the 3' terminal region of human T-cell leukemia virus: evidence for a functional gene. Science 226:57–61

14. Mamoun RZ, Astier-Gin T, Kettmann R, Deschamps J, Rebeyrotte N, Guillemain BJ (1985) The pX region of the bovine leukemia virus is transcribed as a 2.1-kilobase mRNA. J Virol 54:625–629

15. Maniatis T, Fritsch E, Sambrook J (eds) (1982) Molecular cloning. Cold Spring Harbor Lab., Cold Spring Harbor, N.Y.

16. Meeks-Wagner D, Hartwell LH (1986) Normal stoichiometry of histone dimer sets is necessary for high fidelity of mitotic chromosome transmission. Cell 44:43–52

17. Melton D, Krieg P, Rebagliati M, Maniatis T, Zinn K, Green M (1984) Efficient in vitro synthesis of biologically active RNA and RNA hybridization probes from plasmids containing a bacteriophage SP6 promoter. Nucl Acid Res 12:7035–7056

18. Oroszlan S, Sarngadharan MG, Copeland TD, Kalyanaraman VS, Gilden RV, Gallo RC (1982) Primary structure analysis of the major internal protein p24 of human type-C T-cell leukemia virus. Proc Natl Acad Sci USA 79:1291–1294

19. Pelham HRB, Jackson RJ (1976) An efficient mRNA-dependent translation system for reticulocyte lysates. Eur J Biochem 67:247–256

20. Poiesz BJ, Ruscetti FW, Reitz MS, Kalyanaraman VS, Gallo RC (1981) Isolation of a new type-C retrovirus (HTLV) in primary uncultured cells of a patient with Sezary T-cell leukaemia. Nature 294:268–271

21. Renart J, Sandoval IV (1984) Western blots. Methods Enzymol 104:455–460

22. Rice NR, Stephens RM, Burny A, Gilden RV (1985) The gag and pol genes of bovine leukemia virus: nucleotide sequence and analysis. Virology 142:357–377

23. Rice NR, Stephens RM, Couez D, Deschamps J, Kettmann R, Burny A, Gilden RV (1984) The nucleotide sequence of the env and post env region of bovine leukemia virus. Virology 138:82–93

24. Rosen CA, Sodroski JG, Kettmann R, Burny A, Haseltine WA (1985) Transactivation of the bovine leukemia virus long terminal repeat in BLV-infected cells. Science 227:320–322

25. Rosen CA, Sodroski JG, Kettmann R, Haseltine WA (1986) Activation of enhancer sequences in type-II human T-cell leukemia virus and bovine leukemia virus long terminal repeats by virus-associated trans-acting regulatory factors. J Virol 57:738–744

26. Rosen CA, Sodroski JG, Willems L, Kettmann R, Campbell K, Zaya R, Burny A, Haseltine WA (1986) The 3' region of bovine leukemia virus genome encodes a trans-activator protein. EMBO J 5:2585–2589

27. Sagata N, Yasunaga T, Ohishi K, Tsuzuku-Kawamura J, Onuma M, Ikawa Y (1984) Comparison of the entire genomes of bovine leukemia virus and human T-cell leukemia virus and characterization of their unidentified open reading frames. EMBO J 3:3231–3237

28. Sagata N, Tsuzuku-Kawamura J, Nagaioshi-Aia M, Shimizu F, Imagawa KI, Ikawa Y (1985) Identification and some biochemical properties of the major X_{BL} gene product of bovine leukemia virus. Proc Natl Acad Sci USA 82:7879–7882

29. Sagata N, Yasynaga T, Tsuzuku-Kawamura J, Ohishi K, Ogawa Y, Ikawa Y (1985) Complete nucleotide sequence of the genome of bovine leukemia virus: its evolutionary relationship to other retroviruses. Proc Natl Acad Sci USA 82:677–681

30. Seiki M, Hikokoshi A, Taniguchi T, Yoshida M (1985) Expression of the px gene of HTLV-I. General splicing mechanism in the HTLV family. Science 228:1532–1534

31. Slamon DJ, Shimotohno K, Cline MJ, Golde DW, Chen ISY (1984) Identification of the putative transforming protein of the human T-cell leukemia viruses HTLV-I and HTLV-II. Science 226:61–65

32. Slamon DJ, Press MF, Souza LM, Murdock DC, Cline MJ, Golde DW, Gasson JC, Chen ISY (1985) Studies of the putative transforming protein of the type-I human T-cell leukemia virus. Science 228:1247–1430

33. Sodroski J, Rosen C, Goh WC, Haseltine WA (1985) A transcriptional activator protein encoded by the X-LOR region of the human T-cell leukemia virus. Science 228:1430–1432

34. Sodroski JG, Rosen CA, Haseltine WA (1984) Transacting transcriptional activation of the long terminal repeat of human T-lymphotropic viruses in infected cells. Science 225:381–385

35. Taub R, Kirsch I, Morton C, Lenoir G, Swan D, Tronick S, Aaronson S, Leder P (1982) Translocation of the c-myc gene into the immunoglobulin heavy chain locus of human Burkitt lymphoma and murine plasmacytoma cells. Proc Natl Acad Sci USA 79:7837–7841

36. Tsujimoto Y, Finger LR, Yunis J, Nowell PC, Croce C (1984) Cloning of the chromosome breakpoint of neoplastic B cells with the (14;18) chromosome translocation. Science 226:1097–1099

37. Tsujimoto Y, Yunis J, Onorato-Showe L, Erikson J, Nowell PC, Croce C (1984) Molecular cloning of the chromosomal breakpoint of B-cell lymphomas and leukemias with the t (11;14) chromosome translocation. Science 224:1403–1406

Haematology and Blood Transfusion   Vol. 31
Modern Trends in Human Leukemia VII
Edited by Neth, Gallo, Greaves, and Kabisch
© Springer-Verlag Berlin Heidelberg 1987

Monoclonal Antibodies Against the Viral and Human Cellular *myb* Gene Product

H. Bading[1], C. Beutler[1], P. Beimling[1], J. Gerdes[2], H. Stein[2], and K. Moelling[1]

Retroviruses code for oncogenes which cause tumors in animals. The viral oncogenes have evolved from normal cellular proto-oncogenes, to which they are closely related. The viral and cellular oncogenes differ in point mutations and size, the viral genes often being truncated and, in some cases, fused to unrelated cellular genes. These differences may be responsible for the transforming function of the viral oncogenes.

In human tumor cells, activated cellular oncogenes resembling the viral oncogenes have been identified. They also carry mutations and/or deletions, and in many cases are overexpressed from amplified genes. It is of interest to determine whether these activated cellular oncogenes are characteristic of certain tumors and whether their gene products can serve as tumor markers.

To date, nearly two dozen viral oncogenes have been identified. Some of them are closely related to each other, and on the basis of their sequence homology, cellular location, and associated enzymatic activities, they can be roughly classified into three groups. The largest group is the *src* gene family, which consists of tyrosine-specific protein kinases that are predominantly located at the inner side of the plasma membrane. Another group consists of protein kinases which are not tyrosine- but serine-/ threonine-specific and are located in the cytoplasm, such as *mil/raf*. The third group comprises oncogene proteins located in the nucleus, such as *myc, myb*, and *fos*. They presumably play a role in the regulation of gene expression in tumor cells.

The c-*myb* oncogene, the homolog to the transforming gene (v-*myb*) of avian myeloblastosis virus (AMV), is specifically expressed in hematopoietic cells and appears to be tightly regulated during cell differentiation and proliferation [1, 5]. A five- to tenfold amplification of the c-*myb* gene was found in cultured cells of a patient with acute myelogenous leukemia (AML) [3]. Tumor cell lines have been established from AMV-transformed bone marrow cells and from a human immature T-cell line, designated BM-2 and MOLT4, respectively.

To analyze viral and cellular oncogene proteins, antisera are required. They were obtained against bacterially expressed oncogenes. An EcoRI/XbaI DNA fragment which comprises almost the complete viral oncogene *myb* (804 out of 1145 nucleotides) was cloned into pPLc24 expression vector [2]. The bacterially expressed proteins served not only for immunization of rabbits and mice but also for the identification of monoclonal antibodies in enzyme-linked immunoabsorbent assay (ELISA) tests. Monoclonal antibodies against the viral *myb* protein were obtained by standard hybridoma technology. Twenty-one myb-reacting monoclonal antibodies were obtained and subcloned until they were stable and characterized for their reactivities in various assays such as ELISA, Western blots, and indirect radioimmunoprecipitation. For some of the clones,

[1] Max-Planck-Institut für Molekulare Genetik, Abt. Schuster, Ihnestrasse 73, D-1000 Berlin 33, FRG
[2] Institut für Pathologie, Freie Universität Berlin, Klinikum Steglitz, Hindenburgdamm 30, D-1000 Berlin 45, FRG

Table 1. Summary of monoclonal antibody clones isolated against bacterially expressed viral *myb* protein

Clone no.	Clone	ELISA	Titer	Ig class	Blot		RIP	
					BM-2	MOLT4	BM-2	MOLT4
1/10	Lost	+++	10^0		−	−	(+)	−
1/12	+	++	10^{-2}		−	−	(+)	−
1/21	+	+++	10^{-2}		+	−	++	−
2/22	Lost							
3/12	+	+++	10^{-2}		−	−	++	−
3/20	+	+++	10^{-3}	IgG$_{2a}$	+++	−	+++	−
4/10	+	+++	10^{-1}		−	−	+	−
4/14	+	+++	10^{-1}	IgG$_{2b}$	+	+	+++	++
5/18	+	+++	10^{-2}		−	−	++	−
9/ 1	+	++	10^0		−	−	+	−
9/12	+	+++	10^{-1}	IgM	+	−	+	−
9/14	+	+++	10^{-3}	IgG$_1$	++	−	++	−
9/19	+	+++	10^{-3}	IgG$_{2b}$	+++	−	+++	−
10/ 7	Lost						−	−
10/22	Lost						(+)	−
14/14	+	+++	10^{-1}		(+)	−	+	−
15/23	+	+++	10^0		+	−	++	−
18/ 3	+	+++	10^{-1}		+	−	++	−
18/ 9	Lost						−	−
18/24	Lost						−	−
19/16	+	+++	10^{-2}	IgG$_{2a}$	(+)	−	+	−
M 46					++	++	+++	++

The reactivities in various tests were graded by +++, ++, +, and (+), according to the intensities of the signals obtained.

The serum titer was about 1000-fold higher than that of the hybridoma culture supernatants. Isolation of monoclonal antibodies followed standard techniques.

ELISA, enzyme-linked immunoabsorbent assay; RIP, indirect radioimmunoprecipitation; M 46, mouse 46 used for fusion.

their immunoglobulin subgroups were determined and ascites fluid produced. These properties are summarized in Table 1.

Clone 4/14 precipitates the viral and human cellular *myb* gene products from ^{35}S-methionine metabolically labeled BM-2 and MOLT4 cells (Fig. 1). The p48$^{v\text{-}myb}$ and p75$^{hu\text{-}c\text{-}myb}$ proteins are predominantly precipitated (Fig. 1, slot 4, left and right). The specificities of the two precipitations are proven by use of excess bacterial *myb* protein for competition of the antigen-antibody reactions (Fig. 1, slot 5, left and right).

The anti-*myb* monoclonal antibody 3/20 proved useful for the purification of *myb*-specific protein from BM-2 cells. An immunoaffinity column was prepared from ascites fluid, and the immunoglobulin fraction was isolated by protein A chromatography and subsequently coupled to carrier beads. Details of this procedure have been published [2]. The purification of the p48$^{v\text{-}myb}$ protein from ^{35}S-methionine metabolically labeled BM-2 cells is about 3000-fold (Fig. 2). The p75$^{hu\text{-}c\text{-}myb}$ protein can be purified from MOLT4 cells, using an identical approach with clone 4/14 (data not shown). The analysis of human tumor cell lines is hampered by the fact that the level of human *myb* protein expression is about 10-fold lower than that of the avian viral system.

It is of interest to determine the reactivity of the *myb* monoclonal antibody 4/14 with human and avian tumor cells. In order first to establish its specificity in immunoperoxidase staining, clone 4/14 was tested with

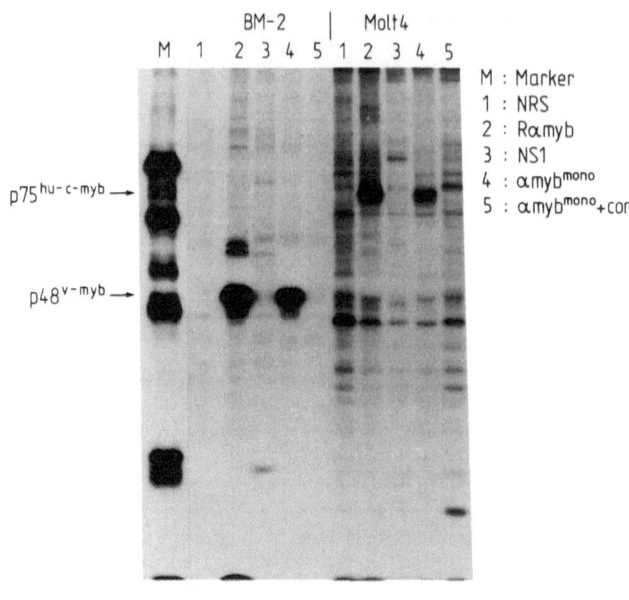

Fig. 1. Indirect immunoprecipitation of *myb* protein from ^{35}S-methionine metabolically labeled avian BM-2 and human MOLT4 cell lines (2×10^6 cells per precipitation labeled with 500 µCi/ml ^{35}S-methionine for 90 min and processed as described in [2]). For precipitation, 5 µl of normal rabbit serum (*slot 1*) and rabbit anti-bacterial *myb* serum (*slot 2*) were used. 1 ml of supernatant from NS-1 myeloma cells (*slot 3*) and from hybridoma clone 4/14 (*slot 4*) were used. Competition of the precipitation reaction was performed using 5 µg of purified *myb* antigen (*slot 5*). *M* indicates marker proteins, from *top* to *bottom:* 92K, 68K, 54K, 45K, and 32K. Exposure time: 1 week

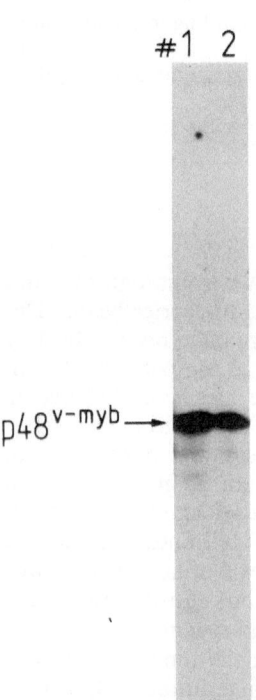

Fig. 2. Immunoaffinity column purification of p48$^{v\text{-}myb}$ protein from ^{35}S-methionine metabolically labeled BM-2 cells, using the monoclonal clone 3/20. The column was prepared according to previously published procedures [2]. 5×10^7 cells labeled with 500 µCi/ml for 90 min were used. An aliquot (5%) of the eluted fractions (2 ml each) was analyzed on sodium dodecyl sulfate polyacrylamide gel and exposed for autoradiography (time: 1 week)

490

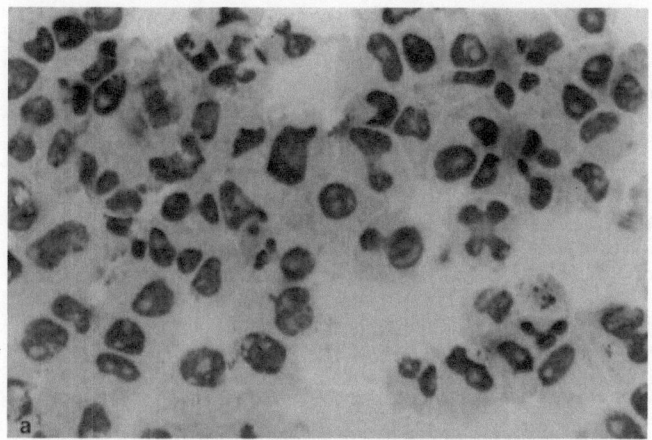

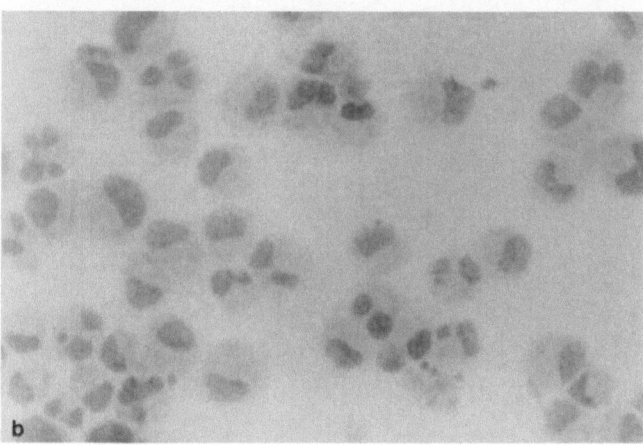

Fig. 3 a, b. Immunoperoxidase staining of BM-2 cells with monoclonal antibody, clone 4/14. Ascites fluid was used at a dilution of 1 : 600 (**a**). Competition by excess of antigen (5 μg) (**b**). Immunoperoxidase staining was performed as described in [4]

BM-2 cells. As is shown in Fig. 3, the monoclonal antibody gives rise to nuclear staining in BM-2 cells. The specificity of the reaction is proven by competition of the antibody binding with excess of antigen, which is shown in Fig. 3 b. Preliminary evidence indicates that the human cellular *myb* gene product can be detected in the human tumor cell line MOLT4 by an identical technique, in spite of the fact that it is expressed at about 10-fold lower levels in those cells (data bot shown).

In summary, of the monoclonal antibodies isolated against v-*myb,* 1 out of 21 recognizes the human cellular *myb* gene product in several experimental approaches. The differences between the viral and cellular *myb* genes are extensive, since besides several point mutations the viral *myb* gene is truncated to about two third the size of the cellular *myb* gene. In spite of this, the cross-reactive monoclonal clone 4/14 suggests the existence of a conserved antigenic site located on an EcoRI/XbaI fragment of v-*myb*. Since the expression of c-*myb* protein may be related to different malignancies, antibody clone 4/14 is a useful tool for investigating whether or not c-*myb* protein can be used as a tumor marker. Such investigations are now under way.

Acknowledgements. The excellent technical assistance of Sabine Richter, Sabine Sukrow, and Silvia Rabe is gratefully acknowledged. This work was supported by the Deutsche Krebshilfe e.V., Stiftung Unterberg, and BMFT.

References

1. Gonda TJ, Metcalf D (1984) Expression of myb, myc and fos proto-oncogenes during the differentiation of a murine myeloid leukaemia. Nature 310:249–251
2. Moelling K, Pfaff E, Beug H, Beimling P, Bunte T, Schaller HE, Graf T (1985) DNA-binding activity is associated with purified myb proteins from AMV and E26 viruses and is temperature-sensitive for E26 ts mutants. Cell 40:983–990
3. Pellici PG, Lanfrancone L, Brathwaite MD, Wolman SR, Dalla-Favera R (1984) Amplification of the c-myb oncogene in a case of human acute myelogenous leukemia. Science 224:1117–1121
4. Stein H, Gerdes J, Schwab U, Lemke H, Mason DY, Ziegler A, Schienle W, Diehl V (1982) Identification of Hodgkin and Sternberg-Reed cells as a unique cell type derived from a newly-detected small-cell population. Int J Cancer 30:445–459
5. Westin EH, Gallo RC, Arya SK, Eva A, Souza LM, Baluda MA, Aaronson SA, Wong-Staal F (1982) Differential expression of the amv gene in human hematopoietic cells. Proc Natl Acad Sci USA 79:2194–2198

Haematology and Blood Transfusion Vol. 31
Modern Trends in Human Leukemia VII
Edited by Neth, Gallo, Greaves, and Kabisch
© Springer-Verlag Berlin Heidelberg 1987

Atavistic Mutations Reflect the Long Life Span of Dispensable Genes

S. Ohno

A. Introduction

It looks as though the list of c-*onc* genes in the mammalian genome has been growing every month: some sharing the tyrosine kinase domain with growth factor receptors, others sharing the domain with steroid hormone receptors. Are they all essential to the development and well-being of the host? From their sheer redundancy alone, I suspect that most of them are not. If they are, more often than not, nonessential, why have they been persisting so long? The evolutionary antiquity of some of them has been well established.

In a previous paper [1], I pointed out that because of the low inherent error rate in vertebrate DNA replication estimated as $10^{-9}/$ base pair per year, the average half-life of genes after they have become dispensable is as long as 45 million years. It would be recalled that the first placental mammals emerged only 75 million years ago. In another previous paper [2] and also in an accompanying paper to this one, I also pointed out the c-*onc* gene coding sequences are still constructed in the manner reminiscent of primordial coding sequences at the very beginning of life on this earth some 3.5 or more billion years ago, the possession of long unused open reading frames giving them a measure of immortality.

In this paper, I shall give an example of the primordial gene evolved before the division of eukaryotes from prokaryotes becom-

Beckman Research Institute of The City of Hope, Duarte, CA 91010, USA

ing dormant in various phylogenetic trees for very, very long time, only to be resurrected later. Before the advent of molecular biology, such resurrections were known as atavistic mutations. A few dramatic examples shall also be given.

B. The Evolutionary Game of Hide- and Emerge Played by Hemoglobin Genes

The ultimate origin of hemoglobin genes is of extreme interest. In vertebrates, hemoglobins are encased in circulating erythrocytes, and the genome of certain teleost fish and upward contains two unlinked sets of genes; one set for α-chain and its allies, and the other for β-chain and its allies. Within vertebrates, hemoglobin polypeptide chains have been changing rather rapidly – a 1% amino acid sequence divergence every 8.3 million years. By contrast, glyceraldehyde 3-phosphate dehydrogenase, one of the sugar-metabolizing enzymes, has been undergoing a 1% amino acid sequence change every 40 million years. Reflecting the above noted rapid evolutionary changes, monomeric hemoglobins of lampreys are already intermediate between myoglobins on one hand and α- and β-chains of jawed vertebrates on the other [3]. Thus, within vertebrates, all the indications were that the gene duplication event that yielded the ancestral hemoglobin gene from a redundant copy of the myoglobin gene must have taken place at the onset of vertebrate evolution 300 million or so years ago. Indeed, at the rate of a 1% amino acid sequence divergence every 8.3 million

years, hemoglobins should have become totally unrecognizable in 830 million years:
100% amino acid sequence divergence.

Yet it had been known for a long time that
hemoglobins appear sporadically not only
among invertebrates (e.g., *Chinoromus*
among dipteran insects, earthworms among
the class *Polychaeta* of the phylum *Annelida*)
but also among the plants (e.g., in nitrogen-
fixing nodules of leguminous plants). A dimeric bacterial hemoglobin from *Vitreoscilla* has recently been sequenced [4]. It
is comprised of 146 amino acid residues and
is therefore of the same length as mammalian β-chains. Furthermore, all the functionally critical residues are present, e.g., a pair
of histidine residues that hold a heme – 46th
phenylalanine, which is invariant in all hemoglobins. This bacterial hemoglobin
shows the greatest sequence homology
(24%) with the pea leghemoglobin which is
153 residue long.

The fascinating evolutionary history of
hemoglobins revealed above again confirms
the view that most of the major innovations
in evolution occurred at the very beginning
of life on this earth before the division of eukaryotes from prokaryotes. In addition, it
reveals yet another evolutionary principle

often overlooked [2]. The gene once invented
might remain dormant for a very, very long
time, only to be resurrected in certain
members. For example, insects as a rule do
not express hemoglobin genes; even among
dipteran insects, the familiar *Drosophila* and
mosquitoes do not, while *Chyronomus* does.
The gene that can be resurrected after a very
long period of dormancy must necessarily be
endowed with the immortal property, being
impervious to normally function-depriving
deleterious mutations that cause premature
chain termination, reading frame shifts, etc.
This is the inherent property of coding sequences endowed with long unused open
reading frames capable of encoding amino
acid sequences similar to that encoded by the
used reading frame of that gene. Such was
the property of primordial coding sequences
of eons ago that were repeats of base
oligomers, the number of bases in oligomeric
units not being a multiple of three [2].

C. A Few of the More Dramatic Examples of Atavistic Mutations

A pair of horns adorning the poll is quite
common among bovids (cattle, sheep, goats,

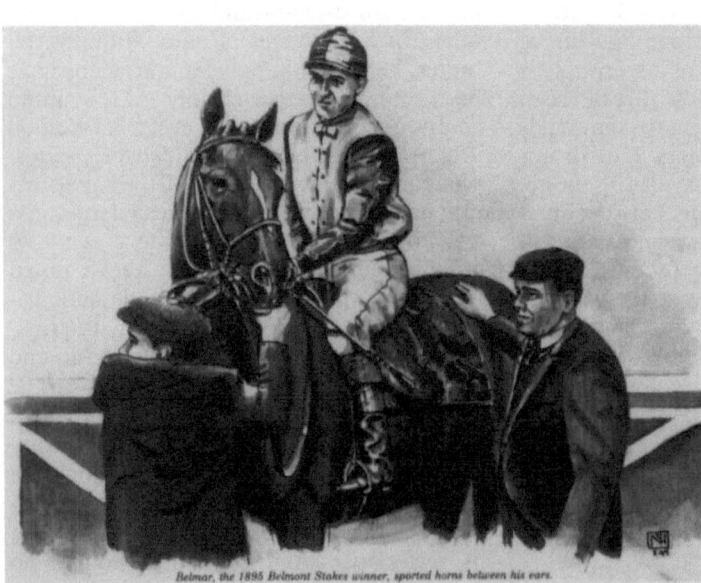

Belmar, the 1895 Belmont Stakes winner, sported horns between his ears.

Fig. 1. A portrait of *Belmar*, the winner of the 1895 Belmont stakes, from a newspaper of the time [5]

494

and antelopes), cervids (deer), and even giraffids of the order *Artiodactyla*. Among members of the order *Perisodactyla*, however, such development apparently has never taken place, although extinct *Brontothelium* sported, and persisting rhinoceroses still sport, a horn or horns on the nose. Yet there have been two documented instances of modern horses growing a pair of horns on the poll. Records of racing thoroughbreds have been kept impeccably. *Marooned* was a popular gelding of the 1930 in the United States. He had small horns growing "pronouncedly" though not "conspicuously." Similarly, the horse who crossed the wire first in the 1895 Belmont Stakes boasted nobs above his forehead (Fig. 1). Belmar, a steel-gray runner of distinction also won the Preakness and Manhattan handicap [5]. It would be recalled that starting with the Kentucky Derby, the Preakness and the Belmont constitute 2nd and 3rd legs of the Triple Crown races for 3-year-olds in the United States.

The characteristic body shape of modern whales was already evident in an Eocene whale (*Zeuglodon*) of some 50 million years ago. This reversion of the body form of tetrapod mammals to the original fish-like body form of ancestral vertebrates was accomplished by transformation of front limbs to a pair of paddles, while pelvic bones became residual, and femur became an internal diminutive cartilaginous vestige, thus eliminating hind limbs. Yet Andrews [6] described a humpback whale, *Megaptera nodosa,* with hind limbs over a meter long. The femur of this whale was external and nearly complete. A number of sperm whales, *Physeter catodon*, have also been discovered which possessed not only the external femur but also partial phalanges [7]. These whales with hind limbs represent the case of an atavistic revision to the tetrapod body form from the previous atavistic reversion to the fish-like form.

D. Summary

Most of the major innovations in evolution occurred at the very beginning of life on this earth some 3.5 billion years ago before the division of eukaryotes from prokaryotes. This initial innovativeness was due, in no small part, to the peculiar construction of primordial coding sequences that were repeats of base oligomers, the number of bases in oligomeric units not being a multiple of three. Such coding sequences are conferred with a measure of immortality. Because of this initial immortality and of long life span of genes after becoming dispensable, the ancient gene may remain silenced in particular phylogenetic trees for a very long time, only to be resurrected later. Hemoglobin genes expressed in exceptional bacteria, plants, worms, insects, as well as in all vertebrates are a good example of this.

Atavistic mutations are more dramatic visible examples of such resurrection of long dormant genes. A few interesting examples are given.

References

1. Ohno S (1985) Dispensable genes. Trends Genet 1:160–164
2. Ohno S (1986) Viral *V-Onc* and host *C-Onc* genes: their dispensability, immortality and active site sequence conservation. Cancer Rev 2:65–85
3. Atlas of Protein Sequence and Structure (1972) Dayhoff MO (ed). Natl Biomed Res Found, Silver Springs
4. Wakabayashi S, Matsubara H, Webster DA (1986) Primary sequence of a dimeric bacterial haemoglobin from *Vitreoscilla*. Nature 322:481–483
5. Fleming M (1984) Wrought by inexact science. Throughbreds of California, June 4–8
6. Andrews RC (1921) A remarkable case of external hind limbs in a humpback whale. Am Mus Novitates 9:1–16
7. Lands R (1978) Evolutionary mechanism of limb loss in tetrapods. Evolution 32:73–92

Haematology and Blood Transfusion   Vol. 31
Modern Trends in Human Leukemia VII
Edited by Neth, Gallo, Greaves, and Kabisch
© Springer-Verlag Berlin Heidelberg 1987

Cancer Genes Generated by Rare Chromosomal Rearrangements Rather than Activation of Oncogenes *

P. H. Duesberg [1]

A. Introduction

In order to understand cancer, it is necessary to identify cancer genes. The search for such genes and for mechanisms that generate such genes must take into consideration that at the cellular level cancer is a very rare event. The kind of cellular transformation that leads to cancer in vivo occurs only in about one out of 2×10^{17} mitoses in humans and animals. The basis for this estimate is that most animal and human cancers are derived from single transformed cells and are hence monoclonal [1–5], that humans and corresponding animals represent about 10^{16} mitoses (assuming 10^{14} cells that go through an average 10^2 mitoses), and that about one person in five dies from tumors [6].

The only proven cancer genes are the transforming (*onc*) genes of retroviruses. These are autonomous transforming genes that are sufficient for carcinogenesis [7, 8]. They transform susceptible cells in culture with the same kinetics as they infect tham, and they cause tumors in animals with single-hit kinetics [7, 8]. Therefore, these viruses are never associated with healthy animals and are by far the most direct and efficient natural carcinogens.

However tumors with retroviruses that contain *onc* genes are very rare in nature, as only less then 50 cases are recorded from which such viruses were isolated [5, 7–9]. Moreover these viruses have never been reported to cause epidemics of cancer. The probable reasons are that viral *onc* genes arise naturally only with great difficulty via two or more illegitimate recombinations, and that once arisen they are very unstable because they are not essential for virus replication [7, 8]. Nonessential genes are readily lost due to spontaneous deletion or mutation. Indeed, *onc* genes were originally discovered by analysis of spontaneous deletions of the *src* gene, the *onc* gene of Rous sarcoma virus (RSV) [10, 11]. Subsequently, about 20 other viral *onc* genes were identified in retroviruses [7–9, 12]. All these viral *onc* genes were originally defined by "transformation-specific" sequences that are different from the known sequences of essential virus genes [13].

Since *onc* genes are unstable, they must also be recent additions to retroviruses. Indeed, the cellular genes from which the transformation-specific sequences of oncogenic retroviruses were transduced have been identified in normal cells. This was initially done by liquid hybridization of transformation-specific viral sequences with cellular DNA [14–18], and later by comparing cloned viral *onc* and corresponding cellular genes [19]. Such cellular genes have since been termed proto-*onc* genes [7].

The cellular origin of the transformation-specific sequences of retroviral *onc* genes is frequently presented as a particular surprise [9, 12]. However, cells are the only known

---

* This manuscript is based on a previous publication [1] and was also presented at the Third International Symposium in Hematology and Oncology: Assessment and Management of Leukemia Cancer Risks in Stockholm, Sweden, May 1987.
[1] Department of Molecular Biology University of California, Berkeley, California

source of genetic material from which viruses could transduce genetic information, and viral transduction has been canonical knowledge since phage λ was first shown by the Lederbergs and Zinder to transduce β-galactosidase in the 1950s [110]. Indeed, viruses are themselves derivatives of cellular genes that have evolved away from their progenitor genes as they acquired their capacity of self-replication.

B. The Oncogene Concept

On the basis of the sequence homology between viral *onc* genes and proto-*onc* genes, viral *onc* genes have been postulated to be transduced cellular cancer genes, and proto-*onc* genes have been postulated to be latent cancer genes or oncogenes [20–29]. According to this view, termed the oncogene concept [29], proto-*onc* genes are not only converted to transforming genes from without by transducing viruses, but also from within the cell by increased dosage or increased function [20–29]. Activation of latent oncogenes from within the cell is postulated to follow one of five prominent pathways: (a) point mutation [30, 31]; (b) chromosomal translocation that brings the latent oncogene under the control of a heterologous enhancer or promoter [24, 32]; (c) gene amplification [28, 29]; (d) activation from a retroviral promoter integrated adjacent to the latent oncogene [9, 23–29]; or (e) inactivation of a constitutive suppressor [33]. Thus, this view predicts that latent cancer genes exist in normal cells. However, the existence of latent cancer genes is a paradox, because such genes would be the most undesirable genes for eukaryotic cells. The very essence of enkaryots is cellular cooperativity, rather than autonomy as is typical of cancer cells and prokaryotes.

The oncogene concept was a revision of Huebner's oncogene hypothesis, which postulated activation of latent oncogenic viruses instead of latent cellular oncogenes as the cause of cancer [34]. Nevertheless, Huebner's hypothesis remained unconfirmed because most human and animal tumors are virus-negative [9, 12]. Moreover, the retroviruses and DNA viruses that have been isolated from tumors are not directly

oncogenic [5], except for the fewer than 50 isolates of animal retroviruses which contain *onc* genes [8, 9, 12].

The oncogene concept was highly attractive at first sight because it derived credibility from the proven oncogenic function of retroviral *onc* genes, the viral derivatives of proto-*onc* genes, and because it promised direct access to the long-sought cellular cancer genes in virus-free tumors with previously defined viral *onc* genes as hybridization probes. Predictably, the hypothesis has focused the search for cellular cancer genes from the 10^5–10^6 genes of eukaryotic cells to the 20 known proto-*onc* genes [8, 9, 23–29, 43].

The hypothesis makes four testable predictions, namely, (a) that viral *onc* genes and proto-*onc* genes are isogenic; (b) that expression of proto-*onc* genes would cause cancer; (c) that proto-*onc* genes from tumors would transform diploid cells as do proviral DNAs of viral *onc* genes; and above all (d) that diploid tumors exist that differ from normal cells only in activated proto-*onc* genes. Despite record efforts in the past 6 years, none of these predictions has been confirmed. On the contrary, in fact, the genetic and biochemical analyses that have defined essential retroviral genes, viral *onc* genes, and proto-*onc* genes during the past 16 years show in reference to (a) that viral *onc* genes and proto-*onc* genes are not isogenic [7, 8] (see below). As regards (b), it turned out that most proto-*onc* genes are frequently expressed in normal cells [8]. Contrary to the expectation in (c), none of the 20 known proto-*onc* genes isolated from tumors functions as a transforming gene when introduced into diploid cells. (The apparent exceptions of proto-*ras* and proto-*myc* are discussed below). By comparison, proviral DNAs of retroviral *onc* genes transform normal cells exactly as the corresponding viruses [9, 12]. And finally, no diploid tumors with activated proto-*onc* genes, as hypothesized in (d), have been found except for those caused by viruses with *onc* genes [35, 36]. Instead of activated oncogenes [8], clonal chromosome abnormalities are a consistent feature of virus-negative tumors [1–4, 37] and also of all those tumors that are infected by retroviruses without *onc* genes [5].

C. Claim that Proto-*ras* Genes Become Cancer Genes Due to Point Mutations

Harvey proto-*ras* is the cellular precursor of Harvey, Balb, and Rasheed murine sarcoma viruses, and Kirsten proto-*ras* is the cellular precursor of the murine Kirsten sarcoma virus [9, 12]. Both proto-*ras* and the viruses encode a colinear protein, termed p21, of 189 amino acids (Fig. 1) [38–44]. In 1982 it was discovered that Harvey proto-*ras* extracted from a human bladder carcinoma cell line, but not from normal cells, would transform the morphology of a few aneuploid murine cell lines, in particular the NIH 3T3 mouse cell line [30, 31]. Subsequently proto-*ras* DNAs from some other cell lines and from some primary tumors [8, 38–40] were also found to transform 3T3 cells. Since such proto-*ras* DNAs behave like dominant and autonomous cancer genes in this morphological assay, they were claimed to be cellular cancer genes [30, 31, 43]. The 3T3 cell transforming function of the Harvey proto-*ras* gene from the bladder carcinoma was reduced to a single point mutation that changed the 12th *ras* codon of p21 from the normal gly to val [30, 31]. In the meantime, more than 50 different point mutations in five different *ras* codons have been identified, all of which activate 3T3 cell transforming function [41, 42, 88]. Since the viral *ras* genes and proto-*ras* genes encode the same p21 proteins, whereas most other viral *onc* genes encode proteins that are different from those encoded by proto-*onc* genes (Fig. 1) [7, 8], this system has been considered a direct support for the hypothesis that viral *onc* genes and proto-*onc* genes are indeed isogenic and hence can become functionally equivalent by point mutations [26–31, 42–44].

However the following arguments cast doubt or the claims that point mutations are indeed necessary or sufficient to convert proto-*ras* to a dominant cancer gene:

1. Although most, but not all (see below), proto-*ras* genes with point mutations have been found in tumors or in certain cell lines, *ras* mutations are very rare in most spontaneous tumors [8, 38–40]. In fact, the gly to val mutation that was originally found in the human bladder carcinoma cell line [30, 31] has never been found in a primary tumor

[43, 88]. Moreover, even in certain chemically induced or spontaneous tumors in which *ras* mutations are relatively frequent a consistent correlation between *ras* mutations and tumors has never been observed [8, 43–45].

Furthermore, it is not known whether in animals the origin of a *ras* mutation coincides with the origin of the tumor. For example, the *ras* mutation of the human bladder carcinoma [30, 31] was only found in a cell line 10 years after this line was derived from the original tumor [46].

On the basis of a numerical argument it is also unlikely that point mutations are sufficient to convert proto-*ras* genes to dominant cancer genes. The frequency of point mutations of eukaryotes is one in 10^8–10^{10} nucleotides per mitosis [47, 48]. Thus, about one in 10^7 mitoses is expected to generate mutant Harvey *ras* genes with dominant transforming function, since the diploid human cell contains about 6×10^9 nucleotides and since 50 different mutations can activate each of two sets of *ras* genes of diploid cells. By contrast, spontaneous transformation that leads to clonal tumors occurs in fewer than one out of about 2×10^{17} mitoses and only a small minority of these contain mutant *ras* genes.

It may be argued, however, that indeed one out of 10^7 mitoses generates a tumor cell with activated proto-*ras* and that the immune system eliminates these cells. However this is unlikely since a point mutation is not an easy target for immunity. Further, animals or humans who are tolerant to *ras* point mutations would be expected to develop tumors at a very early age, if point-mutated proto-*ras* genes were dominant cancer genes, as the 3T3 assay suggests. Instead, spontaneous human tumors with activated proto-*ras* are very rare and all were observed in adults [8, 38–40]. Moreover, the argument that cellular oncogenes exist that can be activated by point mutation and then controlled by immunity is hard to reconcile with the existence of athymic or nude mice which do not develop more spontaneous tumors than other laboratory mice [49]. Furthermore, this view is inconsistent with the evidence that immunosuppressive therapy or thymectomy does not increase the cancer rate of humans [50]. Finally, one would predict that in the absence of immunity, as in cell culture, one out of 10^7 normal cells should spontaneously transform due to point mutation of Harvey proto-*ras* alone and probably the same number due to mutation of Kirsten proto-*ras* [9]. Yet spontaneous transformation of diploid cells in culture is clearly a much less frequent event.

In an effort directly to test the hypothesis that *ras* genes are activated to dominant cancer genes by point mutation, we [41] analyzed whether the transforming function of *ras* genes does indeed depend on point mutations. Using site-directed mutagenesis we have found that point mutations are not necessary for the transforming function of viral *ras* genes and of proto-*ras* genes that had been truncated to be structurally equivalent to viral *ras* genes [41]. (See also Cichutek and Duesberg this volume.)

2. Contrary to expectation, the same proto-*ras* DNAs from human tumors that transform aneuploid 3T3 cells do not transform diploid human [51] or diploid rodent cells [52–54], the initial material of natural tumors. Thus transformation of 3T3 cells does not appear to be a reliable assay for transforming genes of diploid cells. Instead of initiating malignant transformation, mutated proto-*ras* genes merely alter the morphology and enhance tumorigenicity of aneuploid 3T3 cells. Apparently they activate one of the many morphogenic programs of eukaryotic cells. Observations that untreated 3T3 cells are tumorigenic in nude mice [55–57] are consistent with this view. Thus, proto-*ras* genes with point mutations are not sufficient to initiate malignant transformation. They only appear as dominant cancer genes in certain aneuploid cells, such as 3T3 cells, based on unknown biochemical effects that alter the morphology of these cells. Furthermore, morphological transformation of 3T3 cells is not *ras* gene specific. It occurs spontaneously [58] and also upon transfection with several DNA species derived from tumors or tumor cell lines that, like proto-*ras*, do not transform diploid cells [28, 43, 44]. Such DNAs are now widely considered as cellular cancer genes [28, 43, 44], although they are not related to viral *onc* genes and do not transform diploid cells.

3. Assuming that mutated proto-*ras* genes are cancer genes, like viral *onc* genes,

one would expect diploid tumors that differ from normal cells only in *ras* point mutation. Contrary to expectation, chromosome abnormalities are consistently found in those tumors in which proto-*ras* mutations are occasionally found [2, 4]. The human bladder carcinoma cell line, in which the first proto-*ras* mutation was identified, is a convincing example. This cell line contains over 80 chromosomes (instead of 46) and includes rearranged marker chromosomes [46]. In view of such fundamental chromosome alterations, a point mutation seems to be a rather minor event. Indeed among diploid hamster cells transfected with mutated *ras* genes, only those that developed chromosomal abnormalities upon transfection were tumorigenic [59, 60].

Thus, proto-*ras* genes with point mutations are neither sufficient nor proven to be necessary for carcinogenesis and are not autonomous cancer genes as are viral *ras* genes. In addition, there is no kinetic evidence that the origin of the mutation coincides with the origin of the tumors in which it is found. It is consistent with this view that proto-*ras* mutations that register in the 3T3 cell transformation assay have been observed to occur in vivo in benign hyperplasias, as for example in benign murine hepatomas [61] or in benign, purely diploid mouse skin papillomas that differentiate into normal skin cells [62–66]. *Ras* mutations have also been observed to arise after carcinogenesis in aneuploid cancer cells [67–69], rather than to coincide with the origin of cancer. By contrast, viral *ras* genes are sufficient for transformation and thus initiate transformation of diploid cells in vitro and in vivo with single-hit kinetics and concurrent with infection [8, 70, 71].

This then raises the question as to why viral *ras* genes are inevitably carcinogenic under conditions under which proto-*ras* genes with point mutations are not. A sequence comparison between proto-*ras* genes and the known viral *ras* genes has recently revealed a proto-*ras*-specific exon that was not transduced by any of the known retroviruses with *ras* genes [41]. (See also Cichutek and Duesberg this volume.) It follows, that proto-*ras* and viral *ras* genes are not isogenic (Fig. 1). Since four different viral *ras* genes have been shown to lack the same proto-*ras* exon and since point mutations are not necessary for transforming function, we have proposed that proto-*ras* genes derive transforming function for diploid cells by truncation of an upstream exon and recombination with a retroviral promoter ([41], see below).

D. Claim that the Proto-*myc* Gene Becomes a Cancer Gene Under the Influence of a Heterologous Cellular Enhancer

Proto-*myc* is the cellular precursor of four avian carcinoma viruses, termed MC29, MH2, CMII, and OK10, with directly oncogenic *myc* genes [8]. The transforming host range of viral *myc* genes appears to be limited to avian cells, as murine cells are not transformed by cloned proviral DNAs [52, 53, 72]. Nevertheless, it is thought that proto-*myc*, brought under the control of heterologous cellular enhancers or promoters by chromosome translocation, is the cause of human Burkitt's lymphoma or mouse plasmacytoma [32, 64, 73].

The following arguments cast doubt on whether such activated proto-*myc* genes are indeed necessary or sufficient for carcinogenesis:

1. The human proto-*myc* gene is located on chromosome 8. This chromosome is typically rearranged in B cell lines derived from Burkitt's lymphomas [8, 32, 64]. However, although chromosome 8 is subjected to translocations, proto-*myc* is frequently not translocated, and when translocated it is frequently not rearranged [8, 32, 64]. Moreover, no rearrangements of chromosome 8 were observed in about 50% of primary Burkitt's lymphomas; instead, other chromosome abnormalities were recorded [74]. Thus, proto-*myc* translocation is not necessary for lymphomagenesis.

2. Expression of proto-*myc* is not consistently enhanced in lymphomas [8].

3. As yet no proto-*myc* gene isolated from any tumor has been demonstrated to transform any cells [8]. In an effort to assay transforming function in vivo, a proto-*myc* gene that was artificially linked to heterologous enhancers was introduced into the germ line of mice [73]. Several of these transgenic mice developed lymphomas after 1–5 months,

implying that activated proto-*myc* had transformed diploid cells. However, the lymphomas of the transgenic mice were all monoclonal [73]. Thus, if the activated proto-*myc* gene were indeed responsible for the lymphomas, it would be an extremely inefficient carcinogen, because only one of about 10^8 "control" B cells of the same mouse [75] with the same transgenic *myc* gene was transformed. Further, there is no deletion or mutation analysis to show that the activated proto-*myc* indeed played a direct role in the tumors of the transgenic mice [73]. In contrast, viral *myc* genes transform all susceptible cells directly and inevitably [8].

4. If translocated proto-*myc* were the cause of Burkitt's lymphomas, one would expect all tumors to be diploid and to carry only two abnormal chromosomes, namely, number 8 and the chromosome that was subject to reciprocal translocation with number 8. Instead, primary Burkitt's lymphomas exist with two normal chromosomes 8 that carry other chromosome abnormalities [74]. Thus, translocated proto-*myc* genes are not sufficient or proven to be necessary for carcinogenesis.

E. Probability of Spontaneous Transformation In Vivo Is at Least 10^9 Times Lower than Predicted from Proto-*onc* Gene Activation

It was estimated above that the probability of spontaneous transformation that leads to monoclonal tumors in humans is 2×10^{-17} per mitosis. One would expect activation of a preexisting, latent proto-*onc* gene to be a much more frequent event. For a given proto-*onc* gene, the probability of activation per mitosis would be the sum of the probabilities associated with each of the putative pathways [28, 29, 33] of proto-*onc* activation.

1. Since the probability of a point mutation per nucleotide per mitosis is about one in 10^9 [47, 48] per diploid cell, the probability that any one of the 20 known proto-*onc* genes is activated would be $2 \times 20 \times 10^{-9}$, assuming only one activating mutation per proto-*onc* gene. However, it would be 10^{-7} for Harvey-*ras* alone, since 50 different mu-

tations are thought to activate this gene to a dominant cancer gene (see above).

2. The probability of a given proto-*onc* gene to be activated by amplification is about one in 10^8, considering that about one in 10^3–10^5 mitoses leads to gene amplification in vitro and possibly in vivo and that about 10^3 out of the 10^6 kilobases (kb) of eukaryotic DNA are amplified [76, 77]. The probability that any one of the 20 known proto-*onc* genes would be activated by amplification would then be 2×10^{-7}.

3. The probability of oncogene activation by chromosome translocation depends largely on what distances between a proto-*onc* gene and a heterologous enhancer and which enhancers are considered sufficient for activation. Since distances > 50 kb of DNA have been considered sufficient for activation of proto-*myc* [9, 64] and proto-*abl* [9, 78] (the proto-*onc* gene of murine Abelson leukemia virus [9]), and since an enhancer is likely to be found in every 50 kb of cell DNA, nearly every translocation within a 50-kb radius of a proto-*onc* gene should be activating. Thus the probability that a given proto-*onc* gene is activated per translocation would be 5×10^{-5} (50 kb out of 10^6 kb). The probability that one of the 20 known proto-*onc* genes is activated would then be 10^{-3} per translocation.

Translocation frequencies per mitosis are not readily available. In hamster cells, translocations are estimated to occur with a probability of 10^{-6} per mitosis [79, 80]. In cells directly derived from mice and humans, even higher frequencies (0.01–0.3) have been observed upon study in vitro [81–83]. The probability of a translocation per meiotic cell division in humans has been determined to be 10^{-3}–10^{-4}, based on chromosome abnormalities in live births [84]. Assuming one translocation in 10^4 mitoses, the probability that one out of the 20 known proto-*onc* genes is activated per mitosis by translocation would then be about 10^{-7}.

4. The probability that a proto-*onc* gene would be activated from without by the promoter or enhancer of a retrovirus integrated nearby is even higher than those associated with the intrinsic mechanisms. Since retrovirus integration within 1–10 kb of a putative latent cancer gene is considered sufficient for activation [9, 23–29], since retro-

virus integration is not site-specific [10, 12], and since eukaryotes contain about 10^6 kb of DNA, a given proto-*onc* gene would be activated in at least one out of 10^6 infected cells [5, 8]. The probability that any one of the 20 known proto-*onc* genes would be activated would be 2×10^{-5} per infected cell.

The sum of these probabilities should reflect the spontaneous transformation frequency of cells per mitosis in vivo and in vitro. It would be between 10^{-5} and 10^{-7}. However, it should be at least 10^{-7} due to Harvey proto-*ras* mutations alone. Nevertheless, the actual number may be 10 times lower (or about 10^{-8}), depending on whether all or only some of these four putative mechanisms could activate a proto-*onc* gene and depending on whether a given cell is susceptible to transformation by a given *onc* gene or to a given retrovirus. Instead, spontaneous transformation per mitosis that leads to monoclonal tumors is only about 2×10^{-17} in vivo. Thus the expected probability of spontaneous transformation due to activation of preexisting oncogenes differs at least by a factor of 10^9 from that observed in diploid cells in vivo.

Again it may be argued that spontaneous malignant transformation does indeed occur at the above rates but that immunity eliminates nearly all transformants. However in this case athymic or nude mice should not exist and the cancer incidence should increase significantly upon immunosuppressive therapy or thymectomy; yet this is not the case [49, 50]. Moreover, diploid cells in culture have not been observed to transform at the above rates.

5. Certain cancers (e.g., retinoblastomas) are thought to be caused by activation of latent oncogenes that are normally suppressed by two allelic suppressor genes [33]. Cancers caused by such genes would be the product of inactivations of two allelic suppressors and thus very rare [33]. In individuals with genetic defects in one putative suppressor allele tumors such as retinoblastomas should occur due to inactivation of the second suppressor allele with the same frequencies as those estimated above for point mutation, translocation, and retrovirus insertion [33].

However, in over 80% of retinoblastomas that occur in individuals without prior genetic defect the putative suppressor genes appear to be normal as judged by chromosome analysis [33], suggesting that other suppressors inhibit the putative retinoblastoma oncogene or that it does not exist. Instead, other chromosomal abnormalities that are always seen in such tumors [33] may be relevant to carcinogenesis (see below). Further, this activation hypothesis predicts that normal cellular DNA would cure retinoblastoma cells upon experimental transfection. Yet this has not been reported. Likewise, it would be expected that experimental, human-nonhuman heterokaryons that have lost chromosomes with suppressor genes would be transformed. It would also be expected that retinoblasts or other cells from individuals with a genetic defect in one suppressor allele would spontaneously transform with the probability of chromosome nondysjunction. Dysjunction has been observed to occur upon cultivation of biopsied murine [85] and human cells [86] with a probability of one in 10^{-3} (monosomies) to one in 10^{-4} (trisomies) per chromosome and mitosis. However, spontaneous transformations have not been described as occurring at this rate. Thus there is as yet no proof for suppressed cancer genes in normal cells.

F. Hypothesis that Activated Proto-*onc* Genes Require Unknown Complementary Genes for Carcinogenesis

Because of the consistent difficulties in demonstrating oncogenic function of proto-*onc* genes, a further revision of the oncogene concept has recently been favored. It proposes that "activated" proto-*onc* genes, like proto-*ras* or proto-*myc*, are not autonomous *onc* genes like their viral derivatives, but are at least necessary for the kind of carcinogenesis that requires multiple cooperating oncogenes [32, 52, 53, 64, 65, 87, 88]. Thus, activated proto-*onc* genes are proposed to be functionally different, yet structurally equivalent to viral *onc* genes. According to this theory, activated proto-*onc* genes would not be expected to register in transformation assays that detect single-hit carcinogens like viral *onc* genes [7, 8].

However, the hypothesis fails to provide even a speculative explanation as to why activated proto-*onc* genes are no longer to be considered functionally equivalent to viral *onc* genes [8]. Clearly, until the postulated complementary cancer genes are identified, this hypothesis remains unproven [8].

The hypothesis also fails to explain why among certain tumors, such as human carcinomas, individual carcinomas are only distinguishable from each other by the presence or absence of activated, putative oncogenes [8, 38–40, 42–44]. This implies either (a) that unknown oncogenes that do not register in the 3T3 cell assay would cause the same tumors as the putative oncogenes that do, or (b) that the putative oncogenes are not necessary for these tumors.

G. Viral *onc* Genes as Specific Recombinants Between Truncated Viral and Cellular Genes

Genetic and structural analyses of retroviral genes, viral *onc* genes, and proto-*onc* genes and direct comparisons between them have shown that viral *onc* genes and proto-*onc* genes differ both structurally and functionally. Therefore, we have proposed that viral *onc* genes are indeed new genes that do not preexist in normal cells, rather than being transduced cellular genes [7, 8, 13, 19] (Fig. 1). The original basis for this proposal was the definition of the transforming gene of avian carcinoma virus MC29 [89] as a genetic hybrid, rather than a transduced cellular oncogene [90]. It consists of a promoter and coding elements (*Δgag*) from an avian retrovirus linked to 3' coding elements from cellular proto-*myc* (Fig. 1) [90]. Initially this became evident by comparing the structure and map order of MC29 with that of the three essential retrovirus genes, namely 5'*gag-pol-env* 3' (Fig. 1) [91, 92].

Sequence comparison of the viral *Δgag-myc* gene with the chicken proto-*myc* gene provided direct proof that only a truncated proto-*myc* gene was present in MC29. Indeed a complete 5' proto-*myc* exon was missing from the viral *Δgag-myc* gene [19]. This was apparently not an accident since the same 5' proto-*myc* exon was also missing in the three other *myc*-containing avian carcinoma viruses MH2 [93, 94], CMII, and OK10 [8, 95]. Thus a viral and a cellular gene functioned as progenitors or proto-*onc*

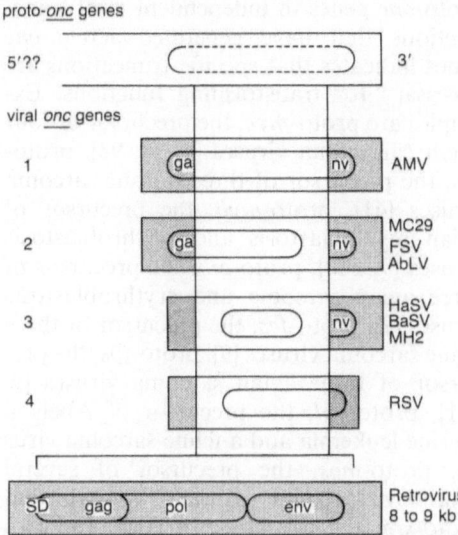

proto-*onc* genes

5'?? ⟞ ⟝ 3'

viral *onc* genes

1 (ga | nv) AMV

2 (ga | nv) MC29 / FSV / AbLV

3 (| nv) HaSV / BaSV / MH2

4 ( ) RSV

SD | gag) | pol) | env) Retrovirus 8 to 9 kb

Fig. 1. The generic, recombinant structures of retroviral *onc* genes and their relationship to viral genes (*stippled*) and cellular proto-*onc* genes (*unshaded*). The genes are compared as transcriptional units, or mRNAs. All known viral *onc* genes are tripartite hybrids of a central sequence derived from a cellular proto-*onc* gene, which is flanked by 5' and 3' elements derived from retroviral "proto-*onc*" genes. Actual size differences, ranging from over 1–7 kb [9], are not recorded. The map order of the three essential retrovirus genes, *gag, pol,* and *env,* and of the splice donor (*SD*) are indicated. Four groups of viral *onc* genes are distinguished based on the origins of their coding sequence (◯): *1*, The coding unit has a tripartite structure of a central proto-*onc*-derived sequence that is initiated and terminated by viral coding sequences; avian myeloblastosis virus (*AMV*) is an example [9, 96]. *2*, The coding unit is initiated by a viral and terminated by a proto-*onc* sequence; the *Δgag-myc* gene of avian carcinoma virus MC29 is an example [8, 9, 19, 90], as are hybrid *onc* genes of avian Fujinami sarcoma virus [97] and murine Abelson leukemia virus [9]. *3*, The coding unit of the viral *onc* gene is colinear with a reading frame of a cellular proto-*onc* gene; the *ras* gene of the murine Harvey and Balb sarcoma viruses [41] and possibly the *myc* gene of the avian carcinoma virus MH2 are examples [93, 94]. *4*, The coding unit is initiated by a proto-*onc* derived domain and terminated by a viral reading frame; the *src* gene of Rous sarcoma virus is an example [7, 9]. The transcriptional starts and 5' untranscribed regulatory sequences (?) of all proto-*onc* genes are as yet not or not exactly known [8, 9]. There is also uncertainty about 5' translational starts and open reading frames in some proto-*onc* genes (?) that are not transduced into viral *onc*

genes of each of the viral recombinant *myc* genes (Fig. 1). More recently, the four known viral *ras* genes were each also shown to lack a 5' proto-*ras* exon [41] (see above; Fig. 1).

Comparisons between the *onc* genes of other retroviruses and the corresponding proto-*onc* genes proved that, defined as transcriptional units, all viral *onc* genes are new genes. They are recombinants of proto-*onc* genes and retroviral genes (Fig. 1) [7–9]. Most but not all viral genes also encode new recombinant proteins. Based on the origin of their coding elements, the viral *onc* genes can be divided into the four groups illustrated in Fig. 1.

1. Those with amino and carboxy terminal domains from retroviruses and central domains from proto-*onc* genes. The *onc* gene avian myeloblastosis virus (AMV) is the prototype [9, 96].
2. Those with amino terminal domains from viral genes and carboxy terminal domains from proto-*onc* genes. The *Δgag-myc* gene of MC29 is the original example (see above). The *onc* genes of Fujinami sarcoma virus [97] and Abelson leukemia virus [9] also have the generic *Δgag*-X structure.
3. Those that are colinear with a reading frame of a proto-*onc* gene. The *ras* genes of Harvey and Balb murine sarcoma virus [41] and possibly the *myc* gene of avian carcinoma virus MH2 [93, 94] are examples.
4. Those with an amino terminal domain from a proto-*onc* gene and a carboxy terminal domain from the virus. The *src* gene of RSV is the prototype [7–9].

Since three of the four groups of recombinant viral *onc* genes also encode recombinant proteins, their specific transforming function can be directly related to their specific structure compared to that of proto-*onc*

genes, as in proto-*myc* [98], proto-*src* [7], or proto-*ras* [41]. It is clear however that proto-*onc*-specific regulatory elements are always replaced by viral promoters and enhancers and that proto-*onc* coding sequences are frequently recombined with viral coding sequences. Thus, all viral *onc* genes are tripartite recombinant genes of truncated viral and proto-*onc* genes

503

gene products. The transforming function of the recombinant *onc* genes of group 3, which encode transforming proteins that are co-linear with proteins encoded by proto-*onc* genes, cannot be explained in this fashion. However, all viral *onc* genes of this group each lack at least one proto-*onc*-specific 5′ exon like the avian carcinoma viruses with *myc* genes [8, 19, 93–95] or the murine sarcoma viruses with *ras* genes [41]. Conceivably elimination of transcribed or untranscribed suppressors or elimination of an upstream proto-*ras* cistron [41] or proto-*myc* cistron [98] and recombination with viral promoters are the mechanisms that generate transforming function (Fig. 1).

It follows that viral *onc* genes and the corresponding proto-*onc* genes are not isogenic. Viral *onc* genes are hybrid genes that consist of truncated proto-*onc* genes recombined with regulatory and frequently with coding elements from truncated retroviral genes. These consistent structural differences must be the reason why viral *onc* genes inevitably transform and why proto-*onc* genes are not transforming although they are present in all and are active in most normal cells [7, 8].

Clearly if cellular oncogenes preexist in normal cells, it would be much more likely to find retroviruses with intact cellular oncogenes than retroviruses with new *onc* genes put together from unrelated and truncated viral and cellular genes by illegitimate recombination. However, it may be argued that proto-*onc* gene truncations reflect packaging restrictions of transducing retroviruses rather than conditions to activate proto-*onc* genes. Such restrictions would have to be mostly sequence-specific, as most retroviruses with *onc* genes can accommodate more RNA – at least 10 kb, as in RSV [99] – than they actually contain, namely 3–8 kb [9]. But there is no evidence that retroviruses discriminate more against certain transduced or artificially introduced sequences [9] than against others, because retroviruses can accommodate very heterogenous sequences, such as the 20 different transformation-specific sequences [7–9, 13]. Yet all nonessential sequences of retroviruses are unstable [7, 8] unless selected for a given function.

Moreover, the fact that the same exons were selectively truncated from several

proto-*onc* genes in independent viral transductions that have generated active *onc* genes indicates that specific truncations are necessary for transforming functions. Examples are proto-*myc*, the precursor of four avian carcinoma viruses [8, 19, 93], proto-*ras*, the precursor of three murine sarcoma viruses [41], proto-*myb*, the precursor of avian myeloblastosis and erythroblastosis viruses [9, 100], proto-*erb*, the precursor of three avian sarcoma and erythroblastosis viruses [9], proto-*fes*, the precursor of three feline sarcoma viruses [9], proto-*fps*, the precursor of three avian sarcoma viruses [9, 101], proto-*abl*, the precursor of Abelson murine leukemia and a feline sarcoma virus [9], proto-*mos*, the precursor of several Moloney sarcoma viruses [9, 102], and proto-*src*, the precursor of RSV and two other avian sarcoma viruses [103]. In some cases of independent transductions, the same proto-*onc* genes were even truncated at exactly the same breakpoints, as for example in two different avian sarcoma viruses derived from proto-*fps* [101].

The existence of at least seven retroviruses containing proto-*onc* sequences that had already been truncated by recombination with other cellular or viral genes prior to transduction lends further independent support to this view. Examples are the *onc* genes of avian carcinoma virus MH2 [8, 93, 94], of avian erythroblastosis and sarcoma virus AEV [9], of avian erythro- and myeloblastosis virus E26 [100], of the feline sarcoma virus GR-FeSV [9, 104], of RSV [7, 9] and of Harvey and Kirsten sarcoma viruses [9, 41]. Certainly the odds against transduction of rare, rearranged proto-*onc* genes instead of normal proto-*onc* genes are overwhelming. Yet seven out of the less than 50 known isolates of retroviruses with *onc* genes [9] contain previously rearranged proto-*onc* sequences, most likely because truncation is necessary for transforming function. Indeed, it may be argued that these viruses have transduced these rearranged proto-*onc* genes from a preexisting tumor that was generated by these rearrangements. Thus, the rearranged proto-*onc* genes of these seven oncogenic retroviruses may be "transduced cellular oncogenes" after all.

Therefore recombination of proto-*onc* genes with retroviral or cellular genes appears to be necessary to convert proto-*onc* genes to transforming genes. A definitive assessment of why viral *onc* genes transform and cellular proto-*onc* genes do not requires more than comparisons of primary structures and transforming tests with DNAs. It will be necessary to know what proto-*onc* genes do and whether they encode proteins that function alone or as complexes with other proteins.

I propose, then, that proto-*onc* genes that are transcriptionally activated or have undergone point mutations but retain a germline structure are not cellular cancer genes. I suggest that the hypothesis that proto-*onc* genes are latent cellular cancer genes that can be converted to active transforming genes by increased dosage or function is an exaggerated interpretation of sequence homology to structural and functional homology with viral *onc* genes.

This proposal readily resolves the paradoxes posed by the hypothesis that proto-*onc* genes are latent cellular cancer genes that can be activated by enhanced expression or point mutation. The proposal accounts for the frequent expression of proto-*onc* genes in normal cells [8]. The proposal is also entirely consistent with the lack of transforming function of "activated" proto-*onc* genes from tumors. The fact that mutated proto-*ras* changes the morphology and enhances tumorigenicity of aneuploid and tumorigenic 3T3 cells is an important observation, but not an exception to the experience that native proto-*onc* genes from tumors analyzed to date do not transform diploid cells. The proposal also provides a rationale for the chromosome abnormalities of tumor cells, as these appear to be microscopic evidence for cancer genes (see below) instead of the "activated" proto-*onc* genes identified to date.

H. Hybrid *onc* Genes of Retroviruses as Models of Cellular Cancer Genes

The proposal that proto-*onc* genes derive transforming function by truncation and recombination with retroviral or cellular genes predicts that recombinations among cellular genes could also generate transforming genes. The view that cellular cancer genes are rare recombinants of normal cellular genes is in accord with the fact that rearranged and abnormal chromosomes are the only consistent, transformation-specific markers of tumor cells [2–5, 37]. Further, the clonality of chromosome alterations, e.g., the marker chromosomes of tumors [2–5, 37], indicates that tumors are initiated with and possibly caused by such abnormalities as originally proposed by Boveri in 1914 [105].

A major difficulty with the view that specific recombination sites among rearranged chromosomes are markers of recombinant cancer genes is that neither the chromosome breakpoints nor the karyotypes of different tumors of the same cell lineage are the same. Although some tumors show typical nonrandom abnormalities, such as the Philadelphia chromosome of chronic myelogenous leukemia and the 8 to 14, 2 and 22 translocations of Burkitt's lymphomas, exceptions are always seen, and the chromosome breakpoints of two different tumors with the same karyotypes are not the same at the nucleotide level [43, 74, 106]. Such heterogeneity of breakpoints, and thus of mutation, among otherwise indistinguishable tumors argues either for different transforming genes in the same tumors or against chromosome breakpoints as markers of transforming genes. However, this argument does not take into consideration that together with the microscopic karyotype alterations other submicroscopic mutations may have occurred that could have produced cancer genes. It is consistent with this that tumor cells contain, in addition to microscopic chromosome abnormalities, submicroscopic deletions and restriction enzyme site alterations [107]. Thus, specific marker chromosomes may only be the tip of an iceberg of multiple chromosomal mutations that may have generated cancer genes as well as mutationally activated or inactivated growth control genes.

The generation of retroviral *onc* genes from viral genes and proto-*onc* genes appears to be a direct model for the process of how cancer genes may be generated by chromosomal rearrangements. Less than 50 isolates of retroviruses with *onc* genes have been recorded in history [8, 9, 12], although both potential parents of retroviral *onc* genes are available in many animal or human cells because retroviruses are widespread in all vertebrates [5, 9, 12]. This extremely low birth rate of retroviruses with *onc* genes must then reflect the low probability of generating de novo an oncogenic retrovirus from a proto-*onc* gene and a retrovirus by truncating and recombining viral and cellular genes via illegitimate recombinations [7, 8, 13]. Clearly, at least two illegitimate recombinations are required (Fig. 1): one to link a 3′ truncated retrovirus with a 5′ truncated proto-*onc* gene, the other to break and then splice the resulting hybrid *onc* gene to the 3′ part of the retroviral vector.

The first of these steps would already generate a "cellular" cancer gene that ought to be sufficient for carcinogenesis. The birth of such a gene would be more probable than that of an oncogenic retrovirus that requires two illegitimate recombinations, but it would be harder to detect than a complete replicating retrovirus with an *onc* gene. Nevertheless even this would be a rare event. Given that such a recombination would have to take place within the 8–9 kb of a retrovirus (Fig. 1) integrated into the 10^6-kb genome of a eukaryotic cell and also within an estimated 1–2 kb of a proto-*onc* gene (Fig. 1), and assuming that translocation or rearrangement occurs with a probability of 10^{-4} (see above), the probability of such a recombination per mitosis would be 8×10^{-6} $2 \times 10^{-6} \cdot 10^{-4}$, or 10^{-15}. That a second illegitimate recombination is required to generate a retrovirus with an *onc* gene would explain why the occurrence of these viruses is much less frequent than spontaneous transformation due to recombinant cancer genes. This probability may, nevertheless, be higher than the square of 10^{-15}, since the two events may be linked and since multiple integrated and unintegrated proviruses exist in most infected cells.

The probability that illegitimate recombination would generate cancer genes from normal cellular genes would also be very low, since most illegitimate recombination would inactivate genes. The above estimates for the probability of spontaneous transformation of 2×10^{-17} per mitosis and of translocation of 10^{-4}, which would be a minimal estimate for illegitimate recombina-

tion, suggest that 10^{13} translocations or rearrangements are needed to generate a transforming gene that causes a monoclonal tumor. This could be either a single autonomous transforming gene that is like a viral *onc* gene or a series of mutually dependent transforming genes [108, 109] that would each arise with a higher probability than an autonomous *onc* gene. The facts that multiple chromosome alterations are typically seen in tumors [2–4, 37, 74] and that as yet no DNAs have been isolated from tumors that transform diploid cells with single-hit kinetics suggest that most cellular cancer genes are indeed not autonomous carcinogens like viral *onc* genes. It is consistent with this view that most cellular genes are also not converted to autonomous cancer genes by retroviral transduction via illegitimate recombination and truncation. Only about 20 cellular genes, the proto-*onc* genes, have been converted to autonomous viral *onc* genes, although viral transduction via illegitimate recombination is a random event that does not benefit from sequence homology between retroviruses and cells [7, 8, 13].

Thus viral *onc* genes have not as yet fingered preexisting cellular cancer genes. No cellular gene is a structural or functional homolog of a viral *onc* gene, but the viral *onc* genes appear to be models for how cancer genes may arise from normal cellular genes by rare truncation and recombination.

Acknowledgments. I would like to thank S. A. Aaronson, S. Blam, M. Kraus, M. Pech, K. Robbins, S. Tronick and others from the Laboratory of Cellular and Molecular Biology, National Cancer Institute, Bethesda, Maryland, for critical and amusing discussions and generous support during a sabbatical leave, and B. Witkop, National Institute of Arthritis, Diabetes and Digestive and Kidney Diseases, Bethesda, Maryland, for asking many of the basic questions that I try to answer in this manuscript. I also thank my colleagues H. Rubin for encouragement and K. Cichutek, R.-P. Zhou, D. Goodrich, S. Pfaff, and W. Phares, University of California, Berkeley, California, for inspiring comments and their work. This research has been supported by (OIG) National Cancer Institute Grant CA-39915A-01 and Council for Tobacco Research Grant 1547 and by a Scholarship-in-Residence of the Fogarty International Center, NIH, Bethesda, Maryland.

References

1. Duesberg PH (1987) Cancer genes: rare recombinants instead of activated oncogenes. Proc Natl Acad Sci USA 84:2117–2124
2. Wolman SR (1983) Karyotypic progression in human tumors. Cancer Metast Rev 2:257–293
3. Rowley JD (1984) Introduction: consistent chromosomal alterations and oncogenes in human tumors. Cancer Surveys 3:355–357
4. Trent JM (1984) Chromosomal alterations in human solid tumors: implications of the stem cell model to cancer cytogenetics. Cancer Surveys 3:393–422
5. Duesberg PH (1987) Retroviruses as carcinogens and pathogens: expectations and reality. Cancer Res 47:1199–1220
6. Silverberg E, Lubera J (1986) Cancer statistics. CA 36:9–25
7. Duesberg PH (1983) Retroviral transforming genes in normal cells? Nature 304:219–226
8. Duesberg PH (1985) Activated proto-*onc* genes: sufficient or necessary for cancer? Science 228:669–677
9. Weiss R, Teich N, Varmus H, Coffin J (eds) (1985) RNA tumor viruses; molecular biology of tumor viruses, 2nd edn. Cold Spring Harbor Press, New York
10. Duesberg PH, Vogt PK (1970) Differences between the ribonucleic acids of transforming and nontransforming avian tumor viruses. Proc Natl Acad Sci USA 67:1673–1680
11. Martin GS, Duesberg PH (1972) The a-subunit on the RNA of transforming avian tumor viruses. I. Occurrence in different virus strains. II. Spontaneous loss resulting in nontransforming variants. Virology 47:494–497
12. Weiss R, Teich N, Varmus H, Coffin J (eds) (1982) RNA tumor viruses; molecular biology of tumor viruses. Cold Spring Harbor Press, New York
13. Duesberg PH (1979) Transforming genes of retroviruses. Cold Spring Harbor Symp Quant. Biol 44:13–27
14. Scolnick EM, Rands F, Williams P, Parks WP (1973) Studies on the nucleic acid sequences of Kirsten sarcoma virus. A model for formation of a mammalian RNA-containing sarcoma virus. J Virol 12:458–463
15. Scolnick EM, Parks WP (1974) Harvey sarcoma virus. A second murine type C sarcoma virus with rat genetic information. J Virol 13:1211–1219
16. Tsuchida N, Gilden RV, Hatanaka M (1974) Sarcoma-virus-related RNA sequences in normal rat cells. Proc Natl Acad Sci USA 71:4503–4507
17. Frankel AE, Fischinger PJ (1976) Nucleotide sequences in mouse DNA and RNA specific for Moloney sarcoma virus. Proc Natl Acad Sci USA 73:3705–3709
18. Stehelin D, Varmus HE, Bishop JM, Vogt PK (1976) DNA related to the transforming gene(s) of avian sarcoma viruses is present in normal avian DNA. Nature 260:170–173
19. Watson DK, Reddy EP, Duesberg PH, Papas TS (1983) Nucleotide sequence analysis of the chicken c-myc gene reveals homologous and unique regions by comparison with the transforming gene of avian myelocytomatosis virus MC29, *Δgag-myc*. Proc Natl Acad Sci USA 80:2146–2150
20. Bishop JM, Courtneidge SA, Levinson AD, Oppermann H, Quintrell N, Sheiness DK, Weiss SR, Varmus HE (1979) Origin and function of avian retrovirus transforming genes. Cold Spring Harbor Symposia Quant. Biol 44:919–930
21. Karess RE, Hayward WS, Hanafusa H (1979) Transforming protein encoded by the cellular information of recovered avian sarcoma viruses. Cold Spring Harbor Symposia Quant. Biol 44:765–771
22. Wang L-H, Snyder P, Hanafusa T, Moscovici C, Hanafusa H (1979) Comparative analysis of cellular and viral sequences related to sarcomagenic cell transformation. Cold Spring Harbor Symposia Quant. Biol 44:755–764
23. Bishop JM (1981) Enemies within: the genesis of retrovirus oncogenes. Cell 23:5–6
24. Klein G (1981) The role of gene dosage and genetic transposition in carcinogenesis. Nature 294:313–318
25. Bishop JM, Varmus H (1982) Functions and origins of retroviral transforming genes in RNA tumor viruses. In: Weiss R, Teich N, Varmus H, Coffin J (eds) RNA tumor viruses; molecular biology of tumor viruses. Cold Spring Harbor Press, New York, pp 999–1108
26. Bishop JM (1982) Oncogenes. Sci Am 246:80–90
27. Bishop JM (1983) Cellular oncogenes and retroviruses. Annu Rev Biochem 52:301–354
28. Varmus H, Bishop JM (1986) Introduction. Biochemical mechanisms of oncogene activity: proteins encoded by oncogenes. Cancer Surv 5:153–158
29. Weiss RA (1986) The oncogene concept. Cancer Rev 2:1–17
30. Tabin CJ, Bradley SM, Bargmann CI, Weinberg RA, Papageorge AG, Scolnick EM,

Dhar R, Lowy DR, Chang EH (1982) Mechanism of activation of a human oncogene. Nature 300:143–149

31. Reddy EP, Reynolds RK, Santos E, Barbacid M (1982) A point mutation is responsible for the acquisition of transforming properties by the T24 human bladder carcinoma oncogene. Nature 300:149–152

32. Leder P, Battey J, Lenoir G, Moulding C, Murphy W, Potter M, Stewart T, Taub R (1983) Translocations among antibody genes in human cancer. Science 227:765–771

33. Knudson AG Jr (1985) Hereditary cancer, oncogenes, and antioncogenes. Cancer Res 45:1437–1443

34. Huebner RJ, Todaro G (1969) Oncogenes of RNA tumor viruses as determinants of cancer. Proc Natl Acad Sci USA 64:1087–1094

35. Pitot HC (1978) Fundamentals of oncology. Dekker, New York

36. Klein G, Ohno S, Rosenberg N, Wiener F, Spira J, Baltimore D (1980) Cytogenic studies on Abelson-virus-induced mouse leukemias. Int J Cancer 25:805–811

37. Levan A (1956) Chromosomes in cancer tissue. Ann NY Acad Sci 63:774–792

38. Feinberg AP, Vogelstein MJ, Droller S, Baylin B, Nelkin BD (1983) Mutation affecting the 12th amino acid of the c-Has-*ras* oncogene product occurs infrequently in human cancer. Science 220:1175–1177

39. Fujita J, Srivastava S, Kraus M, Rhim JS, Tronick SR, Aaronson SA (1985) Frequency of molecular alterations affecting *ras* proto-oncogenes in human urinary tract tumors. Proc Natl Acad Sci USA 82:3849–3853

40. Milici A, Blick M, Murphy E, Gutterman JU (1986) c-K-*ras* codon 12 GGT-CGT point mutation an infrequent event in human lung cancer. Biochem Biophys Res Commun 140:699–705

41. Cichutek K, Duesberg PH (1986) Harvey *ras* genes transform without mutant codons, apparently activated by truncation of a 5' exon (exon-1). Proc Natl Acad Sci USA 83:2340–2344

42. Lowy DR, Willumsen BW (1986) The *ras* gene family. Cancer Surv 5:275–289

43. Marshall C (1985) Human oncogenes. In: Weiss R et al. (eds) RNA tumor viruses; molecular biology of tumor viruses. Cold Spring Harbor Press, New York, pp 487–558

44. Barbacid M (1986) Mutagens, oncogenes and cancer. Trends Gen 2:188–192

45. Needleman SW, Kraus MH, Srivastava SK, Levine PH, Aaronson SA (1986) High frequency of N-*ras* activation in acute myelogenous leukemia. Blood 67:753–757

46. Hastings RJ, Franks LM (1981) Chromosome pattern, growth in agar and tumorigenicity in nude mice of four human bladder carcinoma cell lines. Int J Cancer 27:15–21

47. Wabl M, Burrows PD, Gabain A von, Steinberg A (1984) Hypermutation at the immunoglobulin heavy chain locus in a pre-B cell line. Proc Natl Acad Sci USA 82:479–482

48. Drake JW (1969) Comparative rates of spontaneous mutation. Nature 221:1132

49. Sharkey FE, Fogh J (1984) Considerations in the use of nude mice for cancer research. Cancer Metast Rev 3:341–360

50. Kinlen LJ (1982) Immunosuppressive therapy and cancer. Cancer Surv 1:565–583

51. Sager R, Tanaka K, Lau CC, Ebina Y, Anisowicz A (1983) Resistance of human cells to tumorigenesis induced by cloned transforming genes. Proc Natl Acad Sci USA 80:7601–7605

52. Land H, Parada LF, Weinberg RA (1983) Tumorigenic conversion of primary embryo fibroblasts requires at least two cooperating oncogenes. Nature 304:596–602

53. Land H, Parada LF, Weinberg RA (1983) Cellular oncogenes and multistep carcinogenesis. Science 222:771–778

54. Newbold RF, Overell RW (1983) Fibroblast immortality is a prerequisite for transformation by EJ c-Ha-*ras* oncogene. Nature 304:648–651

55. Boone CW (1975) Malignant hemangioendotheliomas produced by subcutaneous inoculation of BALB/3T3 cells attached to glass beads. Science 188:68–70

56. Littlefield JW (1982) NIH/3T3 cell line. Science 218:214–216

57. Greig RG, Koestler TP, Trayner DL, Corwin SP, Miles L, Kline T, Sweet R, Yokoyama S, Poste G (1985) Tumorigenic and metastatic properties of "normal" and *ras*-transfected NIH/3T3 cells. Proc Natl Acad Sci USA 82:3698–3701

58. Rubin H, Chu BM, Arnstein P (1983) Heritable variations in growth potential and morphology within a clone of Balb/3T3 cells and their relation to tumor formation. J Natl Cancer Inst 71:365–373

59. Spandidos DA, Wilkie NM (1984) In vitro malignant transformation of early passage rodent cells by a single mutated human oncogene. Nature 310:469–475

60. Stenman G, Delorme EO, Lau CC, Sager R (1987) Transfection with plasmid pSV2gptEJ induces chromosome rearrangements in CHEF cells. Proc Natl Acad Sci USA 84:184–188

61. Reynolds SH, Stowers SJ, Maronpot RR, Anderson MW, Aaronson SA (1986) Detection and identification of activated oncogenes in spontaneously occurring benign and malignant hepatocellular tumors of the B6C3F1 mouse. Proc Natl Acad Sci USA 83:33–37

62. Balmain A, Ramsden M, Bowden GT, Smith J (1984) Activation of the mouse cellular Harvey-*ras* gene in chemically induced benign skin papillomas. Nature 307:658–660

63. Balmain A, Pragnell IB (1983) Mouse skin carcinomas induced in vivo by chemical carcinogens have a transforming Harvey-*ras* oncogene. Nature 304:596–602

64. Klein G, Klein E (1984) Oncogene activation and tumor progression. Carcinogenesis 5:429–435

65. Balmain A (1985) Transforming *ras* oncogenes and multistage carcinogenesis. Br J Cancer 51:1–7

66. Burns FJ, Vanderlaan M, Snyder E, Albert RE (1978) Induction and progression kinetics of mouse skin papillomas. In: Slaga TJ, Sivac A, Boutwell RK (eds) Carcinogenesis, vol 2. Mechanisms of tumor promotion and cocarcinogenesis. Raven, New York, pp 91–96

67. Albino AP, Le Strange AI, Oliff MI, Furth ME, Old LJ (1984) Transforming *ras* genes from human melanoma: a manifestation of tumour heterogeneity? Nature 308:69–72

68. Tainsky MA, Cooper GS, Giovanella BC, Vande Woude GF (1984) An activated ras N gene: detected in late but not early passage human teratocarcinoma cells. Science 225:643–645

69. Vousden KH, Marshall CJ (1984) Three different activated *ras* genes in mouse tumors: evidence for oncogene activation during progression of a mouse lymphoma. EMBO J 3:913–917

70. Aaronson SA, Weaver CA (1971) Characterization of murine sarcoma virus (Kirsten) transformation of mouse and human cells. J Gen Virol 13:245–252

71. Hoelzer-Pierce J, Aaronson SA (1982) BALB- and Harvey-murine sarcoma virus transformation of a novel lymphoid progenitor cell. J Exp Med 156:873–887

72. Rapp UR, Cleveland JL, Fredrickson TN, Holmes KL, Morse III HC, Jansen HW, Patschinsky T, Bister K (1985) Rapid induction of hemopoietic neoplasms in newborn mice by a *raf(mil)/myc* recombinant murine retrovirus. J Virol 55:23–33

73. Adams JM, Harris AW, Pinkert CA, Corcoran LM, Alexander WS, Cory S, Palmiter RD, Brinster RL (1985) The c-*myc* oncogene driven by immunoglobulin enhancers induces lymphoid malignancy in transgenic mice. Nature 318:533–538

74. Biggar RJ, Lee EC, Nkrumah FK, Whang-Peng J (1981) Direct cytogenetic studies by needle stick aspiration of Burkitt's lymphoma in Ghana, West Africa. J Natl Cancer Inst 67:769–776

75. Sprent J (1977) Migration and life span of lymphocytes. In: Loor F, Roelants GE (eds) B and T cells in immune recognition. Wiley, New York, pp 59–82

76. Stark GR (1986) DNA amplification in drug resistant cells and in tumours. Cancer Surv 5:1–23

77. Schimke RT, Sherwood SW, Hill AB, Johnston RN (1986) Overreplication and recombination of DNA in higher eukaryotes: potential consequences and biological implications. Proc Natl Acad Sci USA 83:2157–2161

78. Heisterkamp N, Stam K, Groffen J, Klein A De, Grosveld G (1985) Structural organization of the *bcr* gene and its role in the Ph' translocation. Nature 315:758–761

79. Kraemer PM, Ray FA, Brothman AR, Bartholdi MF, Cram LS (1986) Spontaneous immortalization rate of cultured Chinese hamster cells. J Natl Cancer Inst 76:703–709

80. Ray FA, Bartholdi MF, Kraemer PM, Cram LS (1986) Spontaneous in vitro neoplastic evolution: recurrent chromosome changes of newly immortalized Chinese hamster cells. Cancer Genet Cytogenet 21:35–51

81. Terzi M, Hawkins TSC (1975) Chromosomal variation and the establishment of somatic cell lines in vitro. Nature 253:361–362

82. Harnden DG, Benn PA, Oxford JM, Taylor AMR, Webb TP (1976) Cytogenetically marked clones in human fibroblasts cultured from normal subjects. Somatic Cell Genet 2:55–62

83. Martin GM, Smith AC, Ketterer DJ, Ogburn CE, Disteche CM (1985) Increased chromosomal aberrations in first metaphases of cells isolated from the kidneys of aged mice. Israel J Med Sci 21:296–301

84. Hook EB (1985) The impact of aneuploidy upon public health: mortality and morbidity associated with human chromosome abnormalities. In: Dellarco VL, Voytek PE, Hollaender A (eds) Aneuploidy: etiology and mechanisms. Plenum, New York

85. Dzarlieva RT, Fusenig NE (1982) Tumor promoter 12-0-tetradecanoyl-phorbol-13-acetate enhances sister chromatid exchanges and numerical and structural chromosome aberrations in primary mouse epidermal cell cultures. Cancer Lett 16:7–17

509

86. Petersson H, Mitelman F (1985) Nonrandom de novo chromosome aberrations in human lymphocytes and amniotic cells. Hereditas 102:33–38

87. Diamond A, Cooper GM, Ritz J, Lane M-A (1983) Identification and molecular cloning of the human B-*lym* transforming gene activated in Burkitt's lymphomas. Nature 305:112–116

88. Varmus H (1984) The molecular genetics of cellular oncogenes. Annu Rev Genet 18:553–612

89. Duesberg PH, Bister K, Vogt PK (1977) The RNA of avian acute leukemia virus MC29. Proc Natl Acad Sci USA 74:4320–4324

90. Mellon P, Pawson A, Bister K, Martin GS, Duesberg PH (1978) Specific RNA sequences and gene products of MC29 avian acute leukemia virus. Proc Natl Acad Sci USA 75:5874–5878

91. Wang L-H, Duesberg PH, Beemon K, Vogt PK (1975) Mapping RNase T_1-resistant oligonucleotides of avian tumor virus RNAs: sarcoma-specific oligonucleotides are near the poly(A) end and oligonucleotides common to sarcoma and and transformation-defective viruses are at the poly(A) end. J Virol 16:1051–1070

92. Wang L-H (1978) The gene order of avian RNA tumor viruses derived from biochemical analyses of deletion mutants and viral recombinants. Annu Rev Microbiol 32:561–592

93. Kan NC, Flordellis CS, Mark GE, Duesberg PH, Papas TS (1984) Nucleotide sequence of avian carcinoma virus MH2: two potential *onc* genes, one related to avian virus MC29 and the other related to murine sarcoma virus 3611. Proc Natl Acad Sci USA 81:3000–3004

94. Zhou R-P, Kan N, Papas T, Duesberg P (1985) Mutagenesis of avian carcinoma virus MH2: only one of two potential transforming genes (δgag-myc) transforms fibroblasts. Proc Natl Acad Sci USA 82:6389–6393

95. Hayflick J, Seeburg PH, Ohlsson R, Pfeifer-Ohlsson S, watson D, Papas T, Duesberg PH (1985) Nucleotide sequence of two overlapping *myc*-related genes in avian carcinoma virus OK10 and their relation to the *myc* genes of other viruses and the cell. Proc Natl Acad Sci USA 82:2718–2722

96. Duesberg PH, Bister K, Moscovici C (1980) Genetic structure of avian myeloblastosis virus, released from transformed myeloblasts as a defective virus particle. Proc Natl Acad Sci USA 77:5120–5124

97. Lee W-H, Bister K, Pawson A, Robins T, Moscovici C, Duesberg PH (1980) Fujinami sarcoma virus: an avian RNA tumor virus with a unique transforming gene. Proc Natl Acad Sci USA 77:2018–2022

98. Bentley DL, Groudine M (1986) Novel promoter upstream of the human c-*myc* gene and regulation of c-*myc* expression in B-cell lymphomas. Mol Cell Biol 6:3481–3489

99. Duesberg P, Vogt PK, Beemon K, Lai M (1974) Avian RNA tumor viruses: mechanism of recombination and complexity of the genome. Quant Biol 39:847–857

100. Nunn MF, Seeburg PH, Moscovici C, Duesberg PH (1983) Tripartite structure of the avian erythroblastosis virus E26 transforming gene. Nature 306:391–395

101. Pfaff SL, Zhou R-P, Young JC, Hayflick J, Duesberg PH (1985) Defining the borders of the chicken proto-*fps* gene, a precursor of Fujinami sarcoma virus. Virology 146:307–314

102. van der Hoorn A, Neupert B (1986) The repressor sequence upstream of c-*mos* acts neither as polyadenylation site nor as transcription termination region. Nucleic Acids Res 14:8771–8782

103. Ikawa S, Hagino-Yamagishi K, Kawai S, Yamamoto T, Toyoshima K (1986) Activation of the cellular *src* gene by transducing retrovirus. Mol Cell Biol 6:2420–2428

104. Naharro G, Robbins KC, Reddy EP (1984) Gene product of v-*fgr onc:* Hybrid protein containing a portion of actin and a tyrosine-specific protein kinase. Science 223:63–66

105. Boveri T (1914) Zur Frage der Entstehung maligner Tumoren. Fischer, Jena

106. Klein G (1983) Specific chromosomal translocations and the genesis of B-cell-derived tumors in mice and men. Cell 32:311–315

107. Dracopoli NC, Houghton AN, Old LJ (1985) Loss of polymorphic restriction fragments in malignant melanoma: implications for tumor heterogeneity. Proc Natl Acad Sci USA 82:1470–1474

108. Rous P (1967) The challenge to man of the neoplastic cell. Science 157:24–28

109. Cairns J (1978) Cancer, science and society. Freeman, San Francisco

110. Zinder ND (1953) Infective heredity in bacteria. Cold Spring Harbor Symp Quant Biol 18:261–269

Haematology and Blood Transfusion   Vol. 31
Modern Trends in Human Leukemia VII
Edited by Neth, Gallo, Greaves, and Kabisch
© Springer-Verlag Berlin Heidelberg 1987

Repetition as the Essence of Life on this Earth: Music and Genes

S. Ohno [1]

A. Introduction

While it is believed that life on this earth started as long ago as a few billion or more years ago, a number of true innovations in evolution appears to have been rather dismally small. Most of the successful adaptive radiation of living organisms have apparently been accomplished by extensive plagiarization of those preciously few innovations via the mechanism of gene duplication [1]. Furthermore, it appears that most of these true innovations have occurred at the very beginning, before the division of prokaryotes from eukaryotes. For example, nearly all the sugar-metabolizing enzymes appear to have achieved their inviolable functional competence at the above-noted early date. Natural selection has since been spinning wheels in the air.

B. The Story of Glyceraldehyde 3-Phosphate Dehydrogenase

It would be noted in Fig. 1 that the 332-residue-long glyceraldehyde 3-phosphate dehydrogenase of the pig differs from the lobster enzyme only at 86 positions. Inasmuch as vertebrates, or rather chordates diverged from crustaceans roughly 500 million years ago, one can conclude from the above and similar data on additional species that this enzyme has been undergoing 1% amino acid sequence divergence every 20 million years,

thus accumulating 26% amino acid sequence difference in 500 million years. If such a rate calculation can be extended indefinitely, however, even at this snail's pace one still expects this enzyme to have undergone 100% amino acid sequence divergence in 2 billion years. Now 2 billion years ago would have been about the time prokaryotes diverged from eukaryotes. Yet the bacterial amino acid sequence from *Bacillus stearothermophilis,* also shown in Fig. 1, still maintains 177 out of the 332 sites (53%) homology with the pig enzyme, and similar 180 out of 332 sites homology with the lobster enzyme. In fact, there are 19 segments (tripeptidic or longer), comprised of 92 residues in total, that remain invariant in all three species. The longest conserved segment, tridecapeptidic in its length, occupying 144th to 156th position, represents the most critical of the substrate binding sites, 149th Cys forming the thiol linkage with substrate intermediates [2]. Indeed, after achieving the appropriate degree of functional competence 2 billion or more years ago, glyceraldehyde 3-phosphate dehydrogenase has not changed in its essence; evolutionary compatible amino acid substitutions that accompanied successive diversification and speciation merely symbolizing futile spinning of the wheel. Such a futility is also evident in Fig. 1, for at the 14 positions, a eukaryote (the pig) and a prokaryote (*Bacillus stearothermophilis*) share the identical residues, while the other eukaryote (the lobster) is left out as an oddball; e.g., the third position of the pig and the bacillus is Val, while that of the lobster is Ile. At these and many other positions, the game of musical chairs

[1] Beckman Research Institute of the City of Hope Duarte, California 91010, USA

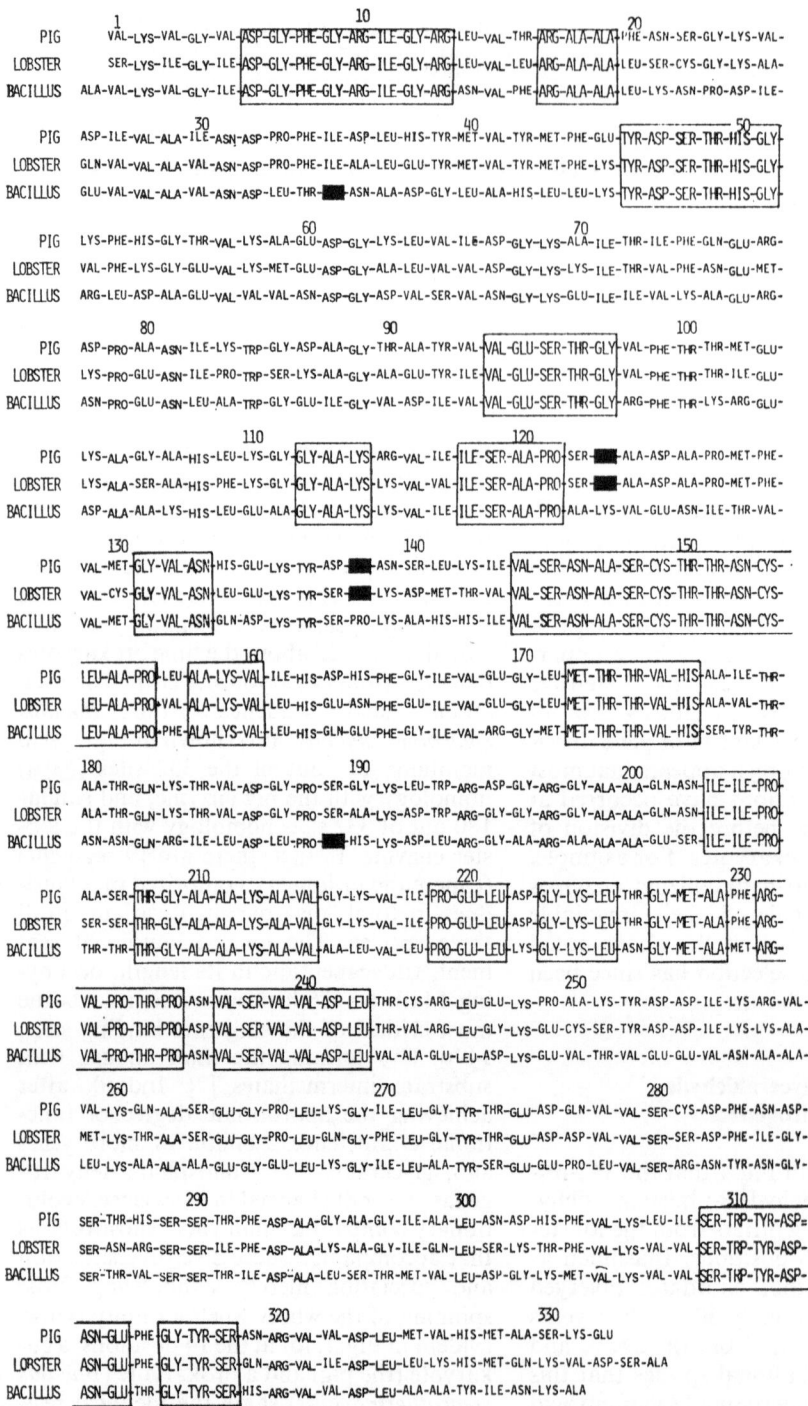

Fig. 1. The amino acid sequences of glyceraldehyde 3-phosphate dehydrogenases from three divergent species are compared. Bacillus refers to *Bacillus stearothermophilis*. Discordant and identical residues are shown slightly displaced from each other; discordant ones are placed little above identical ones. Amino acid residues of tripeptidic or longer conserved segments are shown in *large capital letters* and segments are *boxed in*. Deleted residues are identified as *black boxes*

have apparently been in play among a limited number of functionally compatible amino acids.

Analogous situations have been found with regard to other sugar metabolizing enzymes, e.g., phosphoglycerate kinase, triose isomerase etc. Furthermore, all these sugar-metabolizing enzymes are constructed of the same mould. The amino terminal half and the carboxyl terminal half forming two distinct domains, a cleft between the two accommodating the substrate and the coenzyme. The amino terminal half is for the coenzyme binding and the carboxyl terminal half is for the substrate binding. Furthermore, Rossman [3], among others, has pointed out that in the case of kinases, the mononucleotide (e.g., ATP) binding site of the amino terminal half is comprised of three β-sheet-forming segments and two α-helix-forming segments in the following order from the amino terminus; $\beta\alpha\beta\alpha\beta$. The dinucleotide (NAD or NADP) binding site of dehydrogenases, on the other hand, evolved from the above by duplication; thus, it can be expressed as $2 \times \beta\alpha\beta\alpha\beta$. Inasmuch as the most critical portion of the substrate binding site evolved within the last segment of the duplicate (e.g., 144th to 156th tridecapeptide of Fig. 1), this intrusion of the substrate binding active site into the dinucleotide binding domain froze the dinucleotide binding domain of each enzyme as uniquely its own. Thus, there is no more than 20% amino acid sequence homology between dinucleotide binding sites of different enzymes in spite of the fact that all are made of the same $2 \times \beta\alpha\beta\alpha\beta$ mould. It would be recalled that within the same enzyme, conservation of greater than 50% homology is the rule for the whole enzyme, therefore, the dinucleotide binding amino terminal half.

At any rate, two notable facts emerge from the above. First, coding sequences for sugar-metabolizing enzymes and probably for many other enzymes (e.g., proteases) have already achieved the appropriate degree of functional competence before the division of prokaryotes from eukaryotes. Second, repetitions were the rule of the game from the very onset of life on this earth; the dinucleotide binding site evolving from the mononucleotide binding site by duplication, and that the mononucleotide binding site itself likely to have evolved by 2.5 times duplication of the one $\beta\alpha$ or $\alpha\beta$ unit.

C. Ingeniousness Embodied in the First Set of Coding Sequences that Were Repeats of Base Oligomers

Orgel's group [4] has shown that in the presence of Zn ion, nonenzymatic synthesis of nucleic acids occurs in the proper 3'- to 5' linkage, provided that there is a template. Thus, it would appear that what was in short supply in the prebiotic world, before the emergence of life on this earth was long templates from which copies can be made. Put it more succinctly, the first primordial question is: "How did oligonucleotides manage to extend themselves to become worthy coding sequences?" There is one simple answer: One tandem duplication of the preexisted oligomer assures indefinite extension of that template, as illustrated at the top of Fig. 2. What if the heptameric template CAGCCTG duplicated to become tetradecamer? After completion of its complementary strand, the two might pair in the manner shown; second copy pairing with the first copy of the complementary strand. The paired portion would now serve as the primer for the next round of nucleic acid synthesis. At the completion of the second round, the 14-mer template now becomes 21-mer. In this way, the indefinite extension of the primer is assured a priori, a paired segment always serving as a primer for the next round of nucleic acid synthesis. The above then is the first reason for believing that the first set of coding sequences, or rather all nucleic acids in the prebiotic world that presaged the emergence of life, on this earth were all repeats of various base oligomers.

How accurate was a copying function of the nonenzymatic nucleic acid replication? Of various nucleic acid polymerases known, the most error prone appear to be reverse transcriptase of retroviruses, for their error rate has been estimated as of the order of 10^{-3}/base pair/year [5]. This is one million times higher error rate compared to DNA polymerases of vertebrates, and at this rate, there would be 100% base sequence change every one thousand years. The inherent error rate of prebiotic, therefore, nonen-

```
C-A-G-C-C-T-G
G-T.
     C-G-G.
          A.
           C
```

ONE TANDEM REPLICATION TAKES CARE OF ALL

```
                              C-C-T-G
                          A-G
                       C-
C-A-G-C-C-T-G/C-A-G-C-C-T-G
        G-T-C-G-G-A-C/G-T-C-G-G-A-C
                 G-A-C
G-T-C-G
```

ANCESTRAL REPEATS FOR PHOSPHOGLYCERATE KINASE ?

```
     ARG   SER   CYS   CYS   GLU   ALA   ALA   ALA   LYS   LEU   LEU
     C G A A G C T G C T G/C G A A G C T G C T G/C G A A G C T G C T G   (3 X 11)
        GLU   ALA   ALA   ALA   LYS   LEU   LEU   ARG   SER   CYS   CYS
  ALA   LYS   LEU   LEU   ARG   SER   CYS   CYS   GLU   ALA   ALA
```

Fig. 2. Replication of nucleic acids is based upon the inherent complementarity that exists between two purine-pyrimidine pairs; A pairs with T or U, while G pairs with C. Accordingly, provided that there is a template (the heptamer CAGCCTG shown at the top), mononucleotides would readily assemble themselves in the 3′, 5′ linkage to form a complementary strand in the presence of Zn [4] as shown at the top. What was in short supply in the prebiotic world then were templates of substantial lengths. What if the above noted haptamer repeated itself in tandem or some of the base oligomers were by chance tandem repeats (two copies of the shorter oligomer) to begin with. It and its complementary strand can pair unequally in the manner depicted at the middle. As a paired segment now functions as a primer for the next round of nucleic acid synthesis, infinite extension of templates is now assured. All it takes to start this process is the one tandem duplication.

Of long oligomeric repeats thus formed, those that evolved to be the first set of coding sequences likely started from oligomeric units whose numbers of bases were not multiples of three. There were two distinct advantages: (1) They gave longer periodicities to polypeptide chains; e.g., repeats of the base octamer would have given octapeptidic periodicity while repeat of the base nonamer would have only the tripeptidic periodicity. (2) They would have encoded polypeptide chains of identical periodicity in all three reading frames. Within the periodic unit such repeats could have given both α-helical segment and β-sheet forming segment as shown at the bottom. Such alternating α,β structures gave rise to the mononucleotide binding site (3) which would have been utilized immediately as parts of the primitive nucleic acid polymerase. Later they gave rise to ATP and NAD, NADP binding sites of many enzymes as discussed in the text

zymatic nucleic acid replication is expected to be higher than the above-noted 10^{-3}; as error prone as they are, reverse transcriptases are, after all, the enzyme of a sort. Prebiotic coding sequences had to contend with this very high replication error rate and should still have been able to encode polypeptide chains of potential function. Provided that the number of bases in the oligomeric unit was not a multiple of three, repeats of the base oligomer would have been very stable under this mostly trying circumstance of constant base substitutions, dele-

tions, and insertions. This is also illustrated at the bottom of Fig. 2. Since the monodecamer CGAAGCTGCTG cannot be divided by 3, three consecutive copies of it translated in three different reading frames gives the monodecapeptidic periodicity to a polypeptide chain. Contrast the above to repeats of the base dodecamer, which can give only the tetrapeptidic periodicity to the polypeptide chain. Furthermore, since within a given reading frame three consecutive copies of the monodecamer are to be translated in all three reading frames, such repeats encode polypeptide chains of the identical periodicity in all three reading frames. This openness of all three reading frames give them a great deal of imperviousness to base substitutions, deletions, and insertions. Repeats of the monodecamer shown at the bottom of Fig. 2 encode both potentially α-helix-forming segment and potentially β-sheet-forming segment within one monodecapeptidic unit. In fact, sugar-metabolizing enzymes in general and phosphoglycerate kinase in particular might have originally been encoded by repeats of such a monodecamer, for AAGCTGCTG portion of the monodecameric unit recur in many variations in the modern coding sequence (e.g., of man) for phosphoglycerate kinase as already noted in our previous paper [6].

D. Repetition as the Essence of Coding Sequences and Musical Compositions

Earth on which life has evolved has always been governed by the hierarchy of periodicities. First, earth rotates on its own axis to create days, while the moon's revolution around the earth gives months, with neap tides and spring tides to be topped by years, reflecting the earth's travel around the sun. It is small wonder if life itself was born out of periodicities embodied in repetition of unit base oligomers. Just as man eventually devised seconds, minutes, and hours as arbitrary units of time measurement, one of the periodicities embodied in polypeptide chains encoded by the first set of codeing sequences that were oligomeric repeats must soon have been chosen as the arbitrary time-measuring unit by the ancestral biological clock. It now appears that this arbitrarily chosen unit was the simplest dipeptidic periodicity. The polypeptide chain encoded by *per* locus of *Drosophila merlanogaster,* fundamentally involved in the expression of biological rhythms such as cicardian behaviors and 55-s rhythm of courtship song, is largely comprised of the Gly-Thr dipeptidic repeats interspersed with short stretches of its deviant Gly-Ser dipeptidic repeats, and that the homologous gene encoding the polypeptide chain of the above-noted dipeptidic periodicity is conserved in the mouse as well [7]. Observing the *per* locus coding sequence,

one notices that there have been numerous neutral base substitutions, e.g., free base substitutions at the redundant 3rd base position of glycine codons. Thus, it would appear that the time-keeping was done from the beginning at the polypeptide level rather than at the level of coding sequences, although the initial periodicity of that polypeptide chain had to be the consequence of its coding sequence being repeats of unit base oligomers.

Now we come to the origin shrouded in mist, of the prehistory of musical compositions. Inasmuch as songs of canaries and skylarks are as pleasing to our ears as they must be to their mates as well as to themselves, it is clear that melodies as such are no human invention. Furthermore, the vocal cord and other sound-making apparatuses of our immediate relatives (e.g., *Homo neanderthalensis*) appear to have been rather underdeveloped. Accordingly, I wonder if early *Homo sapiens* were capable even of imitating beautiful bird songs noted above even if they wanted to. I would rather believe that music as such were invented by primitive man as purely rhythmic timekeeping device. For example, a hunting party intent on bringing down a mammoth or two would have to coordinate activities of several cohorts spread over a wide arc surrounding the herd of mammothes. This, I suspect, was done by rhythmic beatings of hollowed tree trunks for example; fast repetitions of a given rhythm conveying an urgent need to close in whereas slow repetitions of the same rhythm meaning cautious approach. It would thus appear that music, too were initally born out of repetitious rendition.

Even today of wonderous melodies, music is still used as a time keeping device, as in dancing and military parades. Rhythm of the latter, marching music are essentially that of our heart beat. Our heart beats slow in slumber and contemplation, while it beats uncontrollably fast in fright. Rhythm of marching music should be somewhere in between to indicate willingness either to go forth against formidable adversaries or to defend against adversaries until death. Because of this homage to the periodicity inherent both in coding sequence construction and musical composition, the way was sought to interconvert the two. The solution

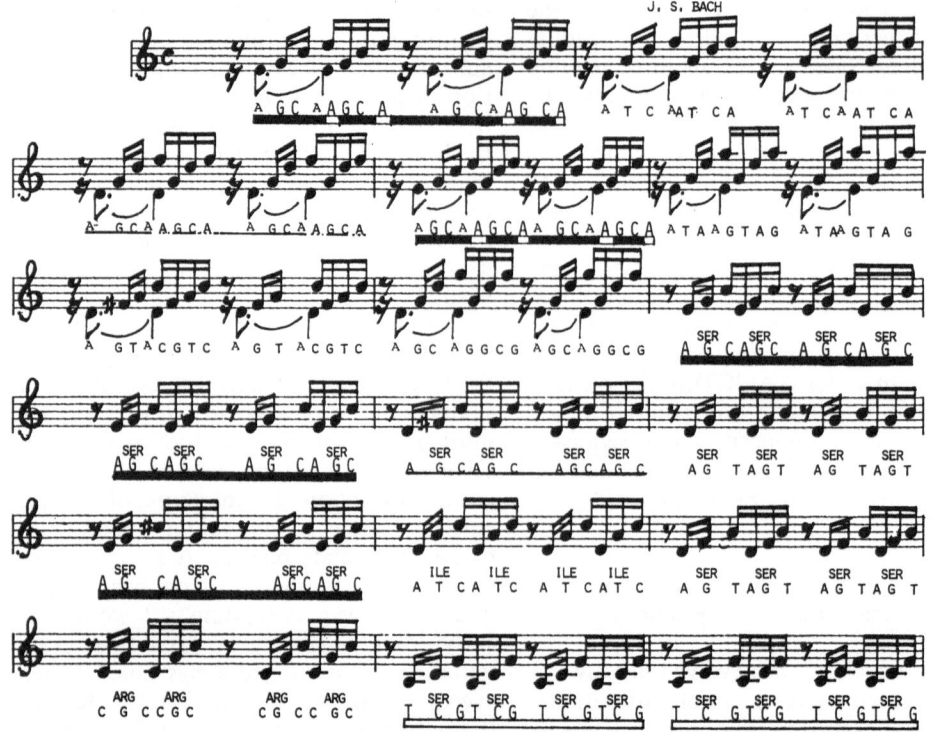

Fig. 3. An initial part of the treble-clef musical score of Prelude No. 1 from well-tempered clavichord by J. S. Bach, accompanied by the base sequence and the amino acid sequence transcribable from that base sequence

that we arrived at is to assign a space and a line on the octave scale to each base in the ascending order of A, G, T, C in such a way so that the classical middle-C position would be occupied by C on the line, A in the space occupying the position immediately above [6].

In Fig. 3, the treble-clef musical score of Prelude No. 1 from well-tempered clavichord by J. S. Bach, the great master of the early Baroque, is accompanied by the base sequence transcribed from it according to the rule stated above. It would be noted that with regard to every 4/4th or 8/8th time signature unit, the second half is the exact repeat of the first half. Furthermore, until the 3rd line, each half is repeats of four notes, the four-note subunit consisting of one 3/16th note and three 1/16th notes followed by one 1/4th note and four 1/16th notes. Translated to base sequence, the first time signature unit is comprised of four exact copies of the AGCA tetramer followed by four copies

of a single-base substituted deviant of the above-noted tetramer ATCA. The AGCA recurrs again 8 times. Since 4 is not a multiple of three, these tetrameric repeats are capable of giving the tetrapeptidic periodicity to a polypeptide chain, but alas. chain terminators TAA and TAG come in pairs at the extreme right of 2nd line. From the 4th line onward, one 3/16th note and a quarter note are relegated to the base clef; therefore, the treble-clef score becomes trimeric repeats. When translated, this portion yields polyserine interspersed with teterailsoleucyne and tetraarginine.

In general, I found musical compositions of the early Baroque period to be repeats of short base oligomers, these oligomers being single-base substituted variants of each other. Indeed, their resemblance to what I conceived as the first set of coding sequences at the very beginning of life on this earth is uncanny (see Fig. 2). Most of the coding sequences possessed by modern organisms

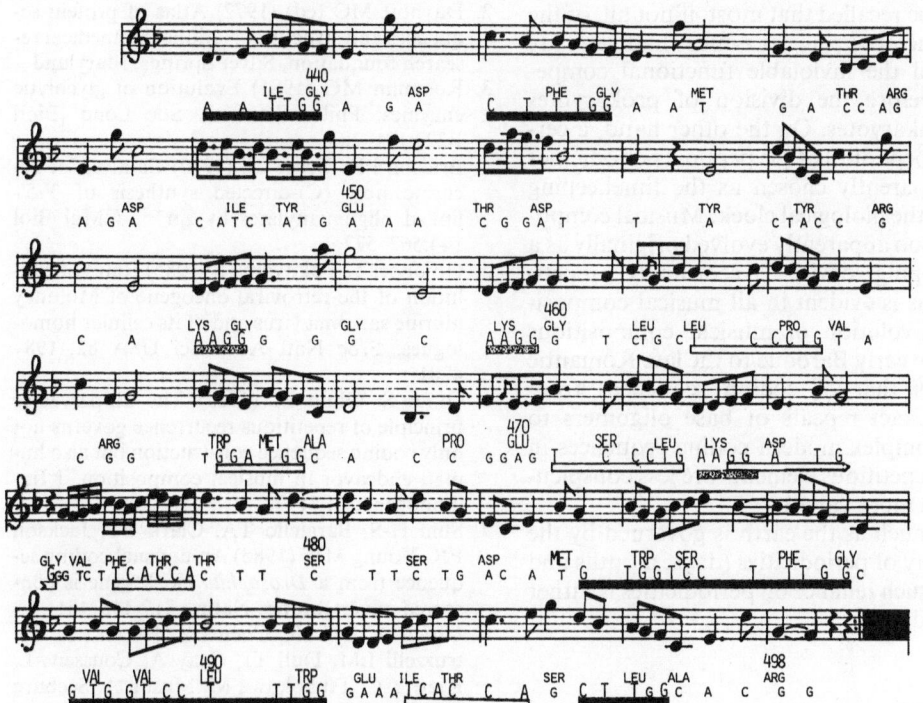

Fig. 4. The heart of the coding segment for tyrosine kinase domain of the human insulin receptor β-chain (8). Amino acid residues of the two active site segments are shown in *large capital let-* *ters*. This musical transformation for violin of the coding segment is in E minor, 4/4th or 8/8th time signature

have endured for hundreds of millions of years. In the case of those for sugar-metabolizing enzymes, 2 billion years or more as already noted. Thus, their original periodicities are obvious only for discerning eyes. Not surprisingly, musical compositions of the late Romantic period resemble these coding sequences. We have previously shown that Frédéric Chopin's nocturne Opus 55, No. 1, resembled the last exon for the largest subunit of RNA polymerase II [6]. In Fig. 4, the musical transformation for violin of the most functionally critical part of the tyrosine kinase domain of the human insulin receptor β-chain [8] is shown. This segment includes two active site segments most critical for the assigned function of tyrosine kinase. Amino acid residues of these two active site oligopeptides are shown in large capital letters. It would be noted that nearly all of the second active site is encoded by tandem repeats of the dodecamer GTGGTCCTTTGG, thickly underlined by solid bars (2nd from the last line of Fig. 4).

Its two truncated derivatives at the top line of Fig. 4 are also underlined by solid bars. Other, more musically pertinent repeats are also underlined by open bars and shaded bars; e.g., the hexamer TCCCTG in 3rd and 4th lines of Fig. 4.

E. Summary

In prebiotic nucleic acid replication, templates appear to have been in short supply. A single round of tandem duplication of existing oligomers assured progressive extension of templates to the length adequate for encoding of polypeptide chains. Thus, the first set of coding sequences had to be repeats of base oligomers encoding polypeptide chains of various periodicities. On one hand, the readiness of these periodical polypeptide chains to assume α-helical and/or β-sheet secondary structures contributed to the extremely rapid initial functional diversification of these polypeptide chains. It would be recalled that most, if not all, of the sugar-metabolizing enzymes had already achieved the inviolable functional competence before the division of prokaryotes from eukaryotes. On the other hand, a certain (dipeptidic?) of the peptidic periodicities was apparently chosen as the timekeeping unit by the biological clock. Musical compositions too apparently evolved originally as a timekeeping device. Accordingly, repetitiousness is evident in all musical compositions. Evolution of musical compositions from the early Baroque to the late Romantic parallels that of coding sequences from rather exact repeats of base oligomers to more complex modern coding sequences in which repetitious elements are less conspicuous and more varied.

Inasmuch as the earth is governed by the hierarchy of periodicities (days, months and years), such reliance on periodicities is rather expected.

References

1. Ohno S (1970) Evolution by gene duplication. Springer-Verlag, Berlin Heidelberg New York

2. Dayhoff MO (ed) (1972) Atlas of protein sequences and structure. National biomedical research foundation, Silver Springs, Maryland

3. Rossman MG (1981) Evolution of glycolytic enzymes. Philos Trans R Soc Lond [Biol] B293:191–203

4. Bridson PK, Orgel LE (1980) Catalysis of accurate poly (C)-directed synthesis of 3'-5'-linked oligoguanylates by Zn^{+2}. J Mol Biol 144:567–577

5. Gojobori T, Yokoyama S (1985) Rates of evolution of the retroviral oncogene of Moloney murine sarcoma virus and of its cellular homologues. Proc Natl Acad Sci USA 82:4198–4201

6. Ohno S, Ohno M (1985) The all-pervasive principle of repetitious recurrence governs not only coding sequence construction but also human endeavor in musical composition. J Immunogenet 24:71–78

7. Shin H-S, Bargiello TA, Clark BT, Jackson FR, Young MW (1985) An unusual coding sequence from a *Drosophila* clock gene is conserved in vertebrates. Nature 317:445–451

8. Ulrich A, Bell JR, Chen EY, Herrera R, Petruzzelli LM, Dull TJ, Gray A, Coussens L, Kiao Y-C, Tsubokawa M, Mason A, Seeburg PH, Gunfeld C, Rosen OM, Ramachandran J (1985) Human insulin receptor and its relationship to the tyrosine kinase family of oncogenes. Nature 313:756–761

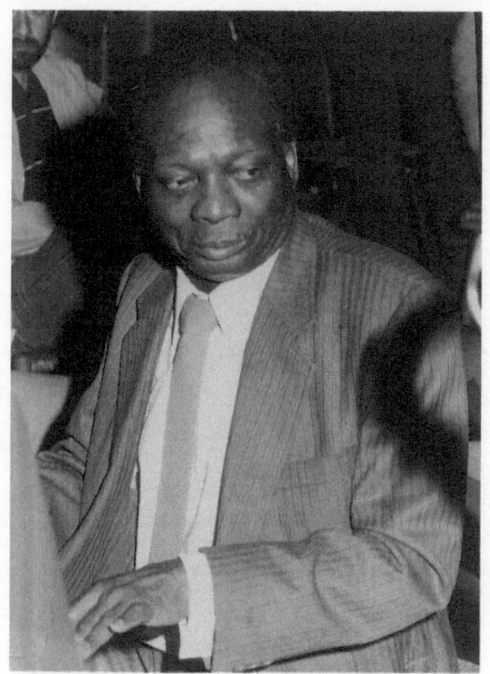

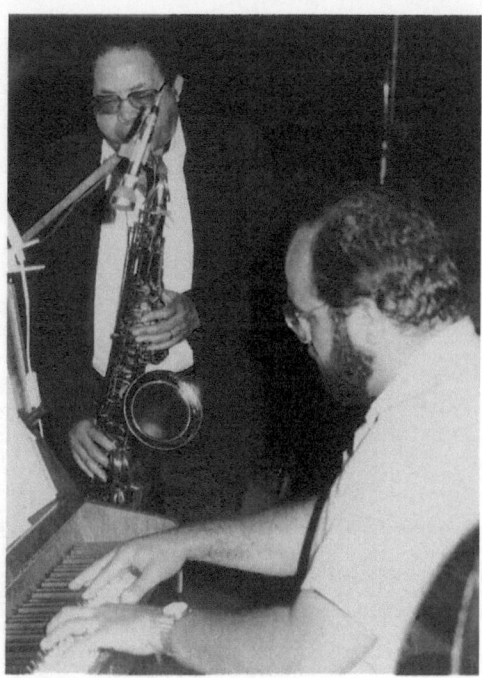

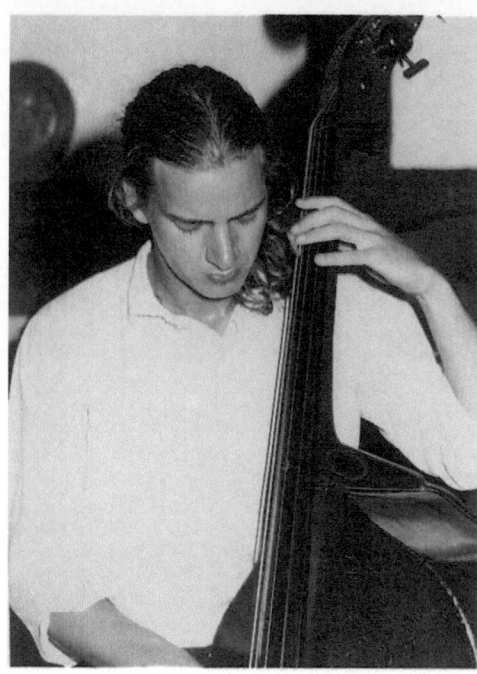

Translation to Human Temparaments
Session in "De Emmenhof"

Fotos Regina Völz

Subject Index